Molecular Advances in Dry Eye Syndrome

Molecular Advances in Dry Eye Syndrome

Guest Editors

Maria Jesus Giráldez-Fernández
Anxo Fernández-Ferreiro

MDPI

Basel • Beijing • Wuhan • Barcelona • Belgrade • Novi Sad • Cluj • Manchester

Guest Editors
Maria Jesus Giráldez-Fernández
Applied Physics Department (Optometry Area)
Universidade de Santiago de Compostela
Santiago de Compostela
Spain

Anxo Fernández-Ferreiro
FarmaCHUSLab
Health Research Institute of Santiago de Compostela (IDIS)
Santiago de Compostela
Spain

Editorial Office
MDPI AG
Grosspeteranlage 5
4052 Basel, Switzerland

This is a reprint of the Special Issue, published open access by the journal *International Journal of Molecular Sciences* (ISSN 1422-0067), freely accessible at: https://www.mdpi.com/journal/ijms/special_issues/G1961F71C3.

For citation purposes, cite each article independently as indicated on the article page online and as indicated below:

Lastname, A.A.; Lastname, B.B. Article Title. *Journal Name* **Year**, *Volume Number*, Page Range.

ISBN 978-3-7258-6784-4 (Hbk)
ISBN 978-3-7258-6785-1 (PDF)
https://doi.org/10.3390/books978-3-7258-6785-1

Contents

About the Editors

Anxo Fernández-Ferreiro

Anxo Fernández-Ferreiro is a researcher coordinator at the FarmaCHUSLab Group of the Health Research Institute of Santiago de Compostela and a clinical pharmacist at the University Clinical Hospital of Santiago de Compostela. His work focuses on translational pharmacology, ocular drug delivery, and the development of innovative therapeutic strategies for ocular diseases. He has led and contributed to multidisciplinary projects involving pharmaceutical formulation, advanced analytical methods, and the application of molecular approaches to optimize treatment outcomes. His scientific contributions include studies on immunomodulatory therapies, pharmacokinetics, and personalized medicine. He has collaborated extensively with clinical and academic partners and has participated in national and international research networks devoted to improving ocular health.

Maria Jesus Giráldez-Fernández

Maria Jesus Giráldez-Fernández is a researcher in the Optometry Group at the Health Research Institute of Santiago de Compostela and a faculty member in the Applied Physics Department at the Universidade de Santiago de Compostela. Her research centers on ocular surface physiology, tear film dynamics, and the development of diagnostic tools for dry eye disease and related disorders. She has directed and participated in collaborative projects integrating clinical assessment, imaging technologies, and molecular analysis to enhance understanding of tear film alterations and visual function. Her work has contributed to the advancement of evidence-based optometric practice and the identification of biomarkers relevant to ocular surface health. She is actively involved in scientific dissemination and the training of students and professionals in optometry and vision science.

Preface

This Reprint, *Molecular Advances in Dry Eye Syndrome*, brings together a curated collection of research articles that deepen our understanding of the biological and molecular foundations of dry eye disease. Its scope encompasses the study of tear film organization, lipid and protein regulation, immune and neurosensory mechanisms, and innovative diagnostic and therapeutic approaches. The aim of this Reprint is to provide an integrated scientific perspective that reflects current progress in the field and highlights emerging concepts with clinical relevance.

This Reprint was motivated by the growing need to bridge molecular discoveries with practical applications that can improve patient care. As interest in dry eye disease continues to expand, consolidating high-quality, multidisciplinary research has become essential for supporting both scientific advancement and translational development. The Reprint is intended for clinicians, researchers, and students seeking a comprehensive overview of the recent advances that are shaping future strategies for diagnosis and therapy.

Prepared by the Guest Editors, it serves as an informative guide to the contributions included in this Reprint and an invitation to further exploration of the molecular pathways that drive dry eye disease.

Maria Jesus Giráldez-Fernández and Anxo Fernández-Ferreiro
Guest Editors

International Journal of
Molecular Sciences

MDPI

Editorial

Special Issue "Molecular Advances in Dry Eye Syndrome"

Anxo Fernández-Ferreiro [1,2,*] and Maria Jesus Giráldez-Fernández [3,4,*]

1 FarmaCHUSLab Group, Health Research Institute of Santiago de Compostela (IDIS), 15706 Santiago de Com-postela, Spain
2 Pharmacy Department, University Clinical Hospital of Santiago de Compostela (SERGAS), 15706 Santiago de Compostela, Spain
3 Applied Physics Department (Optometry Area), Facultade de Óptica e Optometría, Universidade de Santiago de Compostela, 15705 Santiago de Compostela, Spain
4 Optometry Group, Instituto de Investigación Sanitaria Santiago de Compostela (IDIS), 15706 Santiago de Compostela, Spain
* Correspondence: anxordes@gmail.com (A.F.-F.); mjesus.giraldez@usc.es (M.J.G.-F.)

Dry eye disease (DED) is a multifactorial and highly prevalent disorder of the ocular surface, characterized by tear film instability, ocular discomfort, inflammation, and visual fluctuation. Affecting millions worldwide, DED is increasingly recognized as a condition that significantly compromises patients' quality of life and, in advanced stages, can lead to permanent visual impairment. Underlying the clinical manifestations of DED is a complex interplay of molecular, immunological, hormonal, and neurosensory mechanisms that have become the focus of intense research. While current therapies can address certain symptoms, many patients continue to experience persistent ocular surface inflammation, epithelial damage, and neurosensory dysfunction. Therefore, new insights into the molecular basis of DED, the development of improved diagnostic tools, and the identification of innovative pharmacological and biological therapies remain essential. In this Editorial, we summarize the primary findings presented in the articles published in this Special Issue, which aimed to expand current knowledge of DED pathophysiology and introduce new therapeutic perspectives. Recent advances consolidate the TFOS DEWS II framework, which defines DED as a loss of tear film homeostasis driven by tear instability, hyperosmolarity, inflammation, and neurosensory abnormalities. These guidelines emphasize the integration of molecular biomarkers, imaging modalities, and patient-reported outcomes to refine diagnosis and guide therapy, concepts that serve as the foundation for interpreting the mechanistic contributions of this Special Issue [1].

One of the central aspects explored in this Special Issue is the composition and function of the tear film, especially its lipid components. García-Queiruga and colleagues conducted a comprehensive lipidomic analysis of meibum in subjects with evaporative DED. In this study, the authors examined alterations in key lipid species associated with meibomian gland dysfunction. Their findings revealed significant changes in lipid classes relevant to tear film stability, providing molecular insight into the mechanisms that contribute to the evaporative subtype of DED. The detailed lipidomic signatures described by the authors offer potential avenues for future biomarker development and targeted therapeutic interventions, further highlighting the crucial role played by meibomian gland physiology in maintaining tear film homeostasis. Investigations have demonstrated that specific lipid species, such as O-acyl-ω-hydroxy fatty acids (OAHFAs), exhibit liquid-expanded to solid-phase transitions that create highly evaporation-resistant films, while diesters lack this protective capability. The tear film lipid layer serves as the primary barrier against aqueous evaporation, maintains a smooth optical surface, and is essential for ocular surface hydration and tear distribution. Notably, up to 86% of patients with dry eye disease show evidence of meibomian gland dysfunction, and evaporative DED is far more prevalent than pure aqueous deficiency in general clinical cohorts [2,3].

The ocular surface is also influenced by extracellular vesicles naturally present in tear fluids. Oya et al. examined the potential functions of murine tear-derived extracellular vesicles and investigated their effects on corneal epithelial cells in vitro. The authors demonstrated that these vesicles may modulate epithelial cell physiology and participate in intercellular communication. Their findings suggest that vesicles contained in tear fluid might contribute to epithelial repair processes or serve as biomarkers of ocular surface health. Emerging evidence supports the role of tear-derived and cell-derived extracellular vesicles as regulators of inflammation and epithelial repair. Systematic reviews highlight their utility as minimally invasive biomarkers in dry eye and Sjögren-associated keratoconjunctivitis sicca, while preclinical studies suggest that stem cell-derived exosomes may promote nerve regeneration and reduce ocular surface inflammation [4].

A second thematic focus of this Special Issue concerns advances in pharmacological and biological treatments for DED. In an open-label, sequential prospective study, Puente-Iglesias et al. evaluated the clinical effectiveness, safety, and compliance of two compounded formulations of tacrolimus eye drops. Forty patients received sequential treatment with both formulations, and the authors examined ocular surface signs, symptoms, and tolerability. Their results demonstrated notable improvements in clinical parameters and inflammatory signs, with acceptable safety profiles and positive adherence. Calcineurin inhibitors remain key immunomodulatory agents for chronic ocular surface inflammation. Clinical studies indicate that cyclosporine and tacrolimus achieve disease control in 52% and 62% of patients, respectively. Tacrolimus is pharmacodynamically 10–100 times more potent than cyclosporine and exhibits a favorable safety profile. In dry eye disease, it suppresses pro-inflammatory cytokines including IL-2, IFN-γ, and TNF-α, as demonstrated in preclinical models of ocular inflammation [5].

Novel biological approaches were also explored. Lee and colleagues investigated the anti-inflammatory properties of exosomes derived from *Limosilactobacillus fermentum* in a model of benzalkonium chloride-induced inflammation in conjunctival cells. Their work showed that these bacterial exosomes significantly reduced inflammation markers and cellular stress responses. Diquafosol, a well-known P2Y2 receptor agonist, was evaluated in a systematic review and meta-analysis by Serrano-Robles et al. In a randomized double-masked phase III clinical trial involving 287 adults with dry eye disease, 3% diquafosol ophthalmic solution demonstrated non-inferiority to 0.1% sodium hyaluronate and achieved superior improvements in corneal fluorescein staining, tear break-up time, and rose Bengal conjunctival staining. Long-term observational studies support its safety and sustained efficacy in real-world settings [6].

Kaštelan et al. reviewed sex-based differences in lacrimal gland anatomy, function, hormonal regulation, and immune responsiveness. Sexual dimorphism significantly influences lacrimal gland structure and aging. Women exhibit more pronounced degenerative changes—including fibrosis and acinar atrophy—particularly after menopause. Furthermore, androgen deficiency has been implicated in meibomian and lacrimal gland dysfunction, underscoring a hormonal basis for the increased susceptibility to dry eye disease observed in women [7].

Saram and colleagues provided a comprehensive overview of the immunobiology of DED, including the roles played by innate and adaptive immune responses, epithelial damage, cytokine networks, and emerging therapeutic targets. Likewise, Soyfoo et al. focused on the diagnostic and therapeutic challenges of Sjögren disease.

Neurosensory mechanisms also play a pivotal role in DED severity and chronicity. Kahuam-López et al. reviewed the significance of nerve growth factor (NGF) in ocular surface physiology and pathology. NGF is essential for immune modulation, trophic support, epithelial healing, corneal sensitivity, and tear film regulation. Experimental and clinical studies demonstrate that NGF accelerates the regeneration of sub-basal and stromal nerves after LASIK surgery and improves corneal sensitivity and tear stability. These findings support the development of NGF-based therapies such as cenegermin, now approved for neurotrophic keratitis [8]. Environmental exposures such as PHMG-p and air pollutants also contribute to ocular surface disease.

Valencia-Sandonís and colleagues monitored molecular and clinical changes in chronic DED with ocular pain. Growing evidence indicates that a persistent nociceptive input from the ocular surface can induce central sensitization, with alterations in pain pathways and a reduced response to conventional therapies. Patients with neuropathic-like symptoms often require multimodal approaches including neuromodulators and targeted anti-inflammatory strategies [9].

Overall, the contributions to this Special Issue highlight several key insights into dry eye disease: that lipidomic disturbances underpin evaporative DED; that tacrolimus and diquafosol offer promising therapeutic benefits; that microbial- and tear-derived vesicles have regulatory functions in ocular surface biology; that sex differences, immunological mechanisms, and neurosensory factors significantly shape disease presentation; that environmental toxicants may exacerbate ocular surface dysfunction; and that chronic inflammation and pain mechanisms persist in many patients despite treatment. The combination of these findings deepens our understanding of DED from diverse perspectives and paves the way for the performance of future research. In the future, long-term studies of new pharmacological agents, biologically derived therapies, and personalized diagnostic tools should be pursued in larger patient cohorts. Integrating multi-omics approaches, advanced imaging technologies, and artificial intelligence will be essential for identifying reliable biomarkers, refining classification systems, and developing individualized treatment strategies. The advances presented in this Special Issue not only expand our molecular and clinical understanding of DED but also open up new avenues for research and innovation that aims to improve therapeutic outcomes and enhance patients' quality of life.

Funding: This research received no external funding.

Conflicts of Interest: The authors declare no conflicts of interest.

List of Contributions:

1. Garcia-Queiruga, J.; Pena-Verdeal, H.; Sabucedo-Villamarin, B.; Paz-Tarrio, M.; Guitian-Fernandez, E.; Garcia-Resua, C.; Yebra-Pimentel, E.; Giraldez, M.J. Meibum Lipidomic Analysis in Evaporative Dry Eye Subjects. *Int. J. Mol. Sci.* **2024**, *25*, 4782. https://doi.org/10.3390/ijms25094782.
2. Puente-Iglesias, M.; Cuartero-Martínez, A.; Touriño-Peralba, R.; Rodríguez-Ares, M.T.; Giráldez, M.J.; Yebra-Pimentel, E.; García-Quintanilla, L.; García-Otero, X.; González-Barcia, M.; Zarra-Ferro, I.; et al. Clinical Effectiveness, Safety, and Compliance of Two Compounded Formulations of Tacrolimus Eye Drops: An Open-Label, Sequential Prospective Study. *Int. J. Mol. Sci.* **2024**, *25*, 9847. https://doi.org/10.3390/ijms25189847.

3. Lee, K.; Gwon, H.; Kim, J.Y.; Shim, J.J.; Lee, J.H. Exosomes from *Limosilactobacillus fermentum* Ameliorate Benzalkonium Chloride-Induced Inflammation in Conjunctival Cells. *Int. J. Mol. Sci.* **2024**, *25*, 12282. https://doi.org/10.3390/ijms252212282.
4. Kaštelan, S.; Hat, K.; Tomić, Z.; Matejić, T.; Gotovac, N. Sex Differences in the Lacrimal Gland: Implications for Dry Eye Disease. *Int. J. Mol. Sci.* **2025**, *26*, 3833. https://doi.org/10.3390/ijms26083833.
5. Kahuam-López, N.; Hosseini, A.; Ling, J.Y.M.; Chiang, J.; Iovieno, A.; Yeung, S.N. The Role of Nerve Growth Factor on the Ocular Surface: A Review of the Current Experimental Research and Clinical Practices. *Int. J. Mol. Sci.* **2025**, *26*, 6012. https://doi.org/10.3390/ijms26136012.
6. Oya, S.; Higa, K.; Yasutake, T.; Yamazaki-Hokama, R.; Hirayama, M. Potential Roles of Extracellular Vesicles in Murine Tear Fluids in the Physiology of Corneal Epithelial Cells In Vitro. *Int. J. Mol. Sci.* **2025**, *26*, 7559. https://doi.org/10.3390/ijms26157559.
7. Serrano-Robles, J.G.; Pérez-Vázquez, A.K.; Vera-Duarte, G.R.; Navas, A.; Ramirez-Miranda, A.; Graue-Hernandez, E.O.; Kahuam-López, N. Safety and Efficacy of Diquafosol Compared to Artificial Tears for the Treatment of Dry Eye: A Systematic Review and Meta-Analysis. *Int. J. Mol. Sci.* **2025**, *26*, 8113. https://doi.org/10.3390/ijms26178113.
8. Jones, J.; Frenia, K.; Gelman, J.; Beatty, M.; Zhou, M.; Ma, L.; Pieramici, S.; Eger, N.; Dhaliwal, D.; Labriola, L.T.; et al. Translating Biomarker Discovery: From Bench to Bedside in Dry Eye Disease. *Int. J. Mol. Sci.* **2025**, *26*, 8556. https://doi.org/10.3390/ijms26178556.
9. Lee, J.D.; Kim, H.Y.; Oh, S.B.; Goo, H.; Cho, K.J.; Hwang, G.-W.; Kim, S.; Kim, K.-B. Effects of Exposure of PHMG-p, a Humidifier Disinfectant Component, on Eye Dryness: A Study on a Rat Model Based on ^{1}H-NMR Metabolomics. *Int. J. Mol. Sci.* **2025**, *26*, 8660. https://doi.org/10.3390/ijms26178660.
10. Soyfoo, M.; Motulsky, E.; Sarrand, J. Keratoconjunctivitis Sicca in Sjögren Disease: Diagnostic Challenges and Therapeutic Advances. *Int. J. Mol. Sci.* **2025**, *26*, 8824. https://doi.org/10.3390/ijms26188824.
11. Valencia-Sandonís, C.; Calderón-García, A.Á.; Blanco-Vázquez, M.; Valencia-Nieto, L.; Novo-Diez, A.; Vázquez, A.; Calonge, M.; González-García, M.J.; Enríquez-De-Salamanca, A. Long-Term Clinical and Molecular Changes in Dry Eye Disease and Chronic Ocular Pain. *Int. J. Mol. Sci.* **2025**, *26*, 8918. https://doi.org/10.3390/ijms26188918.
12. Saram, S.J.; Thomas, M.N.; Feinberg, L.; Roberts, H.W.; Ramsden, C.M.; Woronkowicz, M.; Skopiński, P. The Immunobiology of Dry Eye Disease: A Review of the Pathogenesis, Regulation and Therapeutic Implications. *Int. J. Mol. Sci.* **2025**, *26*, 10583. https://doi.org/10.3390/ijms262110583.

References

1. Craig, J.P.; Nichols, K.K.; Akpek, E.K.; Caffery, B.; Dua, H.S.; Joo, C.K.; Liu, Z.; Nelson, J.D.; Nichols, J.J.; Tsubota, K.; et al. TFOS DEWS II Definition and Classification Report. *Ocul. Surf.* **2017**, *15*, 276–283. [CrossRef] [PubMed]
2. Garrigue, J.S.; Amrane, M.; Faure, M.O.; Holopainen, J.M.; Tong, L. Relevance of Lipid-Based Products in the Management of Dry Eye Disease. *J. Ocul. Pharmacol. Ther.* **2017**, *33*, 647–661. [CrossRef] [PubMed] [PubMed Central]
3. Bland, H.C.; Moilanen, J.A.; Ekholm, F.S.; Paananen, R.O. Investigating the Role of Specific Tear Film Lipids Connected to Dry Eye Syndrome: A Study on O-Acyl-ω-hydroxy Fatty Acids and Diesters. *Langmuir* **2019**, *35*, 3545–3552. [CrossRef] [PubMed]
4. Fatima, A.; Attem, J.; Esam, S.; Vemuganti, G.K. Extracellular Vesicles of Tears and Ocular Surface: An Enigma. *Curr. Eye Res.* **2025**, *5*, 1–15. [CrossRef] [PubMed]
5. García-Otero, X.; Mondelo-García, C.; González, F.; Perez-Fernandez, R.; Avila, L.; Antúnez-López, J.R.; González-Barcia, M.; Adan, A.; Aguiar, P.; Otero-Espinar, F.J.; et al. Anti-Inflammatory Effect of Tacrolimus/Hydroxypropyl-β-Cyclodextrin Eye Drops in an Endotoxin-Induced Uveitis Model. *Pharmaceutics* **2021**, *13*, 1737. [CrossRef] [PubMed] [PubMed Central]
6. Ohashi, Y.; Munesue, M.; Shimazaki, J.; Takamura, E.; Yokoi, N.; Watanabe, H.; Nomura, A.; Shimada, F. Long-Term Safety and Effectiveness of Diquafosol for the Treatment of Dry Eye in a Real-World Setting: A Prospective Observational Study. *Adv. Ther.* **2020**, *37*, 707–717. [CrossRef] [PubMed] [PubMed Central]
7. Kaštelan, S.; Hat, K.; Tomić, Z.; Matejić, T.; Gotovac, N. Sex Differences in the Lacrimal Gland: Implications for Dry Eye Disease. *Int. J. Mol. Sci.* **2025**, *26*, 3833. [CrossRef] [PubMed] [PubMed Central]

8. Lambiase, A.; Sacchetti, M.; Bonini, S. Nerve growth factor therapy for corneal disease. *Curr. Opin. Ophthalmol.* **2012**, 23, 296–302. [CrossRef] [PubMed]
9. Galor, A.; Moein, H.R.; Lee, C.; Rodriguez, A.; Felix, E.R.; Sarantopoulos, K.D.; Levitt, R.C. Neuropathic pain and dry eye. *Ocul. Surf.* **2018**, *16*, 31–44. [CrossRef] [PubMed] [PubMed Central]

International Journal of
Molecular Sciences

MDPI

Article

Meibum Lipidomic Analysis in Evaporative Dry Eye Subjects

Jacobo Garcia-Queiruga [1,2], Hugo Pena-Verdeal [1,2], Belen Sabucedo-Villamarin [1], Monica Paz-Tarrio [3], Esteban Guitian-Fernandez [3], Carlos Garcia-Resua [1,2], Eva Yebra-Pimentel [1,2] and Maria J. Giraldez [1,2,*]

[1] GI-2092 Optometry, Departamento de Física Aplicada, Facultad de Óptica y Optometría, Universidade de Santiago de Compostela, Campus Vida s/n, 15701 Santiago de Compostela, Spain; jacobogarcia.queiruga@usc.es (J.G.-Q.); hugo.pena.verdeal@usc.es (H.P.-V.); belen.sabucedo@rai.usc.es (B.S.-V.); carlos.garcia.resua@usc.es (C.G.-R.); eva.yebra-pimentel@usc.es (E.Y.-P.)

[2] AC-24 Optometry, Instituto de Investigación Sanitaria de Santiago de Compostela (IDIS), Travesía da Choupana, 15701 Santiago de Compostela, Spain

[3] Mass Spectrometry and Proteomic Unit, Área de Infraestruturas de Investigación, Universidade de Santiago de Compostela, Campus Vida s/n, 15701 Santiago de Compostela, Spain; monica.paz@usc.es (M.P.-T.); esteban.guitian@usc.es (E.G.-F.)

* Correspondence: mjesus.giraldez@usc.es

Abstract: Meibomian Glands (MG) are sebaceous glands responsible for the production of meibum, the main component of the Tear Film Lipid Layer (TFLL). The TFLL facilitates the spread of the tear film over the ocular surface, provides stability and reduces tear evaporation. Alterations in meibum composition lead to different ocular alterations like Meibomian Gland Dysfunction (MGD) and subsequent Evaporative Dry Eye (EDE). The aim of the present study was to investigate the composition and abundance of meibum lipids and their relationship with eyelid margin abnormalities, lipid layer patterns and MG status. The study utilizes a lipidomic approach to identify and quantify lipids in meibum samples using an Elute UHPLC system. This system considered all four dimensions (mass/charge, retention time, ion mobility and intensity) to provide the accurate identification of lipid species. Samples were categorized as healthy or low/no signs of alteration (group 1) or severe signs of alteration or EDE/MGD (group 2). The current investigation found differences in Variable Importance in Projection lipid abundance between both groups for the MGD signs studied. Changes in meibum composition occur and are related to higher scores in eyelid margin hyperaemia, eyelid margin irregularity, MG orifice plugging, MG loss and lipid layer pattern.

Keywords: meibum; tear film lipid layer; eyelid margin abnormalities; meibomian gland; lipid layer pattern

1. Introduction

Meibomian Glands (MG) are sebaceous glands located in the tarsal plates of both superior and inferior eyelids, and which excrete into the eyelid margin where their orifices are located [1]. These glands are responsible for the production of the meibum, which is a lipid secretion and the main component of the Tear Film Lipid Layer (TFLL) [2,3]. Reducing the tear evaporation rate and reducing the surface tension to facilitate the spreading of the tear film on the ocular surface are the main functions of the TFLL, both of which are related to the non-polar and polar lipids that constitute it [3]. The tear film contains water, electrolytes, mucins and a large compound of proteins and lipids, forming a bilayer made of a hydrated mucus layer and a lipid layer [4]. The TFLL is a biphase of non-polar and polar lipids, each with particular characteristics that allow interaction with air (non-polar lipids) and with the muco-aqueous layer (polar lipids) [5]. Changes in the chemical composition of any of the layers can alter the structure, function, or dynamics of the tear film, disrupting the homeostasis of the ocular surface, which may result in dry eye disease (DED) [6–9].

Meibomian Gland Dysfunction (MGD) is the primary cause of Evaporative Dry Eye (EDE), which is the most prevalent type of DED in the entire global population [10]. The diagnosis of EDE due to MGD include a range of clinical tests to identify the presence of symptoms and different signs compatible with eyelid margin abnormalities, alterations in the MG morphology and anormal tear film dynamics [11–15]. These clinical tests evaluate various ocular characteristics of different ocular structures. The features regarding eyelid margin abnormalities include eyelid margin hyperaemia, irregularity, thickening and plugging of the MG orifices [12]. In the case of MG morphology, meibography images captured with infrared cameras allow clinicians to evaluate the MG loss, MG drop out and partial glands [12,13]. Measuring the thickness of the TFLL provides indirect information about the status of the MG secretion, so clinicians analyse Lipid Layer Patterns (LLP) with interferometers to assess it [14,15]. Even though MGD can be present in different forms (highly productive MGD or obstructive MGD), the most prevalent is the obstructive, which is related to the hyper-keratinisation of the MG main duct, the plugging of the MG orifices in the eyelid margin and the destruction of the MGs [1,2]. The obstruction of the MG affects the quantity and quality of the meibum, where thicker secretions are more difficult to spread over the ocular surface, leading to tear film instability [3,4,16].

The meibum is a lipid-rich secretion mainly composed of non-polar lipids such as wax esters, cholesterol esters (CE), triacylglycerols (TG) and polar lipids such as ceramides (Cer), sphingomyelins and phospholipids, among others [2]. The lipidomic profile of the meibum has been studied by performing different techniques in animal and human models, such as thin layer chromatography, gas chromatography, and high-performance liquid chromatography [5,17–21]. Different researchers have found changes in the meibum composition in various states of ocular diseases such as DED and MGD [7,22,23]. It has been observed that changes in meibum composition are not only due to DED, but also to other comorbidities such as diabetes mellitus [21]. In the same way that other ocular physiological aspects such as cataracts or eyelid ptosis are influenced by ageing, changes in the composition of the meibum have also been correlated with older subjects [9]. In addition, researchers have identified a significant negative correlation between the abundance of non-polar lipids and the presence of specific symptoms, including ocular fatigue, blurred vision and decreased visual acuity, among MGD subjects [9]. Specific information on which lipids influence the manifestation of each alteration in the multiple eyelid margin abnormalities, MG features or TFLL has not been found in depth. Paranjpe et al. [7] studied some of these ocular sings of alteration related to different aspects of the MGs, such as MG orifice plugging and MG atrophy or loss. They found an association between these MGD signs and changes in meibum composition, with an increase in sphingomieline and a drop in Cer [7]. In another report, cholesterol esters and wax esters showed no relationship between MGD severity status and precorneal tear film thinning [24].

In response to the demands of researchers in the MGs and meibum field for further research to elucidate the pathophysiology of MGD, the aim of the present study was to determine which lipids are present in high amounts in the different characteristics that should be studied for the proper diagnosis of MGD and the subsequent DED (eyelid margin abnormalities, LLP, and morphological changes in the MG). Also, the lipid identification method performed in the present study is a novel four-dimensional workflow that considered all four dimensions (mass/charge [m/z], retention time, ion mobility and intensity) to provide the most accurate lipid species identification.

2. Results

2.1. Lipidomic Profiling Untargeted Analysis

A total of 44 meibum samples from upper and lower eyelids were analysed using PASEF® MS/MS mode (Online Parallel Accumulation-Serial Fragmentation) for the untargeted analysis [25]. A total of 131 lipids were identified in the data analysis. Among these, 38 lipids were determined in at least 95% of the samples. The number of lipids identified according to their lipid class is listed in Table 1.

Table 1. Number of lipids identified according to their lipid class.

Lipid Class		N° Lipids
Ceramides	(Cer)	15
Hexosyceramides	(HexCer)	1
Monodiacyglycerophosphocholines	(LPC)	8
Diacylglycerophosphocholines	(PC)	15
Diacylglycerophosphoethanolamines	(PE)	2
Diacylglycerophosphoglycerols	(PG)	2
Diacylglycerophosphoinositols	(PI)	1
Ceramide phosphocholenes	(SM)	10
Sphingosines	(SPB)	10
Cholesterol Ester	(CE)	16
Diacyglycerols	(DG)	13
Triacylglycerols	(TG)	38

2.2. Comparison of Meibum Lipids between Groups

A supervised orthogonal partial least squares discriminant analysis (ortho-DA) was performed to discriminate between groups 1 (healthy subjects with no or low levels of alteration in the studied parameters) and 2 (EDE/MGD subjects with severe signs of alteration in the studied parameters) (represented in Figure 1 as purple circles for group 1 and green triangles for group 2) and to graphically observe whether the species present in each group for each characteristic studied were different. The score plot of ortho-DA was performed on the different eyelid margin characteristics studied (Figure 1). Ortho-DA score plots completely distinguished groups 1 and 2 in eyelid margin hyperaemia (Figure 1A), MG orifice plugging (Figure 1B) and eyelid margin irregularity (Figure 1C). Nevertheless, the ortho-DA score plot showed an overlapping of the lipid species between groups for eyelid margin thickening (Figure 1D). A score plot of ortho-DA was also performed for LLP, MG loss, MG drop out and partial glands characteristics. Ortho-DA score plots completely distinguished groups 1 and 2 from the LLPs (Figure 1E) and MG loss (Figure 1F). Nevertheless, they showed an overlapping of lipid species between both groups on MG drop out (Figure 1G) and partial glands (Figure 1H).

The lipids with Variable Importance in Projection (VIP) from the ortho-DA higher than 1.5 (Figure 2) were considered biologically relevant in the LLPs (Figure 2A), eyelid margin hyperaemia (Figure 2B), MG orifice plugging (Figure 2C), eyelid margin irregularity (Figure 2D) and MG loss features (Figure 2E).

The lipid profile of the VIP lipids was studied in detail using a clustering analysis which was represented in a heatmap for each of the ocular features. Heatmaps of the clustering analysis for the different features analysed show graphically which VIP lipids are present or absent in each group (Figures 3–7). Each heatmap shows the VIP lipids in rows and the samples of each eye (secretion collected from both eyelids) analysed in columns. The most similar samples are displayed closely. The first row of boxes represents the group to which samples correspond, with purple for group 1 (healthy subjects with no or low levels of alteration in the studied parameters) and green for group 2 (EDE/MGD subjects with severe signs of alteration in the studied parameters). The colour of each box indicates the high (red) or low (blue) abundance of each VIP lipid.

Heatmaps represent the VIP lipids whose abundance differs between samples according to the ortho-DA analysis. Heatmaps show the differences between group 1 (boxes under the first box purple row) and group 2 (boxes under the first box green row) graphically. While group 1 samples showed high or low abundance of each VIP lipid identified in each ocular parameter analysed (LLPs in Figure 3, eyelid margin hyperaemia in Figure 4, MG orifice plugging in Figure 5, eyelid margin irregularity in Figure 6, and MG loss in Figure 7), group 2 showed the opposite.

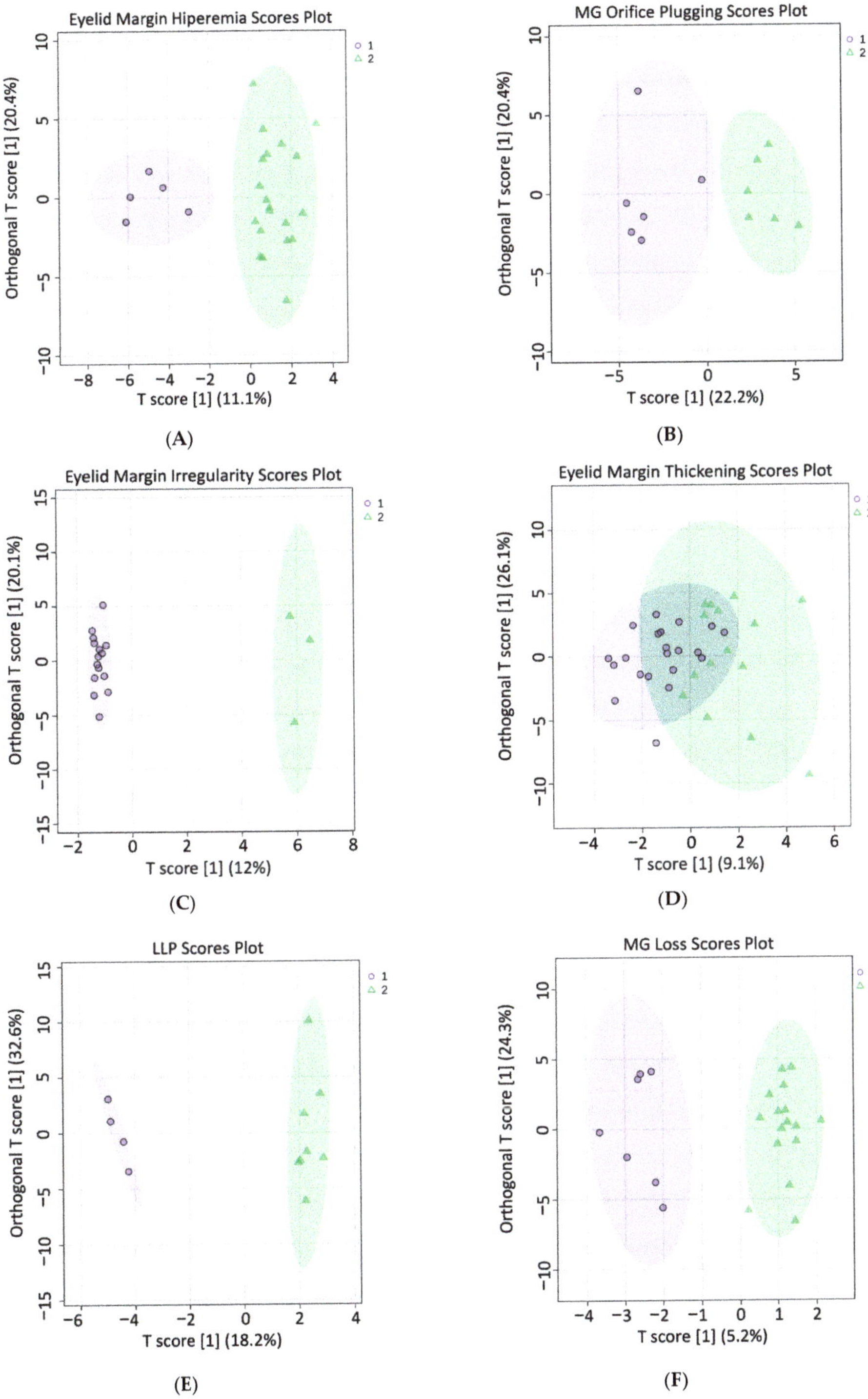

Figure 1. *Cont.*

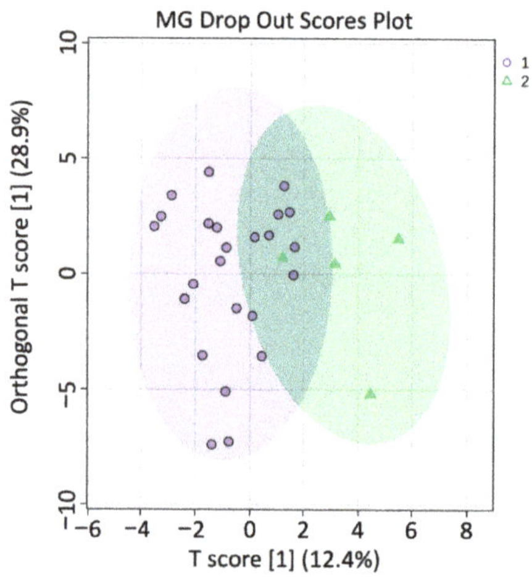

(**G**)

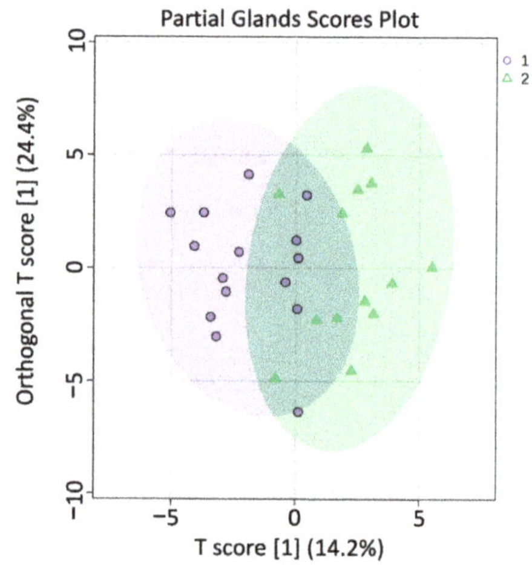

(**H**)

Figure 1. Ortho-DA score plots for eyelid margin abnormalities, LLPs and meibography. (**A**) Hyperaemia ortho-DA; (**B**) MG orifice plugging ortho-DA; (**C**) irregularity ortho-DA; (**D**) eyelid margin thickening ortho-DA; (**E**) LLP ortho-DA; (**F**) MG loss ortho-DA; (**G**) MG drop out ortho-DA; (**H**) partial glands ortho-DA. Score plots are shown for "T score" and "Orthogonal T score." Purple circles and green triangles represents samples from group 1 and group 2, respectively. LLP: lipid layer pattern; MG: meibomian gland; Ortho-DA: supervised orthogonal partial least squares discriminant analysis.

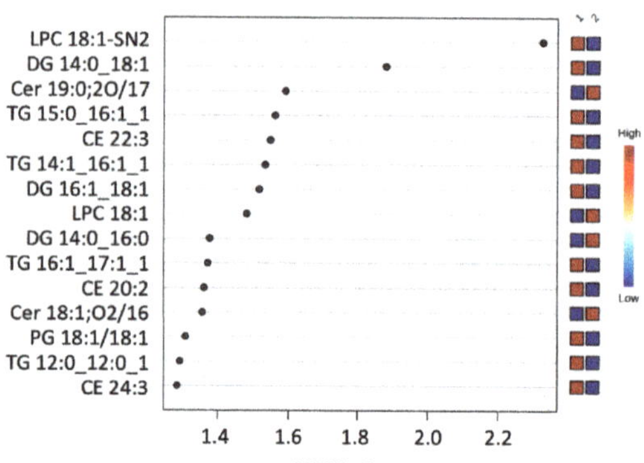

(**A**)

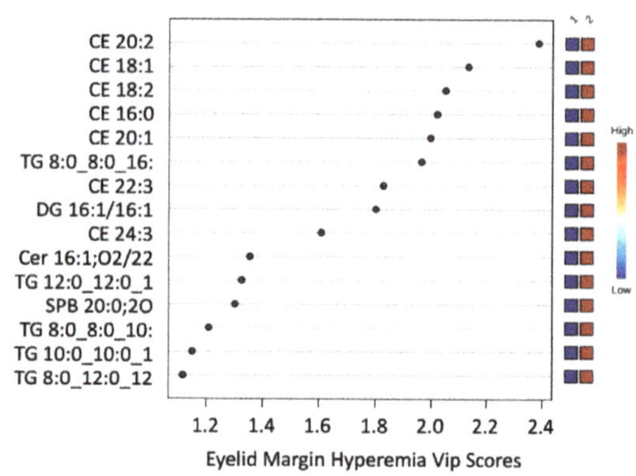

(**B**)

Figure 2. *Cont.*

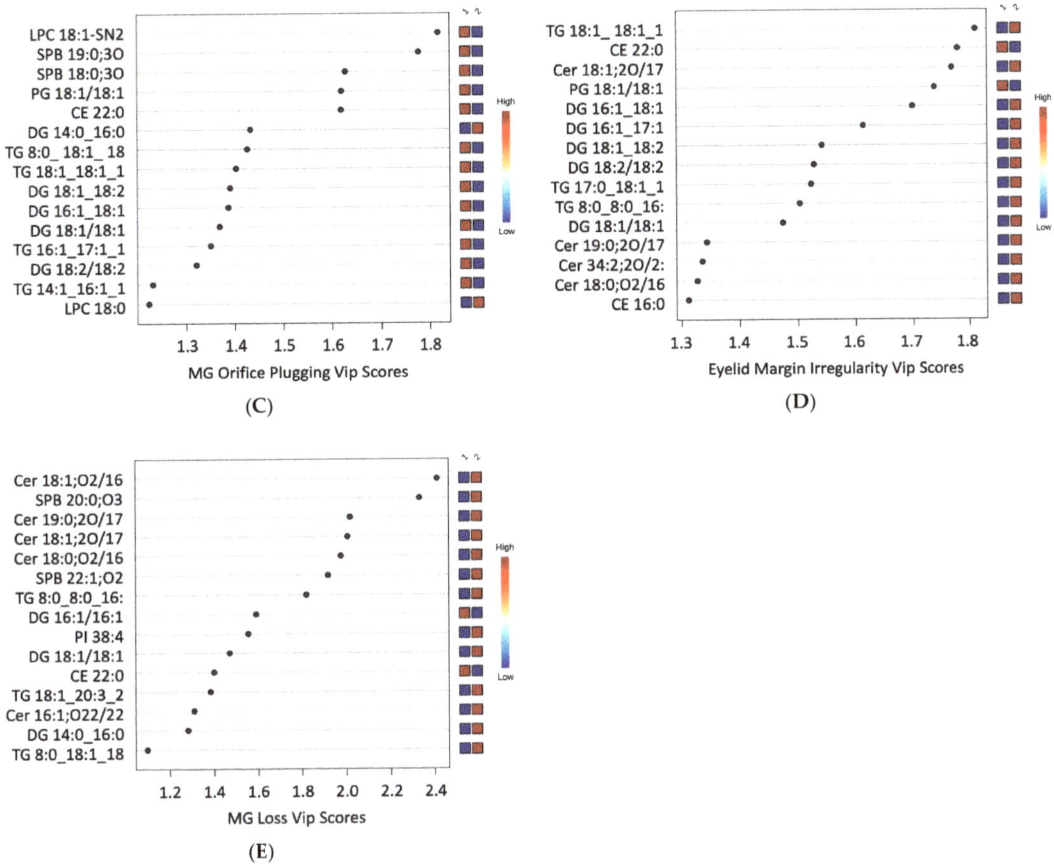

Figure 2. VIP scores of first discriminant function. VIP scores show the top lipid species selected by the ortho-DA analysis for component T. (**A**) VIP scores from LLP study. (**B**) VIP scores from eyelid margin hyperaemia study. (**C**) VIP scores from MG orifice plugging study. (**D**) VIP scores from eyelid margin irregularity study. (**E**) VIP scores from MG loss study. LLP: Lipid Layer Pattern; MG: Meibomian Gland; VIP: Variable Importance in Protection.

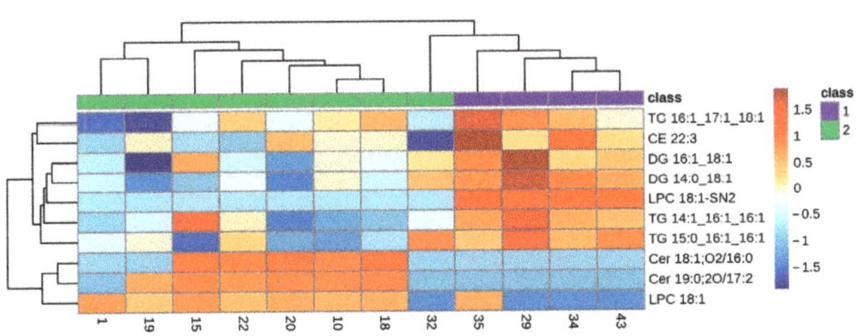

Figure 3. Clustering analysis. Hierarchical clustering analysis from LLP VIP lipids. Clustering analysis of 10 VIP lipid species from the LLP statistical analysis. Each column represents individual samples, and each row represents individual lipids. Blue and red colours represent low and high lipid abundance, respectively. Sample groups are represented by colours purple and green for groups 1 and 2, respectively. LLP: Lipid Layer Pattern; VIP: Variable Importance in Projection.

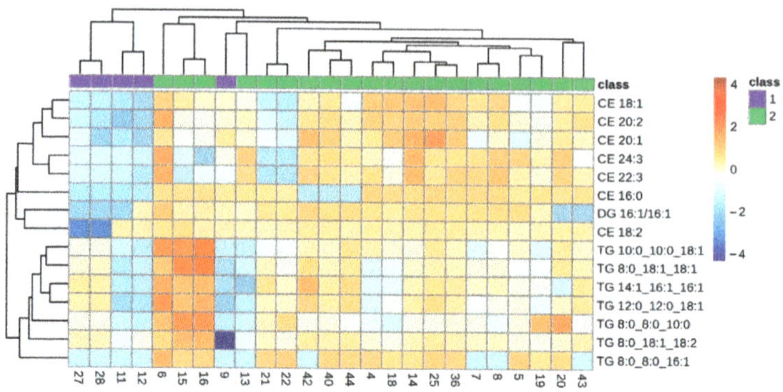

Figure 4. Clustering analysis. Hierarchical clustering analysis from eyelid margin hyperaemia VIP lipids. Clustering analysis of 15 VIP lipid species from the eyelid margin hyperaemia statistical analysis. Each column represents individual samples, and each row represents individual lipids. Blue and red colours represent low and high lipid abundance, respectively. Sample groups are represented by colours purple and green for groups 1 and 2, respectively. VIP: Variable Importance in Projection.

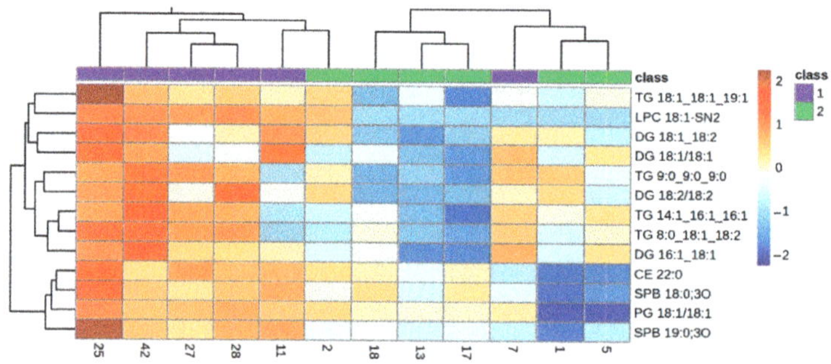

Figure 5. Clustering analysis. Hierarchical clustering analysis from MG orifice plugging VIP lipids. Clustering analysis of 13 VIP lipid species from the MG orifice plugging statistical analysis. Each column represents individual samples, and each row represents individual lipids. Blue and red colours represent low and high lipid abundance, respectively. Sample groups are represented by colours purple and green for groups 1 and 2, respectively. MG: Meibomian Gland; VIP: Variable Importance in Projection.

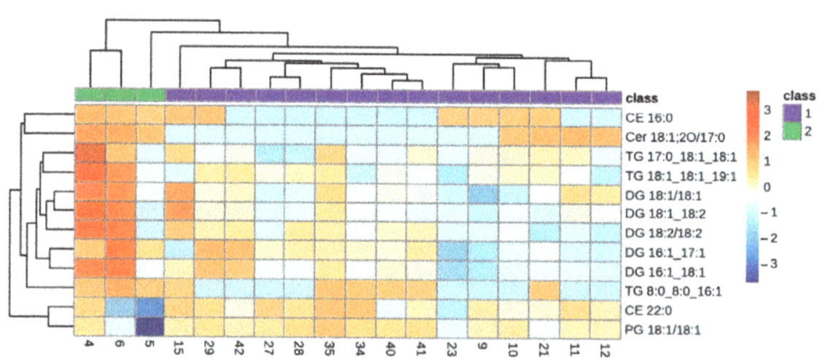

Figure 6. Clustering analysis. Hierarchical clustering analysis from eyelid margin irregularity VIP lipids. Clustering analysis of 12 VIP lipid species from the eyelid margin irregularity statistical analysis. Each column represents individual samples, and each row represents individual lipids. Blue and red colours represent low and high lipid abundance, respectively. Sample groups are represented by colours purple and green for groups 1 and 2, respectively. VIP: Variable Importance in Projection.

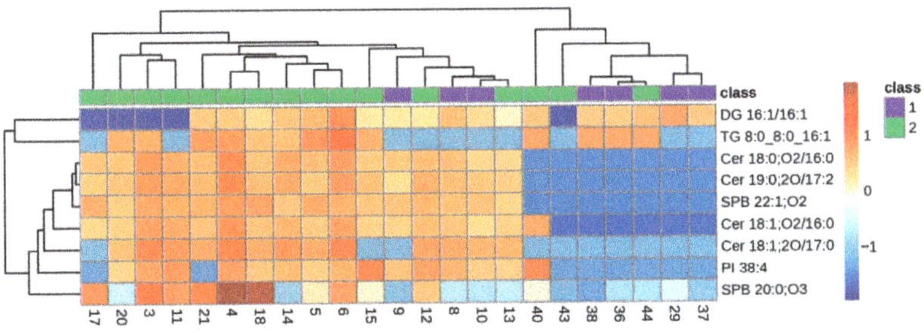

Figure 7. Clustering analysis. Hierarchical clustering analysis from MG loss VIP lipids. Clustering analysis of 9 VIP lipid species from the MG loss statistical analysis. Each column represents individual samples, and each row represents individual lipids. Blue and red colours represent low and high lipid abundance, respectively. Sample groups are represented by colours purple and green for groups 1 and 2, respectively. MG: Meibomian Gland; VIP: Variable Importance in Projection.

3. Discussion

The aim of the present study was to determine which lipids are present in high amounts in those subjects who showed no alteration in the different characteristics of the eyelid margin, of the LLP and of the MG (group 1) compared to those with high degrees of alteration in all studied features (group 2). Only lipids classified as VIP were studied because of their relative presence in the meibum samples and their biological importance [5,26]. Overall, the findings of this study add valuable information to the literature by relating the presence of each lipid and its possible relationship to the severity of ocular disorders.

A total of eight ocular surface features were analysed in the present study, and ortho-DA only found differences in meibum composition due to characteristic alterations in five of them (LLPs, eyelid margin hyperaemia, MG orifice plugging, eyelid margin irregularity and MG loss). The LLPs could be the most representative characteristic of the meibum on the ocular surface because this feature represents the density of the TFLL. The TFLL is a biphase composed of polar and non-polar lipids, and the present study found 64 polar lipids and 67 non-polar lipids in the 44 samples analysed. Among those 131 lipids identified in the meibum samples, 10 of them were characterized as VIP for the LLP. The heatmap (Figure 4) shows an enhancement in the abundance of polar lipids (Cer 18:1;02/16:0, Cer 19:0;2O/17:2 and LPC 18:1) on the samples that presented thinner LLPs (group 2). Additionally, a clear reduction in the abundance of non-polar lipids (CE, TG and DG) is represented in the heatmap (Figure 3). This finding supports the hypothesis stated by different researchers, where thinner TFLL are related to the reduction in meibum production due to MGD, and where a change in the meibum composition, showing an increase in polar lipids, occurs [8,9,27]. Additionally, these findings are in accordance with those supporting the important structural role of the Cer in TFLL, where an increase in concentration leads to an increase in the melting temperature of the meibum, causing the destabilization of the TFLL [16].

In the case of eyelid margin hyperaemia, 15 VIP lipids were identified in the meibum samples of both groups. All those VIP lipids were non-polar species (CE, DG and TG) that showed differences in the ortho-DA between both groups. These non-polar lipids showed a variation in their abundance, from being absent in group 1 to being quite marked in group 2 (Figure 4). This observation could be related to the physiology changes that take place in those MGs from the subjects of the group 2. Those MGs are suffering from altered meibocyte maturation, but they do not stop excreting even though partial hyperkeratinisation occurs in the MG duct [1]. However, a decrease in all VIP lipids analysed from the MG orifice plugging feature in group 1 and group 2 can be observed in the heatmap (Figure 5). Both margin hyperaemia and MG orifice plugging findings in the heatmaps could be interpreted from a clinical perspective, because it is common to find high values of eyelid margin hyperaemia and margin telangiectasia related to high values of MG orifice plugging [6,28]. The decrease in lipid abundance found in the analysed samples between both groups for MG orifice plugging could be explained by the physico-chemical properties of the plug because the plugs are composed of polar species such as diacylglycerols [6]. The present study was not intended to collect the plugs, as it would have been necessary to generate a large force which could cause the lid margin to be scraped off [29]. If the plugs had been included in the samples, an increase in polar lipids would have been observed. However, a lower abundance of the same VIP lipids was found and a high amount of polar lipids was not found because the meibum collected came from those MGs that excreted due to being not plugged.

Eyelid margin irregularity could be found in severe states of MGD and EDE and in elderly populations [30,31]. Due to the small sample analysed in the present study, only 3 meibum samples were from subjects that showed eyelid margin irregularity (group 2), against 15 samples of healthy ones. Nevertheless, ortho-DA was able to discriminate between the two groups in terms of meibum composition (Figure 1C). The samples of group 2 showed higher amounts of non-polar lipids, such as CE, TG and DG, and just Cer formed the group of polar lipids (Figure 6). Two explanations could be attributed to these observations. First, the higher abundance of non-polar lipids observed in those eyelid margins with irregularity could be related to the morphology of those altered eyelid margins that could function as a bigger reservoir. Secondly, Cer is related to destabilization of the TFLL, and so an unstable TFLL could lead to an inefficient tear film that could not be adequately spread over the ocular surface remaining in the eyelid margin reservoir.

The quantification of MG loss by meibography has rapidly become popular for the diagnosis of MGD, but other features of the MGs also play an important role in the pathophysiology of the disease, such as eyelid margin abnormalities [12,32–34]. The ortho-DA analysis performed in the present study was able to discriminate between group 1 and group 2 according to the presence of different lipids species and MG loss. Considerable amounts of SPB 22:1;O2 and SPB 20:0;O3 were found in samples of the group 1, but no sample of group 2 showed the presence of these polar lipids (Figure 7). An MG loss heatmap represented the VIP lipids present among the studied samples, and it showed a decrease in different lipid species for the group 2 samples, with particular emphasis on different Cer. The variation in lipid abundance observed in this study is directly linked to the alteration of the MG morphology. MGs that are reduced in size and number per eyelid produce less meibum compared to healthy and full-length MGs. Also, only digital force was applied during the collection of the meibum; no forceps were used to express the MGs, so meibum samples came primarily from the eyelid margin reservoir. Those subjects that presented severe MG loss had altered MGs, and the main ducts were at some point hyper-keratinised. The lower abundance of Cer shown in the heatmaps could be explained by the absence of a high force applied to force the excretion of the MGs, as their main ducts would be hyper-keratinised and could show high amounts of Cer due to its involvement in the keratinisation process [7,16].

The study of the lipid profile in extracts of complex lipids can be an arduous task that requires a lot of time to perform several types of analyses in database searches and for confident annotation. Lipids are a class of extraordinarily complex compounds, with a wide structural diversity. The work of performing such an annotation can be greatly minimized by applying a 4D workflow (m/z ratio, retention time, ion mobility and intensity). With this 4D workflow, the authors can speed up the annotation process of these lipids using data obtained by mass spectrometry and trapped ion mobility. By using PASEF® [35] MS/MS mode (Online Parallel Accumulation-Serial Fragmentation), the authors could achieve greater coverage in the MS/MS fragmentations performed. Furthermore, by using mobility, the authors managed to clean the MS/MS spectra and improve the matching of the fragmentation rules or spectral libraries. Another third improvement factor is the acquired Collisional Cross Section (CCS) values, which can be used directly to increase confidence in the annotation of the lipids to be searched.

Regarding limitations, the present study used a cross-sectional design, which offers information only at a single time point, potentially overlooking longitudinal changes or causal relationships that may occur during the chronic process of the disease. Moreover, the manual expression technique used for collecting meibum samples may introduce variability in the quantity of samples collected. As other authors have demonstrated, forceps expression could be an alternative to obtain higher amounts of lipids [29], and also from those MG that have been obstructed. However, the use of forceps has the disadvantage that ocular anaesthesia must be applied due to the discomfort of the procedure. Finally, the small sample size, particularly concerning subjects with eyelid margin irregularity, restricts the generalizability of findings, as elderly individuals, potentially presenting with age-related comorbidities, were excluded from the study.

The findings of the present study have many clinical implications, such as offering valuable insights that could provide additional information to clinicians regarding the diagnosis and management of highly prevalent disorders such as MGD and EDE. This interdisciplinary collaboration between basic research and clinical application underscores the transformative power of scientific inquiry in advancing patient care and underscores the critical role of translational research in filling the gap between both areas. First, this investigation could enhance the implementation of meibum analysis by clinical laboratories of hospitals, as occurs with urine, faeces, mucus or blood samples. The implementation of this protocol in hospitals or eye care centres will have a significant clinical impact with a very low economic burden and will produce rapid analysis without being time-consuming. Understanding the correlation between meibum lipid composition and eye conditions will provide eye care professionals with more accurate strategies to treat these disorders and potentially improve the quality of life of affected patients. Second, the current findings have potential for transfer to the pharmaceutical industry, as novel tear substitutes could be developed and customized to each type of DED, focusing on the specific ocular alterations that show those patients suffering from EDE and/or MGD. DED management aims to alleviate ocular symptoms by reducing eye pain and discomfort. Identifying the specific lipids altered in each severity type of EDE/MGD is crucial as it could lead to targeted ocular therapies that restore ocular homeostasis, particularly significant in a chronic condition like DED. Presently, many tear substitutes and liposome sprays may not provide comprehensive relief for EDE/MGD, and in some cases, the compounds they contain might exacerbate patients' conditions. Developing new treatments based on meibum findings holds promise for improving patient outcomes and benefiting pharmaceutical industries.

4. Materials and Methods

4.1. Sample and Study Design

The present cross-sectional study enrolled a total of 22 participants (44 eyes) with mean age 50.8 $\pm$ 14.5 years old (75% women). All the participants were recruited from the Optometry Clinic of the centre, and all signed a written consent form to be included in the study. The protocol adhered to the tenets of the Declaration of Helsinki and was approved by the Bioethics Committee of the institution (Approval Number: USC-40/2020). As the main inclusion criteria, participants could not have a history of eye diseases such as glaucoma, ocular allergy, age-related macular degeneration, ocular trauma or ocular surgery, nor have suffered from any systemic disease [36]. Participants were either healthy subjects or subjects previously diagnosed with EDE/MGD who were offered the opportunity to participate in the study.

In a single appointment, an ocular examination including LLP, eyelid margin exploration, meibography and meibum collection was performed.

4.2. Ocular Procedures

All ocular examinations were performed by the same observer, and all procedures were analysed by a second masked observer. The procedures were performed from least to most invasive to avoid any possible interaction between them [11]. The classification scheme followed for each procedure is summarized in Table 2.

Table 2. Grading scales used to evaluate the ocular parameters related to the meibum.

Procedure		Scheme	Classification Criteria
LLP		Guillon et al. [14]	· Grade 1—Coloured · Grade 2—Amorphous · Grade 3—Fluid · Grade 4—Close Meshwork · Grade 5—Open Meshwork
Eyelid Margin Abnormalities	Hyperaemia	Arita et al. [12]	· Grade 0—No or slight hypaeremia and no telangiectasia · Grade 1—Hyperaemia and no telangiectasia · Grade 2—Hyperaemia and telangiectasia crossing MG in less than half of the full lid margin · Grade 3—Hyperaemia and telangiectasia crossing MG in half or more than half of the full lid margin
	MG orifice plugging	Arita et al. [12]	· Grade 0—No MG orifice plugging · Grade 1—Less than 3 MG plugged · Grade 2—3 or more MG plugged distributed in less than half of the full length of the eyelid margin · Grade 3—3 or more MG plugged distributed in half or more of the full length of the eyelid margin
	Irregularity	Arita et al. [12]	· Grade 0—No irregularity · Grade 1—Less than 3 irregularities · Grade 2—3 or more irregularities
	Eyelid margin thickening	Arita et al. [12]	· Grade 0—No thickening · Grade 1—Thickening with/without rounding · Grade 2—Thickening with diffuse rounding
Meibography	MG loss	Pult et al. [13]	· Grade 1—<25% MG loss · Grade 2—25% to 50% MG loss · Grade 3—50% to 75% MG loss · Grade 4—>75% MG loss
	MG drop out	Arita et al. [12]	· Grade 0—No dropout · Grade 1—Less than 3 dropouts · Grade 2—3 or more dropouts
	Partial glands	Arita et al. [12]	· Grade 0—No partial glands · Grade 1—Less than 3 partial glands · Grade 2—3 or more partial glands and fewer than 3 with loss of half or more of the full MG length · Grade 3—3 or more partial with loss of half or more of the full MG length

LLP: Lipid Layer Pattern; MG: Meibomian Gland.

4.2.1. Lipid Layer Patterns

An EasyTear (Easytear S.R.L, Rovereto, Italy) interferometer was attached to the slit-lamp Topcon SL-D4 (Topcon Corporation, Tokyo, Japan) to observe LLPs [37]. A video of LLPs for each eye was captured by the Topcon DC-4 (Topcon Corporation, Tokyo, Japan) camera mounted on the slit-lamp. LLPs were first described by Guillon and the thickness of the TFLL could be estimated due to the interferometric pattern. Also, Guillon's scheme was followed to categorize LLPs into 5 grades (from thickest to thinnest lipid layer) [14] (Table 2).

4.2.2. Eyelid Margin Abnormalities

Once LLPs had been videotaped, the examination of upper and lower eyelid margins was performed under a Topcon SL-D4 slit-lamp. A video of each eye was captured for its analysis following the Arita et al. [12] grading scale. Several aspects of eyelid margin alterations were assessed, such as hyperemia, MG orifice plugging, irregularity and margin thickening (Table 2).

4.2.3. Meibography

Meibography images were taken with OCULUS Keratograph 5M (OCULUS Optikgeräte GmbH, Wetzlar, Germany), which was used to analyse the in vivo status of the MG. MG loss was calculated by subtracting the total area of the eyelid and the area of the MG [38]. The value obtained was expressed as a percentage, which was used to categorize each eyelid into the grades stated by Pult et al. [13] (Table 2). Also, the total number of partial MG and MG dropout results were classified following Arit et al. [12]'s scheme (Table 2).

4.2.4. Meibum Sample Collection

Participants were requested to position themselves properly in the chinrest of the slit-lamp and to maintain their gaze on the ceiling or to the floor, depending on which eyelid was being examined. A continuous pressure with the thumb for 30 s was applied to the lower and upper eyelids to force the MG to excrete the meibum and reach the MG orifice on the eyelid margin (Figure 8). A clean and sterilized stainless steel spatula was used to collect the meibum, first from the lower and then from the upper eyelid, taking care not scrape the eyelid margins [5]. The samples were placed in a clean topaz HPLC vial filled with 1 mL of chloroform. Each vial contained a sample collected from both lower and upper eyelids. Samples from both eyelids were analysed together because meibum secreted by both eyelids is responsible for tear film dynamics, and one sample can cloud the influence or alter the other due to meibum deposition at the eyelid margin. The samples were stored in a freezer at −30 °C until their later measurement.

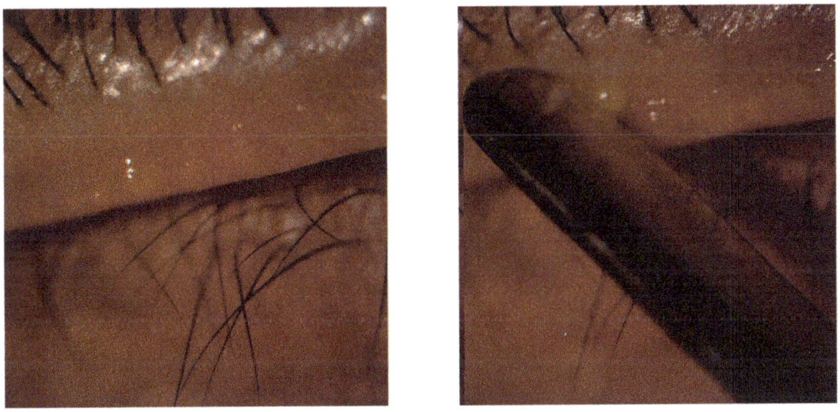

(A) (B)

Figure 8. MG expression and meibum collection. (**A**) Meibum reaching the MG orifices at the eyelid margin; (**B**) sample collection with stainless steel spatula. MG: Meibomian Gland.

4.3. *Materials for Sample Preparation and Liquid Chromatography*

Milli-Q water (Merk KGaA, Darmstadt, Germany), acetonitrile UHPLC-MS (Carlo Erba Reagents, Barcelona, Spain), propano-2-ol for LC/MS (Carlo Erba Reagents, Barcelona, Spain), chloroform HPLC grade (Fisher Chemical, Thermo Fisher Scientific, Waltham, MA,

USA), ammonium formate for LCMS (Carlo Erba Reagents, Barcelona, Spain) and formic acid for LC-MS (Carlo Erba Reagents, Barcelona, Spain) were used in the present study.

4.4. Meibum Sample Preparation

Samples, once collected in topaz vials, were stored in a freezer at −30 °C until their later measurement. Before measuring them, they were evaporated for 30 min in a Speed-Vac Savant SPD121P-230 (Thermo Electron Corporation, Milford, MA, USA), and each sample was resuspended in a methanol–chloroform solution (1:1).

4.5. Liquid Chromatography–Mass Spectrometry Analysis

Reversed phase-based liquid chromatography separation was performed using an Elute® UHPLC system with a Bruker Intensity Solo C18 column (100 × 2.1 mm, 1.8 μm) (Bruker Daltonics GmbH, Billerica, MA, USA).

A volume of 5 μL was injected onto the column. The column compartment was heated to 55 °C, while the autosampler was cooled at 8 °C to avoid sample evaporation. Samples were separated with a binary gradient at a constant flow rate of 0.4 mL/min. The mobile phases were composed of solvent A (acetonitrile/water 60:40, 10 mM NH_4 formate, 0.1% FA) and solvent B (isopropanol/acetonitrile 90:10, 10 mM NH_4 formate, 0.1% FA). A 20 min gradient was used (0 min 40%B, 1 min 43%B, 1.10 min 50%B, 6 min 54%B, 6.10 min 70%B, 9.0 min 99%B, 20.0 min 99%B). Also, 5 min pre-running was employed to re-equilibrate the column for initial conditions.

The mass spectrometry experiment was undertaken in positive VIP-HESI® mode (Vacuum Insulated Probe Heated Electrospray Ionization) using a timsTOF Pro (Bruker Daltonics GmbH & Co. KG., Billerica, MA, USA) mass spectrometer in PASEF MS/MS mode. The transfer parameters were optimized for mass range (100–1350 m/z) and mobility range (0.55–1.87 1/K0), and precursors were fragmented from 100 to 1350 m/z. Mass range was calibrated using the ions of the sodium formate and the ion mobility dimension was calibrated using the ions of the ESI-L Low Concentration Tuning Mix (Agilent Technologies, Santa Clara, CA, USA).

4.6. Lipid Annotation

Resulting data were processed considering all four dimensions (m/z, retention time, ion mobility and intensity) and MS/MS spectra were assigned to them using MetaboScape® 2023b Version 11.0.4 (Bruker Daltonics GmbH & Co. KG., Billerica, MA, USA) in the specified range of 100–1350 m/z. A T-ReX 4D® algorithm (Bruker Daltonics GmbH & Co. KG., Billerica, MA, USA) was used which combined all adducts and isotopes belonging to the same lipid into features. Feature detection was performed using an intensity threshold of 1500 counts. $[M + H]^+$, $[M + Na]^+$ and $[M + NH_4]^+$ ions were selected in the ion configuration settings. The processing algorithm combined all adducts and isotopes belonging to the same lipid.

The features were matched against the open source in-silico MS/MS library LipidBlast (Version 68; http://fiehnlab.ucdavis.edu/projects/LipidBlast; accessed on 15 January 2024) [25,39] and rule-based lipid annotation implemented in MetaboScape (algorithm MCube Lipid Species Annotation). The lipid database implemented in this algorithm is structured according to the lipid maps hierarchy (lipid category > lipid main class > lipid sub class). To distinguish lipid species' accurate m/z ratiod, isotopic pattern (mSigma value) and CCS values of the precursor, as well as MS/MS spectra, were employed.

The tentatively assigned lipids are those that received an annotation by rule-based annotation and LipidBlast assignment, both within 2 mDa precursor mass. Additionally, assignments were filtered, matching with scores greater than 600 MSMS, to ensure that lipids were annotated based on high-quality MS/MS spectra and matching with lower than 3% deviations of CCS measured value vs. the predicted CCS value [26,40,41]. The results were manually inspected and potential false positives removed.

The lipid annotations are listed in Supplementary Materials Table S1 and the total number of identified lipids was 131.

4.7. Statistical Analysis

Statistical analysis was performed to search the changes in relative abundance of lipids in relation to the scores of the LLPs, eyelid margin alterations and morphological characteristics of the MG. All statistical analyses were performed using Metaboanalys 6.0 (https://www.metaboanalyst.ca; accessed on 15 January 2024). Features with more than 50% missing values were removed. The data were transformed using the base-2 logarithm (log2) to correct for non-normal distributions and standardized by the Autoscaling method (mean-centred divided by standard deviations of each variable) [42].

The 44 samples were classified based on the LLPs, eyelid margin abnormalities (eyelid margin hyperaemia, MG orifice plugging, eyelid margin irregularity and eyelid margin thickening) and morphological characteristics of the MG (MG loss, MG drop out and partial glands) (Supplementary Materials Table S2). Upper and lower eyelid scores were combined for every sample, adding both classifications (Table 2). Samples with mild severity grades for each study characteristic have been excluded from the statistical analysis to examine lipidic differences. Finally, the samples that were included were reclassified into two groups (group 1 and group 2) and the classification scores included in every analysis group are listed in Table 3.

Table 3. Clustering criteria for group 1 and group 2 according to the scores assigned to each characteristic studied.

	Scores Range	Scores Included in Statistical Study		n
		Group 1	Group 2	
LLP	1 to 5	=1	≥4	12
Eyelid Margin Hyperaemia	0 to 6	≤1	≥4	25
MG Orifice Plugging	0 to 6	=0	≥4	12
Eyelid Margin Irregularity	0 to 4	=0	≥3	17
Eyelid Margin Thickening	0 to 4	=0	≥2	36
MG Loss	0 to 6	=0	≥3	23
MG Drop Out	0 to 4	=0	≥3	29
Partial Glands	0 to 6	≤2	≥5	28

Score range: the LLP score is the assigned according to Gillon's scheme. Eyelid margin abnormalities and morphological features of the MG are expressed as the sum scores for both eyelids in each sample; n: number of samples included in statistical study. LLP: Lipid Layer Pattern; MG: Meibomian Gland.

A "supervised orthogonal partial least squares discriminant analysis" (ortho-DA) was conducted to identify lipids with the greatest capabilities to separate the sample groups. Those lipids with VIP from the ortho-DA higher than 1.5 were considered biologically relevant in these analyses. A "hierarchical clustering analysis" (heatmap) was performed based on Euclidean distance and the average cluster algorithm to evaluate changes in the VIP lipid datasets and to separate the samples into groups with lipids of similar relative abundance.

5. Conclusions

The study of the lipid profile of the meibum and its relationship with many ocular surface features add valuable information about which lipids enhance or reduce their abundance regarding each sign of alteration. The present study revealed significant variances in lipid abundance between subjects exhibiting no or minimal ocular alterations and those exhibiting higher scores of ocular alterations. The abundance of different lipid species may influence LLPs, eyelid margin hyperaemia, eyelid margin irregularity, MG orifice plugging and MG loss. The current findings have the potential for transfer to the pharmaceutical industry, as novel tear substitutes could be developed and customized for each type of DED. Identifying altered lipids in EDE/MGD could lead to targeted therapies, addressing a critical gap in DED management and potentially benefiting both patients and pharmaceutical industries. The collaboration between basic research and clinical practice showcases how scientific inquiry can enhance patient care. Rapid and cost-effective meibum analysis could revolutionize clinical procedures like routine tests for bodily fluids.

6. Future Perspectives

Future research could address several limitations of the current study, such as by extracting meibum from both eyelids separately, or handling a larger sample with different types of DED subjects (EDE/MGD and Aqueous Deficient Dry Eye) at different severity levels. Studying DED types at different severity levels will add valuable information for understanding the DED pathophysiology related to the MGs. In this sense, researchers could find out which lipids are more involved in the chronification of the disease due to their higher or lower abundance on the ocular surfaces at different levels of severity.

Supplementary Materials: The following supporting information can be downloaded at: https://www.mdpi.com/article/10.3390/ijms25094782/s1.

Author Contributions: Conceptualization, J.G.-Q., H.P.-V., B.S.-V. and M.J.G.; Data Curation, J.G.-Q., H.P.-V. and B.S.-V.; Formal Analysis, J.G.-Q., H.P.-V., M.P.-T. and E.G.-F.; Funding Acquisition, E.Y.-P. and M.J.G.; Investigation, J.G.-Q., H.P.-V., B.S.-V., M.J.G. and E.Y.-P.; Methodology, J.G.-Q., H.P.-V., B.S.-V. and C.G.-R.; Project Administration, J.G.-Q., M.J.G. and E.Y.-P.; Resources, J.G.-Q., H.P.-V., C.G.-R. and M.J.G.; Software, M.P.-T. and E.G.-F.; Supervision, J.G.-Q., C.G.-R., M.J.G. and E.Y.-P.; Validation, J.G.-Q., M.P.-T. and E.G.-F.; Visualization, J.G.-Q., C.G.-R., M.J.G. and E.Y.-P.; Writing—Original Draft, J.G.-Q., H.P.-V., M.P.-T. and E.G.-F.; Writing—Review and Editing, J.G.-Q. and H.P.-V. All authors have read and agreed to the published version of the manuscript.

Funding: This research was funded by the Convocatoria de Axudas para o Uso das Infraestructuras de Investigación da Universidade de Santiago de Compostela, grant number 2021-AD039.

Institutional Review Board Statement: This study was conducted in accordance with the Declaration of Helsinki, and approved by the Ethics Committee Universidade de Santiago de Compostela (USC-40/2020 approved 19 January 2021).

Informed Consent Statement: Informed consent was obtained from all subjects involved in the study.

Data Availability Statement: The raw data supporting the conclusions of this article will be made available by the authors on request.

Conflicts of Interest: The authors declare no conflicts of interest.

References

1. Knop, E.; Knop, N.; Millar, T.; Obata, H.; Sullivan, D.A. The international workshop on meibomian gland dysfunction: Report of the subcommittee on anatomy, physiology, and pathophysiology of the meibomian gland. *Investig. Ophthalmol. Vis. Sci.* **2011**, *52*, 1938–1978. [CrossRef] [PubMed]
2. Butovich, I.A. Meibomian glands, meibum, and meibogenesis. *Exp. Eye Res.* **2017**, *163*, 2–16. [CrossRef] [PubMed]
3. Cwiklik, L. Tear film lipid layer: A molecular level view. *Biochim. Biophys. Acta* **2016**, *1858*, 2421–2430. [CrossRef] [PubMed]
4. Pflugfelder, S.C.; Stern, M.E. Biological functions of tear film. *Exp. Eye Res.* **2020**, *197*, 108115. [CrossRef] [PubMed]
5. Butovich, I.A.; Uchiyama, E.; Di Pascuale, M.A.; McCulley, J.P. Liquid chromatography-mass spectrometric analysis of lipids present in human meibomian gland secretions. *Lipids* **2007**, *42*, 765–776. [CrossRef] [PubMed]
6. Arita, R.; Mori, N.; Shirakawa, R.; Asai, K.; Imanaka, T.; Fukano, Y.; Nakamura, M. Linoleic acid content of human meibum is associated with telangiectasia and plugging of gland orifices in meibomian gland dysfunction. *Exp. Eye Res.* **2016**, *145*, 359–362. [CrossRef] [PubMed]
7. Paranjpe, V.; Tan, J.; Nguyen, J.; Lee, J.; Allegood, J.; Galor, A.; Mandal, N. Clinical signs of meibomian gland dysfunction (MGD) are associated with changes in meibum sphingolipid composition. *Ocul. Surf.* **2019**, *17*, 318–326. [CrossRef]
8. Pucker, A.D.; Haworth, K.M. The presence and significance of polar meibum and tear lipids. *Ocul. Surf.* **2015**, *13*, 26–42. [CrossRef]
9. Suzuki, T.; Kitazawa, K.; Cho, Y.; Yoshida, M.; Okumura, T.; Sato, A.; Kinoshita, S. Alteration in meibum lipid composition and subjective symptoms due to aging and meibomian gland dysfunction. *Ocul. Surf.* **2022**, *26*, 310–317. [CrossRef]
10. Craig, J.P.; Nichols, K.K.; Akpek, E.K.; Caffery, B.; Dua, H.S.; Joo, C.K.; Liu, Z.; Nelson, J.D.; Nichols, J.J.; Tsubota, K.; et al. TFOS DEWS II Definition and Classification Report. *Ocul. Surf.* **2017**, *15*, 276–283. [CrossRef]

11. Wolffsohn, J.S.; Arita, R.; Chalmers, R.; Djalilian, A.; Dogru, M.; Dumbleton, K.; Gupta, P.K.; Karpecki, P.; Lazreg, S.; Pult, H.; et al. TFOS DEWS II Diagnostic Methodology report. *Ocul. Surf.* **2017**, *15*, 539–574. [CrossRef]
12. Arita, R.; Minoura, I.; Morishige, N.; Shirakawa, R.; Fukuoka, S.; Asai, K.; Goto, T.; Imanaka, T.; Nakamura, M. Development of Definitive and Reliable Grading Scales for Meibomian Gland Dysfunction. *Am. J. Ophthalmol.* **2016**, *169*, 125–137. [CrossRef]
13. Pult, H. Relationships Between Meibomian Gland Loss and Age, Sex, and Dry Eye. *Eye Contact Lens* **2018**, *44* (Suppl. S2), S318–S324. [CrossRef] [PubMed]
14. Guillon, J.-P. Non-invasive tearscope plus routine for contact lens fitting. *Contact Lens Anterior Eye* **1998**, *21*, S31–S40. [CrossRef] [PubMed]
15. Arita, R.; Morishige, N.; Fujii, T.; Fukuoka, S.; Chung, J.L.; Seo, K.Y.; Itoh, K. Tear Interferometric Patterns Reflect Clinical Tear Dynamics in Dry Eye Patients. *Investig. Ophthalmol. Vis. Sci.* **2016**, *57*, 3928–3934. [CrossRef]
16. Robciuc, A.; Hyotylainen, T.; Jauhiainen, M.; Holopainen, J.M. Ceramides in the pathophysiology of the anterior segment of the eye. *Curr. Eye Res.* **2013**, *38*, 1006–1016. [CrossRef]
17. Tiffany, J.M. Individual variations in human meibomian lipid composition. *Exp. Eye Res.* **1978**, *27*, 289–300. [CrossRef]
18. Harvey, D.J. Identification by gas chromatography/mass spectrometry of long-chain fatty acids and alcohols from hamster meibomian glands using picolinyl and nicotinate derivatives. *Biomed. Chromatogr.* **1989**, *3*, 251–254. [CrossRef]
19. Shine, W.E.; McCulley, J.P. The role of cholesterol in chronic blepharitis. *Investig. Ophthalmol. Vis. Sci.* **1991**, *32*, 2272–2280.
20. Shine, W.E.; McCulley, J.P. Meibomianitis: Polar lipid abnormalities. *Cornea* **2004**, *23*, 781–783. [CrossRef]
21. Yang, Q.; Li, B.; Sheng, M. Meibum lipid composition in type 2 diabetics with dry eye. *Exp. Eye Res.* **2021**, *206*, 108522. [CrossRef] [PubMed]
22. Eom, Y.; Choi, K.E.; Kang, S.Y.; Lee, H.K.; Kim, H.M.; Song, J.S. Comparison of meibomian gland loss and expressed meibum grade between the upper and lower eyelids in patients with obstructive meibomian gland dysfunction. *Cornea* **2014**, *33*, 448–452. [CrossRef] [PubMed]
23. Galor, A.; Sanchez, V.; Jensen, A.; Burton, M.; Maus, K.; Stephenson, D.; Chalfant, C.; Mandal, N. Meibum sphingolipid composition is altered in individuals with meibomian gland dysfunction-a side by side comparison of Meibum and Tear Sphingolipids. *Ocul. Surf.* **2022**, *23*, 87–95. [CrossRef] [PubMed]
24. Khanal, S.; Bai, Y.; Ngo, W.; Nichols, K.K.; Wilson, L.; Barnes, S.; Nichols, J.J. Human meibum and tear film derived cholesteryl and wax esters in meibomian gland dysfunction and tear film structure. *Ocul. Surf.* **2022**, *23*, 12–23. [CrossRef] [PubMed]
25. Kind, T.; Okazaki, Y.; Saito, K.; Fiehn, O. LipidBlast templates as flexible tools for creating new in-silico tandem mass spectral libraries. *Anal. Chem.* **2014**, *86*, 11024–11027. [CrossRef] [PubMed]
26. Zhou, Z.; Tu, J.; Xiong, X.; Shen, X.; Zhu, Z.J. LipidCCS: Prediction of Collision Cross-Section Values for Lipids with High Precision To Support Ion Mobility-Mass Spectrometry-Based Lipidomics. *Anal. Chem.* **2017**, *89*, 9559–9566. [CrossRef] [PubMed]
27. Borchman, D.; Foulks, G.N.; Yappert, M.C. Confirmation of changes in human meibum lipid infrared spectra with age using principal component analysis. *Curr. Eye Res.* **2010**, *35*, 778–786. [CrossRef] [PubMed]
28. Garcia-Queiruga, J.; Pena-Verdeal, H.; Sabucedo-Villamarin, B.; Giraldez, M.J.; Garcia-Resua, C.; Yebra-Pimentel, E. Meibomian gland secretion quality association with ocular parameters in university students during COVID-19 restrictions. *Int. Ophthalmol.* **2023**, *43*, 2349–2362. [CrossRef]
29. Kunnen, C.M.; Brown, S.H.; Lazon de la Jara, P.; Holden, B.A.; Blanksby, S.J.; Mitchell, T.W.; Papas, E.B. Influence of Meibomian Gland Expression Methods on Human Lipid Analysis Results. *Ocul. Surf.* **2016**, *14*, 49–55. [CrossRef]
30. Ha, M.; Kim, J.S.; Hong, S.Y.; Chang, D.J.; Whang, W.J.; Na, K.S.; Kim, E.C.; Kim, H.S.; Hwang, H.S. Relationship between eyelid margin irregularity and meibomian gland dropout. *Ocul. Surf.* **2021**, *19*, 31–37. [CrossRef]
31. Huang, B.; Fei, F.; Wen, H.; Zhu, Y.; Wang, Z.; Zhang, S.; Hu, L.; Chen, W.; Zheng, Q. Impacts of gender and age on meibomian gland in aged people using artificial intelligence. *Front. Cell Dev. Biol.* **2023**, *11*, 1199440. [CrossRef] [PubMed]
32. Foulks, G.N.; Bron, A.J. Meibomian gland dysfunction: A clinical scheme for description, diagnosis, classification, and grading. *Ocul. Surf.* **2003**, *1*, 107–126. [CrossRef] [PubMed]
33. Pult, H.; Riede-Pult, B.H. Non-contact meibography: Keep it simple but effective. *Contact Lens Anterior Eye J. Br. Contact Lens Assoc.* **2012**, *35*, 77–80. [CrossRef] [PubMed]
34. Tomlinson, A.; Bron, A.J.; Korb, D.R.; Amano, S.; Paugh, J.R.; Pearce, E.I.; Yee, R.; Yokoi, N.; Arita, R.; Dogru, M. The international workshop on meibomian gland dysfunction: Report of the diagnosis subcommittee. *Investig. Ophthalmol. Vis. Sci.* **2011**, *52*, 2006–2049. [CrossRef] [PubMed]
35. Meier, F.; Brunner, A.D.; Koch, S.; Koch, H.; Lubeck, M.; Krause, M.; Goedecke, N.; Decker, J.; Kosinski, T.; Park, M.A.; et al. Online Parallel Accumulation-Serial Fragmentation (PASEF) with a Novel Trapped Ion Mobility Mass Spectrometer. *Mol. Cell Proteom.* **2018**, *17*, 2534–2545. [CrossRef] [PubMed]
36. Garcia-Queiruga, J.; Pena-Verdeal, H.; Sabucedo-Villamarin, B.; Giraldez, M.J.; Garcia-Resua, C.; Yebra-Pimentel, E. A cross-sectional study of non-modifiable and modifiable risk factors of dry eye disease states. *Contact Lens Anterior Eye J. Br. Contact Lens Assoc.* **2023**, *46*, 101800. [CrossRef] [PubMed]
37. Sabucedo-Villamarin, B.; Pena-Verdeal, H.; Garcia-Queiruga, J.; Giraldez, M.J.; Garcia-Resua, C.; Yebra-Pimentel, E. Categorization of the Aqueous Deficient Dry Eye by a Cut-Off Criterion of TMH Measured with Tearscope. *Life* **2022**, *12*, 2007. [CrossRef] [PubMed]

38. Garcia-Queiruga, J.; Pena-Verdeal, H.; Sabucedo-Villamarin, B.; Garcia-Resua, C.; Giraldez, M.J.; Yebra-Pimentel, E. Analysis of the Differences in Ocular Surface Damage and Inflammatory Signs between Healthy and Evaporative Dry Eye Participants. *Ocul. Immunol. Inflamm.* **2023**, *31*, 970–977. [CrossRef] [PubMed]
39. Ma, Y.; Kind, T.; Vaniya, A.; Gennity, I.; Fahrmann, J.F.; Fiehn, O. An in silico MS/MS library for automatic annotation of novel FAHFA lipids. *J. Cheminform* **2015**, *7*, 53. [CrossRef]
40. Zhou, Z.; Luo, M.; Chen, X.; Yin, Y.; Xiong, X.; Wang, R.; Zhu, Z.J. Ion mobility collision cross-section atlas for known and unknown metabolite annotation in untargeted metabolomics. *Nat. Commun.* **2020**, *11*, 4334. [CrossRef]
41. Leaptrot, K.L.; May, J.C.; Dodds, J.N.; McLean, J.A. Ion mobility conformational lipid atlas for high confidence lipidomics. *Nat. Commun.* **2019**, *10*, 985. [CrossRef] [PubMed]
42. Rocha, B.; Illiano, A.; Calamia, V.; Pinto, G.; Amoresano, A.; Ruiz-Romero, C.; Blanco, F.J. Targeted phospholipidomic analysis of synovial fluid as a tool for osteoarthritis deep phenotyping. *Osteoarthr. Cart. Open* **2021**, *3*, 100219. [CrossRef] [PubMed]

International Journal of
Molecular Sciences

MDPI

Article

Potential Roles of Extracellular Vesicles in Murine Tear Fluids in the Physiology of Corneal Epithelial Cells In Vitro

Saya Oya [1], Kazunari Higa [2], Tomohiro Yasutake [1], Risa Yamazaki-Hokama [3] and Masatoshi Hirayama [1,*]

1 Department of Ophthalmology, Faculty of Medicine, Fukuoka University, Fukuoka 814-0180, Japan
2 Department of Ophthalmology, Tokyo Dental College Ichikawa General Hospital, Chiba 272-0824, Japan
3 Department of Ophthalmology, School of Medicine, Keio University, Tokyo 160-8582, Japan
* Correspondence: mhirayama@fukuoka-u.ac.jp; Tel.: +81-92-801-1011

Abstract: Biological extracellular vesicles in tear fluids, such as exosomes, are thought to have physiological functions in the management of healthy ocular surface epithelium, including corneal epithelium. However, the physiological roles of tear extracellular vesicles in the ocular surface remain unclear. In this study, we investigated the physiological function of tear extracellular vesicles in mouse tear fluids in the ocular surface epithelium in vitro. Morphological analysis of the isolated extracellular vesicles from mouse tear fluids was performed using nanoparticle tracking analysis and transmission electron microscopy. The identified particles were characterised by immunoblotting for exosomal markers. After confirming the uptake of tear exosomes in cultured corneal epithelial cells, gene expression changes in mouse cultured corneal epithelial cells after tear exosome treatment were analysed. Immunostaining analysis was performed to confirm cell proliferation in the cultured corneal epithelial cells with tear exosome treatment. Tear fluids from mice contain nanoparticles with exosome-like morphologies, which express the representative exosomal markers CD9 and TSG101. The extracellular vesicles can be taken up by cultivated murine corneal epithelial cells in vitro and induce expression changes in genes related to the cell cycle, cell membranes, microtubules, and signal peptides. Treatment with the tear extracellular vesicles promoted cell proliferation of cultured murine corneal epithelial cells. Our study provides evidence that murine tear fluids contain extracellular vehicles like exosomes and they may contribute to the maintenance of the physiological homeostatic environment of the ocular surface.

Keywords: tear fluid; exosome; extracellular vesicles; dry eye disease; corneal epithelium

1. Introduction

Extracellular vesicles (EVs) have been identified as intercellular signalling factors contained in body fluids that contribute to various cell physiological and pathological processes, including tumour metastasis and neurological diseases [1–4]. EVs represented by exosomes are cell-derived vesicles composed of a lipid bilayer membrane and contain various biological substances, such as nucleic acids [e.g., mRNAs and microRNAs (miRNAs)] [1,5]. EVs are characterised by the expression of various exosomal markers, including membrane proteins, such as CD9, CD63, and multivesicular body synthesis-related proteins, such as TSG101 and Alix [6]. Exosomes are responsible for specific cell–cell communication through uptake into target cells and are involved in the regulation of biological functions of organs and disease-related processes, such as neovascularisation for cancer metastasis [3]. Current exosome research has been diverse and widely used for medical applications.

Researchers have recently focused on the role of EVs in ocular diseases, including glaucoma and retinal diseases [7,8]. For example, EVs and exosomes in anterior chamber fluids, which are derived from cells, have been shown to be involved in the disease mechanism of glaucoma by modulating signalling pathways in trabecular meshwork cells [7]. In ocular surface diseases, studies on corneal damage have suggested the involvement of corneal mesenchymal cell-derived exosomes in the pathological processes of corneal keratitis, such as wound healing and myofibroblastic transformation [9]. EVs and exosomes have been recognised as critical factors that affect the pathological processes of ocular diseases [10]. Elucidation of novel functions of exosomes will lead to a better understanding of the relationship between exosomes and eye diseases and help develop novel clinical treatments and diagnostic methods.

Tear fluids on the ocular surface maintain the homeostatic microenvironment of the ocular surface epithelium, including transparency and barrier function [11]. A sufficient volume of tear fluid must be retained on the ocular surface because the stable tear film forms a smooth optical surface. At the same time, tear fluids are also thought to contain extracellular vesicles, including exosomes that are needed for physiological corneal epithelial cells. However, the existence of exosomes in mouse tear fluids and their physiological roles on the ocular surface are not fully understood.

In this study, we investigated the physiological function of tear exosomes in the ocular surface epithelium in vitro by using mouse tear fluids. We successfully identified EVs isolated from tear fluids and characterised them as tear exosomes by immunoblotting for exosomal markers. After confirming the uptake of tear exosomes in cultured corneal epithelial cells, we revealed a wide range of gene expression changes in mouse cultured corneal epithelial cells after tear exosome treatment. We clarified that the expression of cell proliferation markers increased in the cultured corneal epithelial cells with tear exosome treatment by immunostaining analysis. Our current study thus suggests the importance of exosomes in tear fluids in the cell physiology of the ocular surface epithelium.

2. Results

2.1. Morphological Details of EVs in Tear Fluids

The existence of EVs, including exosomes, has been reported in almost all body fluids, such as blood, saliva, and urine; however, the specific physiological functions of exosomes in tear fluids are unknown. Therefore, we first performed morphological analysis of isolated EVs from tear fluids collected from normal mice by an ultracentrifugation method. Electron microscopic observation revealed spherical structures, which is consistent with previously reported morphological characteristics of exosomes from other cells [12] in tear fluids from mice (Figure 1a). According to nanoparticle tracking analysis (NTA), the average concentration of mouse tear exosomes of the final EV preparation was $2.53 \pm 0.22 \times 10^{12}$ particles/mL, and we confirmed that the diameter of the particles in mouse tear fluids was 134 ± 7.0 nm (Figure 1b) [12]. These results indicate that tear fluids from mice contain extracellular vehicles with exosome-like morphologies.

2.2. Exosomal Marker Expression on EVs in Tear Fluids

Various proteins, such as tetraspanins, are expressed in the lipid bilayer membrane of exosomes, and their expression has been recognised as representative exosomal markers [12,13]. Therefore, we performed Western blotting analysis of EVs in ultracentrifugation pellets using commercially available antibodies against representative exosomal markers, the tetraspanin molecules CD9 and TSG101 for mouse tear EVs, to confirm the exosomal marker expression in the EVs. Western blotting analysis showed the expression of CD9 and

TSG101 in mouse tear EVs (Figure 2). Therefore, we hypothesised that the isolated EVs from mouse tear fluids would contain tear exosomes in this study.

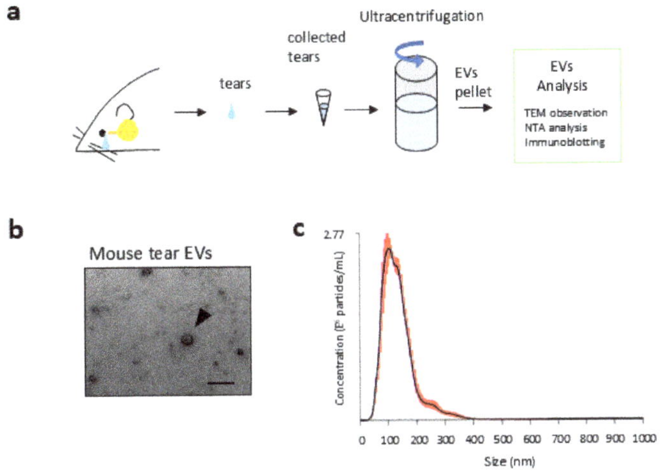

Figure 1. Isolation and morphological analysis of tear extracellular vesicles. (**a**) Schematic representation of the methods used to observe mouse extracellular vesicles from tear fluids. (**b**) Phase-contrast images of the isolated extracellular vesicles derived from mouse tear fluids using electron microscopy (arrowhead) (200 nm, scale bar). (**c**) Size distribution and concentration of extracellular vesicles (EVs) isolated from mouse tear fluid, as determined by nanoparticle tracking analysis (NTA). The *y*-axis indicates particle concentration (particles/mL), and the *x*-axis represents particle diameter (nm). Red error bars indicate ±1 standard error of the mean. The distribution pattern is consistent with small extracellular vesicles, such as exosomes.

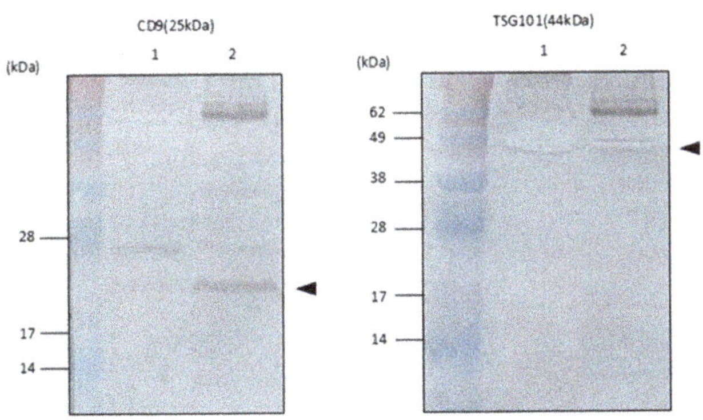

Figure 2. Expression of exosomal markers on EVs in mice tear fluids. (**Left**) CD9 expression in extracellular vesicles from control (lane 1, mouse lacrimal gland extracts as control) and EVs from tear fluids (lane 2, arrowhead). (**Right**) TSG101 expression in extracellular vesicles from control (lane 1, mouse lacrimal gland extracts as control) and EVs from tear fluids (lane 2, arrowhead).

2.3. Uptake of Tear Exosomes in Cultivated Corneal Epithelial Cells In Vitro

Exosomes in body fluids contribute to cell signalling communication between donor cells and recipient cells through an intake mechanism of exosomes [14]. To prove the uptake of tear exosomes in corneal epithelial cells, we cultured corneal epithelial cells using TKE2 cells [15], a mouse corneal epithelial cell line, with culture media and added tear EVs with fluorescein-labelled RNA. Tracing analysis using fluorescein-labelled tear exosomal RNA showed that exosomal RNA were taken up by TKE2 cells at a rate of 89 ± 3.1% (Figure 3a,b). The uptake rate of tear exosomes in cultured C2C12 cells (mouse C3H muscle myoblasts) was also observed; however, the rate was significantly lower (28 ± 1.9%) than that of corneal epithelial cells at the same transduction condition. These results suggest the possibility of cell signalling communication in corneal epithelial cells through EVs in mouse tear fluids.

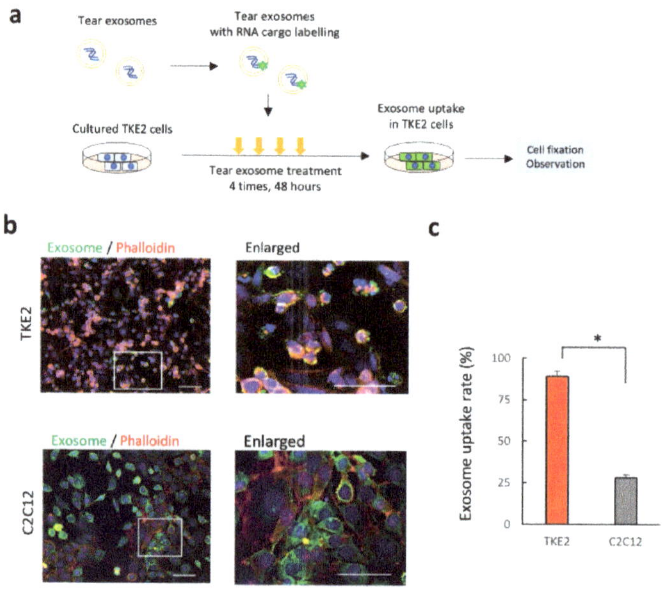

Figure 3. Analysis of uptake in cultured corneal epithelial cells using fluorescein labelled tear exosomes. (**a**) Schematic representation of the methods used to analyse tear exosome uptake in cultured corneal epithelial cells. (**b**) Immunohistochemical analysis of the cultured TKE2 cells (upper panels) and C2C12 cells (lower panels) after a fluorescein-labelled (green) tear exosome treatment. The cells were analysed by immunostaining with specific antibodies for phalloidin (red). Nuclei were stained using DAPI (blue). The boxed area in the left panel is shown at a higher magnification in the right panel. Scale bar, 50 μm. (**c**) The rate of exosome uptake cells in the cultured TKE2 cells and C2C12 cells. The rate of exosome uptake cells in TKE2 cells was significantly higher than in C2C12 cells (* $p = 0.021$, n = 3).

2.4. Gene Expression Changes in Corneal Epithelial Cells After the Uptake of Tear Exosomes

Contents in exosomes, including mRNAs and miRNAs, are taken up into recipient cells and function through various biological pathways [16]. We analysed gene expression changes using a microarray of cells to observe biological changes in cultivated corneal epithelial cells with or without tear EV treatment. We first carried out transcriptome analysis to profile mRNA expression changes in TKE2 cells with or without tear EV treatment, using a DNA microarray containing 23,475 oligonucleotide probes corresponding to mouse genes. The comparison of gene expression between cultured TKE2 cells treated or not treated with EVs revealed that 513 genes were significantly upregulated in the EV-treated cells, while 25 genes were significantly downregulated compared to the untreated control (Figure 4a,b). To explore the biological significance of genes upregulated by tear exosome treatment, we performed functional annotation clustering analysis using DAVID. A total of 513 genes with a fold change ≥2.0 were subjected to this analysis. The results identified six annotation clusters (AC1–AC6) with an enrichment score >1.30 and p-value < 0.05, which were considered significant. These clusters represent functionally related gene groups associated with the cell cycle (AC1), cell membrane (AC2), transmembrane transport (AC3), cytoskeleton and microtubule organisation (AC4), glycoproteins (AC5), and signal peptides (AC6). These findings suggest that tear exosomes may influence a broad range of cellular processes in corneal epithelial cells. Table 1 shows representative GO terms from the six annotation clusters. The following pathway analysis revealed that two pathways, ectodysplasin A (EDA) signalling and steroid biosynthesis, were significantly enriched (Table 2). These results indicate that tear exosomes induce gene expression changes, which are related to various functions, including the cell cycle and microtubule and transmembrane signalling, in cultured corneal epithelial cells.

a

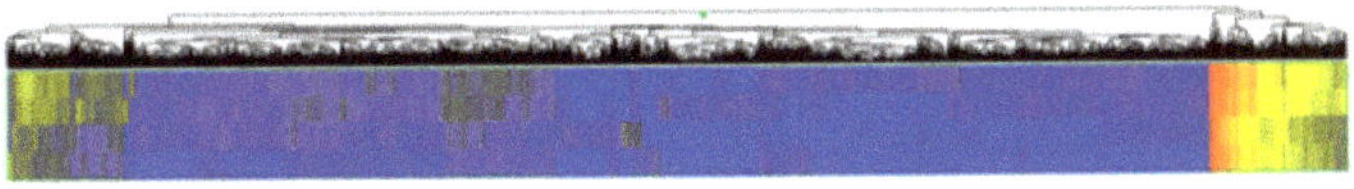

b

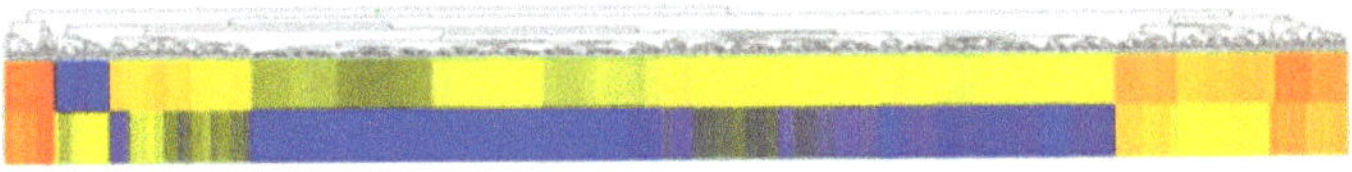

Figure 4. Gene expression changes in cultured corneal epithelial cells with tear exosome treatment. (**a**) Heatmap analysis of all gene expression changes in TKE2 cells with or without tear EV treatment (each kind of sample was duplicated; upper 2 lanes, with the treatment; lower 2 lanes, without the treatment). (**b**) Heatmap analysis of 513 gene expression changes in TKE2 cells, which are increased (fold change $\geq$ 2.0) after tear EV treatment (upper lane, with treatment, lower lane, without treatment).

Table 1. Representative GO terms by functional annotation cluster analysis of the 513 genes, which were increased (fold change $\geq$ 2.0) after tear exosome treatment. AC1, AC2, AC3, and AC5 contain GO terms from AC1–AC6, which represent functional annotation clusters generated by DAVID from 513 upregulated genes (fold change $\geq$ 2.0) following tear exosome treatment [17]. Enrichment score > 1.30 and p-value < 0.05 were considered significant.

AC1 (Enrichment score: 2.77)	
GO Term Biological Process	p-value
GO:0007049 cell cycle	0.007
GO:0051301 cell division	<0.001
GO:0007067 mitotic nuclear division	<0.001
GO:0007059 chromosome segregation	0.009
GO:0000070 mitotic sister chromatid segregation	<0.001
GO Term Cellular Component	p-value
GO:0005694 chromosome	0.041
GO:0000776 kinetochore	<0.001
GO:0000775 chromosome, centromeric region	0.002
GO:0000922 spindle pole	0.001
GO:0000777 condensed chromosome kinetochore	0.001
GO:0000780 condensed nuclear chromosome	0.005

Table 1. *Cont.*

AC2 (Enrichment score: 2.27)	
GO Term Biological Process	*p*-value
GO:0005886 plasma membrane	0.015
AC3 (Enrichment score: 1.86)	
GO Term Cellular Component	*p*-value
GO:0016020 membrane	0.015
GO:0016021 integral component of membrane	0.036
AC5 (Enrichment score: 1.40)	
GO Term Biological Process	*p*-value
GO:0007018 microtubule-based movement	0.073
GO:0007080~mitotic metaphase plate congression	0.031
GO Term Cellular Component	*p*-value
GO:0005819 spindle	0.028
GO:0005871 kinesin complex	0.019
GO:0005876 spindle microtubule	0.044
GO Term Molecular Function	*p*-value
GO:0008017 microtubule binding	0.022
GO:0008574 ATP-dependent microtubule motor activity	0.028

Table 2. Top 10 increased signalling pathways enriched in cells that appear in EVs in mice tear fluids.

Pathway	*p*-Value (Comparison)
Mm_EDA_Signalling_in_Hair_Follicle_Development_WP3652_97556	0.007748972
Mm_Steroid_Biosynthesis_WP55_89970	0.027217017
Mm_Glutathione_metabolism_WP164_85644	0.057912603
Mm_Kit_Receptor_Signaling_Pathway_WP407_69079	0.058914933
Mm_Statin_Pathway_WP1_73346	0.06381421
Mm_Metapathway_biotransformation_WP1251_94721	0.07834384
Mm_Notch_Signaling_Pathway_WP29_79679	0.079050094
Mm_Hedgehog_Signaling_Pathway_WP116_69142	0.08262755
Mm_Chemokine_signaling_pathway_WP2292_97515	0.098608024

2.5. Tear Exosomes Induce the Proliferation of Cultivated Corneal Epithelial Cells

The transparency of the cornea is managed by the proliferation of corneal epithelial cells during wound healing processes after corneal epithelial damage [18]. Especially in DED, corneal epithelial damage occurs due to insufficient tear fluids [18]. According to the results of the gene expression analysis described above, we investigated whether tear EVs contribute to the maintenance of ocular surface homeostasis through the regulation of corneal epithelial cell processes, such as cell proliferation. To analyse the roles of tear exosomes in cell proliferation, we performed immunohistochemical (IHC) analysis using antibodies for cell proliferation markers, such as Ki67 and BrdU. Treatment with tear EVs in cultivated TKE2 cells revealed that the rate of Ki67-positive cells in cultured corneal epithelial cells was significantly higher with the treatment (45.4 ± 6.4%) than without the treatment (3.5 ± 0.4%) (Figure 5a,b) ($p = 0.020$). BrdU staining analysis showed that the BrdU-positive cells in cultured corneal epithelial cells were higher after the treatment

(88.7 ± 0.5%) than without the treatment (53.3 ± 6.5%) ($p = 0.028$) (Figure 5c,d). These results indicate that tear EVs may contribute to the proliferation of cultured corneal epithelial cells.

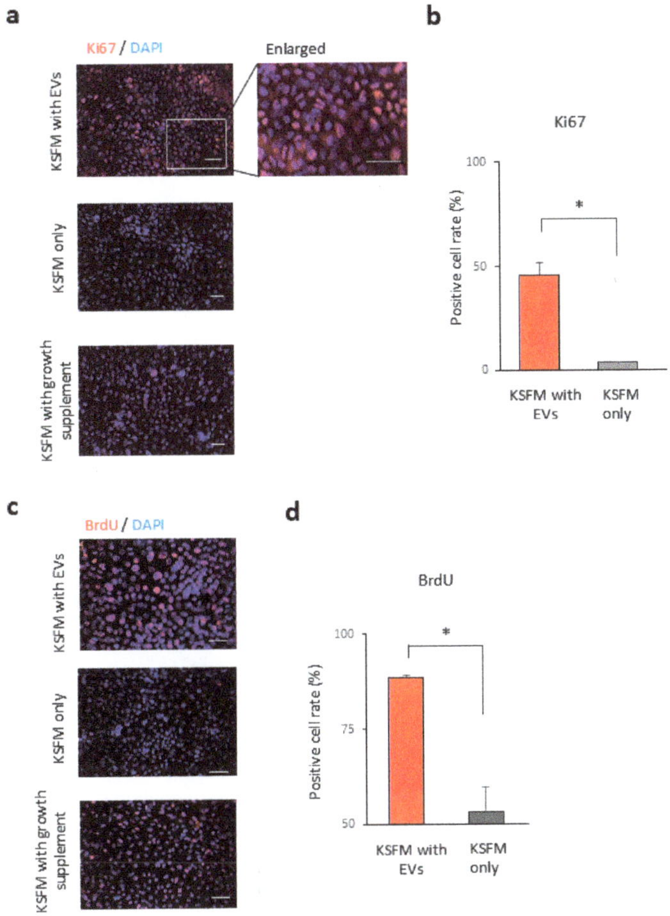

Figure 5. Analysis of cell proliferation in the cultured corneal epithelial cells after tear EV treatment. (**a**) Immunohistochemical analysis of TKE2 cells cultured with basal medium with tear EVs (upper panel and enlarged image), basal medium without tear EVs (middle panel), and medium supplemented with growth factors as a positive control (lower panel). Cells were immunostained with an antibody against Ki67 (red), and nuclei were counterstained with DAPI (blue). Scale bar, 50 μm. (**b**) The rate of Ki67 positive cells in the cultured TKE2 cells. The rate of Ki67 positive cells in TKE2 cells with tear exosome treatment was significantly higher than in TKE2 cells without tear exosome treatment (* $p = 0.020$, n = 3). (**c**) Immunohistochemical analysis of TKE2 cells cultured with basal medium with tear EVs (upper panel), basal medium without tear EVs (middle panel), and medium supplemented with growth factors as a positive control (lower panel). The cells were analysed by immunostaining with specific antibodies for BrdU (red). Nuclei were stained using DAPI (blue). Scale bar, 50 μm. (**d**) The rate of BrdU positive cells in the cultured TKE2 cells. The rate of BrdU positive cells in TKE2 cells with tear EV treatment was significantly higher than in TKE2 cells without the treatment (* $p = 0.028$, n = 3).

3. Discussion

In this study, we revealed that tear fluids of mice and humans contain exosomes expressing representative exosomal markers, and intercellular signalling by mouse tear exosomes has a potential role in regulating physiological functions, including cell proliferation, through various gene expression changes in corneal epithelial cells in vitro. These findings indicate a novel function of tear EVs that contributes to the maintenance of the physiological homeostatic environment of the ocular surface.

Tear fluids are indispensable for the ocular surface epithelium to maintain a smooth optical surface for better visual function [19,20]. A shortage of tear fluids on the ocular surface causes DED, which leads to corneal epithelial damage, resulting in a severe decrease in quality of life due to impaired visual function [18,21]. Artificial tear drops have been developed as alternative aqueous tear water to cure DED [22]. Recent findings revealed that exosomes, which are abundant in body fluids, are responsible for cell–cell communication by delivering proteins and nucleic acids, such as RNA, to recipient cells [1,23]. These concepts predict that EVs and exosomes in tear fluids are involved in the maintenance of homeostasis of the corneal epithelium and disease mechanisms of DED. However, the involvement of tear EVs in corneal epithelial cell physiology is unclear [7]. Our study reported that tear EVs, including exosomes, may be functional substances in tear fluids that may help regulate the proliferation of corneal epithelial cells in vitro.

EVs, including exosomes, which are generally isolated by ultracentrifugation from body fluids, are nanoparticles produced by many different cells [3]. Common features of exosomes include a typical morphology, such as vesicles lined by a lipid bilayer, a homogenous size of approximately 100 nm in diameter, and expression of specific proteins, such as tetraspanins, including CD9 and CD63, and others with endocytic origins, such as TSG101 [2]. Exosomes have been reported in almost all biological fluids, such as blood [24], urine [25], saliva [26], breast milk [27], cerebrospinal fluids [28,29], sperm [30], and malignant effusions [31]. However, details on EVs and exosomes in mouse tear fluids are lacking [32]. In this study, we successfully observed nanoparticles in tear fluids from mice, consistent with similar morphologies of exosomes as described previously [12] and confirmed the expression of exosomal markers, suggesting the existence of exosomes in the tear fluids of mice. Further identification of exosomal marker expression in mouse tear fluids requires the development of available antibodies. Investigation on changes of expression profiles of exosomal markers in tear exosomes in diseased status, such as DED, would provide interesting information as a future study [33].

Exosomes contain a wide range of genetic materials, e.g., functionally active RNAs, such as mRNA and miRNA, for intercellular signalling, which are mostly involved in the cell cycle, angiogenesis, differentiation, and DNA histone modification under both physiological and pathological conditions, including tumorigenesis [14,34,35]. In this study, the labelled RNAs in tear exosomes were transferred to cultured corneal epithelial cells at a high rate, suggesting the possibility of a cell–cell communication network in cells with EVs in tear fluids.

Reliable next-generation sequencing technology for nucleic acids in tear exosomes has been difficult due to the volume limits (small amount) of tear fluids, especially in mice. Our in vitro model using cultured mouse corneal epithelial cells with our purified tear EVs treatment could shed a light on the role of tear EVs on ocular surface by using microarray analysis. Our findings clarify the various gene expression changes in cultured corneal epithelial cells due to tear EV treatments. The EDA signalling pathway, which is significantly enriched in cells treated with tear EVs (Table 1), regulates the induction, morphogenesis and maintenance of epidermal structures, such as teeth, hair follicles, sweat glands, and several other glands, through NF-kB-mediated regulation of Wnt stimulation or inhibition and the sonic hedgehog (SHH) and RelB pathways [36]. Our results indicate that tear EVs, including exosomes, promote cell proliferation of corneal epithelial cells through these signalling pathways. Further analysis of the effects of tear EVs and exosomes on a more physiologically mature cell environment using an in vivo model should be performed. Our in vitro experimental model may be appropriate for analysing the fundamental roles of tear EVs and exosomes on the ocular surface epithelium because it excludes the influence of peripheral tissues, including the corneal stroma. These findings suggest that tear EVs may have a variety of effects on the physiology of corneal epithelial cells.

A limitation of our study is the potential contamination from other tear components during the process of isolating EVs or exosomes, which cannot be completely ruled out. Ultracentrifugation is one of the most reliable methods for isolating EVs from small-volume samples, such as tear fluids. However, to achieve more precise isolation in the future, it will be necessary to compare results using alternative methods, such as adsorption-based techniques. While our study demonstrated a difference in exosome uptake between cell types, the mechanistic basis for this observation remains to be elucidated. The significantly higher uptake of tear exosomes by TKE2 cells may suggest a cell-type-specific mechanism influenced by surface characteristics of both EVs and recipient cells [37–39]. Future studies employing molecular profiling and endocytic pathway inhibition are needed to clarify the receptors or pathways involved in the differential uptake of tear-derived EVs. Further refinement of isolation protocols and additional marker examination are warranted, particularly for isolating EVs from limited sample volumes. Future studies on functional abilities of EVs in tear fluids in vivo to examine whether tear-derived EVs can exert protective or modulatory effects on the ocular surface under physiological or pathological conditions, such as dry eye or corneal injury, will provide interesting information.

4. Materials and Methods

4.1. Ethical Statements

This study was approved by the Animal Care and Experiment Committee of the Tokyo Dental College Ichikawa General Hospital (approval number: 207702). C57BL/6 mice were purchased from Charles River Laboratories (Yokohama, Japan). The care and handling of the animals were performed in accordance with the NIH guidelines.

4.2. Tear Fluid Collection

From the mice, 5 μL of tear fluid was collected from the eyelid margin without touching the eye using a 0.5 μL micropipette (Drummond Scientific, Broomall, PA, USA), 20 min after intraperitoneal injection of 300 μg of pilocarpine kg^{-1} body weight after washing the eye surface with PBS. The samples were pooled as described previously [40]. Each animal was anaesthetised with an intraperitoneal injection of medetomidine (0.15 mg/kg), midazolam (2 mg/kg), and butorphanol (2.5 mg/kg) before the procedures.

4.3. Isolation of EVs

Isolation of EVs from the samples was performed by the differential ultracentrifugation method, as described below [41]. After the addition of 800 μL of PBS, 40 μL of pooled mouse tear samples was centrifuged at 300× *g* for 10 min and 2000× *g* for 10 min. After filtration through a 0.2 μm Millipore filter to remove cell debris, the collected supernatant was centrifuged again at 10,000× *g* for 30 min, and the supernatant was centrifuged in an ultracentrifuge at 100,000× *g* for 70 min to remove proteins and contaminates. After PBS washes, the sample was centrifuged again in an ultracentrifuge at 100,000× *g* for

70 min. All procedures were performed at 4 °C. The pellet containing extracellular vesicles, including exosomes, was used after adding 100 μL of PBS with 1 μL of EV-Save (Fujifilm Wako, Tokyo, Japan) on ice.

4.4. Morphological Analysis of Nanoparticles

Exosome samples were diluted to a concentration of 10^8–10^9 particles/mL in Milli-Q water for analysis. The size and concentration of the exosomes were determined through nanoparticle tracking analysis using a Nano Sight LM10 system (Malvern Panalytical, Ltd., Malvern, UK). Images for analysis of the Brownian motion were obtained five times in 60 s, and the particle size and particle concentration were calculated. Images of the particles were obtained using transmission electron microscopy (H-7600, Hitachi, Tokyo, Japan) and taken using an AMT XR16S-R CCD camera (Hitachi).

4.5. Western Blot Immunoblotting

Isolated EV samples (2.0×10^{10} particles/per lane) were separated on a polyacrylamide gel before being transferred to a PVDF membrane. The blotting membrane was blocked with normal goat serum (Vectastain ABC Kit; Vector Laboratories, Burlingame, CA, USA) and incubated with CD63 antibody (Abcam, Cambridge, UK) and with TSG101 (GeneTex, San Antonio, TX, USA) and CD9 (Abcam), followed by incubation with biotinylated secondary antibody (Vector Laboratories). The proteins were detected using a DAB substrate kit (Vector Laboratories).

4.6. Cell Culture and Analysis of Exosome Uptake

TKE2 is a murine limbal/corneal epithelium progenitor cell line [15]. TKE2 cells were maintained in defined keratinocyte serum-free medium (KSFM; Gibco-Invitrogen Corp., Carlsbad, CA, USA) supplemented with 1% penicillin/streptomycin and growth supplement supplied by the manufacturer until use. C2C12 cells (ECACC catalogue no. 91031101; mouse C3H muscle myoblasts) were cultured in DMEM with 10% FBS supplemented with 1% penicillin/streptomycin. Cell cultures were incubated at 37 °C under 95% humidity and 5% CO_2, and the culture medium was changed every 3 to 4 days. For the assessment of exosome uptake by TKE2 cells, 1×10^4 cells of TKE2 cells and C2C12 cells with KSFM media were cultured on a 4-well Nunc Lab-Tek chamber slide system (Thermo Fisher Scientific, Waltham, MA, USA). Mouse tear EVs (2×10^{12} particles), which were labelled with SYTO RNASelect Green Fluorescent Cell Stain (Thermo Fisher Scientific) according to the manufacturer's protocol, were applied to the culture media every 12 h for 2 days. After exosome treatment, the cells were fixed with 4% paraformaldehyde (PFA) (Wako, Osaka, Japan) for 20 min. After the cells were washed with PBS, they were incubated with 0.1% Triton X-100 for 5 min. After the cells were washed again with PBS, they were incubated with Alexa Fluor 594 phalloidin conjugate (Thermo Fisher Scientific) for 20 min for actin staining according to the manufacturer's protocol. After the samples were stained with 4′,6-diamidino-2-phenylindole (DAPI) (Dojindo Laboratories, Tokyo, Japan), images were obtained using a florescence microscope (Axioplan 2 imaging, Carl Zeiss, Inc., Thornwood, NY, USA). To quantify exosome uptake, images were acquired from three independent experiments (n = 3), and the number of cells showing green fluorescence (SYTO RNASelect-positive) was counted manually under a fluorescence microscope. The total number of cells was determined based on DAPI staining. The uptake ratio was calculated as the percentage of SYTO-positive cells among the total DAPI-positive cells for each image field.

4.7. BrdU Labelling

TKE2 cells (10^4 cells/well) with or without exosome treatment, which were prepared as described above, were incubated with BrdU (final, 10 μM) for 2 h. After fixation with cold acetone at room temperature (RT) for 5 min, the cells were treated with 2 N HCl at RT for 30 min, and BrdU was detected by immunocytochemistry as described below. Ten randomly selected visual fields in each group were photographed, and the rate of BrdU-positive cells was calculated. Three independent experiments were performed.

4.8. Immunostaining

For an assessment of cell proliferation after exosome treatment, we prepared TKE2 and C2C12 cells cultured with DKSFM without growth supplement supplied by the manufacturer. Isolated mouse tear exosomes or PBS was applied to the DKSFM without supplementation every 12 h for 2 days. For comparison, we also prepared TKE2 cells cultured with DKSFM with growth supplement supplied by the manufacturer. The cells treated with or without exosomes were analysed by immunostaining for the proliferation marker Ki67. The treated cells were rinsed with PBS and fixed with cold acetone (Wako) for 5 min. After the cells were blocked with 10% normal donkey serum (Chemicon International, Inc., Temecula, CA, USA) at RT for 1 h, they were incubated with Ki67 [MIB-1 (1:50), Dako Cytomation, Glostrup, Denmark] and 5′-bromo-2′-deoxyuridine (BrdU) (BU1/75 (1:50), Abcam) at RT for 1.5 h. After three washes with phosphate-buffered saline for 5 min, the cells were incubated with a rhodamine-conjugated donkey anti-mouse IgG antibody (1:100; Jackson ImmunoResearch Laboratories, West Grove, PA, USA). After three additional washes with PBS, the cells were incubated with 1 μg/mL DAPI (Dojindo Laboratories) at RT for 5 min. Finally, the cells were washed three times in PBS and coverslipped using aqueous mounting medium (Fluoromount/Blue; Diagnostic BioSystems, Pleasanton, CA, USA). Images were acquired using an Axioplan 2 imaging microscope (Zeiss, Oberkochen, Germany). Ten randomly selected visual fields in each group were photographed, and the rate of Ki67-positive cells was calculated. Three independent experiments were performed.

4.9. Microarray Data Analysis

To assess transcriptomic changes in corneal epithelial cells following EV uptake, total RNA was extracted from TKE2 cells treated or not treated with tear-derived EVs. The extracted RNA samples were analysed using a Mouse Oligo chip 24 k (1-colour array) and scanned with the 3D-Gene Scanner 3000 (Toray, Tokyo, Japan). This oligonucleotide-based DNA microarray includes 23,475 probes representing mouse genes and is used to profile mRNA expression levels. After normalisation, differentially expressed genes were identified by comparing the EV-treated and untreated samples. Genes with a minimum fold change of ≥2.0 were selected for downstream functional analysis. Functional annotation enrichment analysis of these genes was performed using the DAVID Bioinformatics Resources (https://davidbioinformatics.nih.gov/, accessed on 1 May 2025)). Gene Ontology (GO) terms—encompassing molecular function, biological processes, and cellular components—and pathways with a p-value < 0.05 were considered significantly enriched. Annotation clusters with an enrichment score > 1.30 were considered biologically significant and grouped into categories based on DAVID's classification.

4.10. Statistical Analysis

Statistical analysis was performed using BellCurve for Excel (Social Survey Research Information Co., Ltd., Tokyo, Japan). Student's t-test was used for comparative analysis of the rate of exosome uptake and the rate of immunostaining-positive cells. A p value < 0.05 was considered statistically significant.

5. Conclusions

The current study provides novel evidence for the potential roles of EVs in mouse tear fluids in corneal epithelial cell physiology in vitro. Further studies on the identification of miRNA subtypes in tear exosomes using next-generation sequencing and the involvement of tear EVs and exosomes in normal conditions or diseases, such as DED, inflammatory conditions such as Sjogren's syndrome, and ageing in humans, should be conducted in the future.

Author Contributions: Conceptualisation, S.O., T.Y., R.Y.-H. and M.H.; methodology, S.O., K.H. and M.H.; validation, S.O., K.H., T.Y. and R.Y.-H.; resources, K.H., R.Y.-H. and M.H.; writing—original draft preparation, S.O., K.H. and M.H.; writing—review and editing, T.Y. and R.Y.-H.; supervision, M.H. All authors have read and agreed to the published version of the manuscript.

Funding: M.H. received JSPS KAKENHI (Grant Number: 23K09050).

Institutional Review Board Statement: This study was approved by the Animal Care and Experiment Committee of the Tokyo Dental College Ichikawa General Hospital (approval number: 207702).

Informed Consent Statement: Not applicable.

Data Availability Statement: The data that support the findings of this study are available from the corresponding author, M.H., upon reasonable request.

Acknowledgments: The authors have reviewed and edited the output and take full responsibility for the content of this publication.

Conflicts of Interest: The authors declare no conflicts of interest.

Abbreviations

The following abbreviations are used in this manuscript:

EVs	Extracellular Vesicles
DED	Dry Eye Diseases
EDA	Ectodysplasin A

References

1. Valadi, H.; Ekstrom, K.; Bossios, A.; Sjostrand, M.; Lee, J.J.; Lotvall, J.O. Exosome-mediated transfer of mRNAs and microRNAs is a novel mechanism of genetic exchange between cells. *Nat. Cell Biol.* **2007**, *9*, 654–659. [CrossRef]
2. Pegtel, D.M.; Cosmopoulos, K.; Thorley-Lawson, D.A.; van Eijndhoven, M.A.; Hopmans, E.S.; Lindenberg, J.L.; de Gruijl, T.D.; Wurdinger, T.; Middeldorp, J.M. Functional delivery of viral miRNAs via exosomes. *Proc. Natl. Acad. Sci. USA* **2010**, *107*, 6328–6333. [CrossRef] [PubMed]
3. Hoshino, A.; Costa-Silva, B.; Shen, T.L.; Rodrigues, G.; Hashimoto, A.; Tesic Mark, M.; Molina, H.; Kohsaka, S.; Di Giannatale, A.; Ceder, S.; et al. Tumour exosome integrins determine organotropic metastasis. *Nature* **2015**, *527*, 329–335. [CrossRef]
4. Saman, S.; Kim, W.; Raya, M.; Visnick, Y.; Miro, S.; Jackson, B.; McKee, A.C.; Alvarez, V.E.; Lee, N.C.; Hall, G.F. Exosome-associated tau is secreted in tauopathy models and is selectively phosphorylated in cerebrospinal fluid in early Alzheimer disease. *J. Biol. Chem.* **2012**, *287*, 3842–3849. [CrossRef]
5. Pan, B.T.; Johnstone, R.M. Fate of the transferrin receptor during maturation of sheep reticulocytes in vitro: Selective externalization of the receptor. *Cell* **1983**, *33*, 967–978. [CrossRef]
6. van Niel, G.; Porto-Carreiro, I.; Simoes, S.; Raposo, G. Exosomes: A common pathway for a specialized function. *J. Biochem.* **2006**, *140*, 13–21. [CrossRef]
7. Lerner, N.; Avissar, S.; Beit-Yannai, E. Extracellular vesicles mediate signaling between the aqueous humor producing and draining cells in the ocular system. *PLoS ONE* **2017**, *12*, e0171153. [CrossRef] [PubMed]

8. Liu, J.; Jiang, F.; Jiang, Y.; Wang, Y.; Li, Z.; Shi, X.; Zhu, Y.; Wang, H.; Zhang, Z. Roles of Exosomes in Ocular Diseases. *Int. J. Nanomed.* **2020**, *15*, 10519–10538. [CrossRef]
9. Samaeekia, R.; Rabiee, B.; Putra, I.; Shen, X.; Park, Y.J.; Hematti, P.; Eslani, M.; Djalilian, A.R. Effect of Human Corneal Mesenchymal Stromal Cell-derived Exosomes on Corneal Epithelial Wound Healing. *Investig. Ophthalmol. Vis. Sci.* **2018**, *59*, 5194–5200. [CrossRef] [PubMed]
10. Klingeborn, M.; Dismuke, W.M.; Bowes Rickman, C.; Stamer, W.D. Roles of exosomes in the normal and diseased eye. *Prog. Retin. Eye Res.* **2017**, *59*, 158–177. [CrossRef]
11. Mathers, W.D. Why the eye becomes dry: A cornea and lacrimal gland feedback model. *CLAO J.* **2000**, *26*, 159–165. [PubMed]
12. Doyle, L.M.; Wang, M.Z. Overview of Extracellular Vesicles, Their Origin, Composition, Purpose, and Methods for Exosome Isolation and Analysis. *Cells* **2019**, *8*, 727. [CrossRef] [PubMed]
13. Thery, C.; Witwer, K.W.; Aikawa, E.; Alcaraz, M.J.; Anderson, J.D.; Andriantsitohaina, R.; Antoniou, A.; Arab, T.; Archer, F.; Atkin-Smith, G.K.; et al. Minimal information for studies of extracellular vesicles 2018 (MISEV2018): A position statement of the International Society for Extracellular Vesicles and update of the MISEV2014 guidelines. *J. Extracell. Vesicles* **2018**, *7*, 1535750. [CrossRef]
14. Skog, J.; Wurdinger, T.; van Rijn, S.; Meijer, D.H.; Gainche, L.; Sena-Esteves, M.; Curry, W.T., Jr.; Carter, B.S.; Krichevsky, A.M.; Breakefield, X.O. Glioblastoma microvesicles transport RNA and proteins that promote tumour growth and provide diagnostic biomarkers. *Nat. Cell Biol.* **2008**, *10*, 1470–1476. [CrossRef]
15. Kawakita, T.; Shimmura, S.; Hornia, A.; Higa, K.; Tseng, S.C. Stratified epithelial sheets engineered from a single adult murine corneal/limbal progenitor cell. *J. Cell. Mol. Med.* **2008**, *12*, 1303–1316. [CrossRef]
16. Kosaka, N.; Iguchi, H.; Yoshioka, Y.; Takeshita, F.; Matsuki, Y.; Ochiya, T. Secretory mechanisms and intercellular transfer of microRNAs in living cells. *J. Biol. Chem.* **2010**, *285*, 17442–17452. [CrossRef]
17. Gene Ontology Consortium. Gene Ontology Consortium: Going forward. *Nucleic Acids Res.* **2015**, *43*, D1049–D1056. [CrossRef]
18. Tsubota, K.; Satake, Y.; Shimazaki, J. Treatment of severe dry eye. *Lancet* **1996**, *348*, 123. [CrossRef] [PubMed]
19. Mishima, S. Some Physiological Aspects of the Precorneal Tear Film. *Arch. Ophthalmol.* **1965**, *73*, 233–241. [CrossRef]
20. Yokoi, N.; Uchino, M.; Uchino, Y.; Dogru, M.; Kawashima, M.; Komuro, A.; Sonomura, Y.; Kato, H.; Tsubota, K.; Kinoshita, S. Importance of tear film instability in dry eye disease in office workers using visual display terminals: The Osaka study. *Am. J. Ophthalmol.* **2015**, *159*, 748–754. [CrossRef]
21. Uchino, M.; Nishiwaki, Y.; Michikawa, T.; Shirakawa, K.; Kuwahara, E.; Yamada, M.; Dogru, M.; Schaumberg, D.A.; Kawakita, T.; Takebayashi, T.; et al. Prevalence and risk factors of dry eye disease in Japan: Koumi study. *Ophthalmology* **2011**, *118*, 2361–2367. [CrossRef]
22. Ammar, D.A.; Noecker, R.J.; Kahook, M.Y. Effects of benzalkonium chloride- and polyquad-preserved combination glaucoma medications on cultured human ocular surface cells. *Adv. Ther.* **2011**, *28*, 501–510. [CrossRef]
23. Raposo, G.; Nijman, H.W.; Stoorvogel, W.; Liejendekker, R.; Harding, C.V.; Melief, C.J.; Geuze, H.J. B lymphocytes secrete antigen-presenting vesicles. *J. Exp. Med.* **1996**, *183*, 1161–1172. [CrossRef]
24. Caby, M.P.; Lankar, D.; Vincendeau-Scherrer, C.; Raposo, G.; Bonnerot, C. Exosomal-like vesicles are present in human blood plasma. *Int. Immunol.* **2005**, *17*, 879–887. [CrossRef] [PubMed]
25. Pisitkun, T.; Shen, R.F.; Knepper, M.A. Identification and proteomic profiling of exosomes in human urine. *Proc. Natl. Acad. Sci. USA* **2004**, *101*, 13368–13373. [CrossRef]
26. Ogawa, Y.; Kanai-Azuma, M.; Akimoto, Y.; Kawakami, H.; Yanoshita, R. Exosome-like vesicles with dipeptidyl peptidase IV in human saliva. *Biol. Pharm. Bull.* **2008**, *31*, 1059–1062. [CrossRef]
27. Kosaka, N.; Izumi, H.; Sekine, K.; Ochiya, T. microRNA as a new immune-regulatory agent in breast milk. *Silence* **2010**, *1*, 7. [CrossRef] [PubMed]
28. Street, J.M.; Barran, P.E.; Mackay, C.L.; Weidt, S.; Balmforth, C.; Walsh, T.S.; Chalmers, R.T.; Webb, D.J.; Dear, J.W. Identification and proteomic profiling of exosomes in human cerebrospinal fluid. *J. Transl. Med.* **2012**, *10*, 5. [CrossRef]
29. Gui, Y.; Liu, H.; Zhang, L.; Lv, W.; Hu, X. Altered microRNA profiles in cerebrospinal fluid exosome in Parkinson disease and Alzheimer disease. *Oncotarget* **2015**, *6*, 37043–37053. [CrossRef] [PubMed]
30. Madison, M.N.; Roller, R.J.; Okeoma, C.M. Human semen contains exosomes with potent anti-HIV-1 activity. *Retrovirology* **2014**, *11*, 102. [CrossRef]
31. Runz, S.; Keller, S.; Rupp, C.; Stoeck, A.; Issa, Y.; Koensgen, D.; Mustea, A.; Sehouli, J.; Kristiansen, G.; Altevogt, P. Malignant ascites-derived exosomes of ovarian carcinoma patients contain CD24 and EpCAM. *Gynecol. Oncol.* **2007**, *107*, 563–571. [CrossRef]
32. Inubushi, S.; Kawaguchi, H.; Mizumoto, S.; Kunihisa, T.; Baba, M.; Kitayama, Y.; Takeuchi, T.; Hoffman, R.M.; Tanino, H.; Sasaki, R. Oncogenic miRNAs Identified in Tear Exosomes From Metastatic Breast Cancer Patients. *Anticancer Res.* **2020**, *40*, 3091–3096. [CrossRef]

33. Bjordal, O.; Norheim, K.B.; Rodahl, E.; Jonsson, R.; Omdal, R. Primary Sjogren's syndrome and the eye. *Surv. Ophthalmol.* **2020**, *65*, 119–132. [CrossRef]
34. Le, M.T.; Hamar, P.; Guo, C.; Basar, E.; Perdigao-Henriques, R.; Balaj, L.; Lieberman, J. miR-200-containing extracellular vesicles promote breast cancer cell metastasis. *J. Clin. Investig.* **2014**, *124*, 5109–5128. [CrossRef] [PubMed]
35. Lakkaraju, A.; Rodriguez-Boulan, E. Itinerant exosomes: Emerging roles in cell and tissue polarity. *Trends Cell Biol.* **2008**, *18*, 199–209. [CrossRef]
36. Sadier, A.; Viriot, L.; Pantalacci, S.; Laudet, V. The ectodysplasin pathway: From diseases to adaptations. *Trends Genet. TIG* **2014**, *30*, 24–31. [CrossRef]
37. Mulcahy, L.A.; Pink, R.C.; Carter, D.R. Routes and mechanisms of extracellular vesicle uptake. *J. Extracell. Vesicles* **2014**, *3*, 24641. [CrossRef]
38. Svensson, K.J.; Christianson, H.C.; Wittrup, A.; Bourseau-Guilmain, E.; Lindqvist, E.; Svensson, L.M.; Morgelin, M.; Belting, M. Exosome uptake depends on ERK1/2-heat shock protein 27 signaling and lipid Raft-mediated endocytosis negatively regulated by caveolin-1. *J. Biol. Chem.* **2013**, *288*, 17713–17724. [CrossRef]
39. Tkach, M.; Thery, C. Communication by Extracellular Vesicles: Where We Are and Where We Need to Go. *Cell* **2016**, *164*, 1226–1232. [CrossRef] [PubMed]
40. Hirayama, M.; Ogawa, M.; Oshima, M.; Sekine, Y.; Ishida, K.; Yamashita, K.; Ikeda, K.; Shimmura, S.; Kawakita, T.; Tsubota, K.; et al. Functional lacrimal gland regeneration by transplantation of a bioengineered organ germ. *Nat. Commun.* **2013**, *4*, 2497. [CrossRef] [PubMed]
41. Greening, D.W.; Xu, R.; Ji, H.; Tauro, B.J.; Simpson, R.J. A protocol for exosome isolation and characterization: Evaluation of ultracentrifugation, density-gradient separation, and immunoaffinity capture methods. *Methods Mol. Biol.* **2015**, *1295*, 179–209. [PubMed]

International Journal of *Molecular Sciences*

MDPI

Article

Clinical Effectiveness, Safety, and Compliance of Two Compounded Formulations of Tacrolimus Eye Drops: An Open-Label, Sequential Prospective Study

María Puente-Iglesias [1,2,3,†], Andrea Cuartero-Martínez [1,2,3,†], Rosario Touriño-Peralba [4], María Teresa Rodríguez-Ares [4], María Jesús Giráldez [5], Eva Yebra-Pimentel [5], Laura García-Quintanilla [1,2], Xurxo García-Otero [3,6], Miguel González-Barcia [1,2], Irene Zarra-Ferro [1,2], Francisco J. Otero-Espinar [3], Anxo Fernández-Ferreiro [1,2,*] and Ana Castro-Balado [1,2,*]

1 Pharmacy Department, University Clinical Hospital of Santiago de Compostela (SERGAS), 15706 Santiago de Compostela, Spain; andrea.cuartero@rai.usc.es (A.C.-M.)
2 FarmaCHUSLab Group, Health Research Institute of Santiago de Compostela (IDIS), 15706 Santiago de Compostela, Spain
3 Department of Pharmacology, Pharmacy and Pharmaceutical Technology, Faculty of Pharmacy, University of Santiago de Compostela (USC), 15782 Santiago de Compostela, Spain; rancisco.otero@usc.es (F.J.O.-E.)
4 Ophthalmology Department, University Clinical Hospital of Santiago de Compostela (SERGAS), 15706 Santiago de Compostela, Spain; rtourinop2@gmail.com (R.T.-P.)
5 Department of Applied Physics, Optometry, Faculty of Optics and Optometry, University of Santiago de Compostela (USC), 15782 Santiago de Compostela, Spain; mjesus.giraldez@usc.es (M.J.G.)
6 Molecular Imaging Biomarkers and Theragnosis Lab Group, Center for Research in Molecular Medicine and Chronic Diseases (CiMUS), University of Santiago de Compostela (USC), 15782 Santiago de Compostela, Spain
* Correspondence: anxordes@gmail.com (A.F.-F.); ana.castro.balado@gmail.com (A.C.-B.)
† These authors contributed equally to this work.

Abstract: Ophthalmic tacrolimus compounded formulations are usually made from the commercial intravenous presentation, which contains ethanol as a solubilizer due to the low solubility of tacrolimus. The use of cyclodextrins is presented as an alternative to ethanol, an ocular irritant excipient, to avoid its long-term irritant effects. Open-label, sequential, prospective study to compare effectiveness, safety, and adherence of a new formulation of 0.015% tacrolimus with cyclodextrins (TCD) versus 0.03% tacrolimus with ethanol (TE). The ocular evaluation was assessed by ocular signs, corneal staining, subjective questionnaires as Visual Function Questionnaire (VFQ-25) and Visual Analogue Scale (VAS) of symptoms, lacrimal stability, ocular redness, and intraocular pressure. Compliance was assessed by VAS of adherence and empirically (difference between theoretical and actual consumption). Clinical ocular signs and corneal staining score remained stable for most patients 3 months after switching formulations. The TCD formulation did not modify the tear stability and intraocular pressure of the treated patients compared to the TE formulation. TCD eye drops significantly decreased the subjective pain values on VFQ-25 scale and burning sensation on the VAS symptom scale in comparison to TE formulation after 3 months after the change to TCD formulation. The novel tacrolimus in cyclodextrins formulation is a promising alternative for treating inflammatory ocular pathologies refractory to first-line treatments.

Keywords: tacrolimus; hydroxypropyl-β-cyclodextrin; eye drops; efficacy; safety

1. Introduction

Tacrolimus is a cyclic macrolide lactone with immunosuppressive effect which inhibits calcineurin FK506, causing a decrease in the transcription of proinflammatory cytokines. It is commonly used as a prophylactic treatment for organ rejection in solid transplant recipients and for the treatment of allograft rejection resistant to other immunosuppressive drugs [1]. Off-label clinical indications for tacrolimus include the treatment of autoimmune diseases such as atopic dermatitis or psoriasis, among others [2,3]. In ophthalmic pathologies, the use of off-label tacrolimus has been successful in the prevention of corneal rejection, dry eye syndrome, vernal keratoconjunctivitis, atopic keratoconjunctivitis, corneal and conjunctival immune diseases [3–6]. In these ocular pathologies, inflammation has been shown to be a key factor in the pathogenesis, and their treatment include topical corticosteroids, mast cell stabilizers, antihistaminic and immunomodulatory agents [7]. Therapeutic alternatives, such as immunosuppressive drugs as cyclosporine and tacrolimus, are necessary in refractory cases [8].

Tacrolimus eye drops are not commercially available, so they are usually elaborated as a compounded formulation in Hospital Pharmacy Departments (HPDs). The limiting factor in their elaboration is the low water solubility of tacrolimus [9]. One of the most widespread compounded formulation is made by reformulating the intravenous presentation (Prograf®), where tacrolimus is solubilized using ethanol, an irritant excipient for the ocular surface [10,11]. Ophthalmic use of ethanol has been associated with uncomfortable ocular application that can affect adherence, as well as patient safety due to its toxicity when used by this route [12]. Different alternatives have been developed to avoid the use of ethanol in tacrolimus eye drops, but the complexity of the preparation and the need for specific equipment make clinical translation to HPDs difficult [13–15]. Against this background, our group developed an alternative compounded formulation using 2-HydroxyPropil-Beta-Cyclodextrin (HPβCD) as solubilizer [16]. According to the European Medicines Agency (EMA), HPβCD is the safest and most suitable cyclodextrin for use in topical ophthalmic applications [17]. García-Otero et al. developed and characterized the solubility, stability and mucoadhesive properties of this new formulation [16]. The addition of HPβCD resulted in an increase in the solubility and stability of tacrolimus, accompanied by a notable change in the solution's viscosity and adhesiveness. This formulation has been also evaluated in animal models of inflammation, achieving a reduction in leukocytes and cytokines at the ocular level [18]. The new formulation, with greater ocular biopermanence, allows for a reduction in tacrolimus concentration, achieving the desired therapeutic effect and, at the same time, reducing the potential risk of mutagenicity when tacrolimus is used for prolonged periods [19,20].

The elaboration of the new formulation with cyclodextrins was transferred to the HPD in response to demand from prescribing ophthalmologists, with the objective of improving patient safety while maintaining the efficacy. The aim of this study is to evaluate and compare the effectivity, safety, and compliance of 0.015% tacrolimus eye drops with HPβCD (TCD) and the previously used 0.03% tacrolimus eye drops with ethanol (TE) elaborated from Prograf® in the management of ocular inflammatory pathologies.

2. Results

2.1. Population and Treatment Characteristics

The switch to the TCD formulation was made in agreement with the Ophthalmology Department for a total of 56 patients. The median age was 52.5 years (Q_1–Q_3: 18–66), with 25.0% under 18 years old and 16.1% over 70 years old. The proportion of men was slightly higher (64.0%). In terms of diagnosis, tacrolimus was administered to 39.3% of patients for the treatment of conjunctivitis/atopy, 37.5% for prophylaxis/treatment of rejection after corneal transplant, and 9.0% for the treatment of Sjögren's syndrome. The remaining 14.2% of patients suffered from rare diseases such as Lyell or Thyggesson syndrome, or caustic burns.

Patients were instructed to apply the eye drops in the affected eye. However, a considerable proportion of patients exhibited biocular involvement, leading them to apply the eye drops to both eyes. The dosage prior to the start of the study varied between one drop in both eyes (Oculus Uterque, OU) every 6 h and one drop in OU every 48 h, according to the pathology and patient requirements. All patients used artificial tears, 21.4% of patients also received treatment with corticosteroids and 9.0% of patients were treated with autologous serum. The average number of concomitant eye drops prescribed was 2. Between the initial and second visit, 11 patients abandoned treatment (Figure 1), five of them did so before the first month of treatment due to conjunctival hyperemia and a sticky sensation with difficulty blinking after application. In these patients, TE eye drops were reintroduced. The remaining six patients returned to TE eye drops because they had become tolerant to the burning sensation and reported a more satisfactory application due to the lower viscosity of TE eye drops. A total of 9 patients had to change the dosage after switching eye drops: 3 patients needed to increase the dose and 6 had to decrease it. The percentage of patients receiving concomitant corticosteroid treatment decreased from 21.4% to 13.3% after switching from TE to TCD.

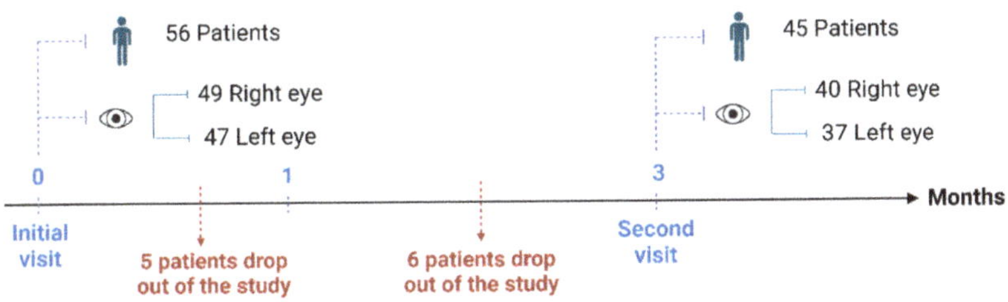

Figure 1. Patient flow and studied eyes during the two study visits. Created in BioRender.

2.2. Clinical Evaluation

For the analysis of clinical ocular parameters, differences between visits were evaluated. Thus, Best Corrected Visual Acuity (BCVA) was analyzed in 69 eyes of which 27.54% had equal BCVA in both visits and the 44.93% had higher BCVA at visit 2 in comparison with visit 1. The remaining 27.54% of the eyes presented a decreased in BCVA with a worsening of only one optotype in most cases (Table 1). The difference between visits in conjunctival integrity, presence of papillae, tranta points on the corneal limbus and corneal integrity were analyzed in 76 eyes (Table 1). In conjunctiva analyses, most eyes had the same (56.58%) or a lower grade (17.11%) at visit 2 compared to the initial one, while 26.32% had a worsening at visit 2. In the papillae evaluation, 63.13% showed no differences between visits, 9.21% showed an improvement and 27.63% worsened. There were no signs of tranta spots in the limbus in any of the patients evaluated. Finally, in the evaluation of corneal signs it was found that 81.58% of the patients obtained the same value at visit 2 compared to the initial visit, while 18.42% improved the integrity of the corneal signs analyzed. No patient had active corneal ulcerations or erosions during the study.

Table 1. Analysis of clinical parameters evaluated for the effectiveness of the new tacrolimus formulation and tear stability parameters (TMH and NIKBUT). Percentage of evaluated eyes maintaining equal, better, or worse values at visit 2 (TCD) compared to visit 1 (TE).

	n (Eyes)	Equal (%)	Improvement (%)	Worsened (%)
BCVA	69	27.54	44.93	27.54
Ocular signs				
Conjunctiva	76	56.58	17.11	26.32
Papillae	76	63.16	9.21	27.63
Tantras points	76	76	-	-
Corneal sign	76	81.58	18.42	0.0
Oxford	76	72.37	25.0	2.63
TMH	73	2.74	54.79	42.47
NIKBUT	65	3.08	44.62	52.31

BCVA: best corrected visual acuity; n: population size; NIKBUT: noninvasive keratograph break up time; TMH: tear meniscus height.

For corneal staining, the difference between visits on the Oxford scale was analyzed (Table 1). Taking this into account, 72.37% of the eyes had no differences between visits.

Within this group, 96.0% were classified as grade 0 at both visits, i.e., they had no corneal staining during the study. A decrease in corneal staining was observed in 25.0% of the eyes analyzed while only 2.63% of the eyes showed an increase in corneal staining. In addition, no symptoms of corneal rejection have been observed in patients who underwent keratoplasty or recurrence of previous pathologies after the change of formulation.

Measurements of Tear Meniscus Height (TMH), Noninvasive Keratograph Break Up Time (NIKBUT) and Ocular Redness (OR) were performed at both visits in the eyes treated with tacrolimus eye drops (Table 2). For the lacrimal stability study, 73 eyes were analyzed in the TMH analysis, of which 54.79% obtained an improvement in the TMH at visit 2, although no significant differences were found. Regarding to NIKBUT analysis, no significant differences were found between tear breakup time measured at each visit. THM and NIKBUT measures of each patient at both visits are shown in Tables S6 and S7 of the Supplementary Material, respectively.

Table 2. Median (Md) and percentiles (Q_1–Q_3) of tear stability parameters (TMH and NIKBUT), ocular redness (OR) and intraocular pressure (IOP) and the comparison between visits.

			TE	TCD	
		n (Eyes)	Md (Q_1–Q_3)	Md (Q_1–Q_3)	*p*-Value
TMH (mm)		73	0.25 (0.19–0.20)	0.26 (0.36–0.39)	0.2404
NIKBUT (s)		65	8.79 (6.26–5.38)	7.66 (15.01–12.70)	0.0922
OR	TB	63	1.0 (0.6–1.6)	1.2 (0.7–1.8)	0.0168
	NB	63	1.2 (0.8–2.1)	1.4 (0.9–2.0)	0.2199
	TL	63	0.5 (0.4–1.1)	0.8 (0.5–1.2)	0.0294
	NL	63	0.6 (0.4–1.4)	0.8 (0.5–1.4)	0.0182
	ORT	63	1.1 (0.7–1.8)	1.3 (0.8–1.8)	0.0829
	AREA (mm^3)	63	10.95 (7.4–13.83)	9.90 (6.9–15.08)	0.8489
IOP (mmHg)		56	14.0 (12.0–16.0)	14.0 (12.0–15.75)	0.7589

AREA: total area analyzed in mm^3; IOP: intraocular pressure; Md: median; n: population size; NB: nasal bulbar area; NIKBUT: noninvasive keratograph break up time; NL: nasal limbal; Q_1: 25th percentile; Q_3: 75th percentile; TB: temporal bulbar area; TCD: tacrolimus 0.015% in cyclodextrin; TE: tacrolimus 0.03% prepared from commercial intravenous presentation Prograf®; TL: temporal limbal; TMH: tear meniscus height; ORT: average ocular redness.

The degree of ocular redness in the bulbar, limbal, and total conjunctiva of 63 eyes was analyzed. In the comparative of OR of the Temporal Bulbar (TB) conjunctiva, Temporal Limbal (TL) and Nasal Limbal (NL), a significant increase in redness was found at visit 2 compared to visit 1 (p_{TB} = 0.0168; p_{TL} = 0.0294; p_{NL} = 0.0182) (Table 2). The comparison in Nasal Bulbar (NB) conjunctiva showed a non-significant difference in OR at visit 2 (p = 0.2199). Finally, in the analysis of average OR measured, non-significant differences were found between visits (p = 0.0829). Descriptive analysis and the multiple comparison between visits of OR are detailed in Table 2. Thus, no significant differences in intraocular pressure (IOP) were found between visit 1 (median = 14.0 mmHg; Q_1–Q_3: 12.0–16.0) and visit 2 (median = 14.0 mmHg; Q_1–Q_3: 12.0–15.75) (p = 0.7589) in 56 evaluated eyes (Table 2).

2.3. *Patient Reported Outcomes and Compliance*

2.3.1. Reported Outcomes

There was a marked increase in the total score on the Visual Function Questionnaire (VFQ-25), with a median of 80.9 (Q_1–Q_3: 66.7–89.7) for TE and 82.8 (Q_1–Q_3: 76.6–92.0) for TCD (p = 0.003), with higher values being associated with more positive results. In the domain-specific analysis, there was a significant improvement in referred pain when switching to the TCD formulation, with a median punctuation of 62.5 (Q_1–Q_3: 56.2–87.5) with TE vs. 75.0 (Q_1–Q_3: 62.5–87.5) with TCD (p = 0.004). The disparity in this variable is evident in Figure 2, which depicts a redial graph representing the total medians obtained for total score and each subcategory studied in the VFQ-25 questionnaire on a scale from 0 to 100. Of the 12 domains assessed, improvement was evident in four of them with the new formulation (near vision, distance vision, role, ocular pain). Eight domains (general health, global vision, social functioning, dependency, mental health, driving difficulties, peripheral vision, color vision) had the same median score, and none of them had a lower score with the initiation of TCD treatment (Table S8 of the Supplementary Material).

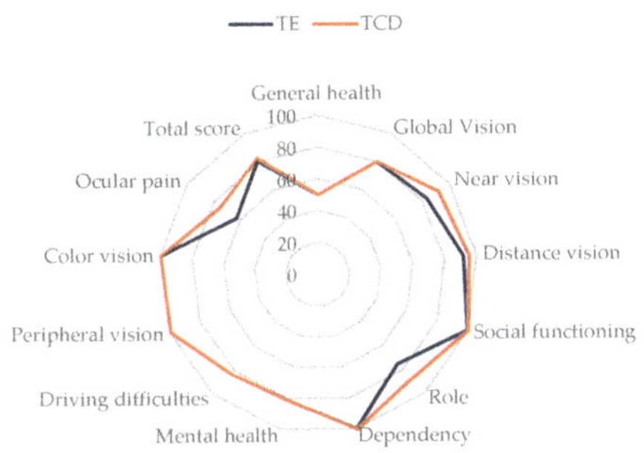

Figure 2. A radial chart showing the subscales examined in the VFQ-25 questionnaire and the medians obtained for TE and TCD. TCD: tacrolimus 0.015% in cyclodextrin; TE: tacrolimus 0.03% prepared from commercial intravenous presentation Prograf®.

VFQ-25 median total scores were also evaluated based on age groups (<18 years, 18–65 years and >65 years), and a clear age dependence was observed, as shown in Table S9 of the Supplementary Material. The analysis concluded that there is a moderately high negative correlation between age and the VFQ score for TE and TCD ($r = -0.647$, $p = 0.001$ for TE, $r = -0.599$, $p = 0.001$ for TCD). A comparison of the medians of the age groups revealed a significant difference in the quality of life between the age groups. As age increases, so does the visual quality of life ($p = 0.001$ for TE, $p = 0.001$ for TCD). It is important to note that the group of patients over the age 65 years showed a mean increase in quality of life of almost 10 points with TCD eye drops.

Regarding the Visual Analogue Scale (VAS) of symptoms, the improvement in burning was statistically significant in both eyes with a decrease from 5.0 (Q_1–Q_3: 1.9–7.0) to 2.0 (Q_1–Q_3: 1.0–3.5) ($p = 0.004$) in the right eye, and from 5.0 (Q_1–Q_3: 2.0–7.0) to 2.5 (Q_1–Q_3: 0.8–4.1) ($p = 0.003$) in the left eye. An improvement in pain perception was only observed in the left eye with a total mean score from 1.3 (Q_1–Q_3: 0.0–3.0) to 0.5 (Q_1–Q_3: 0.0–2.0) ($p = 0.03$). Table S10 of the Supplementary Material shows the comparison of the median scores obtained at the initial visit with TE and at the 3-month follow-up visit with TCD. In the VAS assessment, the 6 symptoms assessed had a lower score for TCD, as shown in the radial graph in Figure 3. This figure shows mean values for both eyes, which are lower for TCD than TE. The greatest differences are observed in the symptoms of burning and photophobia.

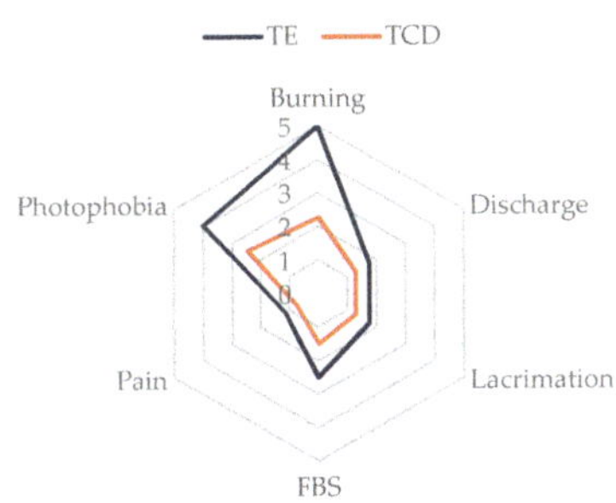

Figure 3. Radial plot of median right and left eye scores for the 6 symptoms examined in the VAS assessment. FBS: foreign body sensation. TCD: tacrolimus 0.015% in cyclodextrin; TE: tacrolimus 0.03% prepared from commercial intravenous presentation Prograf®.

Changes on the VAS symptom scale are shown in Table 3, the percentage of patients reporting improved, worsened, or unchanged symptoms after switching to TCD. An improvement in burning was reported by 51.6% of patients, with 48.5% reducing the intensity of the burning sensation by two or more points on the intensity scale. There was no symptom for which the percentage of worsening was greater than the percentage of improvement.

Table 3. Percentage of patients who improved or worsened in both eyes or in at least one of them, and those who remained with the same symptoms on the VAS of symptoms. The inconclusive section includes those patients who, with both eyes affected, improved in one eye and worsened in the other.

	Burning	Discharge	Lacrimation	FBS	Pain	Photophobia
n	33	35	36	35	33	33
Improved ≥ 2 points	48.5%	22.9%	27.8%	40%	27.3%	27.3%
Improved 1 point	3.1%	11.4%	11.1%	5.7%	6.1%	12.1%
Deterioration ≥ 2 points	15.2%	17.1%	5.6%	17.1%	12.1%	21.2%
Deterioration 1 point	3.1%	5.7%	11.1%	8.6%	9.1%	12.1%
Same symptoms	24.3%	40%	38.8%	25,7%	42.4%	27.3%
Inconclusive	6.1%	2.9%	5.6%	2,9%	3%	-

FBS: foreign body sensation; n: population size.

2.3.2. Compliance

Patient-reported adherence was measured using the VAS adherence scale. Comparing the scales at visit 1 (TE) and visit 2 (TCD), an increase in adherence was observed in 34.3% of patients. It should be noted that 56.6% of the remaining patients continued compliant. Adherence increased significantly from 100.0% (Q_1–Q_3: 80–100) for TE to 100.0% (Q_1–Q_3: 90–100) for TCD (p = 0.003). No association was found between adherence and complexity of dosing.

In the study cohort, only 44 subjects complied with the instructions and returned two TCD bottles. Consequently, the total number of bottles weighed were 88. In terms of the objective measure of adherence, it was concluded that only 23.6% of patients had a difference between actual and theoretical weight of less than 35% in the two returned containers. No correlation was found between actual and subjective adherence.

3. Discussion

Previous studies have analyzed the therapeutic effect of ophthalmic presentations of tacrolimus at different concentrations for different pathologies involving ocular inflammation such as dry eye [21–23], vernal keratoconjunctivitis (VKC) [24,25], shield ulcer and corneal epitheliopathy [26], Sjögren's syndrome dry eye [27], corneal endothelial rejection [28], keratoplastics [29], Thygeson Superficial Punctate Keratitis [30], stromal herpetic keratitis [31]. In the present work, the effectiveness of a tacrolimus 0.015% with cyclodextrins eye drops and how the decrease in concentration could affect in the effectiveness were analyzed using visual acuity to screen for certain ocular pathologies [32], so a positive or neutral variation may demonstrate that there are no negative changes in these patients' condition. Regarding visual acuity analysis, most of the patients showed equal or improved measures. In relation to the clinical signs analyzed, no significant negative changes were observed in most patients after the change of formulation and the cornea was not affected either by alterations in corneal staining or by other structural changes such as stromal edema. These results indicate that the decrease in tacrolimus concentration does not affect the effectiveness of the treatment.

Tacrolimus formulations with concentrations ranging from 0.03 to 0.1% are the most frequently used in clinical practice. Our original formulation (TE) contained 0.03% tacrolimus, which was subsequently replaced with a 0.015% tacrolimus formulation in HPβCD (TCD). This reduction in concentration was made possible by the increased ocular biopermanence provided by cyclodextrins. The new formulation exhibits comparable effectiveness to the previous one, while receiving 50% less immunosuppressant dose. The lower concentration of immunosuppressant implies greater safety of the formulation, given that greater cytotoxic effects of tacrolimus have been reported at higher concentrations. Sella R. et al. reported in a comparative study in human corneal epithelial cell models that cell survival increased as tacrolimus concentration decreased [19]. Despite the absence of a direct causal relationship between topical tacrolimus treatment and the onset of neoplasia in the ophthalmic region, several instances of conjunctival melanoma have been observed in patients who have undergone tacrolimus eye drop therapy (0.03%). It would be beneficial to investigate this potential correlation [20]. However, it is noteworthy that a positive association between topical tacrolimus and cutaneous lymphoma has been documented [33]. In another study, an 0.005% tacrolimus ophthalmic formulation was developed to treat patients with vernal keratoconjunctivitis. According to their study, even with the low tacrolimus concentration, symptom improvement was observed in patients with refractory VKC [34]. These results support the idea of the therapeutic power of tacrolimus in topical formulation and agree with our results as no recurrence or worsening of the ocular pathology was reported after the decrease of tacrolimus concentration in our formulation for any patient.

Regarding the VFQ-25 quality of life questionnaire, the patient's perception of reduced pain may be attributed to the absence of the irritating effect of ethanol. Ethanol has a toxic effect on the corneal epithelium, although it has been used at higher concentrations (13%) in corneal surgeries such as keratectomy to remove the epithelium. Lower concentrations of ethanol are tolerable but are also accompanied by an irritant effect. In a previously published retrospective analysis of 20 mg/mL cyclosporine eye drops containing 25 mg/mL ethanol, 37% of treated patients reported burning sensations after application [19]. Also, the perception of reduced burning and itching sensations associated with data collected on the VAS scale was probably attributed to the removal of ethanol from the composition of the TCD eye drops.

The previous formulation of tacrolimus eye drops was poorly tolerated due to the presence of irritating excipients such as ethanol. To enhance tacrolimus solubility, cyclodextrins were presented as an effective and safe alternative [16]. In vitro studies have previously demonstrated the safety and good tolerability of the ophthalmic administration of cyclodextrins with poorly soluble drugs, such as corticosteroids or econazole [35]. The EMA has determined that 12.5% HPβCD solutions are not toxic or irritating to the eyes of rabbits [17]. García-Otero et al. analyzed the irritation of different cyclodextrins, including HPβCD, though Hen's Egg Test on the Chorioallantois Membrane (HET-CAM) assay and Bovine Corneal Opacity and Permeability test (BCOP) [16]. In addition, ocular biopermanence was verified by in vivo Positron Emission Tomography (PET) [18]. Ex vivo, in vitro and in vivo assays concluded that formulations with HPβCD showed a well toxicity profile and enhanced biopermanence at the ocular level [16,18,19]. There has been an increase in the list of drugs containing cyclodextrins [36]. The main reasons for using these excipients are to reduce the instability of many molecules in aqueous media, e.g., hydrocortisone undergoing hydrolysis, and to reduce ocular irritation, such as pilocarpine which may precipitate and cause eye irritation and damage [37]. Within this context, there are currently 14 ophthalmic cyclodextrin formulations on the market, 8 of them containing HPβCDs [36].

To our knowledge, this is the first study to evaluate tear stability in patients under ophthalmic treatment with tacrolimus eye drops. Ethanol may modify tear stability as it functions as an organic solvent against the lipid layer of the tear [38]. It is known how tear osmolarity affects ocular comfort, with tear hyperosmolarity being one of the causes of discomfort and dry eye [39,40]. Comparing results, in our work it has been found that switching from TE from TCD treatment increased the TMH in at least half of the eyes evaluated. In contrast, the change in treatment produced no change in NIKBUT. All in all, it could be said that tear stability has remained stable, contributing to the effectiveness of the TCD treatment. Concerning the increased in OR after the first 3 months of TCD treatment, when an eye drop is administered, the interaction of the drop with the refractive surface and tear film may produce a slight irritability. In turn, viscosity above the limits may cause blurred vision, foreign body sensation and increased blinking rate, leading to an undesirable irritant effect of the ocular surface [41]. This disturbance would be directly increased by the density and viscosity of the eye drops and may cause some initial discomfort in patients with dryness symptoms or with long term treatments. Even with the objective data on OR, this event has not been correlated with other clinical and tear stability measurements.

The negative effects of steroids on IOP are known [42,43]. According to Miyazaki D. et al., tacrolimus treatment does not raise intraocular pressure although it may be influenced by concomitant use of corticosteroids or poor lid condition [44]. In this work, we studied the variation of intraocular pressure after switching from TE to TCD treatment in patients with concomitant treatments, some of them with corticosteroids. No variations in intraocular pressure were observed between visits, confirming that our 0.015% TCD eye drops do not raise intraocular pressure. These results are in agreement with other studies in which intraocular pressure has been evaluated in different presentations of tacrolimus for ophthalmic treatment [6,45].

In general, adherence to topical ocular treatments is quite low. One study analyzed subjective adherence to eye drops in inflammatory eye disease and concluded that 67% of patients were not adherent [46]. The main cause of lack of adherence is forgetfulness. Adherence questionnaires have significant limitations as subjectivity, memory bias (adherence can only be measured in a recent period), response bias (the patient answers what is expected of him) and the inability to detect unintentional adherence, that is, non-conscious forgetfulness [47]. Therefore, in this study, we attempted to measure adherence objectively by comparing the actual content used by the patient and the theoretical content according to the dosage regimen. Upon implementing this experimental method to calculate the compliance, we observed significant discrepancies in the weights, which could be attributed to a multitude of factors, including poor compliance and unintentional losses. The principal limitation of this analysis was the establishment of a cut-off point to differentiate between adherent and non-adherent patients, given that there is no existing literature on this subject. Finally, a margin of error of 35% was allowed between the actual and estimated weight, to consider accidental losses and evaporation losses. Patients classified as adherent according to the weighing system had reported 100% adherence on the VAS adherence scale.

To facilitate the transfer of this formulation to other centers, it is essential to emphasize that all the raw materials utilized are accessible to any HPD. In addition to this, no special equipment is required for its preparation, being all the apparatus used widely available in HPD.

4. Materials and Methods

4.1. Materials

Tacrolimus was acquired from Guinama® S.L.U. (La Pobla de Vallbona, Spain), 2-hydroxypropyl-β-cyclodextrin Kleptose® HPB (HPβCD; MW = 1399 Da, substitution degree = 0.65 molar ratio) was provided from Roquette Laisa S.A.® (Valencia, Spain), Liquifilm® was purchased from Allergan® Pharmaceuticals Ireland (Mayo, Ireland), Balanced Salt Solution (BSS®) was acquired from Alcon® laboratories (FortWorth, TX, USA) and Prograf® (5 mg/mL, ampoules) was purchased from Astellas Pharma S.A.® (Madrid, Spain).

4.2. Elaboration and Packaging of Tacrolimus Sterile Solutions

Two different tacrolimus formulations were prepared, a 0.03% tacrolimus formulation using intravenous drug presentation (Prograf®) (TE) and a 0.015% tacrolimus formulation (without ethanol) with 40% HPβCD (TCD). Both compounded formulations were elaborated in sterile conditions under a vertical flow cabinet. TE was elaborated following Luaces-Rodriguez et al. previous work [11]. The necessary volume of tacrolimus (Prograf® 5 mg/mL) was added to a luer-lock syringe to reach a concentration of 0.03%. The vehicle used for its preparation was Liquifilm® (LI), an artificial tear based on polyvinyl alcohol 1.4% *w*/*v*. Afterward, the solution was filtered through a 5 µm filter (RoweMed AG—Medical for life, Parchim, Germany) and filled into 5 mL High-Density Polyethylene (HDPE) eye drop containers (Envases Farmacéuticos Sirep, S.L., Tarragona, Spain).

To elaborate TCD compounded formulation, HPβCD was added over 2/3 of the final volume of LI to reach a concentration of 40% under intense magnetic stirring. Later, it was left under agitation at low stirring speed for a total of 24 h to eliminate foam. Tacrolimus was added under intense stirring to obtain a concentration of 0.015%, heating the solution to 40 °C during the addition. The solution was left in agitation for a total of 96 h to achieve maximum tacrolimus solubilization. Finally, it was made up to the final volume with LI and filtered with a 0.22 µm membrane filter (vacuum-driven bottles FPR204250 PES 0.22 µm; Biofil, Alicante, Spain) under vacuum. Both formulations were finally packaged in 5 mL HDPE eye drops containers.

4.3. Study Design and Visits

An open-label, sequential, prospective, single-center, 3-month study was conducted at the Ophthalmology Department of the University Clinical Hospital of Santiago de Compostela. The present study complied with the tenets of the Declaration of Helsinki and was approved by the Institutional Review Board/Ethics Committee of the Ethical Committee of Clinical Research of Galicia (AFF-FOR-2019-01). For inclusion, patients had to have been under treatment with the TE formulation for, at last, 6 months and agree to participate by signing the informed consent form. The only exclusion criteria were that the patient refused to participate or did not sign the informed consent form.

Two visits were planned for the study. At visit 1 (baseline visit), variables related to TE formulations were collected and the new TCD formulation was dispensed. In the second visit, that took place three months after TCD were dispensed, variables regarding TCD eye drops were collected. Study design and visits are shown in Figure 4.

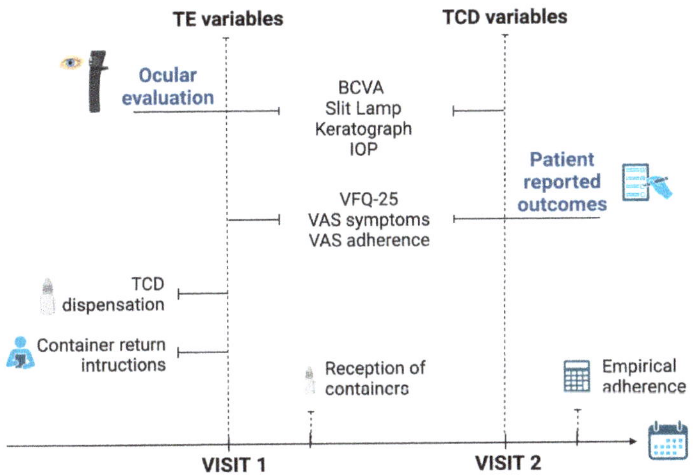

Figure 4. Study design: visits, collected variables and administration of the study medication. BCVA: best-corrected visual acuity; IOP: Intraocular pressure; VFQ-25: Visual Function Questionnaire; TCD: tacrolimus 0.015% in cyclodextrin; TE: tacrolimus 0.03% prepared from commercial intravenous presentation Prograf®; VAS: visual analog scale. Created in BioRender.

4.4. Data Collection and Clinical Evaluation

Demographic (age, gender), clinical (diagnosis, affected eye) and treatment characteristics (dosage regimen, duration, adverse effects, concomitant treatment) were collected through review of medical records and interviews with the patient. To evaluate the effectiveness and safety of TE and TCD eye drops, a clinical examination was performed at each visit, from less invasive tests to more invasive tests to avoid interference. To avoid the influence of diurnal variations in tear and intraocular pressure parameters, all measurements were performed within the same time range for both visits (8:30 a.m.–14:00 p.m.). Clinical evaluation and intraocular pressure were performed only by two ophthalmologists, who in turn employed scales commonly used in this type of studies, in an attempt to reduce subjectivity as much as possible (Tables S1 and S2 of the Supplementary Material). The rest of the clinical tests were carried out by a single optometrist. To avoid bias, data collection and data analyzed was performed by different researchers.

Clinical Evaluation

The ocular evaluation began with the measurement of the BCVA using a Snellen test. If the patient was wearing correction at that moment, the measurement was made with the patient's own spectacles. BCVA improvement was considered when the visual acuity at visit 2 was greater than visual acuity at visit 1, i.e., when patients discerned at least one more optotype line relative to the initial visit. Those patients who only perceived light, with or without projection were excluded, and values were transform in LogMar notation for the correct comparison and analysis [48]. Ocular signs were examined with a slit lamp (Topcon Europe Medical B.V., Barcelona, Spain), consisting of a study of the conjunctiva, presence of papillae, presence of trantas dots on the limbus and presence of corneal signs. For each item, a 4-point classification was performed as shown in Table S1 of the Supplementary Material. For these parameters, a decrease in one grade scale in visit 2 in comparison with visit 1 was considering to be an improvement in the clinical sign evaluated. To assess the corneal fluorescein staining a slit lamp was used and classified using the Oxford corneal staining scheme [49] (Table S2, Supplementary Material). For this analysis, a decrease in Oxford scale between visits was associated with a decrease in corneal staining.

Lacrimal stability and OR were studied using the OCULUS Keratograph 5M® (Oculus, Wetzlar, Germany) and Oculus TF-Scan module (Oculus, Wetzlar, Germany). In the study of lacrimal stability and OR, those eyes whose pathology prevented the proper functioning of the optics of the instruments were excluded. According to our previous work [50], lacrimal stability was measured though the TMH, and the NIKBUT. Both parameters were measured in triplicate. The degree of OR provided by the instrument of the TB and NB area and a TL and NL conjunctiva was measured, as well as the average degree of ocular redness. For TMH and NIKBUT analysis, higher values in visit 2 in comparison with the initial visit were considered an improvement, while improvement in OR was considered if its value decreased over the course of the visits.

With the purpose of verifying that the switch of tacrolimus formulation did not affect the IOP, this was assessed at both visits using Perkins's tonometer (Perkins MK2, Haag-Streig Holding, Harlow, UK). IOP measurements were carried out as the last clinical test to avoid the possible influence in the other parameters since previous administration of a topical anesthetic (Colircusí Fluotest®, Alcon Healthcare, TX, USA) was needed. To minimize instrument variability, the tonometer was calibrated before each visit and the measurement was carried out with the patient in a sitting position. In the analysis of the clinical ocular parameters, those patients who had no measurements at both visits were excluded.

4.5. Patient Reported Outcomes and Compliance

4.5.1. Patient Reported Outcomes

In both initial and second visits patients completed the VFQ-25 (Table S3, Supplementary Material) developed by the National Eye Institute [51], which provides information about items grouped into 12 domains: near vision, difficulty distance vision, social functioning, role limitations due to vision, dependency on others due to vision, mental health symptoms due to vision, driving difficulties, peripheral vision, color vision and ocular pain. Additionally, the VFQ-25 contains a single general health rating question and a single question about global vision. The questionnaire was completed by all patients aged

11 years or older, and those patients who could not complete it themselves received help from companions and research team. The VFQ scale score was established considering that each item has a score range from 0 to 100. A high score indicates excellent functionality and well-being. The overall score was defined by establishing the average per domain and subsequently the scores obtained in each domain were averaged.

Response to treatment perceived by the patient was evaluated using a VAS of symptoms (burning, discharge, tearing, foreign body sensation, pain, photophobia) (Table S4, Supplementary Material) performed at the initial visit (when treated with TE) and at the follow-up visit (when treated with TCD). Patients rated the intensity of these symptoms from 0 to 10 (highest degree of intensity) [52].

4.5.2. Compliance

The level of compliance to treatment was performed at the initial visit (regarding to TE) and three months after the beginning of TCD. Subjective adherence was evaluated through a VAS of adherence questionnaire (Table S5, Supplementary Material) scored from 0 (not adherent) to 10 (fully adherent) [53].

Objective adherence to TCD eye drops was determined by the difference in weight between the bottles before and after use. Patients were instructed at visit 1 to store two containers of used TCD eye drops to return them to the HPD for adherence analysis. Before dispensing to the patient and after use, the two containers of TCD were weighed. In parallel, the theoretical amount used by the patient was calculated based on the dosing regimen and the average weight per drop (0.0444 mg/drop). Finally, the difference between theoretical and actual use was calculated. A margin of error of 35% was assumed to account for the possibility of accidental loss of eye drops.

4.6. Statistical Analysis

The results of the different assays were plotted using Graph Pad Prism® v.9.0.1 software (GraphPad Software, San Diego, CA, USA) and IBM Corp. Released 2021. IBM SPSS Statistics for Windows, Version 28.0. Armonk, NY, USA: IBM Corp. To evaluate the normality of the data, the Kolmogorov Smirnov test was used. To carry out the significance analysis of the data obtained, the Wilcoxon test was performed. Spearman rank correlation was also used to characterize the relationship between two variables. p values < 0.05 were considered statistically significant.

5. Conclusions

The use of cyclodextrins as an excipient of ocular pharmaceutical compounds is a promising alternative to solubilize lipophilic active principles and eliminate irritating excipients, such as those used in the preparation of the ophthalmic tacrolimus compounded formulation. The administration of TCD eye drops for a period of three months resulted in the maintenance of stable ocular clinical signs, tear stability and intraocular pressure. Furthermore, the patient-reported damage was also favorable, particularly in terms of pain and burning. Decreasing the concentration of tacrolimus in our formulation may be a appropriate alternative to reduce the dose of immunosuppression, allowing to mitigate the mutagenic risk of the drug in long-term use. Further studies with larger populations and longer study periods are needed to confirm these findings.

Supplementary Materials: The following supporting information can be downloaded at: https://www.mdpi.com/article/10.3390/ijms25189847/s1.

Author Contributions: Conceptualization, L.G.-Q., X.G.-O., M.G.-B. and A.F.-F.; methodology, L.G.-Q., X.G.-O. and A.C.-B.; software, M.P.-I., A.C.-M. and A.F.-F.; validation, R.T.-P., M.T.R.-A., M.J.G. and E.Y.-P.; formal analysis, M.P.-I. and A.C.-M.; investigation, M.P.-I., A.C.-M., R.T.-P. and M.T.R.-A.; resources, M.J.G., E.Y.-P., I.Z.-F. and F.J.O.-E.; data curation, M.P.-I. and A.C.-M.; writing—original draft preparation, M.P.-I. and A.C.-M.; writing—review and editing, L.G.-Q., M.G.-B. and A.C.-B.; visualization, M.T.R.-A., M.J.G. and M.G.-B.; supervision, R.T.-P., M.T.R.-A., X.G.-O. and A.C.-B.;

project administration, M.J.G., E.Y.-P., I.Z.-F., F.J.O.-E., A.F.-F. and A.C.-B.; funding acquisition, I.Z.-F., F.J.O.-E., A.F.-F. and A.C.-B. All authors have read and agreed to the published version of the manuscript.

Funding: This research was funded by Fundación Española de Farmacia Hospitalaria (FEFH), grant number Ayudas Investigación FEFH 2021-2022 (FEFH2021). This work was supported by Xunta de Galicia (GAIN) IN607A2023/04.

Institutional Review Board Statement: The study was conducted in accordance with the Declaration of Helsinki and approved by Institutional Review Board/Ethics Committee of the Ethical Committee of Clinical Research of Galicia (AFF-FOR-2019-01, 2019/204).

Informed Consent Statement: Informed consent was obtained from all subjects involved in the study.

Data Availability Statement: Data are contained within the article and Supplementary Materials.

Acknowledgments: The authors would like to thank the collaboration in the study of researchers associated with FarmaCHUSLab, Antonio Cañizo-Outeiriño, Diana Carolina Castro-Fernández and Olga Tellería-Barcia, and the team associated with the Faculty of Optics and Optometry of the University of Santiago de Compostela, Hugo Pena-Verdeal and Jacobo García-Queiruga.

Conflicts of Interest: The authors declare no conflicts of interest.

References

1. Kino, T.; Hatanaka, H.; Hashimoto, M.; Nishiyama, M.; Goto, T.; Okuhara, M.; Kohsaka, M.; Aoki, H.; Imanaka, H. FK-506, a Novel Immunosuppressant Isolated from a Streptomyces. I. Fermentation, Isolation, and Physico-Chemical and Biological Characteristics. *J. Antibiot.* **1987**, *40*, 1249–1255. [CrossRef]
2. Hernandez, T.D.; Aleman, S.J.; Bao-Loc-Trung, M.; Forte, M.V.; Brandt, W.; Armstrong, C.; Howard, J.; Mosieri, C.N.; Ahmadzadeh, S.; Varrassi, G.; et al. Advancing Treatment in Atopic Dermatitis: A Comprehensive Review of Clinical Efficacy, Safety, and Comparative Insights Into Corticosteroids, Calcineurin Inhibitors, and Phosphodiesterase-4 Inhibitors as Topical Therapies. *Cureus* **2024**, *16*, e55393. [CrossRef] [PubMed]
3. Zhao, M.; Huang, F.; Tang, L.; Zhou, X.; Zhang, M.; Liao, M.; Liu, L.; Huang, M. Case Report: Successful Treatment of Acute Generalized Pustular Psoriasis with Multiple Comorbidities with Oral Tacrolimus. *Front. Immunol.* **2024**, *15*, 1354578. [CrossRef]
4. Bernardes, L.; Costa, E.; Tavares, C.; Rosa, A.; Quadrado, M.; Murta, J. Topical Tacrolimus in High-Risk Corneal Transplants. *Eur. J. Ophthalmol.* **2023**, *34*, 140–145. [CrossRef] [PubMed]
5. Erdinest, N.; Noyman, D.B.E.; London, N.; Lavy, I.; Levinger, N.; Landau, D.; Solomon, A.; Morad, Y.; Naroo, S.A. Applications of Topical Immunomodulators Enhance Clinical Signs of Vernal Keratoconjunctivitis (VKC) and Atopic Keratoconjunctivitis (AKC): A Meta-Analysis. *Int. Ophthalmol.* **2024**, *44*, 157. [CrossRef] [PubMed]
6. Yazu, H.; Fukagawa, K.; Shimizu, E.; Sato, Y.; Fujishima, H. Long-Term Outcomes of 0.1% Tacrolimus Eye Drops in Eyes with Severe Allergic Conjunctival Diseases. *Allergy Asthma Clin. Immunol. Off. J. Can. Soc. Allergy Clin. Immunol.* **2021**, *17*, 11. [CrossRef] [PubMed]
7. Leonardi, A.; Silva, D.; Perez Formigo, D.; Bozkurt, B.; Sharma, V.; Allegri, P.; Rondon, C.; Calder, V.; Ryan, D.; Kowalski, M.L.; et al. Management of Ocular Allergy. *Allergy* **2019**, *74*, 1611–1630. [CrossRef] [PubMed]
8. Mazet, R.; Yaméogo, J.B.G.; Wouessidjewe, D.; Choisnard, L.; Gèze, A. Recent Advances in the Design of Topical Ophthalmic Delivery Systems in the Treatment of Ocular Surface Inflammation and Their Biopharmaceutical Evaluation. *Pharmaceutics* **2020**, *12*, 570. [CrossRef]
9. Prajapati, M.; Eiriksson, F.F.; Loftsson, T. Stability Characterization, Kinetics and Mechanism of Tacrolimus Degradation in Cyclodextrin Solutions. *Int. J. Pharm.* **2020**, *586*, 119579. [CrossRef]
10. Agencia Española de Medicamentos y Productos Sanitarios (AEMPS). Ficha Técnica Prograf 5 mg/mL Concentrado Para Solución Para Perfusión. Available online: https://cima.aemps.es/cima/dochtml/ft/61004/FT_61004.html (accessed on 1 April 2024).
11. Luaces-Rodríguez, A.; Touriño-Peralba, R.; Alonso-Rodríguez, I.; García-Otero, X.; González-Barcia, M.; Rodríguez-Ares, M.T.; Martínez-Pérez, L.; Aguiar, P.; Gómez-Lado, N.; Silva-Rodríguez, J.; et al. Preclinical Characterization and Clinical Evaluation of Tacrolimus Eye Drops. *Eur. J. Pharm. Sci. Off. J. Eur. Fed. Pharm. Sci.* **2018**, *120*, 152–161. [CrossRef]
12. Oh, J.Y.; Yu, J.M.; Ko, J.H. Analysis of Ethanol Effects on Corneal Epithelium. *Investig. Opthalmology Vis. Sci.* **2013**, *54*, 3852–3856. [CrossRef] [PubMed]
13. Zeng, W.; Li, Q.; Wan, T.; Liu, C.; Pan, W.; Wu, Z.; Zhang, G.; Pan, J.; Qin, M.; Lin, Y.; et al. Hyaluronic Acid-Coated Niosomes Facilitate Tacrolimus Ocular Delivery: Mucoadhesion, Precorneal Retention, Aqueous Humor Pharmacokinetics, and Transcorneal Permeability. *Colloids Surf. B Biointerfaces* **2016**, *141*, 28–35. [CrossRef] [PubMed]
14. Wang, Y.; Wang, C.; Fu, S.; Liu, Q.; Dou, D.; Lv, H.; Fan, M.; Guo, G.; Luo, F.; Qian, Z. Preparation of Tacrolimus Loaded Micelles Based on Poly(ε-Caprolactone)–Poly(Ethylene Glycol)–Poly(ε-Caprolactone). *Int. J. Pharm.* **2011**, *407*, 184–189. [CrossRef] [PubMed]

15. Janicki, J.; Chancellor, M.; Kaufman, J.; Gruber, M.; Chancellor, D. Potential Effect of Liposomes and Liposome-Encapsulated Botulinum Toxin and Tacrolimus in the Treatment of Bladder Dysfunction. *Toxins* **2016**, *8*, 81. [CrossRef]
16. García-Otero, X.; Díaz-Tomé, V.; Varela-Fernández, R.; Martín-Pastor, M.; González-Barcia, M.; Blanco-Méndez, J.; Mondelo-García, C.; Bermudez, M.A.; Gonzalez, F.; Aguiar, P.; et al. Development and Characterization of a Tacrolimus/Hydroxypropyl-β-Cyclodextrin Eye Drop. *Pharmaceutics* **2021**, *13*, 149. [CrossRef]
17. EMA European Medicines Agency. Questions and Answers on Cyclodextrins Used as Excipients in Medicinal Products for Human Use. Available online: https://www.ema.europa.eu/en/cyclodextrins (accessed on 26 October 2023).
18. García-Otero, X.; Mondelo-García, C.; González, F.; Perez-Fernandez, R.; Avila, L.; Antúnez-López, J.R.; González-Barcia, M.; Adan, A.; Aguiar, P.; Otero-Espinar, F.J.; et al. Anti-Inflammatory Effect of Tacrolimus/Hydroxypropyl-β-Cyclodextrin Eye Drops in an Endotoxin-Induced Uveitis Model. *Pharmaceutics* **2021**, *13*, 1737. [CrossRef]
19. Sella, R.; Cohen-Tayar, Y.; Noguchi, T.; Finburgh, E.N.; Lian, R.R.; Abbas, A.A.; Hakim, D.F.; Bu, J.J.; Zhao, J.; Shaw, P.; et al. The Effect of Anti-Inflammatory Topical Ophthalmic Treatments on In Vitro Corneal Epithelial Cells. *Transl. Vis. Sci. Technol.* **2022**, *11*, 16. [CrossRef]
20. Kwitko, S.; Marafon, S.B.; Simao, M.F.; Giacomini, F.; Marinho, D.R. Conjunctival Melanoma Following Cornea Transplant from a Cancer Donor: A Case Report. *Am. J. Ophthalmol. Case Rep.* **2023**, *29*, 101809. [CrossRef]
21. Sanz-Marco, E.; Udaondo, P.; García-Delpech, S.; Vazquez, A.; Diaz-Llopis, M. Treatment of Refractory Dry Eye Associated with Graft versus Host Disease with 0.03% Tacrolimus Eyedrops. *J. Ocul. Pharmacol. Ther. Off. J. Assoc. Ocul. Pharmacol. Ther.* **2013**, *29*, 776–783. [CrossRef]
22. Moscovici, B.K.; Holzchuh, R.; Chiacchio, B.B.; Santo, R.M.; Shimazaki, J.; Hida, R.Y. Clinical Treatment of Dry Eye Using 0.03% Tacrolimus Eye Drops. *Cornea* **2012**, *31*, 945–949. [CrossRef]
23. Liu, S.W.; Zhao, Y.H.; Ma, J.; Shen, Z.; Hu, B.H.; Peng, R.M.; Hong, J. [Efficacy evaluation of 0.05% cyclosporine A and 0.1% tacrolimus eye drops in the treatment of severe dry eye associated with chronic graft-versus-host disease]. *Zhonghua Yan Ke Za Zhi Chin. J. Ophthalmol.* **2023**, *59*, 805–813. [CrossRef]
24. Albarry, M.A.; Parekh, M.; Ferrari, S.; Eltahir, H.M.; Shehata, A.M.; Shaker, M.A.; Elbadawy, H.M. Incremental Concentrations of Tacrolimus Eye Drops as a Strategy for the Management of Severe Vernal Keratoconjunctivitis. *Front. Pharmacol.* **2022**, *13*, 798998. [CrossRef] [PubMed]
25. Eltagoury, M.; Abou Samra, W.; Ghoneim, E. Safety and Efficacy of Topical Tacrolimus 0.03% in the Management of Vernal Keratoconjunctivitis: A Non-Randomized Controlled Clinical Trial. *Med. Hypothesis Discov. Innov. Ophthalmol. J.* **2022**, *11*, 52–63. [CrossRef] [PubMed]
26. Miyazaki, D.; Fukushima, A.; Ohashi, Y.; Ebihara, N.; Uchio, E.; Okamoto, S.; Shoji, J.; Takamura, E.; Nakagawa, Y.; Namba, K.; et al. Steroid-Sparing Effect of 0.1% Tacrolimus Eye Drop for Treatment of Shield Ulcer and Corneal Epitheliopathy in Refractory Allergic Ocular Diseases. *Ophthalmology* **2017**, *124*, 287–294. [CrossRef]
27. Moawad, P.; Shamma, R.; Hassanein, D.; Ragab, G.; El Zawahry, O. Evaluation of the Effect of Topical Tacrolimus 0.03% versus Cyclosporine 0.05% in the Treatment of Dry Eye Secondary to Sjogren Syndrome. *Eur. J. Ophthalmol.* **2022**, *32*, 673–679. [CrossRef]
28. Ghaffari, R.; Ghassemi, H.; Zarei-Ghanavati, M.; Latifi, G.; Dehghani, S.; Haq, Z.; Djalilian, A.R. Tacrolimus Eye Drops as Adjunct Therapy in Severe Corneal Endothelial Rejection Refractory to Corticosteroids. *Cornea* **2017**, *36*, 1195–1199. [CrossRef]
29. Li, X.; Zhang, Y.N.; Yin, M.Y.; Pan, Z.Q. [The effectiveness and safety of topical 0.1% tacrolimus after high-risk penetrating keratoplasty]. *Zhonghua Yan Ke Za Zhi Chin. J. Ophthalmol.* **2019**, *55*, 419–427. [CrossRef]
30. Shoughy, S.S.; Tabbara, K.F. Topical Tacrolimus in Thygeson Superficial Punctate Keratitis. *Cornea* **2020**, *39*, 742–744. [CrossRef]
31. Akbari, M.; Soltani Moghadam, R.; Elmi, R.; Nosrati, A.; Taghiabadi, E.; Aghdami, N. Topical Tacrolimus as an Adjunct to Conventional Therapy for Stromal Herpetic Keratitis: A Randomized Clinical Trial. *J. Ophthalmic Vis. Res.* **2019**, *14*, 400–411. [CrossRef]
32. Naël, V.; Moreau, G.; Monfermé, S.; Cougnard-Grégoire, A.; Scherlen, A.-C.; Arleo, A.; Korobelnik, J.-F.; Delcourt, C.; Helmer, C. Prevalence and Associated Factors of Uncorrected Refractive Error in Older Adults in a Population-Based Study in France. *JAMA Ophthalmol.* **2019**, *137*, 3–11. [CrossRef]
33. Castellsague, J.; Kuiper, J.G.; Pottegård, A.; Anveden Berglind, I.; Dedman, D.; Gutierrez, L.; Calingaert, B.; Van Herk Sukel, M.P.; Hallas, J.; Sundström, A.; et al. A Cohort Study on the Risk of Lymphoma and Skin Cancer in Users of Topical Tacrolimus, Pimecrolimus, and Corticosteroids (Joint European Longitudinal Lymphoma and Skin Cancer Evaluation – JOELLE Study). *Clin. Epidemiol.* **2018**, *10*, 299–310. [CrossRef] [PubMed]
34. Kheirkhah, A.; Zavareh, M.K.; Farzbod, F.; Mahbod, M.; Behrouz, M.J. Topical 0.005% Tacrolimus Eye Drop for Refractory Vernal Keratoconjunctivitis. *Eye* **2011**, *25*, 872–880. [CrossRef] [PubMed]
35. Díaz-Tomé, V.; Luaces-Rodríguez, A.; Silva-Rodríguez, J.; Blanco-Dorado, S.; García-Quintanilla, L.; Llovo-Taboada, J.; Blanco-Méndez, J.; García-Otero, X.; Varela-Fernández, R.; Herranz, M.; et al. Ophthalmic Econazole Hydrogels for the Treatment of Fungal Keratitis. *J. Pharm. Sci.* **2018**, *107*, 1342–1351. [CrossRef]
36. Puskás, I.; Szente, L.; Szőcs, L.; Fenyvesi, É. Recent List of Cyclodextrin-Containing Drug Products. *Period. Polytech. Chem. Eng.* **2023**, *67*, 11–17. [CrossRef]
37. Palem, C.R.; Chopparapu, K.S.C.; Subrahmanyam, P.V.R.S.; Yamsani, M.R. Cyclodextrins and Their Derivatives in Drug Delivery: A Review. *Curr. Trends Biotechnol. Pharm.* **2012**, *6*, 255–279; ISSN 0973-8916.

38. McCulley, J.P.; Shine, W.E. The Lipid Layer: The Outer Surface of the Ocular Surface Tear Film. *Biosci. Rep.* **2001**, *21*, 407–418. [CrossRef] [PubMed]
39. Suzuki, M.; Massingale, M.L.; Ye, F.; Godbold, J.; Elfassy, T.; Vallabhajosyula, M.; Asbell, P.A. Tear Osmolarity as a Biomarker for Dry Eye Disease Severity. *Investig. Opthalmology Vis. Sci.* **2010**, *51*, 4557–4561. [CrossRef]
40. Bron, A.J.; de Paiva, C.S.; Chauhan, S.K.; Bonini, S.; Gabison, E.E.; Jain, S.; Knop, E.; Markoulli, M.; Ogawa, Y.; Perez, V.; et al. TFOS DEWS II Pathophysiology Report. *Ocul. Surf.* **2017**, *15*, 438–510. [CrossRef]
41. Ishioka, M.; Kato, N.; Takano, Y.; Shimazaki, J.; Tsubota, K. The Quantitative Detection of Blurring of Vision after Eyedrop Instillation Using a Functional Visual Acuity System. *Acta Ophthalmol.* **2009**, *87*, 574–575. [CrossRef]
42. Fini, M.E.; Schwartz, S.G.; Gao, X.; Jeong, S.; Patel, N.; Itakura, T.; Price, M.O.; Price, F.W.; Varma, R.; Stamer, W.D. Steroid-Induced Ocular Hypertension/Glaucoma: Focus on Pharmacogenomics and Implications for Precision Medicine. *Prog. Retin. Eye Res.* **2017**, *56*, 58–83. [CrossRef]
43. Senthil, S.; Thakur, M.; Rao, H.L.; Mohamed, A.; Jonnadula, G.B.; Sangwan, V.; Garudadri, C.S. Steroid-Induced Glaucoma and Blindness in Vernal Keratoconjunctivitis. *Br. J. Ophthalmol.* **2020**, *104*, 265–269. [CrossRef] [PubMed]
44. Miyazaki, D.; Tominaga, T.; Kakimaru-Hasegawa, A.; Nagata, Y.; Hasegawa, J.; Inoue, Y. Therapeutic Effects of Tacrolimus Ointment for Refractory Ocular Surface Inflammatory Diseases. *Ophthalmology* **2008**, *115*, 988–992. [CrossRef] [PubMed]
45. Magalhaes, O.A.; Marinho, D.R.; Kwitko, S. Topical 0.03% Tacrolimus Preventing Rejection in High-Risk Corneal Transplantation: A Cohort Study. *Br. J. Ophthalmol.* **2013**, *97*, 1395–1398. [CrossRef]
46. Javidi, H.; Poonit, N.; Patel, R.P.; Barry, R.J.; Rauz, S.; Murray, P.I. Adherence to Topical Medication in Patients with Inflammatory Eye Disease. *Ocul. Immunol. Inflamm.* **2021**, *29*, 890–895. [CrossRef]
47. Nguyen, T.-M.-U.; Caze, A.L.; Cottrell, N. What Are Validated Self-Report Adherence Scales Really Measuring?: A Systematic Review: Systematic Review on Validated Medication Adherence Measurement Scales. *Br. J. Clin. Pharmacol.* **2014**, *77*, 427–445. [CrossRef]
48. Holladay, J.T. Proper Method for Calculating Average Visual Acuity. *J. Refract. Surg.* **1997**, *13*, 388–391. [CrossRef]
49. Figueroa-Ortiz, L.C.; Rodríguez, E.; García-Ben, A.; García-Campos, J. Estudio de La Función Lagrimal y La Superficie Conjuntival En Pacientes Diabéticos. *Arch. Soc. Esp. Oftalmol.* **2011**, *86*, 107–112. [CrossRef]
50. Castro-Balado, A.; Cuartero-Martínez, A.; Pena-Verdeal, H.; Hermelo-Vidal, G.; Schmidt, A.; Montero, B.; Hernández-Blanco, M.; Zarra-Ferro, I.; González-Barcia, M.; Mondelo-García, C.; et al. Cysteamine Eye Drops in Hyaluronic Acid Packaged in Innovative Single-Dose Systems, Part II: Long-Term Stability and Clinical Ocular Biopermanence. *Pharmaceutics* **2023**, *15*, 2589. [CrossRef] [PubMed]
51. Mangione, C.M.; Lee, P.P.; Gutierrez, P.R.; Spritzer, K.; Berry, S.; Hays, R.D. National Eye Institute Visual Function Questionnaire Field Test Investigators Development of the 25-Item National Eye Institute Visual Function Questionnaire. *Arch. Ophthalmol.* **2001**, *119*, 1050–1058. [CrossRef]
52. Klimek, L.; Bergmann, K.-C.; Biedermann, T.; Bousquet, J.; Hellings, P.; Jung, K.; Merk, H.; Olze, H.; Schlenter, W.; Stock, P.; et al. Visual Analogue Scales (VAS): Measuring Instruments for the Documentation of Symptoms and Therapy Monitoring in Cases of Allergic Rhinitis in Everyday Health Care: Position Paper of the German Society of Allergology (AeDA) and the German Society of Allergy and Clinical Immunology (DGAKI), ENT Section, in Collaboration with the Working Group on Clinical Immunology, Allergology and Environmental Medicine of the German Society of Otorhinolaryngology, Head and Neck Surgery (DGHNOKHC). *Allergo J. Int.* **2017**, *26*, 16–24. [CrossRef]
53. ADHEFAR. Grupo de Trabajo Sobre Adherencia Recursos. EVA—Escala Analógica Visual de Adherencia. Available online: https://gruposdetrabajo.sefh.es/adhefar/infografias-que-sabes-sobre-adherencia/25-recursos (accessed on 9 September 2024).

International Journal of
Molecular Sciences

MDPI

Article

Exosomes from *Limosilactobacillus fermentum* Ameliorate Benzalkonium Chloride-Induced Inflammation in Conjunctival Cells

Kippeum Lee, Hyeonjun Gwon, Joo Yun Kim *, Jae Jung Shim and Jae Hwan Lee

R&BD Center, Hy Co., Ltd., 22 Giheungdanji-ro 24 Beon-gil, Giheung-gu, Yongin-si 17086, Republic of Korea; joy4917@hanmail.net (K.L.); hjgwon@hy.co.kr (H.G.); jjshim@hy.co.kr (J.J.S.); jaehwan@hy.co.kr (J.H.L.)
* Correspondence: monera@hy.co.kr

Abstract: Dry eye is characterized by persistent instability and decreased tear production, which are accompanied by epithelial lesions and inflammation on the surface of the eye. In our previous paper, we reported that supplementation with *Limosilactobacillus fermentum* HY7302 (HY7302) could inhibit corneal damage in a benzalkonium chloride (BAC)-induced mouse model of dry eye, through its effects in gut microbiome regulation. The aim of this study was to determine what functional extracellular substances can alter the inflammatory response of conjunctival cells. We isolated exosomes from HY7302 probiotic culture supernatant, analyzed their morphological characteristics, and found that their average size was 143.8 ± 1.1 nm, which was smaller than the exosomes from the *L. fermentum* KCTC 3112 strain. In addition, HY7302-derived exosomes significantly reduced the levels of genes encoding pro-inflammatory cytokines, including *interleukin (IL)-20*, *IL-8*, *IL-6*, and *IL-1B*, in BAC-treated human conjunctival cells. Moreover, HY7302-derived exosomes significantly increased the levels of genes encoding tight junction proteins, including *TJP1*, *TJP2*, and *occludin-1*, in Caco-2 cells. Lastly, the HY7302 exosomes reduced mRNA expression levels of *IL1B*, *IL20*, *IL6*, *IL8*, and *NFAT5* in a transwell coculture system. Our findings indicate that HY7302 exosomes have potential for use in the treatment of ocular inflammation-related dry eye disease, through gut–eye axis communication via exosomes.

Keywords: conjunctiva cell; exosomes; exosomes; ocular inflammation; *Limosilactobacillus fermentum* HY7302

1. Introduction

Dry eye disease (DED) is a multifactorial eye disorder characterized by symptoms of ocular dryness, dysfunctional tear production, somatosensory abnormalities, and ocular surface inflammation [1,2]. DED, also known as keratoconjunctivitis sicca, is a persistent issue that can compromise eye health and quality of life [3,4] The worldwide prevalence of DED ranges from 5% to 50%, and the condition impacts life quality, vision, ocular function, and work productivity, as well as causing considerable pain [5,6]. DED can be caused by various environmental factors, including dry and windy conditions, air pollution, and exposure to digital screens for extended periods, which contribute to the accelerated evaporation of tears [7,8]. These environmental factors cause changes in the conjunctiva and ocular surfaces, which disrupt the tear film, leading to dryness and epithelial stress [9]. DED can be a natural part of the aging process, or attributable to various health conditions, such as chronic disease, diabetes, and long-term wearing of contact lenses or exposure to preservatives contained in artificial tear drops, such as benzalkonium chloride (BAC) [10,11]. In particular, since the effect of artificial tear drops and their side effects is only temporary, various alternative approaches to ameliorate the symptoms of dry eyes through dietary adjustment have been attempted [12]. For example, foods rich in omega-3 fatty acids, such as fish, flaxseed, and walnuts, can help improve tear production and relieve DED symptoms [13–15].

DED often results in an inflammatory reaction accompanied by pink eye, which is usually caused by an inflammatory response of the conjunctiva, a transparent membrane between the eyelids and the eyeball [16]. Conjunctival inflammation often leads to conjunctival edema, which significantly disrupts the ocular surface. Moreover, persistent inflammatory stimulation of conjunctival tissue can activate adaptive immune responses, resulting in chronic inflammation [9,17]. Further, it is reported that production of the inflammatory cytokines, interleukin (IL)-1, IL-6, and IL-8, in the tear membrane is increased in patients with dry eyes [18,19]. However, despite investigation of the correlation between DED and inflammation for the past 40 years, the underlying cellular and molecular level mechanisms involved have yet to be fully elucidated [9].

Extracellular vesicles (EVs) are small membrane-bound compartments released by cells, including microbes, that have important roles in intracellular and intercellular communication [20,21]. Structurally, EVs are surrounded by phospholipid bilayer membranes, and can contain proteins, lipids, DNA, mRNA, and miRNA [22,23]. Although EVs were considered "cell dust" in the past, there is now strong evidence that nanoscale EVs have pivotal roles in inter-microbial communication, as well as host-to-bacteria interactions, by mediating the diffusion of signaling molecules [24,25]. EVs are mainly distinguished by their size, and can be further delineated by their composition and function [26]. Several studies have shown that EVs are divided into the three major types of apoptotic bodies, microvesicles, and exosomes [22]. These EV subclassifications are distinguished by their size or biosynthetic characteristics, but ultimately lead to confusion in nomenclature, duplication, and confusion [27]. In particular, EVs of 30–160 nm, derived from a specific intracellular biosynthesis process, are referred to as exosomes [28,29]. The importance and biomedical effects of exosomes are established and widely described in the literature [27,30]. There is a growing appreciation of the functional importance of gut microbiota in health and disease, and the roles of microorganism-derived exosomes in tissue-to-tissue communication, horizontal gene transfer, the distribution of nutrients among communities, and inflammatory control have become the focus of considerable research attention [20,31]. In addition, exosomes secreted by non-pathogenic microorganisms, including probiotics, are reported to have various health promoting effects, for example, in skin care and aging prevention, inflammation, cardiovascular disease, and cancer [32–34]. Therefore, exosomes are rapidly becoming recognized as promising treatment platforms [35].

Probiotics are living microorganisms which, when ingested, can improve or restore physiological intestinal microbial composition, thereby providing health benefits [36,37]. Probiotics are mainly Gram-positive bacteria, including various species of the genera, *Lactobacillus* and *Bifidobacterium* [38]. In particular, lactic acid bacteria (LAB) are generally distributed as natural microbiota in various fermented foods, such as kimchi, as well as dairy products, beverages, meats, wine, fruits, and plants [39,40]. LAB can have several health benefits, along with nutritional advantages, including reduction in body fat and cholesterol, prevention and control of infections, and control of certain cancers, among other conditions [41,42]. *Limosilactobacillus fermentum* is an important LAB with probiotic properties [43], and is commonly recognized as a safe bacterium, and thus used to trigger food fermentation. Further, *L. fermentum* offers technological advantages, such as enhancing the flavor and texture of food products, as well as having probiotic benefits, including anti-infection and anti-inflammatory properties [44]. In our previous study, we found that *L. fermentum* HY7302 (HY7302; 1×10^9 colony forming units (CFU)/kg/day) significantly suppressed the corneal fluorescence score (CFS), as well as activating tear production and tear break time (TBUT) in Balb/c mice with BAC-induced corneal damage [45]. In addition, HY7302 increased microbiota beta diversity and altered the microbiome composition in dry eye model mice [46]; however, the underlying effects of HY7302 on ocular health remains unclear. In this study, we explored the effects of HY7302 exosomes on human conjunctiva cells. The aim of the present study was to explore whether exosomes isolated from HY7302 can improve BAC-induced inflammation in the human conjunctival cell line, clone 1-5c-4.

2. Results

2.1. Isolation of Exosomes from HY7302

In this study, the exosomes were isolated from HY7302 culture supernatant using a standard optimized high-speed centrifugation method (Figure 1A) [47], and their morphological properties were analyzed by electron microscopy. As shown in Figure 1B, HY7302 exosomes were spheroid, measured approximately 50–150 nm, and exhibited a central depression, which is a characteristic of exosomes. In addition, although the internal structure and cargo of the exosomes could not be detected, the fact that they were formed of lipid bilayers supported the inference that these particles were exosomes.

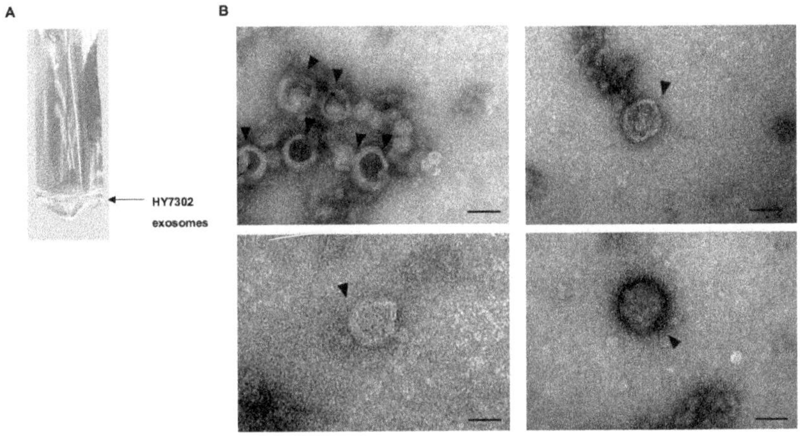

Figure 1. Images showing the morphology of exosomes from *Limosilactobacillus fermentum* HY7302 (HY7302). (**A**) HY7302 exosomes isolated by high-speed centrifugation. (**B**) Negative staining transmission electron microscopy images of exosomes isolated from *L. fermentum* HY7302. Scale bar, 50 nm. Arrowheads, exosomes.

2.2. Physiological Properties of Exosomes Isolated from HY7302

To investigate the size distribution of exosomes, including exosomes isolated from HY7302 and *L. fermentum* Korean Collection for Type Cultures (KCTC) strain 3112 (KCTC3112), we conducted nanoparticle tracking analysis (NTA) (Figure 2). Exosome suspension samples from HY7302 contained $3.32 \pm 0.35 \times 10^{11}$ particles/mL, with a size range of 89–231 nm, while those from KCTC contained $2.90 \pm 0.32 \times 10^{10}$ particles/mL, and ranged in size from 100 to 231 nm. Mean HY7302 exosome size was 143.8 ± 1.1 nm, while that of KCTC3112 exosomes was 151.2 ± 5.8 nm. These data suggest that exosomes isolated from the same *L. fermentum* species by high-speed centrifugation may differ in mean size, distribution, and concentration. We also quantified exosome yield using a pseudo-Lowry assay method, which is an indirect quantification technique used to infer the concentration of exosomes based on exosome membrane proteins. The protein concentration of HY7302 exosomes was 21.37 μg/μL, while that of KCTC3112 exosomes was 6.51 μg/μL suggesting that the HY7302 exosomes can effectively and stably produce exosomes at a high concentration.

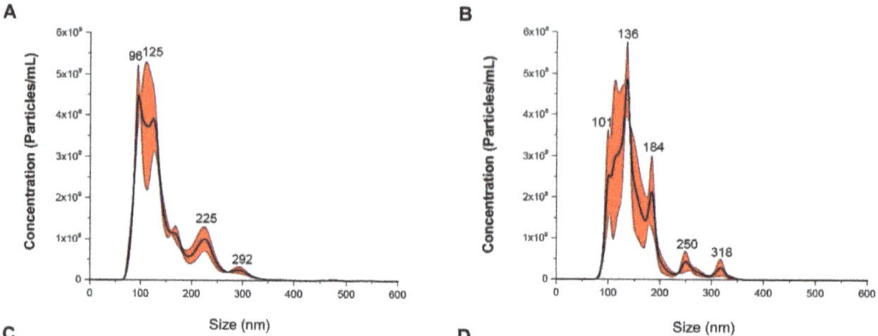

C

Results	Mean ± SD
Mean (nm)	143.8 ± 1.1
D10 (nm)	92.3 ± 2.8
D50 (nm)	125.3 ± 1.6
D90 (nm)	227.7 ± 3.6
Concentration (Particles/mL)	3.32 ± 0.35 X 10^{11}

D

Results	Mean ± SD
Mean (nm)	151.2 ± 5.8
D10 (nm)	106.4 ± 5.8
D50 (nm)	137.7 ± 3.7
D90 (nm)	210.2 ± 20.8
Concentration (Particles/mL)	2.90 ± 0.32 X 10^{10}

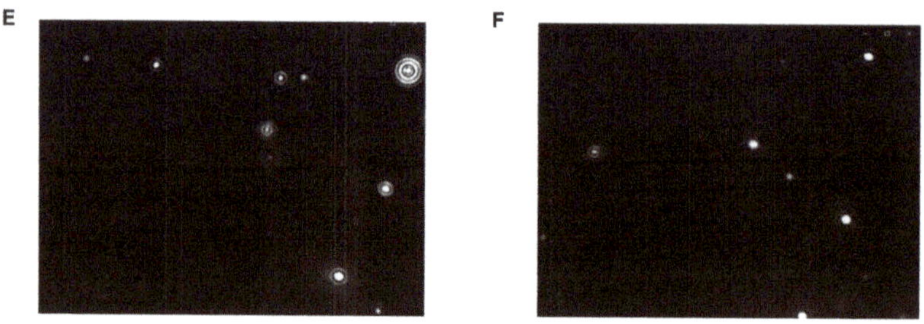

Figure 2. Characterization of exosomes from *Limosilactobacillus fermentum*. Nanoparticle tracking analysis of exosomes isolated from *L. fermentum* HY7302 (**A**) and KCTC3112 (**B**). Table box below show size distribution data obtained using a Malvern NanoSight NS300 and NanoSight NTA 3.4 Analytical software exosomes isolated from *L. fermentum* HY7302 (**C**) and KCTC3112 (**D**). Nanoparticle image of the isolated exosome from (**E**) HY7302 and (**F**) KCTC3112 were obtained using NTA analysis.

2.3. Cytotoxicity of Exosomes Isolated from HY7302

Cells from the human conjunctival line, clone 1-5c-4 (10^4/well), were treated with 0.01–5 μg/mL of HY7302 exosomes, followed by evaluation using lactate dehydrogenase (LDH) and 3-(4,5-dimethylthiazol-2-yl)-2,5-diphenyltetrazolium bromide (MTT) assays, to test for cytotoxicity. The results of the LDH assay showed no significant cytotoxicity of HY7302 exosomes up to 5 μg/mL, whereas MTT test data showed that HY7302 exosomes had no cytotoxicity up to 1 μg/mL (Figure 3A,B). We also examined the protective effect of HY7302 exosomes against BAC cytotoxicity, which induces dry eye in human conjunctiva cells. Cells were pre-treated with HY7302 exosomes (0.01–5 μg/mL) for 24 h and then treated with 0.0005% (*v*/*v*) BAC for 3 h. LHD test showed that BAC treatment increased cytotoxicity in human conjunctival cells to 37.03%, compared with 12.96% in control cells, while HY7302 exosomes significantly reduced this cytotoxicity in a concentration-dependent manner, with a reduction of 28.55% at 1 μg/mL relative to the BAC group (Figure 3C). Further, the MTT test data showed that BAC treatment dramatically decreased conjunctival cell viability from 100% to 19.67% (Figure 3D); however, cell viability slightly increased to 26.65% when cells were treated with HY7302 exosomes at 1 μg/mL.

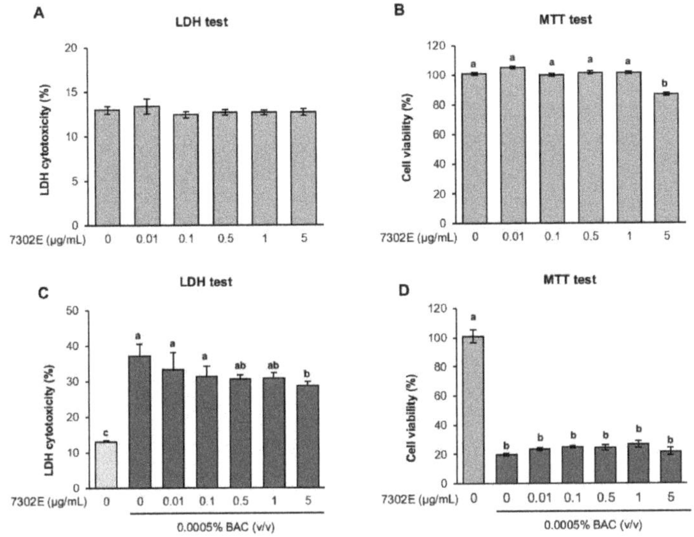

Figure 3. Effect of exosomes from *Limosilactobacillus fermentum* HY7302 (7302E) on cytotoxicity. (**A**,**C**) Lactate dehydrogenase (LDH) release cytotoxicity assay and (**B**,**D**) 3-(4,5-dimethylthiazol-2-yl)-2,5-diphenyltetrazolium bromide (MTT) test. Control cells or cells exposed to 0.0005% benzalkonium chloride (BAC) for 3 h were treated with *L. fermentum* HY7302 exosomes (7302E; 0, 0.01, 0.1, 0.5, 1.0, or 5.0 μg/10^4 cells). Data are expressed as mean ± standard deviation (SD) (n = 3). Different letters indicate significantly different values ($p < 0.05$) (a > ab > b > c).

2.4. Effects of Exosomes Isolated from HY7302 on Tight Junction Molecules

To assess the ability of HY7302 to modulate the gut–eye axis, we next evaluated the effect of HY7302 exosomes on regulation of intestinal tight junctions in differentiated human intestinal Caco-2 cells. Before investigating the effect of HY7302 exosomes, cells were treated with cell pellets and supernatants of 10^6 CFU/mL HY7302 cultured in de Man Rogosa and Sharpe (MRS) broth and the effects were compared with those of MRS broth alone, as a control. As shown in Figure 4A,B, quantitative real-time polymerase chain reaction (qRT-PCR) analysis indicated that treatment with HY7302 culture supernatant increased the expression of genes (*TJP1* and *occludin-1*) encoding two tight junction proteins higher than the response to MRS medium or HY7302 cell pellet. In cells treated with HY7302 supernatant, *TJP1* and *occludin-1* mRNA levels were significantly increased by 2.00-fold and 1.35-fold, respectively, while they were upregulated by 1.92-fold and 1.19-fold in Caco-2 cells treated with HY7302 cell pellets. Subsequently, we assessed whether HY7302 exosomes had regulatory effects on epithelial intestinal cells by treating confluent CaCo-2 cells with increasing concentrations of HY7302 exosomes (0.5–1 μg/mL HY7302 probiotics as a positive control. Levels of *TJP1* and *TJP2* mRNA were 1.14-fold higher in both HY7302 groups than those in the control group, and were significantly higher (by 1.19- and 1.15-fold, respectively) in the group treated with 1 μg/mL HY7302 exosomes. In addition, HY7302 exosome-treated cells exhibited dose-dependent upregulation of the expression of both genes. By contrast, a non-significant increase (1.16-fold) in levels of *OCLN* was detected following HY7302 treatment, while its expression was significantly increased by 1.45-fold after addition of HY7302 exosomes.

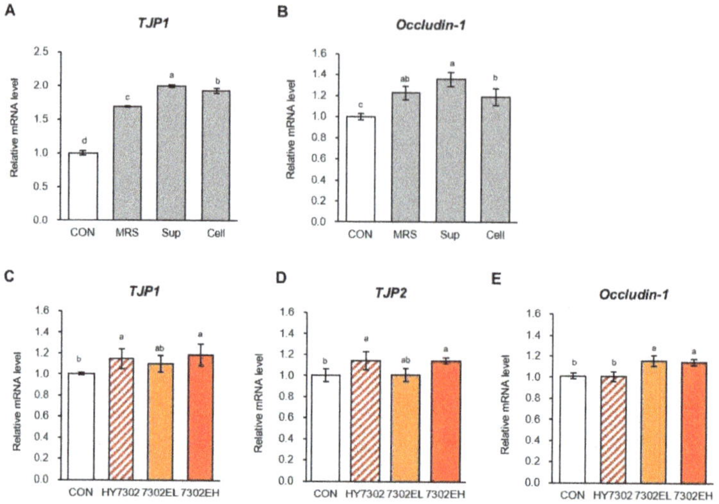

Figure 4. Effect of *Limosilactobacillus fermentum* HY7302 exosomes on tight junction molecules in Caco-2 cells. (**A**) Tight junction protein 1 (*TJP1*) and (**B**) occludin-1 were normalized to those of *GAPDH* and relative fold changes in their levels calculated. Levels of mRNA encoding (**C**) *TJP1*, (**D**) *TJP2*, and (**E**) occludin-1 were normalized to those of *GAPDH* and relative fold changes in their levels calculated. CON, control; HY7302, 10^6 CFU/mL HY7302; 7302EL, 0.5 μg/mL of HY7302 exosomes; 7302EH, 1 μg/mL of HY7302 exosomes. Data are expressed as mean ± standard deviation (SD) (n = 3). Different letters indicate significantly different values ($p < 0.05$) (a > ab > b > c > d).

2.5. Anti-Inflammatory Effect of Exosomes Isolated from HY7302

In a previous study, we found that the abundance of inflammatory cytokines increased significantly after treatment of human conjunctiva cell lines with 0.0005% (v/v) of the dry eye-inducing substance, BAC [45], while treatment with 10^6 or 10^7 CFU/mL HY7302 probiotics could inhibit these pro-inflammatory responses in conjunctival cells treated with BAC. In this study, to determine whether the exosomes isolated from HY7302 LAB had functional effects, we analyzed the anti-inflammatory efficacy of 1 μg of exosomes isolated from HY7302 probiotics and 10^6 CFU of HY7302 LAB. In addition, the effects of 1 μg exosomes isolated from 10^6 CFU KCTC3112 or HY7302 were compared with those of HY7302 probiotics. As illustrated in Figure 5, BAC treatment increased the expression of pro-inflammatory cytokine genes, including *IL20*, *IL1B*, and *IL6*, by 47.1, 11.2, and 46.3-fold, respectively, while levels of the inflammatory chemokine, *IL8*, increased by > 700-fold. Treatment of HY7302 probiotics to BAC-treated cells slightly decreased *IL8*, *IL20*, *IL1B*, and *IL6* mRNA levels by 0.83-, 0.79-, 0.37-, and 0.60-fold, respectively. However, treatment with HY7302 exosomes significantly reduced *IL8*, *IL20*, *IL1B*, and *IL6* mRNA levels by 0.66-, 0.60-, 0.25-, and 0.64-fold relative to BAC-only treated cells. Meanwhile, treatment with KCTC3112 reduced levels of the corresponding cytokines by 0.78-, 0.78-, 0.66-, and 0.61-fold, which was similar to the effects of HY7302 probiotics, except for the difference in the effect on IL1B. However, the levels of IL20 (0.95-fold) in cells treated with KCTC3112 exosomes and BAC did not differ significantly from those of cells treated with HY7302 exosomes. Meanwhile, KCTC3112 exosomes showed a significant difference from HY7302 exosomes, as there was no significant difference from the BAC treatment group for IL8 and IL6. Levels of nuclear factor of activated T cells 5 (*NFAT5*) and nuclear factor kappa-light-chain-enhancer of activated B cells (*NFKB1*) mRNAs, which encode proteins that stimulate the expression of various pro-inflammatory cytokines, were also investigated. *NFAT5* and *NFKB1* levels were significantly higher following BAC treatment, rising by 4.24- and

6.47-fold; meanwhile, among the treatments tested, only HY7302 exosomes significantly reduced their levels by 0.67- and 0.64-fold.

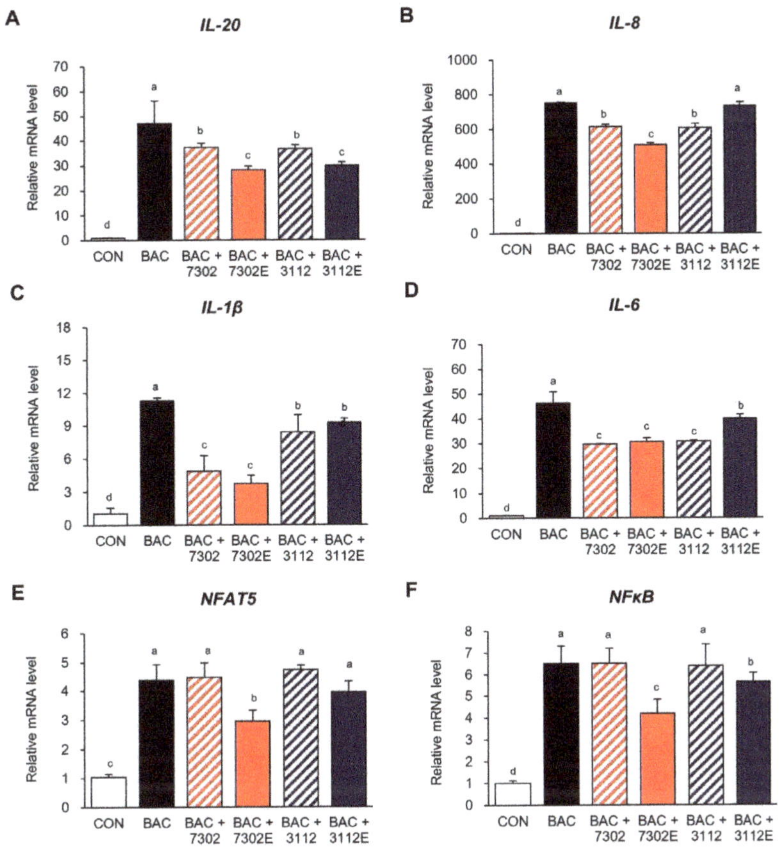

Figure 5. Effects of *Limosilactobacillus fermentum* HY7302 extracellular vesicles (7302E) on pro-inflammatory factors in conjunctival cell lines treated using 0.0005% BAC. Levels of (**A**) interleukin-20 (*IL20*), (**B**) *IL8*, (**C**) *IL1B*, (**D**) *IL6*, (**E**) nuclear factor of activated T cells 5 (*NFAT5*), and (**F**) nuclear factor kappa B subunit 1 (*NFKB1*) mRNA were normalized to those of *GAPDH* and calculated as relative fold-change values. CON, control; BAC, 0.0005% (v/v) BAC; 7302, 10^6 CFU/mL HY7302; 7302E, 1 μg/mL of HY7302 exosomes; 3112, 10^6 CFU/mL KCTC3112; 3112E, 1 μg/mL of KCTC3112 exosomes. Data are expressed as mean ± SD (n = 3). Different letters indicate significant differences ($p < 0.05$) (a > b > c > d).

2.6. Exosomes Isolated from HY7302 Are Taken Up by Conjunctival Cells in a Transwell System

Next, analysis was performed using transwell plates consisting of two culture chambers separated by porous membrane filters. We investigated whether exosomes isolated from HY7302 LAB acted as regulators of cell-to-cell communication. To determine whether the exosomes added to Caco-2 intestinal cells could migrate and affect the conjunctival cells, we used membrane filters with 0.4 μm pores. As shown in Figure 6A, exosomes were added to Caco-2 cell culture medium, and conjunctival cells were treated by incubation with 0.0005% BAC for the last 3 h of the experiment. Levels of mRNAs encoding the inflammatory cytokines, IL-1b, IL-20, IL-6, and *IL-8* were significantly higher (3.42-, 15.17-, 11.62-fold, and 51.66-fold, respectively) in the BAC-treated group than those in the control group. Low concentrations of HY7302 exosomes (0.5 μg/mL) only significantly reduced levels of *IL1B* mRNA (1.81-fold), but did not alter those of *IL6*, *IL20*, and *IL6*; however, levels of *IL1B*, *IL20*, *IL6*, and *IL8* mRNA were significantly lower following treatment with a high concentration of HY7302 exosomes (1 µg/mL) than those in BAC-treated cells (1.38-, 10.88-, 8.36-, and 25.79-fold, respectively). Treatment with 10^6 CFU/mL HY7302 probiotics as a control also led to significantly lower expression levels of *IL1B*, *IL6*, and *IL8* (1.86-, 9.76-, 30.54-fold, respectively), but not those of *IL20*. Finally, levels of the gene encoding NFAT5 in cells treated with HY7302 or both concentrations of HY7302 exosomes (0.5 and 1 µg/mL) were significantly lower than those in the BAC group, but did not differ significantly from one another. In summary, our data show that 1 µg/mL HY7302 exosomes could significantly attenuate BAC-induced pro-inflammatory cytokine expression in conjunctival cells, and were more effective than the HY7302 probiotic.

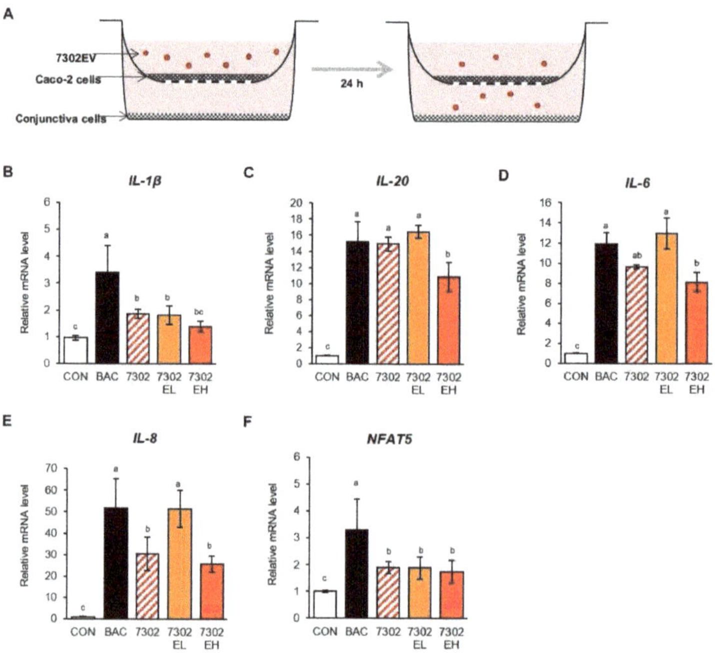

Figure 6. (**A**) Schematic of the experimental protocol to test the effect of exosomes of *Limosilactobacillus fermentum* HY7302 (7302E) on pro-inflammatory cytokines production. Clone 1-5c-4 cells were seeded in transwell plates and, once they reached confluence, exposed to Caco-2 cells. Caco-2 cells were co-cultured either with or without exosomes, using transwells, and culture medium samples of conjunctiva cell collected for analysis. Levels of (**B**) *IL1B*, (**C**) *IL20*, (**D**) *IL6*, (**E**) *IL8*, and (**F**) *NFAT5* mRNA in cells were normalized to those of *GAPDH* and relative fold-change values calculated. CON, control; BAC, 0.0005% (*v*/*v*) BAC; 7302, 10^6 CFU/mL HY7302; 7302E, 1 µg/mL of HY7302 exosomes; 3112, 10^6 CFU/mL KCTC3112; 3112E, 1 µg/mL of KCTC3112 exosomes. Data are expressed as mean ± SD (n = 3). Different letters indicate significant differences ($p < 0.05$) (a > ab > b > bc > c).

3. Discussion

Exosomes are biological extracellular EV that are naturally secreted by mammalian and plant cells [48], with diameters of 30–160 nm and densities of 1.1–1.2 g/mL [49]. Exosomes comprise a lipid bilayer structure enclosing small molecule components, such as proteins, nucleic acids, lipids, and secondary metabolites [50,51]. The release of these intracellular cargoes can induce physiological, phenotypic, and functional changes in recipient cells [28]. Interestingly, exosomes were previously considered to be a means of transport for removal of waste from cells [52]; however, it has since been established that they act as regulators of cell-to-cell communication through gene expression regulation, as well as by delivering biologically active substances [53].

Numerous studies have focused on exosomes as novel biomarkers or potential therapeutics [54,55]. For example, plant-derived exosomes can have protective effects in immunity against pathogen invasion [56]. In addition, microbial-derived exosomes can also act as natural antipathogens or food preservatives, as well as having anti-inflammation, anti-obesity, anti-alcoholic-related liver disease, and anti-gut barrier dysfunction effects [31,57,58]. *Bifidobacterium longum* NCC2705 releases numerous nanoparticles, made up of lipid bilayers, into the extracellular environment [59]. Further, *B. longum* AO44 secretes exosomes, which can promote intestinal bacterial immunomodulatory and anti-inflammatory effects on the host through IL-10 and IL-17 [60]. Additionally, exosomes from *Lactiplantibacillus plantarum* regulate skin aging by inhibiting wrinkle formation and pigmentation, and reduce mRNA expression levels of *MMP1*, an inflammatory factor [32]. Hence, various gut microbes have the potential to impact health in numerous ways, among which important mechanisms related to probiotic-induced therapeutic effects include communication to influence inflammation and the immune system [36,61]; however, the immunomodulatory molecules involved in this mode of symbiotic LAB–host communication remain largely unknown.

DED, or keratoconjunctivitis sicca, is a multifactorial ocular surface disease, characterized by decreased tear production [3]. Ocular inflammation is a critical factor in DED, which is accompanied by eye irritation, hyperemia, glare, eye fatigue, and blurred vision [2,62]. Inflammation of the ocular epithelial cells induces these complications through a cascade of increased cytokines [63]. Traditionally, lubricating eye drops and ointments have been used to treat dry eye, as well as topical anti-inflammatory therapies; however, common ocular anti-inflammatory drugs, such as corticosteroid eye drops or cyclosporine, have various side effects in patients with dry eye, making them generally difficult to use [64,65]. Therefore, research on functional health foods, with the aim of identifying novel, safe, and effective anti-inflammatory therapies for DED, has attracted attention. In this study, we aimed to provide a basis for a therapeutic approach in which HY7302-derived exosomes can regulate the production of inflammatory cytokines in the pathogenesis of inflammatory eye disease. In our previous paper, we observed that HY7302 intake could suppress corneal damage and improve the function-related tear production in BAC-induced dry eye model mice. Further, the HY732 probiotic altered the microbiota composition by influencing beta diversity and increasing the abundance of *Bifidobacterium pseudolongum* [46]; however, there are no previous reports on which functional molecules of *L. fermentum* affect eye health. Therefore, we investigated whether HY7302 exosomes could exert specific functional effects that alter the inflammatory response of conjunctival cells by acting on the gut–ocular axis. In particular, the conjunctival tissue is rich in blood vessels, lymphatic vessels, and nerve fibers [66]. In addition, conjunctival cells are closely related to tear secretion because the secretions from the lacrimal glands flow into the conjunctival sac, and are drained by the lacrimal ducts of the upper and lower eyelids [67]. Therefore, we suggest that the exosomal functional components of probiotics can circulate to the conjunctival tissue, which may ultimately act directly to improve dry eye and corneal damage.

It is established in the literature that it is important to isolate exosomes of high purity and with high yield in a state close to that occurring in vivo. There are various methods for isolating and purifying exosomes, such as high-speed centrifugation and polymer precipitation [68,69]. In this study, we used high-speed centrifugation to isolate high-purity exosomes from HY7302 culture supernatant, which is the most commonly used method for isolating exosomes by size. Moreover, we isolated exosomes from both HY7302 and KCTC3112 in the same way and compared their physiological properties. Data generated by NTA showed that the number of extracellular particles isolated from HY7302 differed from that isolated from KCTC3112 visible in the same optical area. We concluded that smaller exosomes were actively produced by HY7302, as the average sizes of particles extracted from HY7302 in each size range were smaller than those from KCTC3112, except among the top 10% of total exosome particle size. In addition, HY7302-derived exosomes were observed via transmission electron microscopy (TEM), which is a basic method used to characterize particle size. The diameters of the HY7302 particles inferred to be exosomes, based on their double-membrane structure observed in TEM images, were approximately 50–150 nm.

Tight junctions are cell–cell adhesion complexes that are strongly developed in intestinal tissues and form intercellular barriers [70]. When tight junctions leak, due to external invasion or imbalance of the intestinal microbiome, inflammatory cytokines can escape into other tissues and induce immune and inflammatory responses [71]. The tight junction proteins, TJP1 and TJP2, are cytoplasmic peripheral membrane proteins with multiple domains specialized for protein interaction that are required for assembly of both adherences and tight junctions [72]. Occludin-1 is also an essential tight junction component, which seals the paracellular space and prevents unrestricted leakage [73]. To confirm that exosomes play an important role in the effects of HY7302 on eye health via the gut–eye axis, we evaluated their effects on the regulation of tight junctions in human intestinal Caco-2 cells. Our data demonstrate a potentially important effect of HY7302 supernatant in enhancing tight junction barrier gene levels in the cells. Indeed, we established that the anti-inflammatory bioactive effect of culture supernatant was stronger than that of the bacterial cells themselves. Relative to the controls treated only with HY7302, cell pellets, or MRS, culture supernatant substantially increased levels of *TJP1* and *OCLN*. We inferred from these findings that the active substance derived from HY7302 is present in the culture supernatant or bacterial cells, and therefore investigated the effect of isolated HY7302 exosomes in the supernatant in Caco-2 cells on gut junction molecules. Both low (0.5 μg/mL) and high (1 μg/mL) concentrations of HY7302 exosomes were used to treat confluent Caco-2 cells for 24 h; HY7302 probiotics served as a positive control. Levels of mRNAs encoding TJP1, TJP2, and occludin-1 were significantly higher after treatment with 0.5 and 1 μg/mL HY7302 exosomes than those in untreated or probiotic-treated cells. Based on the above results, it is most likely that HY7302-derived exosomes enhance the integrity of intercellular junctions by regulating the expression of junction molecules, leading to enhanced tight junction interactions between endothelial cells.

As understanding of the role of inflammation in DED increases, improvement in the changes to the ocular surface through the consumption of functional foods is becoming a focus of attention as an alternative to use of tear replacements [74]. Ocular epithelial cells exposed to certain concentrations of BAC exhibit increased inflammatory cytokine production [11]. In addition, BAC-induced DED has been reported to be accompanied by increased production of inflammatory chemokines in several studies. For example, increases in the concentrations of inflammatory cytokines, such as IL-1B, Il-6, IL-8, and tumor necrosis factor-α (TNF-α), in tears are correlated with clinical indices of dry eye [19]. In addition, IL-20 was significantly increased in the tears of animal models with BAC-induced dry eye; as IL-20 can induce an inflammatory response, including infiltration and activation of macrophages, it has been suggested that it is a potential treatment target in patients with dry eyes [75]. Moreover, the expression of these pro-inflammatory cytokines can be regulated by NF-κB and NFAT5. NF-κB is a member of a family of inducible transcription factors that regulate numerous genes involved in various immune and inflammatory response processes [63]. In addition, NFAT5 is an important regulator of the expression of NF-κB, which is a key inflammatory response modulator [76]. In this study, we found that the mRNA levels of IL-20, IL-8, and IL-1B of the cell treated with 1 μg/mL HY7302 exosomes significantly lower than those of the cell treated with 10^6 CFU/mL HY7302 probiotics. In this study, we found that treatment of cells induced with inflammation by BAC with 1 μg/mL HY7302 exosomes significantly reduced the mRNA levels of IL-20, IL-8, and IL-1B as much as when treated with 10^6 CFU/mL HY7302 probiotics. In addition, *NFAT5* and *NFKB1* mRNA expression levels were strongly induced by BAC treatment, but dramatically decreased in cells treated with HY7302 exosomes, with levels much lower than those in cells treated with KCTC3112 exosomes. Together, our data show that HY7302 exosomes have the potential to prevent BAC-induced multifactorial ocular dysfunction by reducing inflammatory cytokine expression. We also investigated the anti-inflammatory responses of intestinal and ocular conjunctival cells to HY7302 exosomes, by the coculture of both types of cell line in a transwell system. Treatment of Caco-2 cells with 0.5 and 1 μg/mL HY7302 exosomes significantly reduced transcription of all the intercellular cytokines tested, with levels of *IL20*, *IL6*, and *IL8* markedly lowered. These results indicate that exosomes derived from HY7302 probiotic can migrate to ocular epithelial cells and suppress BAC-related inflammation. Furthermore, our findings confirm that these exosomes can act as anti-inflammatory regulators between gut and ocular tissues, suggesting that exosomes are functional agents of *L. fermentum* HY 7302.

The number of patients with dry eye has increased dramatically over the past few decades. Dry eye disease can cause inflammatory responses in ocular and conjunctiva tissues. In our previous study, we analyzed changes in the intestinal microbiome and changes in inflammatory markers in intestinal tissue, among several factors that may affect distant organs when orally consumed probiotics. In this study, we demonstrated that the exosomes of HY7302 can pass through differentiated enterocytes and directly reach and affect conjunctival cells. This provides clues to how HY7302 acts (MOA) to directly improve dry eye syndrome in addition to regulating the microbiome and intestinal immunity. Further investigations to clarify the physiological characteristics of the extracellular particles involved, by revealing which proteins, DNA, RNA, or organic acids, etc., are present in exosomes from HY7302 probiotics, are warranted. These extracellular secreted exosomes are important factors in host–microbe interactions; however, it will also be necessary to determine whether they act as specific factors that enable HY7302 attachment and survival in the gastrointestinal tract. Our results highlight the importance of HY7302 exosomes and their potential for development as a future therapeutic approach for dry eye and conjunctival inflammation. Furthermore, the data suggest that certain exosomes isolated from HY7302, which have been proven to be safe, may be utilized as effective materials of potential value as treatments for dry eyes or functional health foods. It is easily applicable in clinical practice and would help establish new clinical trials for dry eye using supplementation with HY7302 probiotics

4. Materials and Methods

4.1. HY7302 Cell Culture and Exosome Isolation

L. fermentum HY7302 was isolated from raw milk obtained from Korean farms. *L. fermentum* type strain KCTC 3112 was obtained from KCTC. Both *L. fermentum* strains were cultured in MRS medium (BD Difco, Detroit, MI, USA; KisanBio, Seoul, Republic of Korea) at 37 °C for 18 h. For in vitro studies, *L. fermentum* cultures were centrifuged (2000× *g*, 20 min), and then culture supernatant medium was centrifuged again (2000× *g*, 4 °C, 20 min). After centrifugation, cell pellets were washed twice with PBS, and then resuspended in PBS. Culture supernatant and cell pellet samples were prepared to a final concentration of 1×10^6 CFU/mL and used for in vitro experiments.

Exosomes were isolated from culture supernatants by sequential high-speed centrifugation using a total exosome isolation commercial kit (Cat no. 4478359, Thermo Fisher Scientific, Waltham, MA, USA). Briefly, HY7302 and KCTC3112 cell supernatant samples were centrifuged (2000× *g*, 20 min, 4 °C) and cell debris removed. Supernatants were transferred to new tubes and then mixed with kit reagents at a 1:2 ratio before incubation overnight at 4 °C. Exosome pellets were washed with PBS and subjected to high-speed centrifugation (10,000× *g*, 60 min, 4 °C). HY7302 and KCTC3112 exosomes samples were resuspended in PBS, aliquoted, and stored at −80 °C until further use.

4.2. Detection of Total Protein Content in HY7302 Exosomes

Protein concentrations in exosomes were measured using a DC Protein Analysis Kit (BIO-RAD, Hercules, CA, USA), according to the manufacturer's instructions; absorbance was measured at 750 nm on an ELISA microreader (BioTek, Winooski, VT, USA). Based on the results of this analysis, 50 μg/mL stock solutions of HY7302- and KCTC3112-derived exosomes were prepared in PBS, and added to cells at final concentrations of 0.5 or 1 μg/mL for 24 h.

4.3. Cell Culture

The human conjunctival epithelial cell line, clone 1-5c-4, was seeded at 1×10^5 cells/mL and cultured in Dulbecco's modified Eagle's medium (DMEM)/F-12 containing 10% *v/v* fetal bovine serum (FBS; Gibco, Thermo Fisher Scientific, Waltham, MA, USA) and 1% antibiotic/antimycotic in a 5% CO_2 humidified air atmosphere at 37 °C. For treatments, 1×10^9 cells/mL stock solutions of HY7302 or KCTC3112 were prepared in PBS, and added to cells at a final concentration of 1×10^6 CFU/mL. HY7302 and KCTC3112 exosomes were prepared in PBS and added to cells at final concentrations of 0.5 and 1 μg/mL for 24 h. To generate a dry eye model, clone 1-5c-4 cells were treated with 0.0005% (*v*/*v*) BAC for the last 3 h.

Caco-2 cells were also seeded at 1×10^5 cells/mL and maintained in DMEM containing 10% *v/v* FBS and 1% antibiotic/antimycotic in a 5% CO_2 humidified air atmosphere at 37 °C. Cells were cultured and fully differentiated for 21 days. Caco-2 cells were treated with culture supernatants and cell pellets of HY7302 and KCTC3112 probiotics at 1×10^6 CFU/mL for 24 h.

4.4. Cell Viability Protection and Toxicity Assays

The effects of HY7302 exosomes on cell viability were determined using MTT and LDH assays. Conjunctival epithelial cells were seeded in 96-well plates at 1×10^4 cells/mL and incubated in serum-free medium, then treated with various concentrations of HY7302 exosomes (0.01, 0.1, 1, 0.5, and 5 μg/mL) for 24 h. For the MTT test, 0.5 mg/mL MTT stock solution was added and incubated for 4 h. After MTT-containing medium was aspirated, 200 μL of DMSO was added for elution of formazan crystals. Then, absorbance values at 590 nm were measured using a microreader (BioTek, Winooski, VT, USA). Cytoplasmic LDH activity was detected in cell-free supernatant samples from HY7302 exosome-treated cells using an LDH assay kit (G1780; Promega, Madison, WI, USA), according to the manufacturer' instructions. LDH assay results are expressed as percentage cell viability relative to that of positive control-treated controls, which was set at 100%.

4.5. NTA of HY7302 Exosomes

The exosome size distributions and concentrations were detected using a Nanosight NS300 instrument (Malvern Panalytical Ltd., Malvern, UK, version no. 3.4). Fractions were diluted 1:100 or 1:1000 with sterile PBS, to ensure that the number of detectable particles was within the optimal range of 106–109 particles/mL. NanoSight NTA 3.4 analytical software was used to accurately quantify the size and concentration of exosomes in samples; each sample was analyzed in triplicate.

4.6. TEM Analysis of HY7302 Exosomes

Exosomes freshly isolated from HY7302 culture supernatants were resuspended in Dulbecco's PBS. HY7302 exosomes were fixed using 4% (*v*/*v*) paraformaldehyde, then dropped onto a copper grid and stored at room temperature for 1 min before removal of the liquid using filter paper. Samples were then treated with uranyl acetate for 1 min and then remaining liquid was removed with filter paper. Prepared samples were then dried at room temperature for further observation. TEM was conducted using a JEM-1400 (JEOL Co., Ltd., Tokyo, Japan). The exosome sizes were determined using RADIUS software (EMSIS, Version 3.0.26).

4.7. Transwell Coculture of Caco-2 and Clone 1-5c-4 Cells

Briefly, fully differentiated Caco-2 cells (1×10^5 cells/well) and 0.5 or 1.0 μg/mL HY7302 exosomes were seeded in the upper chambers of 6-well 24 mm transwell plates with 0.4 μm pore filters (Costar, Washington, DC, USA). Conjunctival clone 1-5c-4 cells without exosomes were added to the lower chambers. After incubation for 24 h, cells in the lower chamber were exposed to 0.0005% (v/v) BAC for 3 h. Aliquots of medium and harvested cells were collected from the lower chamber and stored at −80 °C until further use. Each experiment was repeated three times.

4.8. qRT-PCR

RNA was extracted using Trizol reagent (iNtRON Biotechnology, Seongnam-si, Republic of Korea) according to the manufacturer's instructions, and cDNA synthesized from 600 ng total RNA using a commercial kit (Maxime RT PreMix Kit; iNtRON Biotechnology). Then, cDNA was analyzed by qRT-PCR using the TaqMan Probe-Based Gene expression assay system (Applied Biosystems, Carlsbad, CA, USA) and TaqMan Gene Expression Master Mix (Applied Biosystems, Waltham, MA, USA). Quantification of *TJP1* (Hs01551871_m1), *TJP2* (Hs00910543_m1), occludin-1 (Hs05465837_g1), *IL20* (Hs00218888_m1), *IL1B* (Hs01555410_m1), *IL8* (Hs00174103_m1), *IL6* (Hs00174131_m1), *NFAT5* (Hs00232437_m1), and *NFKB1* (Hs00765730_m1) transcripts was performed using gene-specific primers. All mRNA data were normalized to *GAPDH* (Hs99999905_m1) levels. To compare levels between samples, relative mRNA levels were calculated using the $2^{(-\Delta\Delta CT)}$ method.

4.9. Statistical Analysis

At least three independent NTA analyses were performed, and data on particle amounts and diameters are presented as mean ± standard deviation (SD) values. Cell toxicity, viability data, qRT-PCR and ELISA data were analyzed using one-way ANOVA and Duncan's test (SPSS, version 18.0, Chicago, IL, USA) and are presented as mean ± SD. $p < 0.05$ was considered significant.

5. Conclusions

Although gut–eye axis communication provides an attractive perspective for interpretation of mechanisms occurring in health and disease, the role of L. fermentum in this context has remained relatively unexplored. In the present study, we identified the properties and activities of functional substances from HY7302 probiotics, which have previously been shown to improve dry eyes using in vivo experiments. We observed that HY7302 produced exosomes were of a smaller mean particle size and present in larger amounts than those from a standard strain of the same species, KCTC3112. In addition, we provide evidence that HY7302-derived exosomes both enhance tight junction barriers in intestinal cells, and reduce the expression levels of inflammatory cytokines in ocular epithelial cells. Overall, our data suggest that HY7302 probiotics could significantly improve gut–eye axis communication through exosome-mediated anti-inflammatory regulation.

Author Contributions: Conceptualization, K.L. and J.Y.K.; methodology, K.L.; software, K.L. and H.G.; validation, K.L.; formal analysis, K.L.; investigation, K.L.; data curation, K.L.; writing—original draft preparation, K.L.; writing—review and editing, J.Y.K. and J.H.L.; visualization, K.L.; project administration, K.L., J.J.S. and J.H.L. All authors have read and agreed to the published version of the manuscript.

Funding: This research received no external funding.

Institutional Review Board Statement: Not applicable.

Informed Consent Statement: Not applicable.

Data Availability Statement: Data are contained within the article.

Conflicts of Interest: The authors Kippeum Lee, Hyeonjun Gwon, Jae Jung Shim, Joo Yun Kim and Jae Hwan Lee were employed by the company Hy Co., Ltd. The authors declare that the research was conducted in the absence of any commercial or financial relationships that could be construed as potential conflicts of interest.

References

1. Stevenson, W.; Chauhan, S.K.; Dana, R. Dry eye disease: An immune-mediated ocular surface disorder. *Arch. Ophthalmol.* **2012**, *130*, 90–100. [CrossRef] [PubMed]
2. Yamaguchi, T. Inflammatory response in dry eye. *Investig. Ophthalmol. Vis. Sci.* **2018**, *59*, DES192–DES199. [CrossRef] [PubMed]
3. Phadatare, S.P.; Momin, M.; Nighojkar, P.; Askarkar, S.; Singh, K.K. A comprehensive review on dry eye disease: Diagnosis, medical management, recent developments, and future challenges. *Adv. Pharm.* **2015**, *2015*, 704946. [CrossRef]
4. Uchino, M.; Schaumberg, D.A. Dry eye disease: Impact on quality of life and vision. *Curr. Ophthalmol. Rep.* **2013**, *1*, 51–57. [CrossRef] [PubMed]
5. Boboridis, K.G.; Messmer, E.M.; Benítez-del-Castillo, J.; Meunier, J.; Sloesen, B.; O'Brien, P.; Quadrado, M.J.; Rolando, M.; Labetoulle, M. Patient-reported burden and overall impact of dry eye disease across eight European countries: A cross-sectional web-based survey. *BMJ Open* **2023**, *13*, e067007. [CrossRef]
6. Stapleton, F.; Alves, M.; Bunya, V.Y.; Jalbert, I.; Lekhanont, K.; Malet, F.; Na, K.-S.; Schaumberg, D.; Uchino, M.; Vehof, J. Tfos dews ii epidemiology report. *Ocul. Surf.* **2017**, *15*, 334–365. [CrossRef]
7. Al-Dossary, S.K. Environmental and Occupational Triggers of Dry Eye Symptoms in the Ahsa Region of Saudi Arabia: A Cross-Sectional Study. *Clin. Ophthalmol.* **2024**, *18*, 2427–2438. [CrossRef]
8. Idarraga, M.A.; Guerrero, J.S.; Mosle, S.G.; Miralles, F.; Galor, A.; Kumar, N. Relationships between short-term exposure to an indoor environment and dry eye (DE) symptoms. *J. Clin. Med.* **2020**, *9*, 1316. [CrossRef]
9. Rao, S.K.; Mohan, R.; Gokhale, N.; Matalia, H.; Mehta, P. Inflammation and dry eye disease—Where are we? *Int. J. Ophthalmol.* **2022**, *15*, 820. [CrossRef]
10. Kitazawa, K.; Inomata, T.; Shih, K.; Hughes, J.-W.B.; Bozza, N.; Tomioka, Y.; Numa, K.; Yokoi, N.; Campisi, J.; Dana, R. Impact of aging on the pathophysiology of dry eye disease: A systematic review and meta-analysis. *Ocul. Surf.* **2022**, *25*, 108–118. [CrossRef]
11. Thacker, M.; Sahoo, A.; Reddy, A.A.; Bokara, K.K.; Singh, S.; Basu, S.; Singh, V. Benzalkonium chloride-induced dry eye disease animal models: Current understanding and potential for translational research. *Indian J. Ophthalmol.* **2023**, *71*, 1256–1262. [CrossRef] [PubMed]
12. Kim, M.; Lee, Y.; Mehra, D.; Sabater, A.L.; Galor, A. Dry eye: Why artificial tears are not always the answer. *BMJ Open Ophthalmol.* **2021**, *6*, e000697. [CrossRef] [PubMed]
13. Wang, W.-X.; Ko, M.-L. Efficacy of Omega-3 Intake in Managing Dry Eye Disease: A Systematic Review and Meta-Analysis of Randomized Controlled Trials. *J. Clin. Med.* **2023**, *12*, 7026. [CrossRef] [PubMed]
14. Downie, L.E.; Ng, S.M.; Lindsley, K.B.; Akpek, E.K. Omega-3 and omega-6 polyunsaturated fatty acids for dry eye disease. *Cochrane Database Syst. Rev.* **2019**, *12*, CD011016. [CrossRef]
15. Zhang, G.; Fu, W.; Xu, J.; Hu, P.; Zhang, Y.; Sang, Z.; Wu, W.; Zheng, K.; Wu, L.; Liu, Z. Moxibustion with Walnut Shell Spectacles Could Improve the Objective Symptoms and Tear Film Stability of Patients with Dry Eye Disease: A Randomized Controlled Trial. *Evid.-Based Complement. Altern. Med.* **2022**, *2022*, 1773444. [CrossRef]
16. Mahoney, M.J.; Bekibele, R.; Notermann, S.L.; Reuter, T.G.; Borman-Shoap, E.C. Pediatric conjunctivitis: A review of clinical manifestations, diagnosis, and management. *Children* **2023**, *10*, 808. [CrossRef]
17. Soifer, M.; Azar, N.S.; Mousa, H.M.; Perez, V.L. Ocular surface inflammatory disorders (OSID): A collective of systemic etiologies which cause or amplify dry eye syndrome. *Front. Med.* **2022**, *9*, 949202. [CrossRef]
18. Enríquez-de-Salamanca, A.; Castellanos, E.; Stern, M.E.; Fernández, I.; Carreño, E.; García-Vázquez, C.; Herreras, J.M.; Calonge, M. Tear cytokine and chemokine analysis and clinical correlations in evaporative-type dry eye disease. *Mol. Vis.* **2010**, *16*, 862.
19. Na, K.-S.; Mok, J.-W.; Kim, J.Y.; Rho, C.R.; Joo, C.-K. Correlations between tear cytokines, chemokines, and soluble receptors and clinical severity of dry eye disease. *Investig. Ophthalmol. Vis. Sci.* **2012**, *53*, 5443–5450. [CrossRef]
20. Kumar, M.A.; Baba, S.K.; Sadida, H.Q.; Marzooqi, S.A.; Jerobin, J.; Altemani, F.H.; Algehainy, N.; Alanazi, M.A.; Abou-Samra, A.-B.; Kumar, R. Extracellular vesicles as tools and targets in therapy for diseases. *Signal Transduct. Target. Ther.* **2024**, *9*, 27. [CrossRef]
21. Maas, S.L.; Breakefield, X.O.; Weaver, A.M. Extracellular vesicles: Unique intercellular delivery vehicles. *Trends Cell Biol.* **2017**, *27*, 172–188. [CrossRef] [PubMed]
22. Di Bella, M.A. Overview and update on extracellular vesicles: Considerations on exosomes and their application in modern medicine. *Biology* **2022**, *11*, 804. [CrossRef] [PubMed]
23. O'Brien, K.; Breyne, K.; Ughetto, S.; Laurent, L.C.; Breakefield, X.O. RNA delivery by extracellular vesicles in mammalian cells and its applications. *Nat. Rev. Mol. Cell Biol.* **2020**, *21*, 585–606. [CrossRef]
24. Askenase, P.W. Exosome carrier effects; resistance to digestion in phagolysosomes may assist transfers to targeted cells; II transfers of miRNAs are better analyzed via systems approach as they do not fit conventional reductionist stoichiometric concepts. *Int. J. Mol. Sci.* **2022**, *23*, 6192. [CrossRef]
25. Jeong, M.H.; Han, H.; Lagares, D.; Im, H. Recent advances in molecular diagnosis of pulmonary fibrosis for precision medicine. *ACS Pharmacol. Transl. Sci.* **2022**, *5*, 520–538. [CrossRef]
26. Mohieldin, A.M.; Pala, R.; Beuttler, R.; Moresco, J.J.; Yates, J.R., III; Nauli, S.M. Ciliary extracellular vesicles are distinct from the cytosolic extracellular vesicles. *J. Extracell. Vesicles* **2021**, *10*, e12086. [CrossRef]
27. Yáñez-Mó, M.; Siljander, P.R.-M.; Andreu, Z.; Bedina Zavec, A.; Borràs, F.E.; Buzas, E.I.; Buzas, K.; Casal, E.; Cappello, F.; Carvalho, J. Biological properties of extracellular vesicles and their physiological functions. *J. Extracell. Vesicles* **2015**, *4*, 27066. [CrossRef]

28. Kalluri, R.; LeBleu, V.S. The biology, function, and biomedical applications of exosomes. *Science* **2020**, *367*, eaau6977. [CrossRef]
29. Ruzycka-Ayoush, M.; Nowicka, A.M.; Kowalczyk, A.; Gluchowska, A.; Targonska, A.; Mosieniak, G.; Sobczak, K.; Donten, M.; Grudzinski, I.P. Exosomes derived from lung cancer cells: Isolation, characterization, and stability studies. *Eur. J. Pharm. Sci.* **2023**, *181*, 106369. [CrossRef]
30. Herrmann, I.K.; Wood, M.J.A.; Fuhrmann, G. Extracellular vesicles as a next-generation drug delivery platform. *Nat. Nanotechnol.* **2021**, *16*, 748–759. [CrossRef]
31. Zhang, B.; Zhao, J.; Jiang, M.; Peng, D.; Dou, X.; Song, Y.; Shi, J. The potential role of gut microbial-derived exosomes in metabolic-associated fatty liver disease: Implications for treatment. *Front. Immunol.* **2022**, *13*, 893617. [CrossRef] [PubMed]
32. Jo, C.S.; Myung, C.H.; Yoon, Y.C.; Ahn, B.H.; Min, J.W.; Seo, W.S.; Lee, D.H.; Kang, H.C.; Heo, Y.H.; Choi, H. The effect of Lactobacillus plantarum extracellular vesicles from Korean women in their 20s on skin aging. *Curr. Issues Mol. Biol.* **2022**, *44*, 526–540. [CrossRef]
33. Yang, G.H.; Lee, Y.B.; Kang, D.; Choi, E.; Nam, Y.; Lee, K.H.; You, H.-J.; Kang, H.J.; An, S.H.; Jeon, H. Overcome the barriers of the skin: Exosome therapy. *Biomater. Res.* **2021**, *25*, 22. [CrossRef]
34. Krzyżek, P.; Marinacci, B.; Vitale, I.; Grande, R. Extracellular vesicles of probiotics: Shedding light on the biological activity and future applications. *Pharmaceutics* **2023**, *15*, 522. [CrossRef]
35. Grangier, A.; Branchu, J.; Volatron, J.; Piffoux, M.; Gazeau, F.; Wilhelm, C.; Silva, A.K. Technological advances towards extracellular vesicles mass production. *Adv. Drug Deliv. Rev.* **2021**, *176*, 113843. [CrossRef]
36. Plaza-Diaz, J.; Ruiz-Ojeda, F.J.; Gil-Campos, M.; Gil, A. Mechanisms of action of probiotics. *Adv. Nutr.* **2019**, *10*, S49–S66. [CrossRef]
37. Mazziotta, C.; Tognon, M.; Martini, F.; Torreggiani, E.; Rotondo, J.C. Probiotics mechanism of action on immune cells and beneficial effects on human health. *Cells* **2023**, *12*, 184. [CrossRef]
38. Fijan, S. Microorganisms with claimed probiotic properties: An overview of recent literature. *Int. J. Environ. Res. Public Health* **2014**, *11*, 4745–4767. [CrossRef]
39. Wang, Y.; Wu, J.; Lv, M.; Shao, Z.; Hungwe, M.; Wang, J.; Bai, X.; Xie, J.; Wang, Y.; Geng, W. Metabolism characteristics of lactic acid bacteria and the expanding applications in food industry. *Front. Bioeng. Biotechnol.* **2021**, *9*, 612285. [CrossRef]
40. Tamang, J.P.; Watanabe, K.; Holzapfel, W.H. Diversity of microorganisms in global fermented foods and beverages. *Front. Microbiol.* **2016**, *7*, 377.
41. Das, T.K.; Pradhan, S.; Chakrabarti, S.; Mondal, K.C.; Ghosh, K. Current status of probiotic and related health benefits. *Appl. Food Res.* **2022**, *2*, 100185. [CrossRef]
42. Kim, J.-E.; Kim, J.-Y.; Lee, K.-W.; Lee, H.-J. Cancer chemopreventive effects of lactic acid bacteria. *J. Microbiol. Biotechnol.* **2007**, *17*, 1227–1235. [PubMed]
43. Hossain, T.J. Functional genomics of the lactic acid bacterium Limosilactobacillus fermentum LAB-1: Metabolic, probiotic and biotechnological perspectives. *Heliyon* **2022**, *8*, e11412. [CrossRef] [PubMed]
44. Pakroo, S.; Tarrah, A.; Takur, R.; Wu, M.; Corich, V.; Giacomini, A. Limosilactobacillus fermentum ING8, a potential multifunctional non-starter strain with relevant technological properties and antimicrobial activity. *Foods* **2022**, *11*, 703. [CrossRef]
45. Lee, K.; Jeong, J.W.; Shim, J.J.; Hong, H.S.; Kim, J.Y.; Lee, J.L. Lactobacillus fermentum HY7302 improves dry eye symptoms in a mouse model of benzalkonium chloride-induced eye dysfunction and human conjunctiva epithelial cells. *Int. J. Mol. Sci.* **2023**, *24*, 10378. [CrossRef]
46. Lee, K.; Gwon, H.; Shim, J.J.; Kim, J.Y.; Lee, J.H. Consumption of Limosilactobacillus fermentum Inhibits Corneal Damage and Inflammation in Dry Eye Disease Mouse Model through Regulating the Gut Microbiome. *Int. J. Mol. Sci.* **2024**, *25*, 3528. [CrossRef]
47. Brennan, K.; Martin, K.; FitzGerald, S.; O'sullivan, J.; Wu, Y.; Blanco, A.; Richardson, C.; Mc Gee, M. A comparison of methods for the isolation and separation of extracellular vesicles from protein and lipid particles in human serum. *Sci. Rep.* **2020**, *10*, 1039. [CrossRef]
48. Sall, I.M.; Flaviu, T.A. Plant and mammalian-derived extracellular vesicles: A new therapeutic approach for the future. *Front. Bioeng. Biotechnol.* **2023**, *11*, 1215650. [CrossRef]
49. Rajput, A.; Varshney, A.; Bajaj, R.; Pokharkar, V. Exosomes as new generation vehicles for drug delivery: Biomedical applications and future perspectives. *Molecules* **2022**, *27*, 7289. [CrossRef]
50. Tenchov, R.; Sasso, J.M.; Wang, X.; Liaw, W.-S.; Chen, C.-A.; Zhou, Q.A. Exosomes—Nature's lipid nanoparticles, a rising star in drug delivery and diagnostics. *ACS Nano* **2022**, *16*, 17802–17846. [CrossRef]
51. Jeppesen, D.K.; Zhang, Q.; Franklin, J.L.; Coffey, R.J. Extracellular vesicles and nanoparticles: Emerging complexities. *Trends Cell Biol.* **2023**, *33*, 667–681. [CrossRef] [PubMed]
52. Gurunathan, S.; Kang, M.-H.; Jeyaraj, M.; Qasim, M.; Kim, J.-H. Review of the isolation, characterization, biological function, and multifarious therapeutic approaches of exosomes. *Cells* **2019**, *8*, 307. [CrossRef] [PubMed]
53. Liu, S.-L.; Sun, P.; Li, Y.; Liu, S.-S.; Lu, Y. Exosomes as critical mediators of cell-to-cell communication in cancer pathogenesis and their potential clinical application. *Transl. Cancer Res.* **2019**, *8*, 298. [CrossRef] [PubMed]
54. Song, Y.; Kim, Y.; Ha, S.; Sheller-Miller, S.; Yoo, J.; Choi, C.; Park, C.H. The emerging role of exosomes as novel therapeutics: Biology, technologies, clinical applications, and the next. *Am. J. Reprod. Immunol.* **2021**, *85*, e13329. [CrossRef]

55. Liu, Q.; Li, S.; Dupuy, A.; Mai, H.l.; Sailliet, N.; Logé, C.; Robert, J.-M.H.; Brouard, S. Exosomes as new biomarkers and drug delivery tools for the prevention and treatment of various diseases: Current perspectives. *Int. J. Mol. Sci.* **2021**, *22*, 7763. [CrossRef]
56. Subha, D.; Harshnii, K.; Madhikiruba, K.; Nandhini, M.; Tamilselvi, K. Plant derived exosome-like Nanovesicles: An updated overview. *Plant Nano Biol.* **2023**, *3*, 100022. [CrossRef]
57. Manzaneque-López, M.C.; Sánchez-López, C.M.; Pérez-Bermúdez, P.; Soler, C.; Marcilla, A. Dietary-derived exosome-like nanoparticles as bacterial modulators: Beyond MicroRNAs. *Nutrients* **2023**, *15*, 1265. [CrossRef]
58. Díez-Sainz, E.; Milagro, F.I.; Riezu-Boj, J.I.; Lorente-Cebrian, S. Effects of gut microbiota–derived extracellular vesicles on obesity and diabetes and their potential modulation through diet. *J. Physiol. Biochem.* **2022**, *78*, 485–499. [CrossRef]
59. Nishiyama, K.; Takaki, T.; Sugiyama, M.; Fukuda, I.; Aiso, M.; Mukai, T.; Odamaki, T.; Xiao, J.-z.; Osawa, R.; Okada, N. Extracellular vesicles produced by Bifidobacterium longum export mucin-binding proteins. *Appl. Environ. Microbiol.* **2020**, *86*, e01464-20. [CrossRef]
60. Mandelbaum, N.; Zhang, L.; Carasso, S.; Ziv, T.; Lifshiz-Simon, S.; Davidovich, I.; Luz, I.; Berinstein, E.; Gefen, T.; Cooks, T. Extracellular vesicles of the Gram-positive gut symbiont Bifidobacterium longum induce immune-modulatory, anti-inflammatory effects. *npj Biofilms Microbiomes* **2023**, *9*, 30. [CrossRef]
61. Zhou, P.; Chen, C.; Patil, S.; Dong, S. Unveiling the therapeutic symphony of probiotics, prebiotics, and postbiotics in gut-immune harmony. *Front. Nutr.* **2024**, *11*, 1355542. [CrossRef] [PubMed]
62. Patel, S.; Mittal, R.; Kumar, N.; Galor, A. The environment and dry eye—Manifestations, mechanisms, and more. *Front. Toxicol.* **2023**, *5*, 1173683. [CrossRef] [PubMed]
63. Henrioux, F.; Navel, V.; Belville, C.; Charnay, C.; Antoine, A.; Chiambaretta, F.; Sapin, V.; Blanchon, L. Inflammation of Dry Eye Syndrome: A Cellular Study of the Epithelial and Macrophagic Involvement of NFAT5 and RAGE. *Int. J. Mol. Sci.* **2023**, *24*, 11052. [CrossRef]
64. Lee, J.S.; Kim, Y.H.; Park, Y.M. The toxicity of nonsteroidal anti-inflammatory eye drops against human corneal epithelial cells in vitro. *J. Korean Med. Sci.* **2015**, *30*, 1856–1864. [CrossRef]
65. Hossain, P. Cyclosporine in ocular surface inflammation. *Eye* **2017**, *31*, 665–667. [CrossRef]
66. Subileau, M.; Vittet, D. Lymphatics in eye fluid homeostasis: Minor contributors or significant actors? *Biology* **2021**, *10*, 582. [CrossRef]
67. Machiele, R.; Lopez, M.J.; Czyz, C.N. *Anatomy, Head and Neck, Eye Lacrimal Gland*; StatPearls Publishing: Treasure Island, FL, USA, 2018.
68. Liangsupree, T.; Multia, E.; Riekkola, M.-L. Modern isolation and separation techniques for extracellular vesicles. *J. Chromatogr. A* **2021**, *1636*, 461773. [CrossRef]
69. Gao, J.; Li, A.; Hu, J.; Feng, L.; Liu, L.; Shen, Z. Recent developments in isolating methods for exosomes. *Front. Bioeng. Biotechnol.* **2023**, *10*, 1100892. [CrossRef]
70. Chelakkot, C.; Ghim, J.; Ryu, S.H. Mechanisms regulating intestinal barrier integrity and its pathological implications. *Exp. Mol. Med.* **2018**, *50*, 1–9. [CrossRef]
71. Usuda, H.; Okamoto, T.; Wada, K. Leaky gut: Effect of dietary fiber and fats on microbiome and intestinal barrier. *Int. J. Mol. Sci.* **2021**, *22*, 7613. [CrossRef]
72. Fanning, A.S.; Anderson, J.M. Zonula occludens-1 and-2 are cytosolic scaffolds that regulate the assembly of cellular junctions. *Ann. N. Y. Acad. Sci.* **2009**, *1165*, 113–120. [CrossRef] [PubMed]
73. Horowitz, A.; Chanez-Paredes, S.D.; Haest, X.; Turner, J.R. Paracellular permeability and tight junction regulation in gut health and disease. *Nat. Rev. Gastroenterol. Hepatol.* **2023**, *20*, 417–432. [CrossRef] [PubMed]
74. Tavakoli, A.; Flanagan, J.L. The case for a more holistic approach to dry eye disease: Is it time to move beyond antibiotics? *Antibiotics* **2019**, *8*, 88. [CrossRef]
75. Wang, H.-H.; Chen, W.-Y.; Huang, Y.-H.; Hsu, S.-M.; Tsao, Y.-P.; Hsu, Y.-H.; Chang, M.-S. Interleukin-20 is involved in dry eye disease and is a potential therapeutic target. *J. Biomed. Sci.* **2022**, *29*, 36. [CrossRef]
76. Ouyang, W.; Wu, Y.; Lin, X.; Wang, S.; Yang, Y.; Tang, L.; Liu, Z.; Wu, J.; Huang, C.; Zhou, Y. Role of CD4+ T helper cells in the development of BAC-induced dry eye syndrome in mice. *Investig. Ophthalmol. Vis. Sci.* **2021**, *62*, 25. [CrossRef]

International Journal of
Molecular Sciences

MDPI

Review

Sex Differences in the Lacrimal Gland: Implications for Dry Eye Disease

Snježana Kaštelan [1,*,†], Koraljka Hat [2,†], Zora Tomić [3], Tomislav Matejić [4] and Nikola Gotovac [5]

[1] Department of Ophthalmology, Clinical Hospital Dubrava, School of Medicine, University of Zagreb, 10000 Zagreb, Croatia
[2] Department of Maxillofacial Surgery, Clinical Hospital Dubrava, University of Zagreb School of Dental Medicine, 10000 Zagreb, Croatia
[3] Health Centre of the Croatian Department of Internal Affairs, 10000 Zagreb, Croatia
[4] Surgery Clinic, Clinical Hospital Sveti Duh, 10000 Zagreb, Croatia
[5] Department of Clinical Radiology, General Hospital Požega, Faculty of Dental Medicine and Health, J. J. Strossmayer University of Osijek, 31000 Osijek, Croatia
* Correspondence: snjezana.kastelan@mef.hr
† These authors contributed equally to this work.

Abstract: Sexual dimorphism significantly impacts the lacrimal gland's structure, function, and ageing processes, playing an important role in dry eye disease (DED) pathophysiology. This multifactorial disorder, characterised by tear film instability, inflammation, and visual impairment, disproportionately affects women, especially after menopause. It highlights the interplay between sex steroid hormones, lacrimal gland function, and environmental factors. Systemic and local androgens are vital for maintaining lacrimal gland health and tear production, while the role of oestrogens remains less clear. Evidence suggests dose and context-dependent effects on inflammation and glandular function. Histopathological and molecular studies reveal significant sex differences in the lacrimal gland, with women exhibiting more pronounced age-related degenerative changes, including fibrosis and acinar atrophy, contributing to their increased susceptibility to DED. Despite these findings, the underlying mechanisms connecting sex steroid hormones, receptor expression, and local tissue regulation to these disparities remain poorly understood, highlighting the need for further research. This review synthesises the current knowledge of sex-specific differences in the lacrimal gland, emphasising the importance of integrating systemic and local biomarkers, histological data, and molecular insights into personalised therapeutic strategies. By tailoring treatments to patients' unique hormonal and molecular profiles, personalised medicine has the potential to transform DED management, addressing unmet clinical needs and improving outcomes.

Keywords: sexual dimorphism; lacrimal gland; dry eye disease; sex steroid hormones; androgens; oestrogens; tear film; personalised treatment

1. Introduction

Sexual dimorphism is evident across various species, encompassing distinctions between males and females beyond reproductive functions. These differences manifest in secondary sexual characteristics and are observed at genetic, cellular, and systemic levels, profoundly affecting health, disease susceptibility, and life expectancy. The emergence of sex differences is shaped by the interplay of genes, chromosomes, sex steroid hormones

(SSHs), and environmental factors, though their precise contributions remain under investigation. The contemporary understanding of the development of sex differences involves a complex interplay of chromosomes, genes, SSHs, and the individual's environment. However, the precise roles and contributions in this process remain unclear. A thorough understanding of the biology of both sexes and the development of reliable, practical knowledge requires conducting separate studies for each sex [1,2].

Dry eye disease (DED) is a multifactorial disorder affecting the tears and the ocular surface. It results in tear film instability and symptoms such as discomfort and visual disturbances. This condition can potentially damage the ocular surface and is marked by elevated tear film osmolarity and inflammation of the ocular surface [3].

Current research shows that women have a 50–70% higher risk of developing DED compared to men [4], and this risk becomes even more pronounced after menopause, suggesting that female sex and advanced age are significant risk factors for DED [5,6]. As age increases, levels of SSH decline, indicating that systemic and local levels of androgens and oestrogens may play a significant role in the pathophysiology of lacrimal gland dysfunction. Optimal androgen levels for normal lacrimal and Meibomian gland function have been established [7–9]. However, the role of oestrogen remains unclear: some studies suggest it has a pro-inflammatory effect, while others point to an anti-inflammatory effect. At the same time, some report no significant impact on the lacrimal gland [10–12]. Oestrogens and progestogens most likely play a less prominent role than androgens in driving sex differences in gene expression and lacrimal gland sexual dimorphism. Additional research is necessary for a clearer understanding of their roles and to improve our knowledge of the underlying mechanisms [13,14].

DED's significant public health burden has encouraged extensive research into its genetic, hormonal, biochemical, and molecular foundations [15]. While studies have highlighted sex- and age-related differences in the structure and function of the lacrimal gland, research involving human subjects remains limited, resulting in insufficient data. Only a few investigations have specifically addressed the sex- and age-related differences in the human lacrimal gland [16–24]. Observations across various animal models, including mice, rats, and rabbits, have demonstrated sex-based variations in morphology, immunological responses, hormonal regulation, and secretory activity [10,25–32]. Similarly, studies on the human lacrimal gland indicate sex-related differences in age-associated degenerative changes and the expression of SSH receptors [16–22] (Figure 1).

This review provides a novel and comprehensive perspective on the role of sex differences in the lacrimal gland, encompassing structural characteristics, hormonal regulation, immune responses, and gene expression in the development and progression of DED. While many previous reviews have described DED as a multifactorial disease, few have specifically focused on how biological sex affects lacrimal gland function and contributes to the differences in disease prevalence and severity between sexes. By connecting the findings from experimental models and clinical studies, we aim to highlight how a deeper understanding of sex-based mechanisms may guide the development of more personalised approaches to diagnosis and treatment. This includes the potential use of sex-specific biomarkers for early detection, hormone-targeted therapies, and improved patient stratification in clinical settings.

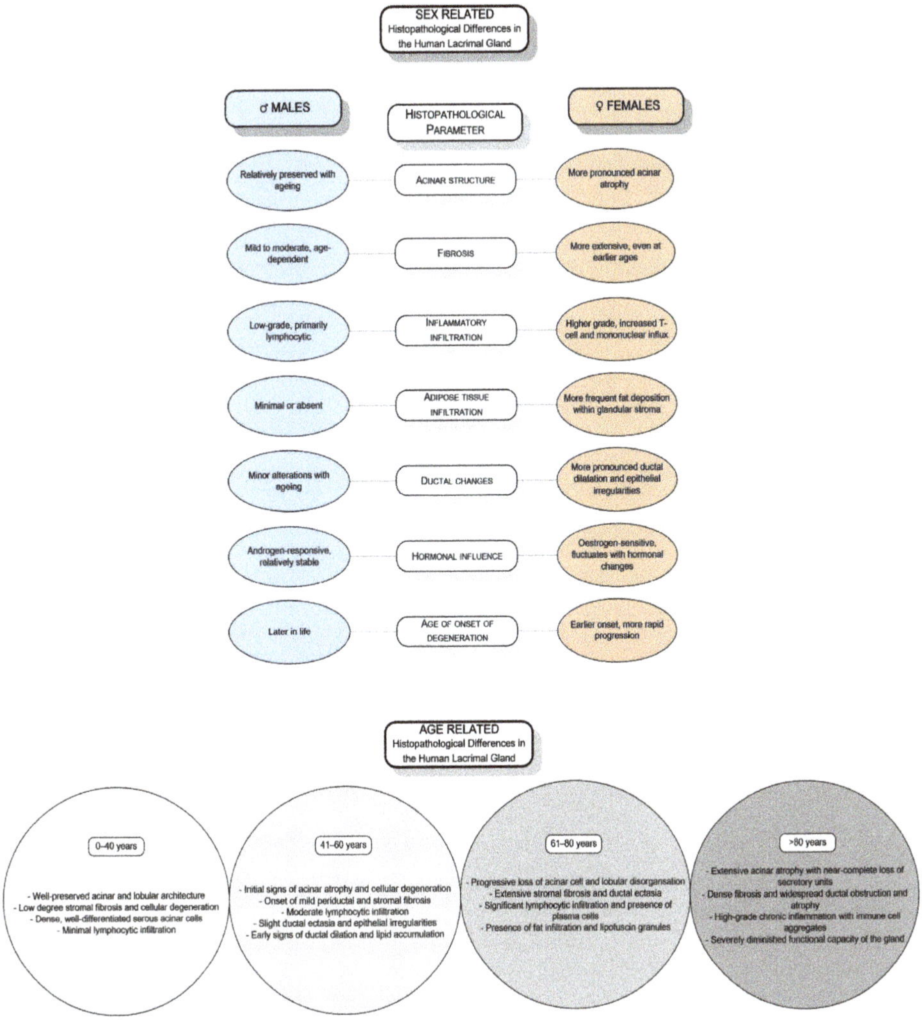

Figure 1. Sex- and age-related histopathological differences of the human lacrimal gland.

2. The Lacrimal Functional Unit

Tear production involves complex interactions among the nervous, muscular, endocrine, vascular, and immune systems [33]. The lacrimal gland is the primary source of tear film fluid, electrolytes, and proteins. Along with the accessory lacrimal glands, meibomian glands, conjunctiva, cornea, and neural reflex arc, it constitutes the lacrimal functional unit (LFU) [34]. The proper functioning of all LFU components is crucial for efficient ocular lubrication and the maintenance of ocular surface integrity [35]. Disruptions in any part of the LFU, often due to systemic or local inflammation, can lead to DED [34,36].

2.1. The Lacrimal Gland

Lacrimal glands are paired exocrine seromucous glands, essential components of the LFU [34], and histologically are classified as tubuloalveolar glands [18]. Tear secretion is a complex, multi-step process. Initially, acinar cells produce a primary fluid, an ultrafiltrate of plasma made of water and ions. As this fluid moves through the canal system, it is altered by ductal epithelial cells incorporating potassium and modifying the protein composition [37]. The final composition of tears includes sodium, potassium, magnesium, calcium, chloride, bicarbonate, and phosphate ions, all of which contribute to tear osmolarity. Ductal cells, which contain numerous secretory granules, play a crucial role in regulating the protein content of tears [33]. The tear film comprises diverse proteins; 491 have been identified, including lipocalin, lipophilin, lactoferrin, lysozyme, serum albumins, and IgA [38–41].

2.2. Tear Film

The tear film acts as a vital barrier, nourishing corneal layers, enabling gas exchange, and supplying nutrients to the avascular cornea. Additionally, the tear film protects the eye's surface from pathogens, aids wound healing, and enhances eye comfort and visual clarity [40,42]. The quality, quantity, and stability of the tear film are vital for preserving the optical quality, maintaining corneal transparency, and ensuring the integrity of the anterior eye surface [3,43,44]. Disorders affecting components of the LFU, predominantly due to systemic or local inflammation [34,36], often result in DED.

The tear film was traditionally described as having a tri-layered structure consisting of lipid, aqueous, and mucin layers. However, it is now recognised as being more intricately organised. The outer layer is primarily made of lipids along with intercalated proteins. The middle layer contains water, electrolytes, proteins, and mucins. Finally, the inner layer is viscous and connects the tear film to the corneal surface epithelial cells through transmembrane glycoproteins and mucins [45–47].

The precorneal tear film acts as a dynamic, integrated unit with distinct layers [48].

The 40 nm thick lipid layer is a critical component of the tear film, playing a vital role in maintaining ocular surface health by reducing evaporation, providing a smooth optical surface, lowering surface tension, preventing tear film collapse, and enabling the tear film to spread evenly across the eye's surface [43,49–54]. Understanding its composition and function is essential for addressing conditions like DED [55]. The lipid layer consists of two main phases: a thin polar phase adjacent to the aqueous layer and a thicker nonpolar phase at the air interface. The polar lipids, such as phospholipids, form a structural base with surfactant properties, while the nonpolar lipids, including wax esters and cholesteryl esters, provide barrier functions [53,56]. Lipids from the meibomian glands play a key role in preventing the collapse of the aqueous layer, with smaller contributions from Zeiss's and Moll's glands. Sex hormones, particularly androgens, significantly modulate the lipid profile of the meibomian glands, which are essential for maintaining the tear film's lipid layer. They primarily act by regulating lipid production and gene expression. Deficiency or dysfunction in androgen signalling can lead to significant meibomian gland dysfunction and contribute to DED [9,57–59]. Oestrogen receptors are present in the meibomian glands, indicating that oestrogens also influence these glands' function, primarily through the modulation of lipid production [60–62]. Oestrogen receptors are present in the meibomian glands, indicating that oestrogens also influence these glands' function, primarily through the modulation of lipid production. The effects of oestrogen on lipid layer formation remain controversial. Most studies suggest that oestrogens promote inflammation, decrease secretion from the meibomian glands, and inhibit lipogenesis, potentially contributing to DED symptoms, especially in postmenopausal women [63–66], while others suggest a protective role [67]. However, the direct impact of these hormonal changes on the stability and function of the lipid layer of the tear film remains unclear and warrants further investigation.

The aqueous and mucin layers together form a gel-like mucoaqueous layer. Most of the aqueous component is secreted by the lacrimal gland, with approximately 10% originating from accessory lacrimal glands [68,69]. Corneal and conjunctival epithelium also contribute to the aqueous component by secreting electrolytes, water, and mucins [33,34,70].

3. Dry Eye Disease

Dry eye disease, known as keratoconjunctivitis sicca, is a multifactorial condition characterised by instability and tear film deficiency. This leads to discomfort and visual impairment and is often associated with varying degrees of ocular surface epitheliopathy, inflammation, and neurosensory abnormalities [71–73]. The key diagnostic criteria for DED include tear film instability, inflammation, ocular discomfort, and visual impairment [73,74].

The pathophysiology of DED primarily involves evaporative water loss, which leads to hyperosmolar damage to the ocular tissues. This damage results in the loss of epithelial and goblet cells, directly or through induced inflammation [75]. The reduction in ocular surface moisture accelerates the tear film's rupture and further increases hyperosmolarity, creating a vicious cycle [43,74]. Persistent inflammation and epithelial breakdown expose nociceptive receptors on the eye's surface, triggering sensory nerve activation and causing discomfort. Additionally, the instability of the tear film disrupts its optical properties, contributing to visual impairment [44,73–79].

Mechanical abrasions due to lid margin disorders, such as the obstruction of meibomian gland openings and conjunctivochalasis, can cause micro-trauma of the ocular surface during blinking and affect tear dynamics. Eyelid abnormalities, including lagophthalmos, incomplete or reduced blinking, and poor eyelid-to-eye adhesion, can further contribute to tear film instability [74].

3.1. Classification of Dry Eye Disease

Dry eye disease is characterised by inadequate production or excessive evaporation of tears, leading to altered tear osmolarity and increased osmotic stress on the ocular surface [72,73]. DED can be categorised into two primary subtypes based on aetiology: aqueous tear-deficient dry eye and lipid-layer-deficient evaporative dry eye. It is not uncommon for patients to display features of both subtypes simultaneously [77]. Typically, meibomian gland dysfunction is associated with evaporative dry eye, while lacrimal gland dysfunction primarily relates to aqueous tear-deficient dry eye. It is now widely accepted that meibomian gland dysfunction can be classified into two categories based on gland secretion: the hyposecretory (or obstructive) subtype and the hypersecretory subtype [78]. More broadly, DED can be categorised into four subtypes: (1) lipid-deficient dry eye, resulting from abnormalities in the tear film's lipid layer; (2) aqueous-deficient dry eye, characterised by insufficient tear production, including cases of primary mucin deficiency; (3) dry eye induced by allergies or environmental irritants; and (4) dry eye associated with eyelid surface anomalies, including primary epitheliopathy and structural abnormalities of the eyelids. Dry eye with a lipid anomaly and dry eye with aqueous tear deficiency are the most common subcategories [62].

3.2. Prevalence of Dry Eye Disease

The prevalence of dry eye symptoms and tear film dysfunction increases with age, affecting between 5% and 34% of the population, depending on the diagnostic criteria and demographic factors [80]. In the United States, 6.8% of the adult population meets the diagnostic criteria for DED. The condition is notably more prevalent among older adults, with 2.7% of those aged 18–34 affected compared to 18.6% of those over 75. Furthermore, women are more frequently affected than men, with 8.8% of women and 4.5% of men experiencing dry eye symptoms [81].

Albietz et al. reported a dry eye prevalence of approximately 10.8%, with notably higher rates in individuals over the age of 40 (18.1%) compared to those under 40 (7.3%) [82]. The study identified lipid-anomaly dry eye as the most common subtype, occurring in 4.0% of the population, followed by allergic and toxic dry eye at 3.1%, lid-surfacing anomalies dry eye at 1.8%, and aqueous tear deficiencies at 1.7%. Notably, aqueous tear deficiencies exhibited a significant gender disparity, being more prevalent in women. Lipid-anomaly dry eye and aqueous tear deficiencies were significantly more common in individuals over 40 [79]. Since women face a 50–70% higher risk of developing DED, with the risk increasing further after menopause [4], both female gender and ageing are key risk factors for DED [4,36,79].

3.3. Risk Factors and Pathophysiology of Dry Eye Disease

Numerous factors influencing the development and progression of dry eye have been identified and can be categorised into intrinsic and extrinsic factors [83] (Figure 2). Intrinsic factors include autoimmune disorders [83–88], hormonal imbalances [75,89–91], systemic diseases such as diabetes mellitus [92,93], hereditary disorders [94,95], nerve damage [96,97], and intestinal dysbiosis [98,99].

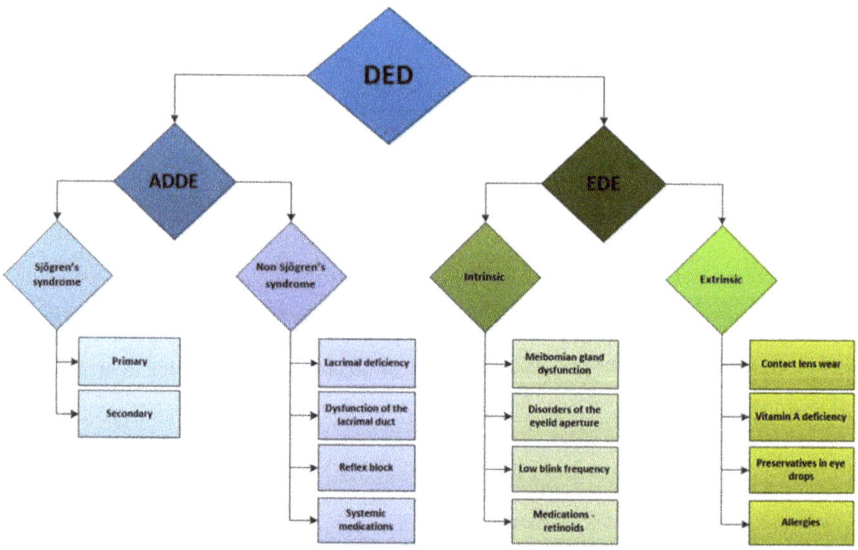

Figure 2. Schematic presentation of dry eye disease subtypes and etiological factors contributing to its development. DED: dry eye disease; ADDE: aqueous tear-deficient dry eye; EDE: evaporative dry eye.

Extrinsic factors encompass environmental influences affecting lacrimal function [100,101]. These include behaviours and habits such as smoking and excessive screen time [102–105], contact lens wearing [106], laser eye surgery [107–109], the use of certain systemic and ocular medications such as antidepressants, antipsychotics, beta-blockers, diuretics, oral contraceptives, and topical beta-blockers for glaucoma [110], and diets low in omega-3 fatty acids [111,112].

The most prevalent autoimmune disorder associated with DED is Sjögren's syndrome, which primarily affects the lacrimal and salivary glands and has a significant female predominance, with over 90% of patients being women [93]. Other autoimmune disorders, such as sarcoidosis and Graves' disease, can also cause non-infectious dacryoadenitis and DED. Less commonly, dry eye may arise from other chronic inflammatory conditions, including IgG4-related disease, inflammatory orbital pseudotumor, chronic graft-versus-host disease, and diabetes, as well as from radiation and infections such as HIV, CMV, and hepatitis C [3,111].

Emerging evidence underscores the significant role of chronic inflammation in DED. Research indicates that chronic inflammation and autoimmunity are primary etiological factors contributing to DED. Elevated levels of inflammatory mediators, including IL-1β, IL-6, IL-8, TNF-α, IL-17, and IFN-γ, have been found in the conjunctiva and tear fluid of patients with dry eye compared to healthy controls [9,112,113]. Furthermore, DED is associated with several pathological changes, including an increased production of matrix metalloproteinases, heightened levels of chemokines and oxidative stress markers, and exacerbated squamous metaplasia of the ocular surface epithelium. These changes are accompanied by a loss of goblet cells and increased endoplasmic reticulum stress [40,114].

With ageing, the immune system becomes dysregulated, leading to changes in antibodies and cytokines and a decline in immunity, with an increase in autoimmunity. The lacrimal gland also undergoes functional changes, such as reduced innervation and secretory activity [115]. Structural changes include atrophy of acini and fibrosis, periductal fibrosis, ductal dilation and proliferation, lymphocytic infiltration, and fatty infiltration [17]. These structural changes correlate with a decline in the gland's secretory function [17,33].

4. The Role of Sex Steroid Hormones in the Development of Sex Differences in Dry Eye Disease

SSHs, particularly androgens and oestrogens, significantly influence the structure and function of the human lacrimal gland, which is crucial for tear production and ocular health. These hormones interact with specific receptors in the lacrimal gland, affecting its physiology and potentially contributing to conditions like dry eye disease. Sex differences mainly develop throughout complex interactions of SSHs at the local and systemic levels, such as receptor expression and gene regulation, but this complex mechanism has not been elucidated [1,2,6,9,23,57,59,62].

SSHs are a subset of steroid hormones derived from cholesterol. They play a crucial role in regulating various physiological processes related to sexual development and reproduction. In humans, SSHs are classified into three main groups: androgens, oestrogens, and gestagens [13,116–118]. Androgens, often classified as male hormones, are present in both males and females. Key androgens include dehydroepiandrosterone sulphate, dehydroepiandrosterone, androstenedione, testosterone, and dihydrotestosterone. Oestrogens, primarily known as female hormones, also have a significant role in males. Key oestrogens include estrone, 17-β-estradiol, and estriol. Gestagens are involved in regulating the menstrual cycle and maintaining pregnancy. Key gestagens are progesterone and 17α-hydroxyprogesterone. Each of these hormones has specific functions, but they often interact with each other to maintain hormonal balance and support various bodily functions [116–118].

4.1. Synthesis of Sex Steroid Hormones

The synthesis of SSHs in the human body shows gender-specific patterns, including differences in hormone levels, predominant types, and secretion rhythms. Women primarily produce β-estradiol, whereas men have higher testosterone levels.

Steroidogenesis is the process by which cholesterol is converted into biologically active steroid hormones. This conversion occurs in the gonads, adrenal cortex, and various tissues throughout the body. The regulatory control of steroidogenesis is exerted by trophic hormones from the anterior lobe of the pituitary gland, namely follicle-stimulating hormone, luteinising hormone, and adrenocorticotropic hormone. Within the target cell, steroidogenesis is facilitated by enzymes found in the mitochondria and the smooth endoplasmic reticulum.

The initial step involves the transfer of cholesterol to the inner mitochondrial membrane, a process regulated by the steroidogenic acute regulatory protein. Cholesterol is then converted into pregnenolone, the precursor for all mineralocorticoids, glucocorticoids, and SSHs, through the action of the cytochrome P450 SCC enzyme CYP11A1. Pregnenolone is converted into either progesterone or 17-hydroxypregnenolone. Progesterone is a mineralocorticoid precursor, while 17-hydroxypregnenolone is a precursor for androgens, oestrogens, and glucocorticoids. Oestrogens are produced from androgens through aromatisation, and dihydrotestosterone is formed from testosterone by the action of 5α-reductase [119] (Figure 3).

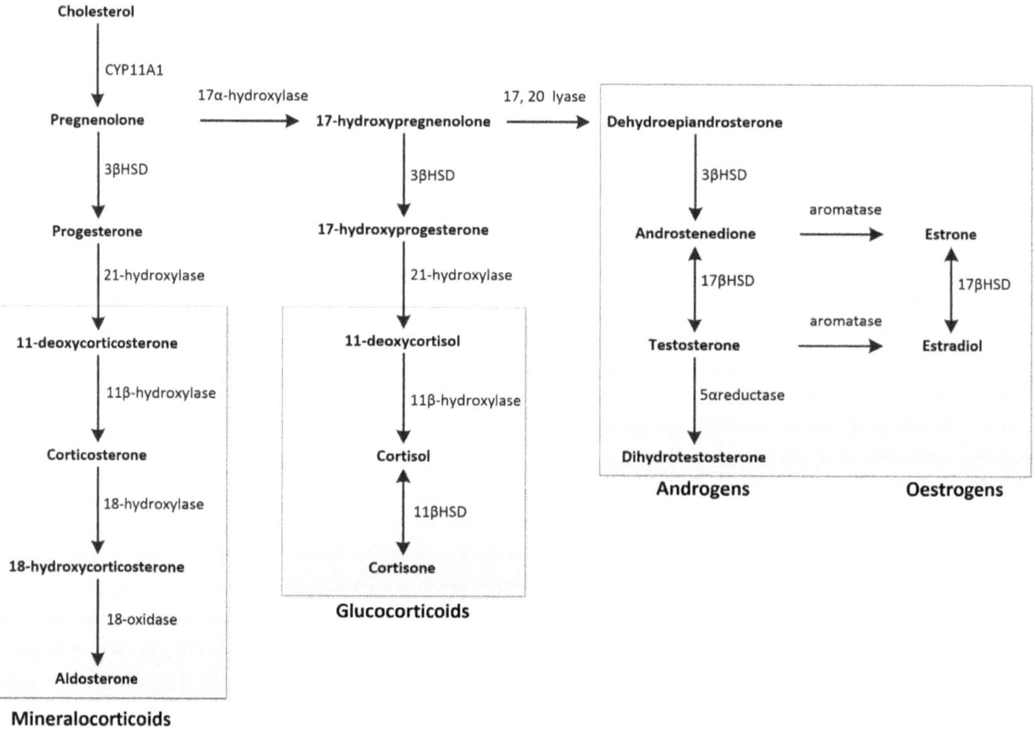

Figure 3. Schematic overview of steroidogenesis: Steroidogenesis begins with cholesterol, converted into pregnenolone, the precursor for all mineralocorticoids, glucocorticoids, and sex steroids. Pregnenolone can be metabolised into either progesterone or 17-hydroxypregnenolone. Progesterone serves as the primary precursor for mineralocorticoids. 17-hydroxypregnenolone acts as the precursor for all androgens, oestrogens, and glucocorticoids. Androgens can undergo aromatisation to form oestrogens, while testosterone can be converted into dihydrotestosterone through 5α-reductase action.

In the testicles, Leydig cells, located in the interstitium between seminiferous tubules, predominantly synthesise testosterone [120]. SSHs are synthesised in small amounts in the third layer (zona reticularis) within the adrenal gland cortex, with androstenedione being the primary product. In the ovary, granulosa cells predominantly produce progesterone and 17-β-estradiol, while theca cells produce androgens, and luteal cells produce progesterone [119].

Recent studies have demonstrated that various tissues express enzymes capable of activating steroid precursors, a process known as extra-glandular steroid activation, and synthesising active steroids de novo through a mechanism of extracrine steroidogenesis. As a result, many tissues and organs previously considered non-steroidogenic are now recognised for their ability to biosynthesise steroids. Local steroid hormone synthesis is well-established in the brain [121,122], spinal cord [123], and peripheral nerves [124], where these hormones are collectively referred to as neurosteroids [124–127]. Moreover, the extra-glandular steroidogenesis of SSHs has been identified in various tissues, including adipose tissue [128], skin [129], exocrine glands [130], the small intestine [131], and the kidneys [130]. Furthermore, the local synthesis of glucocorticoids has been documented in the intestinal mucosa [126,130] and thymus [127,132–137]. SSHs, along with genetic and environmental factors, play a crucial role in the development of sexual differences. The biological significance of extra-glandular steroidogenesis is associated with paracrine, autocrine, or intracrine signalling being mediated by these locally produced molecules [122]. Furthermore, the synthesis of these steroids is often regulated by complex multifactorial systems independent of hypothalamic and pituitary control. Therefore, measuring local steroid levels is frequently a more precise indicator of steroid action within specific tissues when compared to systemic levels [123].

4.2. Steroid Hormone Receptors

Steroid hormone receptors belong to the nuclear receptor superfamily and function as ligand-dependent transcription factors [124]. This superfamily encompasses androgen receptor (AR), oestrogen receptor (ER), progesterone receptor (PR), glucocorticoid, and mineralocorticoid receptors [128,133], in addition to retinoic acid and thyroid hormone receptors [124].

The role of SSHs in shaping sexual differences is intricate, as research has shown that specific hormones exert sexually distinct, tissue-specific, and cell-specific effects [138–140]. SSHs and genetic and environmental factors are essential in developing gender differences. mRNA for AR, ER, and PR is present in various ocular tissues, including the lacrimal and meibomian glands, eyelids, palpebral and bulbar conjunctiva, cornea, iris, ciliary body, lens, retina, choroid, and retinal pigment epithelial cells in rats, rabbits, and humans [140–143].

It is recognised that sex-related differences in the prevalence of DED are predominantly linked to the influences of SSHs, the hypothalamic–pituitary axis, corticosteroids, insulin, IGF-1, pineal hormones, along with sex chromosomes, sex-specific autosomal factors, and epigenetic factors [4]. As ageing causes a reduction in SSH levels, both androgen and oestrogen become vital in the pathophysiology of lacrimal gland dysfunction. Importantly, androgens are significant, and their deficiency is connected with dysfunction in the meibomian and lacrimal glands, which contributes to DED [7–9,13,63,142,143].

Experimental studies involving castration or androgen antagonist exposure in mice have shown considerable changes in the anatomy and physiology of the lacrimal gland. These changes include degenerative alterations such as reduced growth, loss of glandular tissue, diminished size of acini and nuclei, nuclear polymorphism, increased connective tissue proliferation, disruptions in protein levels, changes in enzyme activity, modifications in fluid and protein secretion, and altered gland morphology, leading to feminisation of the male gland [142].

4.3. Androgens

Androgens regulate the expression of over 2200 genes in the lacrimal gland of mice and approximately 3000 genes in the human meibomian gland and conjunctival epithelial cells [28,144]. These genes are involved in various functions, including cell growth, proliferation, metabolism, cell communication and transport, nucleic acid binding, signal transduction, and receptor activity. Thus, androgens exert a multi-faceted influence on the structure and function of the lacrimal gland at multiple levels [7,10,25,29,145–147]. Androgen deficiency has also been noted in women with Sjögren's syndrome, suggesting that androgens may facilitate disease progression rather than cause it directly [141,148].

Androgen receptors have been identified in acinar and epithelial cells of the lacrimal ducts [26,149]. Androgens also affect the expression of their receptors in the lacrimal gland, increasing androgen receptor protein levels while decreasing androgen receptor mRNA levels. In a mouse model, androgen administration significantly increases the number of cells containing androgen receptors and the density of these receptors within the nuclei of epithelial cells in the lacrimal gland. This regulatory effect is specific to androgens, as similar effects are not observed with oestrogen, glucocorticoids, or cyclophosphamide. Importantly, cessation of androgen therapy leads to a substantial decrease in AR expression [26,150–152].

4.4. Oestrogens

Previous research on the effects of oestrogen on the lacrimal glands has yielded inconsistent results [4,13,27,29,153]. Hormone replacement therapy, including oestrogen and medroxyprogesterone acetate, has been shown to enhance tear production, although it does not necessarily improve tear quality [154,155]. Reduced lacrimal gland function has been noted in postmenopausal or ovariectomised women, as well as in women using oral contraceptives, despite fluctuations in oestrogen levels [156,157].

Oestrogen has demonstrated an anti-inflammatory effect in mouse models of Sjögren's syndrome, which contrasts with the findings from studies showing that hormone replacement therapy in postmenopausal women is associated with an increased risk of DED [11]. This discrepancy may arise from the differential effects of high versus low doses of oestrogen on inflammation [10,11]. Research suggests that lower doses of oestrogen can promote cell survival and provide protective effects against inflammation in exocrine glands, whereas higher doses may exacerbate inflammatory responses [12,158–160].

Recent research suggests that oestrogen and progesterone have a relatively minor influence on sex-related differences in gene expression and structural variations in the lacrimal gland compared to androgens [161,162]. However, Hat et al., in their analysis of 35 human lacrimal gland tissue samples from 19 cornea donors, observed significantly higher ERα mRNA expression than AR and ERβ [163]. Furthermore, antiandrogenic therapy in men does not appear to affect tear secretion, emphasising a sex-specific role of androgens in lacrimal gland function. While testosterone and dihydrotestosterone have shown efficacy in rat models, the current evidence is insufficient to justify their use in human clinical trials [164]. The presence of mRNAs for steroidogenic enzymes in the human lacrimal gland indicates the potential for intracrine synthesis and metabolism of sex steroids, offering valuable insights into the complex relationship between systemic sex hormone levels and DED [130].

5. Sexual Dimorphism and the Development of Sexual Differences

Sexual dimorphism is any structural difference between male and female individuals of the same species [165], excluding differences directly related to reproduction. It broadly encompasses sex differences across the genome, transcriptome, proteome, metabolome, and phenotype [166]. Most sexually dimorphic traits evolved through sexual selection to enhance reproductive success, with a smaller proportion shaped by natural selection [167,168]. Natural, sexual, and environmental selections interact as individuals and are influenced by their surroundings [169,170]. In sexually reproducing species, differences between males and females typically reflect sexual dimorphism, ranging from subtle to pronounced depending on the species.

In mammals, sex is categorised as binary, distinguishing between male and female individuals. The process of sex differentiation involves a series of events during foetal development that shape an individual's sex, including the formation of gonads and the secretion of sex hormones. This process is sequentially divided into three phases: the determination of chromosomal sex at fertilisation, the establishment of gonadal sex, and the development of primary sexual characteristics. Postnatally, the deepening of sex differences is mainly influenced by sex hormone levels and environmental and behavioural factors, with the most pronounced changes occurring during puberty [116,171]. The factors impacting the development of sex differences are schematically illustrated in Figure 4.

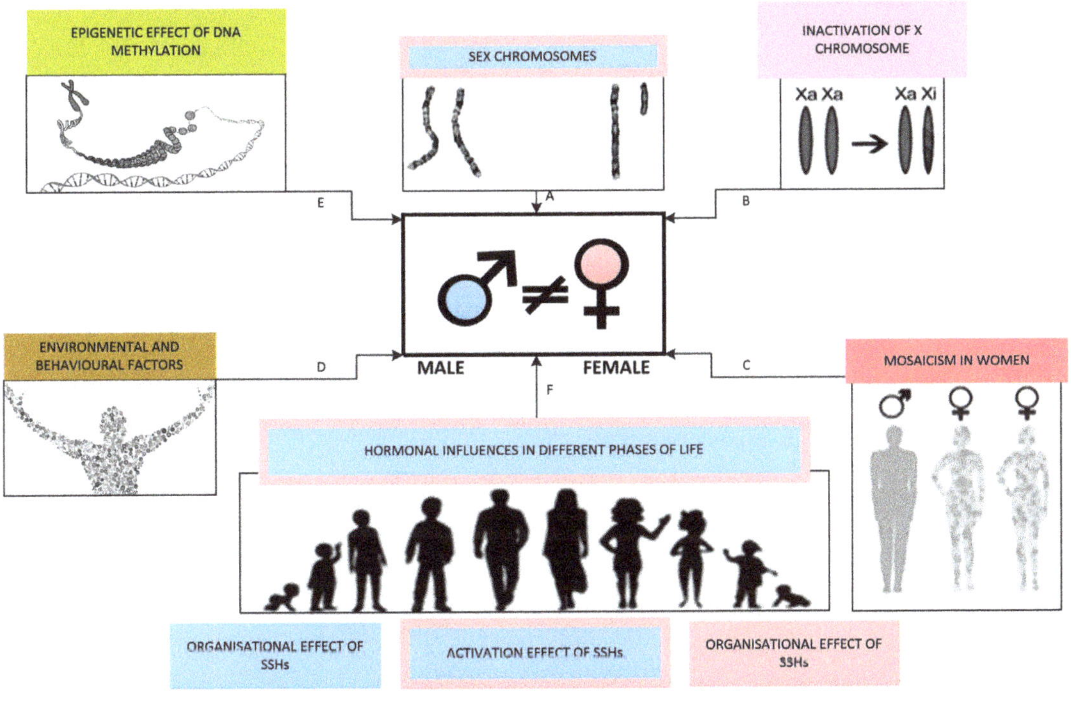

Figure 4. Factors influencing the development of sex differences: (**A**) Sex chromosomes determine chromosomal sex, with the Y chromosome facilitating male gonadal differentiation through the *sex-determining region Y gene*. (**B**) Different extents of X chromosome inactivation contribute to sex differences. (**C**) Mosaicism occurs in various tissues in females. (**D**) Environmental and behavioural factors directly impact sex steroid hormone receptors as endocrine disruptors and induce epigenetic changes. (**E**) Epigenetic influences are primarily mediated through DNA methylation. (**F**) Levels of SSHs at various life stages play a crucial role in shaping and enhancing sex differences.

6. Sexual Dimorphism of the Lacrimal Gland

The public health burden of DED prompted numerous studies focused on the genetic, hormonal, pathophysiological, biochemical, and molecular basis of this disorder [15]. In the mid-20th century, interest in the histological features of the lacrimal gland increased significantly due to its crucial role in maintaining ocular surface homeostasis. Various animal models have been developed to elucidate the physiology and pathophysiology of lacrimal gland dysfunction and its contribution to DED. As a result, most of the current research has been conducted using these animal models [10,23,24,32,172]. Studies involving human subjects are comparatively rare [16,17,149,163,173–176].

6.1. Sexual Dimorphism of the Lacrimal Gland in Animal Models

Previous research has confirmed the presence of sex differences across various mammalian species. However, interpreting these results requires careful consideration of the structural differences in the lacrimal glands among different laboratory animals [173,177,178], such as mice, rats, rabbits, and hamsters. Most research on animal models highlights substantial structural changes in the lacrimal gland, including inflammatory infiltration, loss of innervation, and the progression of degenerative changes in glandular tissue with age. These changes lead to functional impacts on the quantity and composition of tears [177].

The most commonly observed structural alterations include acinar degeneration, connective tissue proliferation, periductal and periacinar fibrosis, lymphocytic infiltration, proliferation of excretory ducts, and ductal dilation, with thinning of their walls [179,180]. Research indicates that acini undergo a progressive transition with age, shifting from serous to seromucous and eventually to mucous acini, which leads to decreased protein and increased mucus production [181]. These structural alterations in the lacrimal glands of older rats have been linked to reduced tear production, lower protein content in tears, and changes in the corneal epithelium [16,142,176,180,182–184]. In the rat model, female lacrimal glands have a smaller surface area but higher acinar density when compared with male glands, with more pronounced differences in older age groups [180]. Similar findings were observed in prostaglandin receptor knockout mice (PRLR -/-) [185], suggesting more significant acinar atrophy in females. In older female samples, periacinar fibrosis was markedly more pronounced [180]. Additionally, females exhibited more extensive proliferation of excretory ducts, while males showed more significant lymphocytic infiltration and females more mast cell infiltration [180,185].

Sex, SSHs, and environmental factors are recognised as key regulators of the ocular surface and adnexal tissues, influencing the prevalence of DED between sexes [4]. Beyond the well-documented physiological differences in SSH levels between males and females, research has revealed sex-specific variations in the regulation of gene expression activated by these hormones. For instance, sex differences in AR expression have been identified in rat lacrimal glands [150]. In ovariectomised mice, testosterone, estradiol, and progesterone regulate the expression of thousands of genes in the lacrimal and meibomian glands. Although many genes regulated by testosterone in female tissues are similar to those in males, distinct sex-specific differences in gene activation have been observed. In some cases, androgens have even opposite effects on the same gene depending on the sex, highlighting how these sex differences in gene regulation contribute to sexual dimorphism [28,32,180].

While current research confirms the presence of sex differences in various mammalian species, it is essential to consider the differences in lacrimal gland structure across different species of laboratory animals when interpreting the results [173,186–188]. Studies using various animal models have significantly advanced our understanding of the molecular, endocrine, and immunological mechanisms underlying sex-related differences in the structure and function of the lacrimal gland [25,27,29,31,139,147,172,182]. However, species-specific anatomical and physiological characteristics limit the direct translation of these findings to human biology. Bridging this gap requires validation through human-focused research to ensure accurate interpretation and clinical relevance of the sex-based differences observed in preclinical studies.

6.2. Sexual Dimorphism of the Human Lacrimal Gland

Sex differences have been observed in various ocular structures, including the meibomian gland, lacrimal gland, conjunctiva, cornea, anterior chamber, iris, ciliary body, lens, vitreous body, retina, nasolacrimal duct, and tear film. The influence of SSHs on these structures has also been documented [4,16,152,179,181,183,184,187,189–191]. Research on human eye tissues and the lacrimal apparatus has confirmed sex differences in tissue morphology, gene expression, protein and lipid synthesis, secretory activity, immune function, cell density, epithelial dynamics, permeability, immune response, tear film stability, blink rate, and visual acuity [4,26,28]. These sex-related differences play a significant role in the onset and progression of various eye diseases, such as DED, refractive errors, myopia, glaucoma, cataracts, age-related macular degeneration, diabetic retinopathy, vernal keratoconjunctivitis, impaired vision, and blindness [192–197].

A limited number of studies on human lacrimal gland tissue have primarily focused on age-related pathohistological changes, with only a few addressing sex differences (Table 1). The most frequently observed pathohistological changes include reductions in gland weight, fibrosis, atrophy of acini, alterations in ductal structures, and lymphocytic infiltration [6,16,17,19–21,23,149,157,173–176,185,198,199].

Table 1. Studies on sexual dimorphism of the human lacrimal gland.

Author (Year)	Sample	Methodology	Main Findings and Conclusions
Waterhouse et al. (1963) [19]	Human cadaveric lacrimal glands (238 autopsy specimens: 159 females, 67 males)	Histopathological examination: Focal adenitis (inflammatory foci) in lacrimal gland tissue was identified	A higher prevalence of focal adenitis in female lacrimal glands, particularly in women over 45 years old
Damato et al. (1984) [173]	Human cadaveric lacrimal glands (99 specimens: 52 males, 47 females)	Histopathology and immunohistochemistry: Assessed acinar atrophy, periductal fibrosis, lymphocytic infiltration, and ductal changes. Investigated B lymphocyte subpopulations in 35 cases	Identified progressive acinar atrophy, fibrosis, and inflammation with age Chronic inflammation leads to ductal obstruction and lacrimal gland dysfunction No significant sex differences in B lymphocyte subpopulations
Cornell-Bell et al. (1985) [16]	Human cadaveric lacrimal glands (10 specimens: 5 males, 5 females)	Stereology, histology: Measured acinar surface area	Found a 21% difference in acinar size (larger in males: 2.18 mm^2 vs. 1.80 mm^2 in females) Suggested sex differences in lacrimal gland structure may be linked to androgen levels
Roen JL (1985) [164]	Human cadaveric lacrimal glands (32 specimens)	Histopathology: Examined lacrimal gland tissue for degenerative changes and inflammatory markers	Chronic inflammation and periductal fibrosis were found in 75% of samples, more common in individuals over 50. Fibrosis likely contributes to lacrimal gland dysfunction with age

Table 1. *Cont.*

Author (Year)	Sample	Methodology	Main Findings and Conclusions
Obata et al. (1995) [17]	Human cadaveric lacrimal glands (80 specimens)	Histopathology: Fibrosis, acinar atrophy, periductal fibrosis, ductal proliferation, and lymphocytic infiltration in the palpebral and orbital lobes were analysed	Diffuse fibrosis and acinar atrophy are more frequent in older women, particularly in the orbital lobe. Findings suggest these degenerative changes contribute to dry eye disease in postmenopausal women
Smith et al. (1999) [149]	Human lacrimal glands	Immunohistochemistry: Identified the location and distribution of androgen receptors in lacrimal gland tissue	ARs identified in the nuclei and cytoplasm of lacrimal acinar and ductal cells. Staining intensity and number of AR-positive cells varied among specimens. ARs are also detected in interstitial and inflammatory cells surrounding acinar units. Androgens likely play a regulatory role in lacrimal gland function. Presence of ARs in interstitial and immune cells suggests a broader role in immune modulation and glandular homeostasis
Rocha et al. (2000) [6]	Human lacrimal glands (2 specimens: 1 male, 1 female)	RT-PCR, immunohistochemistry: Analysed mRNA and protein expression of sex steroid receptors	Confirmed mRNA expression of ARs, ERs, and PRs in lacrimal gland tissue, suggesting local hormonal regulation of gland function
Wickham et al. (2000) [23]	Human lacrimal glands (3 specimens)	RT-PCR, agarose gel electrophoresis, Southern blot hybridisation: Detected mRNA for ARs, ERs, and PRs	Identified AR, ER, and PR mRNAs, suggesting lacrimal glands act as target organs for sex steroids.
Spelsberg et al. (2004) [199]	Human cadaveric lacrimal glands (20 samples from 13 cornea donors)	RT-PCR, immunohistochemistry: Detected ERs (ERα and Erβ) in lacrimal tissues.	ERα mRNA: found in 10 lacrimal gland tissue samples. ERβ mRNA: found in 9 lacrimal gland tissue samples. Postmortem time: no influence on the expression grade of ERα and ERβ. Immunohistochemical evaluation for ERα: weak staining was observed in 2 lacrimal gland samples, likely due to the thermolability of ERs and small sample sizes. Suggested potential role of estrogens in keratoconjunctivitis sicca

Table 1. *Cont.*

Author (Year)	Sample	Methodology	Main Findings and Conclusions
Lorber and Vidić (2009) [20]	Human cadaveric lacrimal glands (45 specimens: 22 males, 23 females)	Morphometric analysis: Measured lacrimal gland size and weight	Male lacrimal glands had greater absolute size and weight than female glands, suggesting structural sex differences
Gligorijević et al. (2011) [198]	Human lacrimal glands (20 specimens: 10 males, 10 females)	Immunohistochemistry: Stained for ERs and PRs	ER and PR are present in both sexes but are significantly higher in females ($p < 0.001$). The highest expression in women aged 30–50 indicates age- and sex-related differences in receptor expression.
Bukhari et al. (2014) [21]	MRI of lacrimal glands (998 lacrimal glands from 499 patients)	MRI study: Measured lacrimal gland volume across age groups, sexes, and racial backgrounds. Imaging Technique: Fat-saturated fluid-attenuated inversion recovery (FLAIR) images Volume Calculation: TeraRecon iNtuition viewer software	Lacrimal glands were larger in women. Maximum gland volume observed in the second decade of life
Hat et al. (2023) [174]	Human lacrimal glands (81 specimens: 34 females, 47 males)	Histopathology, stereology: Assessed degenerative changes and volume densities of glandular components	Acinar atrophy is significantly more prevalent in females, and ductal dilation more common in males. Females had higher fat/connective tissue volume, suggesting greater susceptibility to age-related changes
Hat et al. (2023) [163]	Human lacrimal glands (35 specimens from 19 donors: 10 females, 9 males)	qPCR: Quantification of mRNA expression for AR, ERα, and ERβ IHC Staining: Performed on selected samples to evaluate protein expression of the receptors	ERα mRNA expression was significantly higher than AR and Erβ, with no significant differences in receptor expression between sexes or correlation with age, suggesting ERα dominance in the human lacrimal gland function

RT-PCR: reverse transcriptase-polymerase chain reaction; AR: androgen receptor; ER: oestrogen receptor; PR: progesterone receptor; MRI: magnetic resonance imaging; qPCR: quantitative polymerase chain reaction; IHC: immunohistochemical.

Prager A. 1966 first described senile alterations in the lacrimal gland, noting reductions in gland weight, fibrosis, and acinar atrophy [176]. Similar age-related changes were also reported in a study of 99 cadaveric glands conducted by Damato et al. [173]. They identified several key changes: acinar atrophy, excretory duct obstruction, and periductal fibrosis, accompanied by the infiltration of lymphocytes and polymorphonuclear cells. They also observed mild vasculitis of the periductal blood vessels, which could contribute to chronic inflammation in this region. Their findings suggest that acinar atrophy and fibrosis can begin before middle age but become significantly more pronounced with advancing age [173]. These findings highlight the importance of ductal changes, proposing that repeated episodes of subclinical inflammation over a lifetime may lead to obstruction of the excretory ducts. This obstruction can result in periductal fibrosis that progressively extends into the lobules. The resulting obstruction and subsequent dilation and tortuosity of the ducts, sometimes reaching the point of cystic formation, can lead to variability in the acinar atrophy among different lobules [173].

Supporting these observations from Damato et al. [173], Roen JL and colleagues [185] studied 32 cadaveric lacrimal glands. They found that 75% exhibited microscopic abnormalities, with chronic inflammation and periductal fibrosis being the most common histopathological features. Notably, 52% of glands from individuals over 50 showed periductal fibrosis, while 74% exhibited ductal changes.

While current research has provided valuable insights into age-related changes in the lacrimal gland, research on sex differences in the human lacrimal gland regarding structure and function remains limited. Until now, few studies have investigated the sex differences in the human lacrimal gland. In 1963, Waterhouse reported a higher incidence of focal adenitis in the female lacrimal glands [19]. The first systematic investigation into sex differences in the structure of the human lacrimal gland was published by Cornell-Bell and colleagues in 1985 [16]. Using stereology software, they measured the surface area of 50 acini, revealing a 21% difference between sexes, with average acinus areas of 2.18 mm^2 in men and 1.80 mm^2 in women. This study was conducted on a sample of five glands per sex. Additionally, they measured acinar diameter in a lacrimal gland in rats, mice, guinea pigs, and rabbits, identifying significant interspecies differences, suggesting a potential correlation between sex differences and androgen levels [16].

The most comprehensive investigation of the pathohistological features of the human lacrimal gland and sex-related differences was conducted by Obata et al. [17]. They analysed 80 donor cadaveric lacrimal glands and thoroughly examined eight pathohistological features: fibrosis, acinar atrophy, periductal fibrosis, interlobular ductal dilation, interlobular ductal proliferation, lymphocytic foci, periductal lymphocytic infiltration, and fatty infiltration in both the orbital and palpebral lobes. The study found a statistically significant higher prevalence of diffuse fibrosis and diffuse acinar atrophy in women over 60. The findings suggest notable sex differences in pathohistological features and propose a potential link between specific pathohistological changes and DED [17]. Additionally, research into sex differences in lacrimal gland weight has indicated that male glands tend to have greater absolute weight [20]. A magnetic resonance imaging study showed that the thickness and area of the lacrimal gland decreased with age in women but not in men [200].

In a recent study, Hat et al. [174] investigated the pathohistological features of the ageing human lacrimal gland and found notable differences based on sex. Their research demonstrated that the connective tissue and fat volume density within the lacrimal gland of female subjects increases with age. In contrast, no significant correlation between age and these parameters was observed in male subjects, suggesting that age-related connective and fatty degeneration is more pronounced in women. The study also highlighted that, in males, intralobular fibrosis becomes more prominent with age, as indicated by a significant increase in the volume density of intralobular connective tissue. However, the volume density of intralobular adipose tissue did not exhibit a statistically significant correlation with age in either gender, indicating it is not a major factor in age-related degenerative changes [174]. According to the research by Hat et al. [174], periacinar fibrosis does not seem to depend on age or sex, which contrasts with the findings by Obata et al. [17], who found a significant positive correlation between acinar atrophy and age in both sexes, with a notably higher prevalence in women. The predominance of interlobular ductal dilation in the palpebral lobes suggests obstruction of tear outflow in the conjunctival fornix [17]. In contrast, Hat et al. [174] reported a significantly higher frequency of ductal dilation in male glands, probably caused by the unequal representation of palpebral and orbital lobes in their samples. Additionally, their study observed lymphocytic infiltration in 69% of subjects, with no gender differences, which is consistent with earlier findings [173,175].

It is believed that chromosomes, genes, and SSHs are key factors driving the development of sex differences. However, their specific contributions to the structure and function of the lacrimal gland remain incompletely understood. The impact of SSHs on the human lacrimal gland is particularly noteworthy due to its role in the development of DED [142,185]. Despite the established presence of SSH receptors in various eye tissues [196], research on this subject is limited [23,150,197].

Previous studies by Smith et al. [149] and Rocha et al. [6] reported the immunohistochemical identification of androgen receptor protein in the human lacrimal gland. On the other hand, Rocha et al. found AR in two human lacrimal gland samples with mRNA for 5α-reductase, suggesting local regulation of androgen levels in the lacrimal gland [6]. Further, two studies have reported immunohistochemical detection of ER in the human lacrimal gland. One study showed weak staining in a small number of acinus cells in 12 out of 20 cadaveric lacrimal gland samples; another study detected ERβ in 9 out of 10 samples and a weak ERα signal outside the cell nucleus in 2 out of 10 samples [198].

Wickham et al. detected androgen, oestrogen, and progesterone receptor mRNA expression in a sample from three human lacrimal glands. However, their study did not quantify the results or examine the differences between the sexes. Additionally, their research found mRNA for these receptors in lacrimal gland acinar epithelial cells, meibomian glands, the eyelid and bulbar conjunctiva, the cornea, the iris/ciliary body, the lens, the retina/uvea, and retinal pigment cells in rat, rabbits, and human samples [23]. Similarly, Spelsberg et al. detected mRNA for ERα and ERβ in several ocular tissues, including the lacrimal gland, using samples from ten donor lacrimal glands but did not quantify the results or investigate sex differences [199].

The first study to quantify the mRNA expression of SSH receptors (AR, ERα, and ERβ) in the human lacrimal gland was conducted by Hat et al. [163]. This study not only quantified and compared the relative mRNA expression of these receptors but also performed immunohistochemical verification and quantification of the corresponding proteins, offering new insights into the complex factors contributing to sex differences in the human lacrimal gland. This study confirmed the presence of AR, ERα, and ERβ mRNA in the human lacrimal gland using quantitative polymerase chain reaction and, for the first time, quantified their relative mRNA expression levels. It was found that the relative mRNA expression of ERα was significantly higher than that of AR and ERβ. No sex-related differences were observed in the relative mRNA expression of these sex hormone receptors, nor was there any correlation between mRNA expression and age. Immunohistochemical analysis further demonstrated that the protein expression levels of ERα and AR corresponded with their mRNA expression levels [163], suggesting more complex mechanisms of regulation of SSH receptor expression.

7. Perspective and Conclusions

Many sex differences emerge from hormonal influences and genetic variations between the sexes. Advances in molecular biology have highlighted that "every cell has a gender", underscoring the importance of studying sex differences at the cellular and molecular levels. This approach enhances our understanding of how genes drive biological organisation across cells, organs, and organ systems. Furthermore, it sheds light on the roles of sex chromosomes, hormones, and epigenetic mechanisms in shaping physiological differences and their implications for health and disease.

The lacrimal gland has garnered increasing research interest over recent decades due to its critical role in maintaining tear film homeostasis. This attention has led to the development of animal models to explore its physiology, pathophysiology, and contributions to DED [23,24,172,201].

Despite this growing interest, research on human lacrimal glands remains sparse, leaving many questions unanswered. Existing studies have confirmed sex-related differences in the ocular tissues' morphology, physiology, and pathology, including the lacrimal gland. These differences are primarily shaped by sex chromosomes, genes, SSHs, and environmental factors [10,14,16,17]. However, sex differences in this area often receive insufficient attention.

While it is evident that sex differences arise from a complex interplay of genetic, hormonal, and environmental factors, the specific contributions of each remain unclear [116]. Most documented differences are linked to gene expression variations, heavily influenced by SSHs [29,32,180]. Studies have shown that sex chromosomes alone cannot induce sex differences in the lacrimal glands without the influence of SSHs [31]. Sex significantly affects gene expression in the lacrimal glands, with females showing an increased expression of the genes related to inflammation and immune responses in certain autoimmune conditions like Sjögren syndrome. Over 490 genes in the mouse lacrimal gland show sex-related differential expression, affecting various biological processes and molecular functions [29,32]. The presence of androgen and oestrogen receptors in the lacrimal gland suggests a genetic basis for the hormonal regulation of these differences [163,202]. In the absence of sex hormones, as seen in SF-1 knockout mice, sexual dimorphism in the lacrimal gland is absent, indicating that sex chromosomes alone cannot induce sex differences in lacrimal glands without the influence of SSHs [31]. Additionally, studies on animal models, including ovariectomised and orchiectomised rats, have shown that although androgen receptor expression levels are similar in both sexes, intact male rats exhibit significantly higher androgen receptor levels. This indicates that androgens can independently regulate their receptor expression [7,8]. Additionally, imbalances in steroid hormone levels, either in excess or deficiency, modulate receptor activity through up- and down-regulation processes [203].

In men, serum testosterone levels naturally decline between the ages of 35 and 40, decreasing by approximately 0.5–2% annually [204]. Significant reductions are typically observed in older age, with about 20% of men over 60 and 50% over 80 experiencing testosterone levels below the normal range for younger men [205]. In women, testosterone levels decrease from the fourth decade of life, falling to about 50% of premenopausal levels by menopause and further decreasing over the subsequent 2–5 years [206]. Daily, cyclical, and seasonal fluctuations in serum SSH levels, alongside various physiological and psychological factors, add complexity to hormonal regulation [196]. Individual variations in SSH receptor expression within ocular tissues further complicate this dynamic [196]. The presence of enzymes for steroid synthesis in the lacrimal gland suggests a role for intracrine signalling in modulating its function. These complexities underscore the intricate relationship between systemic SSH levels and local receptor expression, with no apparent differences between sexes [130,206].

Research indicates that SSH receptor expression alone does not fully account for the observed sex differences in the human lacrimal gland. Most studies have found no significant differences in the relative mRNA expression levels of AR, ERα, or ERβ between sexes. This suggests that additional factors play pivotal roles in shaping sex differences in the lacrimal gland.

Future studies on sex differences in the lacrimal gland should address the current limitations by involving living participants of all ages and sexes. Such studies should integrate systemic and local biomarkers, including SSH levels, receptor expression, and tear film quality, with histological evaluations of lacrimal gland tissues. This comprehensive approach could illuminate how sex differences influence glandular function and contribute to DED. Furthermore, it could pave the way for personalised therapeutic strategies to improve outcomes for individuals affected by this condition.

In conclusion, this review highlights the crucial yet often overlooked role of sexual dimorphism in lacrimal gland biology as a key factor in the pathophysiology of dry eye disease. Integrating sex-specific molecular profiles, hormone receptor expression patterns, and immune response characteristics from experimental and clinical studies highlights the urgent need to move beyond conventional "one-size-fits-all" approaches to DED management. A key innovation proposed by this synthesis lies in identifying sex-informed diagnostic and prognostic biomarkers, such as androgen-responsive tear proteins, sex-specific inflammatory mediators, and lacrimal gland morphometric parameters that may enhance early detection and disease monitoring. Furthermore, therapeutic strategies targeting hormonal pathways, including selective androgen receptor modulators and oestrogen antagonists or strategies aimed at modulating sex-biased immune responses, represent promising avenues for future research and clinical application. Recognising and leveraging these sex-based differences not only deepens our understanding of DED pathogenesis but also paves the way for more personalised and effective ocular surface therapies. Ultimately, incorporating sex as a fundamental biological variable in both basic and translational research is essential to improving clinical outcomes and optimising therapeutic efficacy for individuals affected by DED.

Author Contributions: Conceptualisation, S.K. and K.H.; data curation, T.M., Z.T., N.G. and K.H.; original draft preparation and writing, S.K. and K.H.; review and editing, S.K., N.G. and K.H.; visualisation, Z.T. and T.M.; supervision, S.K. and K.H. All authors have read and agreed to the published version of the manuscript.

Funding: This research received no external funding.

Institutional Review Board Statement: Not applicable.

Acknowledgments: We acknowledge Angela Budimir, University Hospital Dubrava, for proofreading the manuscript.

Conflicts of Interest: The authors declare no conflicts of interest.

References

1. Arnold, A.P. A General Theory of Sexual Differentiation. *J. Neurosci. Res.* **2017**, *95*, 291–300. [CrossRef] [PubMed]
2. Szadvári, I.; Ostatníková, D.; Babková Durdiaková, J. Sex Differences Matter: Males and Females Are Equal but Not the Same. *Physiol. Behav.* **2023**, *259*, 114038. [CrossRef] [PubMed]
3. Kaštelan, S.; Tomić, M.; Salopek-Rabatić, J.; Novak, B. Diagnostic Procedures and Management of Dry Eye. *BioMed Res. Int.* **2013**, *2013*, 309723. [CrossRef] [PubMed]
4. Sullivan, D.A.; Rocha, E.M.; Aragona, P.; Clayton, J.A.; Ding, J.; Golebiowski, B.; Hampel, U.; McDermott, A.M.; Schaumberg, D.A.; Srinivasan, S.; et al. TFOS DEWS II Sex, Gender, and Hormones Report. *Ocul. Surf.* **2017**, *15*, 284–333. [CrossRef]
5. De Paiva, C.S. Effects of Aging in Dry Eye. *Int. Ophthalmol. Clin.* **2017**, *57*, 47–64. [CrossRef]
6. Rocha, E.M.; Wickham, L.A.; Yu, F.-S.; Toda, I.; Sullivan, B.D.; Sullivan, D.A. Identification of Androgen Receptor Protein and 5 -Reductase mRNA in Human Ocular Tissues. *Br. J. Ophthalmol.* **2000**, *84*, 76–84. [CrossRef]

7. Sullivan, D.A.; Wickham, L.A.; Rocha, E.M.; Kelleher, R.S.; da Silveira, L.A.; Toda, I. Influence of Gender, Sex Steroid Hormones, and the Hypothalamic-Pituitary Axis on the Structure and Function of the Lacrimal Gland. *Adv. Exp. Med. Biol.* **1998**, *438*, 11–42. [CrossRef]
8. Sullivan, D.A.; Edwards, J.A.; Wickham, L.A.; Pena, J.D.O.; Gao, J.; Ono, M.; Kelleher, R.S. Identification and Endocrine Control of Sex Steroid Binding Sites in the Lacrimal Gland. *Curr. Eye Res.* **1996**, *15*, 279–291. [CrossRef]
9. Sullivan, D.A.; Sullivan, B.D.; Evans, J.E.; Schirra, F.; Yamagami, H.; Liu, M.; Richards, S.M.; Suzuki, T.; Schaumberg, D.A.; Sullivan, R.M.; et al. Androgen Deficiency, Meibomian Gland Dysfunction, and Evaporative Dry Eye. *Ann. N. Y. Acad. Sci.* **2002**, *966*, 211–222. [CrossRef]
10. Toda, I.; Sullivan, B.D.; Rocha, E.M.; Da Silveira, L.A.; Wickham, L.A.; Sullivan, D.A. Impact of Gender on Exocrine Gland Inflammation in Mouse Models of Sjögren's Syndrome. *Exp. Eye Res.* **1999**, *69*, 355–366. [CrossRef]
11. Schaumberg, D.; Buring, J.; Sullivan, D.; Dana, M. Hormone replacement therapy and dry eye syndrome. *JAMA* **2001**, *286*, 2114–2119. [CrossRef] [PubMed]
12. Fairweather, D.; Petri, M.A.; Coronado, M.J.; Cooperr, L.T. Autoimmune Heart Disease: Role of Sex Hormones and Autoantibodies in Disease Pathogenesis. *Expert Rev. Clin. Immunol.* **2012**, *8*, 269–284. [CrossRef] [PubMed]
13. Truong, S.; Cole, N.; Stapleton, F.; Golebiowski, B. Sex Hormones and the Dry Eye. *Clin. Exp. Optom.* **2014**, *97*, 324–336. [CrossRef] [PubMed]
14. Oprea, L.; Tiberghien, A.; Creuzot-Garcher, C.; Baudouin, C. Influence des hormones sur le film lacrymal. *J. Fr. Ophtalmol.* **2004**, *27*, 933–941. [CrossRef]
15. Miljanović, B.; Dana, R.; Sullivan, D.A.; Schaumberg, D.A. Impact of Dry Eye Syndrome on Vision-Related Quality of Life. *Am. J. Ophthalmol.* **2007**, *143*, 409–415.e2. [CrossRef]
16. Cornell-Bell, A.H.; Sullivan, D.A.; Allansmith, M.R. Gender-Related Differences in the Morphology of the Lacrimal Gland. *Investig. Ophthalmol. Vis. Sci.* **1985**, *26*, 1170–1175.
17. Obata, H.; Yamamoto, S.; Horiuchi, H.; Machinami, R. Histopathologic Study of Human Lacrimal Gland. *Ophthalmology* **1995**, *102*, 678–686. [CrossRef]
18. Obata, H. Anatomy and Histopathology of the Human Lacrimal Gland. *Cornea* **2006**, *25*, S82–S89. [CrossRef]
19. Waterhouse, J.P. Focal Adenitis in Salivary and Lacrimal Glands. *Proc. R. Soc. Med.* **1963**, *56*, 911–918. [CrossRef]
20. Lorber, M.; Vidić, B. Measurements of Lacrimal Glands from Cadavers, With Descriptions of Typical Glands and Three Gross Variants. *Orbit* **2009**, *28*, 137–146. [CrossRef]
21. Bukhari, A.A.; Basheer, N.A.; Joharjy, H.I. Age, Gender, and Interracial Variability of Normal Lacrimal Gland Volume Using MRI. *Ophthal. Plast. Reconstr. Surg.* **2014**, *30*, 388–391. [CrossRef]
22. Huang, S.; Juniat, V.; Satchi, K.; Cohen, L.M.; Davis, G.; Rootman, D.B.; McNab, A.; Selva, D. Bilateral Lacrimal Gland Disease: Clinical Features and Outcomes. *Eye* **2022**, *36*, 2163–2171. [CrossRef] [PubMed]
23. Wickham, L.A.; Gao, J.; Toda, I.; Rocha, E.M.; Ono, M.; Sullivan, D.A. Identification of Androgen, Estrogen and Progesterone Receptor mRNAs in the Eye. *Acta Ophthalmol. Scand.* **2000**, *78*, 146–153. [CrossRef] [PubMed]
24. Ding, C.; Huang, J.; MacVeigh-Aloni, M.; Lu, M. Not All Lacrimal Epithelial Cells Are Created Equal—Heterogeneity of the Rabbit Lacrimal Gland and Differential Secretion. *Curr. Eye Res.* **2011**, *36*, 971–978. [CrossRef] [PubMed]
25. Gao, J.; Lambert, R.W.; Wickham, L.A.; Banting, G.; Sullivan, D.A. Androgen Control of Secretory Component mRNA Levels in the Rat Lacrimal Gland. *J. Steroid Beachem. Mol. Biol.* **1995**, *52*, 239–249. [CrossRef]
26. Ono, M.; Rocha, F.; Sullivan, D. Immunocytochemical Location and Hormonal Control of Androgen Receptors in Lacrimal Tissues of the Female MRL/Mp-Lpr/Lpr Mouse Model of Sjögren's Syndrome. *Exp Eye Res.* **1995**, *61*, 659–666. [CrossRef]
27. Rahimi Darabad, R.; Suzuki, T.; Richards, S.M.; Jakobiec, F.A.; Zakka, F.R.; Barabino, S.; Sullivan, D.A. Does Estrogen Deficiency Cause Lacrimal Gland Inflammation and Aqueous-Deficient Dry Eye in Mice? *Exp. Eye Res.* **2014**, *127*, 153–160. [CrossRef]
28. Richards, S.M.; Liu, M.; Jensen, R.V.; Schirra, F.; Yamagami, H.; Lombardi, M.J.; Rowley, P.; Treister, N.S.; Suzuki, T.; Sullivan, B.D.; et al. Androgen Regulation of Gene Expression in the Mouse Lacrimal Gland. *J. Steroid Biochem. Mol. Biol.* **2005**, *96*, 401–413. [CrossRef]
29. Richards, S.M.; Jensen, R.V.; Liu, M.; Sullivan, B.D.; Lombardi, M.J.; Rowley, P.; Schirra, F.; Treister, N.S.; Suzuki, T.; Steagall, R.J.; et al. Influence of Sex on Gene Expression in the Mouse Lacrimal Gland. *Exp. Eye Res.* **2006**, *82*, 13–23. [CrossRef]
30. Schechter, J.E.; Warren, D.W.; Mircheff, A.K. A Lacrimal Gland Is a Lacrimal Gland, But Rodent's and Rabbit's Are Not Human. *Ocul. Surf.* **2010**, *8*, 111–134. [CrossRef]
31. Šemanjski, K.; Majdič, G.; Kozina, V.; Ježek, D. Sexual Dimorphism of the Extraorbital Lacrimal Glands in SF-1 Knockout Mice. *Acta Histochem.* **2021**, *123*, 151669. [CrossRef] [PubMed]

32. Tellefsen, S.; Morthen, M.K.; Richards, S.M.; Lieberman, S.M.; Rahimi Darabad, R.; Kam, W.R.; Sullivan, D.A. Sex Effects on Gene Expression in Lacrimal Glands of Mouse Models of Sjögren Syndrome. *Investig. Opthalmol. Vis. Sci.* **2018**, *59*, 5599–5614. [CrossRef] [PubMed]
33. Conrady, C.D.; Joos, Z.P.; Patel, B.C.K. Review: The Lacrimal Gland and Its Role in Dry Eye. *J. Ophthalmol.* **2016**, *2016*, 7542929. [CrossRef] [PubMed]
34. Stern, M.E.; Gao, J.; Siemasko, K.F.; Beuerman, R.W.; Pflugfelder, S.C. The Role of the Lacrimal Functional Unit in the Pathophysiology of Dry Eye. *Exp. Eye Res.* **2004**, *78*, 409–416. [CrossRef]
35. Rolando, M.; Zierhut, M. The Ocular Surface and Tear Film and Their Dysfunction in Dry Eye Disease. *Surv. Ophthalmol.* **2001**, *45*, S203–S210. [CrossRef]
36. Wei, Y.; Asbell, P.A. The Core Mechanism of Dry Eye Disease Is Inflammation. *Eye Contact Lens. Sci. Clin. Pract.* **2014**, *40*, 248–256. [CrossRef]
37. Tóth-Molnár, E.; Ding, C. New Insight into Lacrimal Gland Function: Role of the Duct Epithelium in Tear Secretion. *Ocul. Surf.* **2020**, *18*, 595–603. [CrossRef]
38. Chang, A.Y.; Purt, B. Biochemistry, Tear Film. In *StatPearls*; StatPearls Publishing: Treasure Island, FL, USA, 2025.
39. Kaštelan, S.; Braš, M.; Pjevač, N.; Bakija, I.; Tomić, Z.; Pjevač Keleminić, N.; Gverović Antunica, A. Tear Biomarkers and Alzheimer's Disease. *Int. J. Mol. Sci.* **2023**, *24*, 13429. [CrossRef]
40. Pflugfelder, S.C.; Stern, M.E. Biological Functions of Tear Film. *Exp. Eye Res.* **2020**, *197*, 108115. [CrossRef]
41. Zhou, L.; Beuerman, R.W. The Power of Tears: How Tear Proteomics Research Could Revolutionize the Clinic. *Expert Rev. Proteomics* **2017**, *14*, 189–191. [CrossRef]
42. Purt, B.; Chang, A.Y. Biochemistry, Tear Film. In *StatPearls [Internet]*; StatPearls Publishing: Treasure Island, FL, USA, 2023.
43. Willcox, M.D.P.; Argüeso, P.; Georgiev, G.A.; Holopainen, J.M.; Laurie, G.W.; Millar, T.J.; Papas, E.B.; Rolland, J.P.; Schmidt, T.A.; Stahl, U.; et al. TFOS DEWS II Tear Film Report. *Ocul. Surf.* **2017**, *15*, 366–403. [CrossRef] [PubMed]
44. Wolff, E. The Muco-Cutaneous Junction of the Lid Margin and the Distribution of the Tear Fluid. *Trans. Ophthalmol. Soc. UK* **1946**, *66*, 291–308.
45. Holly, F.J.; Lemp, M.A. Tear Physiology and Dry Eyes. *Surv. Ophthalmol.* **1977**, *22*, 69–87. [CrossRef]
46. Herbaut, A.; Liang, H.; Denoyer, A.; Baudouin, C.; Labbé, A. Tear Film Analysis and Evaluation of Optical Quality: A Review of the Literature. *J. Fr. Ophtalmol.* **2019**, *42*, e21–e35. [CrossRef]
47. Tiffany, J.M. The Normal Tear Film. In *Developments in Ophthalmology*; Geerling, G., Brewitt, H., Eds.; KARGER: Basel, Switzerland, 2008; Volume 41, pp. 1–20. ISBN 978-3-8055-8376-3.
48. Arita, R.; Fukuoka, S.; Morishige, N. Functional Morphology of the Lipid Layer of the Tear Film. *Cornea* **2017**, *36*, S60–S66. [CrossRef]
49. Yokoi, N.; Bron, A.J.; Georgiev, G.A. The Precorneal Tear Film as a Fluid Shell: The Effect of Blinking and Saccades on Tear Film Distribution and Dynamics. *Ocul. Surf.* **2014**, *12*, 252–266. [CrossRef]
50. King-Smith, P.E.; Hinel, E.A.; Nichols, J.J. Application of a Novel Interferometric Method to Investigate the Relation between Lipid Layer Thickness and Tear Film Thinning. *Investig. Opthalmol. Vis. Sci.* **2010**, *51*, 2418–2423. [CrossRef]
51. Millar, T.; Schuett, B. The real reason for having a meibomian lipid layer covering the outer surface of the tear film—A review. *Exp. Eye Res.* **2015**, *137*, 125–138. [CrossRef]
52. Xu, X.; Li, G.; Zuo, Y. Biophysical properties of tear film lipid layer I. Surface tension and surface rheology. *Biophys. J.* **2022**, *121*, 439–450. [CrossRef]
53. Paananen, R.; Viitaja, T.; Olżyńska, A.; Ekholm, F.; Moilanen, J.; Cwiklik, L. Interactions of polar lipids with cholesteryl ester multilayers elucidate tear film lipid layer structure. *Ocul. Surf.* **2020**, *18*, 545–553. [CrossRef]
54. Georgiev, G.; Eftimov, P.; Yokoi, N. Structure-function relationship of tear film lipid layer: A contemporary perspective. *Exp. Eye Res.* **2017**, *163*, 17–28. [CrossRef] [PubMed]
55. Cwiklik, L. Tear film lipid layer: A molecular level view. *Biochim. Biophys. Acta* **2016**, *1858*, 2421–2430. [CrossRef] [PubMed]
56. McCulley, J.; Shine, W. A compositional based model for the tear film lipid layer. *Trans. Am. Ophthalmol. Soc.* **1997**, *95*, 79–88, discussion 88–93.
57. Sullivan, D.; Sullivan, B.; Ullman, M.; Rocha, E.; Krenzer, K.; Cermak, J.; Toda, I.; Doane, M.; Evans, J.; Wickham, L. Androgen influence on the meibomian gland. *Investig. Ophthalmol. Vis. Sci.* **2000**, *41*, 3732–3742.
58. Sullivan, B.; Evans, J.; Cermak, P.; Krenzer, O.; Dana, P.; Moore, A. Complete androgen insensitivity syndrome: Effect on human meibomian gland secretions. *Arch. Ophthalmol.* **2002**, *120*, 1689–1699. [CrossRef]
59. Wang, L.; Deng, Y. Androgen and meibomian gland dysfunction: From basic molecular biology to clinical applications. *Int. J. Ophthalmol.* **2021**, *14*, 915–922. [CrossRef]

60. Suzuki, T.; Schirra, F.; Richards, S.; Jensen, R.; Sullivan, D. Estrogen and progesterone control of gene expression in the mouse meibomian gland. *Investig. Ophthalmol. Vis. Sci.* **2008**, *49*, 1797–1808. [CrossRef]
61. Esmaeli, B.; Harvey, J.; Hewlett, B. Immunohistochemical evidence for estrogen receptors in meibomian glands. *Ophthalmology* **2000**, *107*, 180–184. [CrossRef]
62. Auw-Haedrich, C.; Feltgen, N. Estrogen receptor expression in meibomian glands and its correlation with age and dry-eye parameters. *Graefes Arch. Clin. Exp. Ophthalmol.* **2003**, *241*, 705–709. [CrossRef]
63. Nuzzi, R.; Caselgrandi, P. Sex hormones and their effects on ocular disorders and pathophysiology: Current aspects and our experience. *Int. J. Mol. Sci.* **2022**, *23*, 3269. [CrossRef]
64. Grasso, A.; Di Zazzo, A.; Giannaccare, G.; Sung, J.; Inomata, T.; Shih, K.; Micera, A.; Gaudenzi, D.; Spelta, S.; Romeo, M.; et al. Sex hormones related ocular dryness in breast cancer women. *J. Clin. Med.* **2021**, *10*, 2620. [CrossRef] [PubMed]
65. Sullivan, D.; Schaumberg, D.; Suzuki, T.; Schirra, F.; Liu, M.; Richards, S.; Sullivan, R.; Dana, M.; Sullivan, B. Sex steroids, meibomian gland dysfunction and evaporative dry eye in Sjögren's syndrome. *Lupus* **2002**, *11*, 667. [CrossRef] [PubMed]
66. Suzuki, T.; Sullivan, B.; Liu, M.; Schirra, F.; Richards, S.; Yamagami, H.; Sullivan, D. Estrogen and progesterone effects on the morphology of the mouse meibomian gland. *Adv. Exp. Med. Biol.* **2002**, *506*, 483–488. [CrossRef] [PubMed]
67. Jin, X.; Lin, Z.; Liu, Y.; Lin, L.; Zhu, B. Hormone replacement therapy benefits meibomian gland dysfunction in perimenopausal women. *Medicine* **2016**, *95*, e4268. [CrossRef]
68. Cher, I. A New Look at Lubrication of the Ocular Surface: Fluid Mechanics Behind the Blinking Eyelids. *Ocul. Surf.* **2008**, *6*, 79–86. [CrossRef]
69. Mishima, S.; Gasset, A.; Klyce, S., Jr.; Baum, J. Determination of Tear Volume and Tear Flow. *Invest. Ophthalmol.* **1966**, *5*, 264–276.
70. Braun, R.J. Dynamics of the Tear Film. *Annu. Rev. Fluid Mech.* **2012**, *44*, 267–297. [CrossRef]
71. Research in Dry Eye: Report of the Research Subcommittee of the International Dry Eye WorkShop (2007). *Ocul. Surf.* **2007**, *5*, 179–193. [CrossRef]
72. Rouen, P.A.; White, M.L. Dry Eye Disease: Prevalence, Assessment, and Management. *Home Healthc. Now* **2018**, *36*, 74–83. [CrossRef]
73. Tsubota, K.; Pflugfelder, S.C.; Liu, Z.; Baudouin, C.; Kim, H.M.; Messmer, E.M.; Kruse, F.; Liang, L.; Carreno-Galeano, J.T.; Rolando, M.; et al. Defining Dry Eye from a Clinical Perspective. *Int. J. Mol. Sci.* **2020**, *21*, 9271. [CrossRef]
74. Craig, J.P.; Nichols, K.K.; Akpek, E.K.; Caffery, B.; Dua, H.S.; Joo, C.-K.; Liu, Z.; Nelson, J.D.; Nichols, J.J.; Tsubota, K.; et al. TFOS DEWS II Definition and Classification Report. *Ocul. Surf.* **2017**, *15*, 276–283. [CrossRef] [PubMed]
75. Bron, A.J.; De Paiva, C.S.; Chauhan, S.K.; Bonini, S.; Gabison, E.E.; Jain, S.; Knop, E.; Markoulli, M.; Ogawa, Y.; Perez, V.; et al. TFOS DEWS II Pathophysiology Report. *Ocul. Surf.* **2017**, *15*, 438–510. [CrossRef] [PubMed]
76. Kaštelan, S.; Gabrić, K.; Mikuličić, M.; Mrazovac Zimak, D.; Karabatić, M.; Gverović Antunica, A. The Influence of Tear Film Quality on Visual Function. *Vision* **2024**, *8*, 8. [CrossRef] [PubMed]
77. McMonnies, C.W. Aqueous Deficiency Is a Contributor to Evaporation-Related Dry Eye Disease. *Eye Vis.* **2020**, *7*, 6. [CrossRef]
78. Messmer, E.M. The Pathophysiology, Diagnosis, and Treatment of Dry Eye Disease. *Dtsch. Ärztebl. Int.* **2015**, *112*, 71–81. [CrossRef]
79. Doctor, M.B.; Basu, S. Lacrimal Gland Insufficiency in Aqueous Deficiency Dry Eye Disease: Recent Advances in Pathogenesis, Diagnosis, and Treatment. *Semin. Ophthalmol.* **2022**, *37*, 801–812. [CrossRef]
80. Singh, S.; Donthineni, P.R.; Srivastav, S.; Jacobi, C.; Basu, S.; Paulsen, F. Lacrimal and Meibomian Gland Evaluation in Dry Eye Disease: A Mini-Review. *Indian J. Ophthalmol.* **2023**, *71*, 1090–1098. [CrossRef]
81. McCann, L.C.; Tomlinson, A.; Pearce, E.I.; Diaper, C. Tear and Meibomian Gland Function in Blepharitis and Normals. *Eye Contact Lens Sci. Clin. Pract.* **2009**, *35*, 203–208. [CrossRef]
82. Albietz, J.M. Prevalence of dry eye subtypes in clinical optometry practice. *Optom Vis Sci.* **2000**, *77*, 357–363. [CrossRef]
83. De Paiva, C.; Coursey, T. Managing Sjögren's Syndrome and non-Sjögren Syndrome dry eye with anti-inflammatory therapy. *Clin. Ophthalmol.* **2014**, *8*, 1447–1458. [CrossRef]
84. Abd-Allah, N.M.; Hassan, A.A.; Omar, G.; Hamdy, M.; Abdelaziz, S.T.A.; Abd El Hamid, W.M.; Moussa, R.A. Dry Eye in Rheumatoid Arthritis: Relation to Disease Activity. *Immunol. Med.* **2020**, *43*, 92–97. [CrossRef] [PubMed]
85. Huang, R.; Su, C.; Fang, L.; Lu, J.; Chen, J.; Ding, Y. Dry Eye Syndrome: Comprehensive Etiologies and Recent Clinical Trials. *Int. Ophthalmol.* **2022**, *42*, 3253–3272. [CrossRef]
86. Liu, K.C.; Huynh, K.; Grubbs, J.; Davis, R.M. Autoimmunity in the Pathogenesis and Treatment of Keratoconjunctivitis Sicca. *Curr. Allergy Asthma Rep.* **2014**, *14*, 403. [CrossRef] [PubMed]
87. Stern, M.E.; Schaumburg, C.S.; Pflugfelder, S.C. Dry Eye as a Mucosal Autoimmune Disease. *Int. Rev. Immunol.* **2013**, *32*, 19–41. [CrossRef] [PubMed]

88. Yumori, J.W.; Trinh, D.; Lee, E.; Escobedo, T.; Hollands, G.; Gordon, R.; Wang, C.-T.; Le, T.; Hou, A.; Finley, M. Prevalence of Dry Eye Disease in Rheumatoid Arthritis Patients. *Investig. Ophthalmol. Vis. Sci.* **2015**, *56*, 4437.
89. Gorimanipalli, B.; Khamar, P.; Sethu, S.; Shetty, R. Hormones and Dry Eye Disease. *Indian J. Ophthalmol.* **2023**, *71*, 1276–1284. [CrossRef]
90. Peck, T.; Olsakovsky, L.; Aggarwal, S. Dry Eye Syndrome in Menopause and Perimenopausal Age Group. *J. Life Health* **2017**, *8*, 51–54. [CrossRef]
91. Versura, P.; Giannaccare, G.; Campos, E.C. Sex-Steroid Imbalance in Females and Dry Eye. *Curr. Eye Res.* **2015**, *40*, 162–175. [CrossRef]
92. De Freitas, G.R.; Ferraz, G.A.M.; Gehlen, M.; Skare, T.L. Dry Eyes in Patients with Diabetes Mellitus. *Prim. Care Diabetes* **2021**, *15*, 184–186. [CrossRef]
93. Zhang, X.; Zhao, L.; Deng, S.; Sun, X.; Wang, N. Dry Eye Syndrome in Patients with Diabetes Mellitus: Prevalence, Etiology, and Clinical Characteristics. *J. Ophthalmol.* **2016**, *2016*, 8201053. [CrossRef]
94. Gold-von Simson, G.; Axelrod, F.B. Familial Dysautonomia: Update and Recent Advances. *Curr. Probl. Pediatr. Adolesc. Health Care* **2006**, *36*, 218–237. [CrossRef] [PubMed]
95. Mendoza-Santiesteban, C.E.; Hedges, T.R.; Norcliffe-Kaufmann, L.; Warren, F.; Reddy, S.; Axelrod, F.B.; Kaufmann, H. Clinical Neuro-Ophthalmic Findings in Familial Dysautonomia. *J. Neuroophthalmol.* **2012**, *32*, 23–26. [CrossRef] [PubMed]
96. Belmonte, C.; Nichols, J.J.; Cox, S.M.; Brock, J.A.; Begley, C.G.; Bereiter, D.A.; Dartt, D.A.; Galor, A.; Hamrah, P.; Ivanusic, J.J.; et al. TFOS DEWS II Pain and Sensation Report. *Ocul. Surf.* **2017**, *15*, 404–437. [CrossRef] [PubMed]
97. Galor, A.; Levitt, R.C.; Felix, E.R.; Martin, E.R.; Sarantopoulos, C.D. Neuropathic Ocular Pain: An Important yet Underevaluated Feature of Dry Eye. *Eye* **2015**, *29*, 301–312. [CrossRef]
98. Moon, J.; Choi, S.H.; Yoon, C.H.; Kim, M.K. Gut Dysbiosis Is Prevailing in Sjögren's Syndrome and Is Related to Dry Eye Severity. *PLoS ONE* **2020**, *15*, e0229029. [CrossRef]
99. Tsigalou, C.; Stavropoulou, E.; Bezirtzoglou, E. Current Insights in Microbiome Shifts in Sjogren's Syndrome and Possible Therapeutic Interventions. *Front. Immunol.* **2018**, *9*, 1106. [CrossRef]
100. Alves, M.; Novaes, P.; Morraye, M.D.A.; Reinach, P.S.; Rocha, E.M. Is Dry Eye an Environmental Disease? *Arq. Bras. Oftalmol.* **2014**, *77*, 193–200. [CrossRef]
101. Mandell, J.T.; Idarraga, M.; Kumar, N.; Galor, A. Impact of Air Pollution and Weather on Dry Eye. *J. Clin. Med.* **2020**, *9*, 3740. [CrossRef]
102. Akkaya, S.; Atakan, T.; Acikalin, B.; Aksoy, S.; Ozkurt, Y. The Effect of Long Term Computure Use on Dry Eye. *North. Clin. Istanb.* **2018**, *5*, 319–322. [CrossRef]
103. Erginturk Acar, D.; Acar, U.; Ozen Tunay, Z.; Ozdemir, O.; Germen, H. The Effects of Smoking on Dry Eye Parameters in Healthy Women. *Cutan. Ocul. Toxicol.* **2017**, *36*, 1–4. [CrossRef]
104. Khalil, H.E.M.; Aboud, S.A.; Azzab, M.A. Comparative Study between Smokers and Nonsmokers Regarding Dry Eye. *Delta J. Ophthalmol.* **2018**, *19*, 9–13. [CrossRef]
105. Xu, L.; Zhang, W.; Zhu, X.-Y.; Suo, T.; Fan, X.-Q.; Fu, Y. Smoking and the Risk of Dry Eye: A Meta-Analysis. *Int. J. Ophthalmol.* **2016**, *9*, 1480–1486. [CrossRef] [PubMed]
106. Koh, S. Contact Lens Wear and Dry Eye: Beyond the Known. *Asia-Pac. J. Ophthalmol.* **2020**, *9*, 498–504. [CrossRef] [PubMed]
107. Khoo, P.; Groeneveld, T.; Boyle, F.; O'Neill, S.; Forster, B.; Watson, S.L. Dry Eye Signs and Symptoms in Patients on Aromatase Inhibitor Therapy. *Eye* **2022**, *36*, 766–772. [CrossRef] [PubMed]
108. Shtein, R.M. Post-LASIK Dry Eye. *Expert Rev. Ophthalmol.* **2011**, *6*, 575–582. [CrossRef]
109. Wong, A.H.Y.; Cheung, R.K.Y.; Kua, W.N.; Shih, K.C.; Chan, T.C.Y.; Wan, K.H. Dry Eyes After SMILE. *Asia-Pac. J. Ophthalmol.* **2019**, *8*, 397–405. [CrossRef]
110. Apostol, S.; Filip, M.; Dragne, C.; Filip, A. Dry Eye Syndrome. Etiological and Therapeutic Aspects. *Oftalmol. Buchar. Rom.* **2003**, *59*, 28–31.
111. Britten-Jones, A.C.; Wang, M.T.M.; Samuels, I.; Jennings, C.; Stapleton, F.; Craig, J.P. Epidemiology and Risk Factors of Dry Eye Disease: Considerations for Clinical Management. *Medicine* **2024**, *60*, 1458. [CrossRef]
112. Downie, L.E.; Ng, S.M.; Lindsley, K.B.; Akpek, E.K. Omega-3 and Omega-6 Polyunsaturated Fatty Acids for Dry Eye Disease. *Cochrane Database Syst. Rev.* **2019**, *12*, CD011016. [CrossRef]
113. Oydanich, M.; Maguire, M.G.; Pistilli, M.; Hamrah, P.; Greiner, J.V.; Lin, M.C.; Asbell, P.A. Effects of Omega-3 Supplementation on Exploratory Outcomes in the Dry Eye Assessment and Management Study. *Ophthalmology* **2020**, *127*, 136–138. [CrossRef]
114. Solomon, A.; Dursun, D.; Liu, Z.; Xie, Y.; Macri, A.; Pflugfelder, S.C. Pro- and Anti-Inflammatory Forms of Interleukin-1 in the Tear Fluid and Conjunctiva of Patients with Dry-Eye Disease. *Investig. Ophthalmol. Vis. Sci.* **2001**, *42*, 2283–2293. [PubMed]

115. Lam, H.; Bleiden, L.; De Paiva, C.S.; Farley, W.; Stern, M.E.; Pflugfelder, S.C. Tear Cytokine Profiles in Dysfunctional Tear Syndrome. *Am. J. Ophthalmol.* **2009**, *147*, 198–205.e1. [CrossRef] [PubMed]
116. Blencowe, M.; Chen, X.; Zhao, Y.; Itoh, Y.; McQuillen, C.N.; Han, Y.; Shou, B.L.; McClusky, R.; Reue, K.; Arnold, A.P.; et al. Relative Contributions of Sex Hormones, Sex Chromosomes, and Gonads to Sex Differences in Tissue Gene Regulation. *Genome Res.* **2022**, *32*, 807–824. [CrossRef]
117. Pillerová, M.; Borbélyová, V.; Hodosy, J.; Riljak, V.; Renczés, E.; Frick, K.M.; Tóthová, Ľ. On the Role of Sex Steroids in Biological Functions by Classical and Non-Classical Pathways. *Update. Front. Neuroendocrinol.* **2021**, *62*, 100926. [CrossRef]
118. Varticovski, L.; Stavreva, D.A.; McGowan, A.; Raziuddin, R.; Hager, G.L. Endocrine Disruptors of Sex Hormone Activities. *Mol. Cell. Endocrinol.* **2022**, *539*, 111415. [CrossRef]
119. Saldanha, C.J. Brain-Derived Steroids and Behaviors. In *Oxford Research Encyclopedia of Neuroscience*; Oxford University Press: Oxford, UK, 2019; ISBN 978-0-19-026408-6.
120. Heinlein, C.A.; Chang, C. The Roles of Androgen Receptors and Androgen-Binding Proteins in Nongenomic Androgen Actions. *Mol. Endocrinol.* **2002**, *16*, 2181–2187. [CrossRef]
121. Hu, J.; Zhang, Z.; Shen, W.-J.; Azhar, S. Cellular Cholesterol Delivery, Intracellular Processing and Utilization for Biosynthesis of Steroid Hormones. *Nutr. Metab.* **2010**, *7*, 47. [CrossRef]
122. Miller, W.L. Steroidogenesis: Unanswered Questions. *Trends Endocrinol. Metab.* **2017**, *28*, 771–793. [CrossRef]
123. Li, J.; Papadopoulos, V.; Vihma, V. Steroid Biosynthesis in Adipose Tissue. *Steroids* **2015**, *103*, 89–104. [CrossRef]
124. King, S.R.; Manna, P.R.; Ishii, T.; Syapin, P.J.; Ginsberg, S.D.; Wilson, K.; Walsh, L.P.; Parker, K.L.; Stocco, D.M.; Smith, R.G.; et al. An Essential Component in Steroid Synthesis, the Steroidogenic Acute Regulatory Protein, Is Expressed in Discrete Regions of the Brain. *J. Neurosci.* **2002**, *22*, 10613–10620. [CrossRef]
125. King, S.R. Emerging Roles for Neurosteroids in Sexual Behavior and Function. *J. Androl.* **2008**, *29*, 524–533. [CrossRef] [PubMed]
126. Melcangi, R.C.; Giatti, S.; Pesaresi, M.; Calabrese, D.; Mitro, N.; Caruso, D.; Garcia-Segura, L.M. Role of Neuroactive Steroids in the Peripheral Nervous System. *Front. Endocrinol.* **2011**, *2*, 104. [CrossRef] [PubMed]
127. Mensah-Nyagan, A.G.; Kibaly, C.; Schaeffer, V.; Venard, C.; Meyer, L.; Patte-Mensah, C. Endogenous Steroid Production in the Spinal Cord and Potential Involvement in Neuropathic Pain Modulation. *J. Steroid Biochem. Mol. Biol.* **2008**, *109*, 286–293. [CrossRef] [PubMed]
128. Meseguer, A.; Puche, C.; Cabero, A. Sex Steroid Biosynthesis in White Adipose Tissue. *Horm. Metab. Res.* **2002**, *34*, 731–736. [CrossRef]
129. Slominski, A.; Zbytek, B.; Nikolakis, G.; Manna, P.R.; Skobowiat, C.; Zmijewski, M.; Li, W.; Janjetovic, Z.; Postlethwaite, A.; Zouboulis, C.C.; et al. Steroidogenesis in the Skin: Implications for Local Immune Functions. *J. Steroid Biochem. Mol. Biol.* **2013**, *137*, 107–123. [CrossRef]
130. Schirra, F.; Suzuki, T.; Dickinson, D.P.; Townsend, D.J.; Gipson, I.K.; Sullivan, D.A. Identification of Steroidogenic Enzyme mRNAs in the Human Lacrimal Gland, Meibomian Gland, Cornea, and Conjunctiva. *Cornea* **2006**, *25*, 438–442. [CrossRef]
131. Bouguen, G.; Dubuquoy, L.; Desreumaux, P.; Brunner, T.; Bertin, B. Intestinal Steroidogenesis. *Steroids* **2015**, *103*, 64–71. [CrossRef]
132. Quinkler, M.; Bumke-Vogt, C.; Meyer, B.; Bähr, V.; Oelkers, W.; Diederich, S. The Human Kidney Is a Progesterone-Metabolizing and Androgen-Producing Organ. *J. Clin. Endocrinol. Metab.* **2003**, *88*, 2803–2809. [CrossRef]
133. Davey, R.A.; Grossmann, M. Androgen Receptor Structure, Function and Biology: From Bench to Bedside. *Clin. Biochem. Rev.* **2016**, *37*, 3–15.
134. Saito, K.; Cui, H. Estrogen Receptor Alpha Splice Variants, Post-Translational Modifications, and Their Physiological Functions. *Cells* **2023**, *12*, 895. [CrossRef]
135. Talaber, G.; Jondal, M.; Okret, S. Local Glucocorticoid Production in the Thymus. *Steroids* **2015**, *103*, 58–63. [CrossRef]
136. Vacchio, M.S.; Papadopoulos, V.; Ashwell, J.D. Steroid Production in the Thymus: Implications for Thymocyte Selection. *J. Exp. Med.* **1994**, *179*, 1835–1846. [CrossRef] [PubMed]
137. Yaşar, P.; Ayaz, G.; User, S.D.; Güpür, G.; Muyan, M. Molecular Mechanism of Estrogen–Estrogen Receptor Signaling. *Reprod. Med. Biol.* **2017**, *16*, 4–20. [CrossRef] [PubMed]
138. Chighizola, C.; Meroni, P.L. The Role of Environmental Estrogens and Autoimmunity. *Autoimmun. Rev.* **2012**, *11*, A493–A501. [CrossRef] [PubMed]
139. Gray, L.E.; Ostby, J.S.; Kelce, W.R. Developmental Effects of an Environmental Antiandrogen: The Fungicide Vinclozolin Alters Sex Differentiation of the Male Rat. *Toxicol. Appl. Pharmacol.* **1994**, *129*, 46–52. [CrossRef]
140. Toppari, J. Environmental Endocrine Disrupters and Disorders of Sexual Differentiation. *Semin. Reprod. Med.* **2002**, *20*, 305–312. [CrossRef]
141. Konttinen, Y.T.; Porola, P.; Konttinen, L.; Laine, M.; Poduval, P. Immunohistopathology of Sjögren's Syndrome. *Autoimmun. Rev.* **2006**, *6*, 16–20. [CrossRef]

142. Sullivan, D.A. Tearful Relationships? Sex, Hormones, the Lacrimal Gland, and Aqueous-Deficient Dry Eye. *Ocul. Surf.* **2004**, *2*, 92–123. [CrossRef]
143. Sullivan, D.A.; Krenzer, K.L.; Sullivan, B.D.; Tolls, D.B.; Toda, I.; Dana, M.R. Does Androgen Insufficiency Cause Lacrimal Gland Inflammation and Aqueous Tear Deficiency? *Investig. Ophthalmol. Vis. Sci.* **1999**, *40*, 1261–1265.
144. Khandelwal, P.; Liu, S.; Sullivan, D.A. Androgen Regulation of Gene Expression in Human Meibomian Gland and Conjunctival Epithelial Cells. *Mol. Vis.* **2012**, *18*, 1055–1067.
145. Ranganathan, V.; De, P.K. Androgens and Estrogens Markedly Inhibit Expression of a 20-kDa Major Protein in Hamster Exorbital Lacrimal Gland. *Biochem. Biophys. Res. Commun.* **1995**, *208*, 412–417. [CrossRef] [PubMed]
146. Richards, S.M.; Liu, M.; Sullivan, B.D.; Sullivan, D.A. Gender-Related Differences in Gene Expression of the Lacrimal Gland. In *Lacrimal Gland, Tear Film, and Dry Eye Syndromes 3: Basic Science and Clinical Relevance Part A and B*; Sullivan, D.A., Stern, M.E., Tsubota, K., Dartt, D.A., Sullivan, R.M., Bromberg, B.B., Eds.; Springer US: Boston, MA, USA, 2002; pp. 121–127. ISBN 978-1-4615-0717-8.
147. Toda, I.; Wickham, L.A.; Sullivan, D.A. Gender and Androgen Treatment Influence the Expression of Proto-Oncogenes and Apoptotic Factors in Lacrimal and Salivary Tissues of MRL/lprMice. *Clin. Immunol. Immunopathol.* **1998**, *86*, 59–71. [CrossRef] [PubMed]
148. Nikolov, N.P.; Illei, G.G. Pathogenesis of Sjögren's Syndrome. *Curr. Opin. Rheumatol.* **2009**, *21*, 465–470. [CrossRef] [PubMed]
149. Smith, R.E.; Taylor, C.R.; Rao, N.A.; Young, L.L.; Rife, L.L. Immunohistochemical Identification of Androgen Receptors in Human Lacrimal Glands. *Curr. Eye Res.* **1999**, *18*, 300–309. [CrossRef]
150. Rocha, F.J.; Wickham, L.A.; Pena, J.D.; Gao, J.; Ono, M.; Lambert, R.W.; Kelleher, R.S.; Sullivan, D.A. Influence of Gender and the Endocrine Environment on the Distribution of Androgen Receptors in the Lacrimal Gland. *J. Steroid Biochem. Mol. Biol.* **1993**, *46*, 737–749. [CrossRef]
151. Sullivan, D.A. Sex Hormones and Sjögren's Syndrome. *J. Rheumatol. Suppl.* **1997**, *50*, 17–32.
152. Wickham, L.A.; Rocha, E.M.; Gao, J.; Krenzer, K.L.; Da Silveira, L.A.; Toda, I.; Sullivan, D.A. Identification and Hormonal Control of Sex Steroid Receptors in the Eye. In *Lacrimal Gland, Tear Film, and Dry Eye Syndromes 2*; Sullivan, D.A., Dartt, D.A., Meneray, M.A., Eds.; Advances in Experimental Medicine and Biology; Springer US: Boston, MA, USA, 1998; Volume 438, pp. 95–100. ISBN 978-1-4613-7445-9.
153. Sullivan, D.A.; Wickham, L.A.; Rocha, E.M.; Krenzer, K.L.; Sullivan, B.D.; Steagall, R.; Cermak, J.M.; Dana, M.R.; Ullman, M.D.; Sato, E.H.; et al. Androgens and Dry Eye in Sjögren's Syndrome. *Ann. N. Y. Acad. Sci.* **1999**, *876*, 312–324. [CrossRef]
154. Affinito, P.; Sardo, A.D.S.; Di Carlo, C.; Sammartino, A.; Tommaselli, G.A.; Bifulco, G.; Loffredo, A.; Loffredo, M.; Nappi, C. Effects of Hormone Replacement Therapy on Ocular Function in Postmenopause. *Menopause* **2003**, *10*, 482–487. [CrossRef]
155. Feng, Y.; Feng, G.; Peng, S.; Li, H. The Effects of Hormone Replacement Therapy on Dry Eye Syndromes Evaluated by Schirmer Test Depend on Patient Age. *Contact Lens Anterior Eye* **2016**, *39*, 124–127. [CrossRef]
156. Chen, S.P.; Massaro-Giordano, G.; Pistilli, M.; Schreiber, C.A.; Bunya, V.Y. Tear Osmolarity and Dry Eye Symptoms in Women Using Oral Contraception and Contact Lenses. *Cornea* **2013**, *32*, 423–428. [CrossRef]
157. Mathers, W.D.; Stovall, D.; Lane, J.A.; Zimmerman, M.B.; Johnson, S. Menopause and Tear Function: The Influence of Prolactin and Sex Hormones on Human Tear Production. *Cornea* **1998**, *17*, 353–358. [CrossRef] [PubMed]
158. Villa, A.; Rizzi, N.; Vegeto, E.; Ciana, P.; Maggi, A. Estrogen accelerates the resolution of inflammation in macrophagic cells. *Sci. Rep.* **2015**, *5*, 15224. [CrossRef] [PubMed]
159. Pepe, G.; Braga, D.; Renzi, T.; Villa, A.; Bolego, C.; D'Avila, F.; Barlassina, C.; Maggi, A.; Locati, M.; Vegeto, E. Self-renewal and phenotypic conversion are the main physiological responses of macrophages to the endogenous estrogen surge. *Sci. Rep.* **2017**, *7*, 44270. [CrossRef]
160. Mohammad, I.; Starskaia, I.; Nagy, T.; Guo, J.; Yatkin, E.; Väänänen, K.; Watford, W.; Chen, Z. Estrogen receptor α contributes to T cell–mediated autoimmune inflammation by promoting T cell activation and proliferation. *Sci. Signal.* **2018**, *11*, eaap9415. [CrossRef]
161. Suzuki, T.; Schirra, F.; Richards, S.; Treister, N.; Lombardi, M.; Rowley, P.; Jensen, R.; Sullivan, D. Estrogen's and progesterone's impact on gene expression in the mouse lacrimal gland. *Investig. Ophthalmol. Vis. Sci.* **2006**, *47*, 158–168. [CrossRef]
162. Srikantan, S.; Paliwal, A.; Quintanar-Stephano, A.; De, P. Estrogen and androgen repression of two female specific lacrimal lipocalins in hamster: Pituitary independent and sex hormone receptor mediated action. *Gen. Comp. Endocrinol.* **2007**, *151*, 172–179. [CrossRef]
163. Hat, K.; Planinić, A.; Ježek, D.; Kaštelan, S. Expression of Androgen and Estrogen Receptors in the Human Lacrimal Gland. *Int. J. Mol. Sci.* **2023**, *24*, 5609. [CrossRef]
164. Sullivan, D.A.; Kelleher, R.S.; Vaerman, J.P.; Hann, L.E. Androgen Regulation of Secretory Component Synthesis by Lacrimal Gland Acinar Cells in Vitro. *J. Immunol. Baltim.* **1990**, *145*, 4238–4244. [CrossRef]

165. Sivapathasundharam, B.; Prabhakar, M. Sexual Dimorphism. *J. Oral Maxillofac. Pathol.* **2019**, *23*, 152–153. [CrossRef]
166. Lau, E.S.; Binek, A.; Parker, S.J.; Shah, S.H.; Zanni, M.V.; Van Eyk, J.E.; Ho, J.E. Sexual Dimorphism in Cardiovascular Biomarkers: Clinical and Research Implications. *Circ. Res.* **2022**, *130*, 578–592. [CrossRef]
167. Berns, C.M. The Evolution of Sexual Dimorphism: Understanding Mechanisms of Sexual Shape Differences. In *Sexual Dimorphism*; Moriyama, H., Ed.; InTech: Rijeka, Croatia, 2013; ISBN 978-953-51-1075-0.
168. Ralls, K.; Mesnick, S. Sexual Dimorphism. In *Encyclopedia of Marine Mammals*, 2nd ed.; Perrin, W.F., Würsig, B., Thewissen, J.G.M., Eds.; Academic Press: London, UK, 2009; pp. 1005–1011.
169. Gates, K.; Sandoval-Castillo, J.; Brauer, C.J.; Unmack, P.J.; Laporte, M.; Bernatchez, L.; Beheregaray, L.B. Environmental Selection, Rather than Neutral Processes, Best Explain Regional Patterns of Diversity in a Tropical Rainforest Fish. *Heredity* **2023**, *130*, 368–380. [CrossRef] [PubMed]
170. Maan, M.E.; Seehausen, O. Ecology, Sexual Selection and Speciation: Ecology, Sexual Selection and Speciation. *Ecol. Lett.* **2011**, *14*, 591–602. [CrossRef] [PubMed]
171. Hayashi, S.; Abe, T.; Igawa, T.; Katsura, Y.; Kazama, Y.; Nozawa, M. Sex Chromosome Cycle as a Mechanism of Stable Sex Determination. *J. Biochem.* **2024**, *176*, 81–95. [CrossRef]
172. Ubels, J.L.; Hoffman, H.M.; Srikanth, S.; Resau, J.H.; Webb, C.P. Gene Expression in Rat Lacrimal Gland Duct Cells Collected Using Laser Capture Microdissection: Evidence for K+ Secretion by Duct Cells. *Investig. Opthalmol. Vis. Sci.* **2006**, *47*, 1876–1885. [CrossRef]
173. Damato, B.E.; Allan, D.; Murray, S.B.; Lee, W.R. Senile Atrophy of the Human Lacrimal Gland: The Contribution of Chronic Inflammatory Disease. *Br. J. Ophthalmol.* **1984**, *68*, 674–680. [CrossRef]
174. Hat, K.; Kaštelan, S.; Planinić, A.; Muller, D.; Ježek, D. Pathohistological Features of the Aging Human Lacrimal Gland. *Croat. Med. J.* **2023**, *64*, 307–319. [CrossRef]
175. Nasu, M.; Matsubara, O.; Yamamoto, H. Post-mortem Prevalence of Lymphocytic Infiltration of the Lacrymal Gland: A Comparative Study in Autoimmune and Non-autoimmune Diseases. *J. Pathol.* **1984**, *143*, 11–15. [CrossRef]
176. Prager, A. [Macroscopic and microscopic investigations on senile atrophy of the lacrimal gland (preliminary report)]. *Bibl. Ophthalmol. Suppl. Ad Ophthalmol.* **1966**, *69*, 146–158.
177. Christensen, F.; Dam, H. A Sexual Dimorphism of the Harderian Glands in Hamsters. *Acta Physiol. Scand.* **1953**, *27*, 332–336. [CrossRef]
178. Sullivan, D.A.; Hann, L.E.; Yee, L.; Allansmith, M.R. Age- and Gender-related Influence on the Lacrimal Gland and Tears. *Acta Ophthalmol.* **1990**, *68*, 188–194. [CrossRef]
179. Chew, C.K.S.; Hykin, P.G.; Jansweijer, C.; Dikstein, S.; Tiffany, J.M.; Bron, A.J. The Casual Level of Meibomian Lipids in Humans. *Curr. Eye Res.* **1993**, *12*, 255–259. [CrossRef] [PubMed]
180. Sullivan, D.A.; Jensen, R.V.; Suzuki, T.; Richards, S.M. Do Sex Steroids Exert Sex-Specific and/or Opposite Effects on Gene Expression in Lacrimal and Meibomian Glands? *Mol. Vis.* **2009**, *15*, 1553–1572. [PubMed]
181. Suzuki, T.; Richards, S.M.; Liu, S.; Jensen, R.V.; Sullivan, D.A. Influence of Sex on Gene Expression in Human Corneal Epithelial Cells. *Mol. Vis.* **2009**, *15*, 2554–2569.
182. Ferrara, D.; Monteforte, R.; Baccari, G.C.; Minucci, S.; Chieffi, G. Androgen and Estrogen Receptors Expression in the Rat Exorbital Lacrimal Gland in Relation to "Harderianization". *J. Exp. Zoolog. A Comp. Exp. Biol.* **2004**, *301*, 297–306. [CrossRef]
183. Goto, T.; Klyce, S.D.; Zheng, X.; Maeda, N.; Kuroda, T.; Ide, C. Gender- and Age-Related Differences in Corneal Topography. *Cornea* **2001**, *20*, 270–276. [CrossRef]
184. Sullivan, D.A.; Hann, L.E. Hormonal Influence on the Secretory Immune System of the Eye: Endocrine Impact on the Lacrimal Gland Accumulation and Secretion of IgA IgG. *J. Steroid Biochem.* **1989**, *34*, 253–262. [CrossRef]
185. Roen, J.L.; Stasior, O.G.; Jakobiec, F.A. Aging Changes in the Human Lacrimal Gland: Role of the Ducts. *C LAO J. Off. Publ. Contact Lens Assoc. Ophthalmol. Inc* **1985**, *11*, 237–242.
186. Lorber, M. Gross Characteristics of Normal Human Lacrimal Glands. *Ocul. Surf.* **2007**, *5*, 13–22. [CrossRef]
187. Boyce, R.W.; Dorph-Petersen, K.-A.; Lyck, L.; Gundersen, H.J.G. Design-Based Stereology: Introduction to Basic Concepts and Practical Approaches for Estimation of Cell Number. *Toxicol. Pathol.* **2010**, *38*, 1011–1025. [CrossRef]
188. Weibel, E.R.; Kistler, G.S.; Scherle, W.F. Practical stereological methods for morphometric cytology. *J. Cell Biol.* **1966**, *30*, 23–38. [CrossRef]
189. Cruz-Orive, L.M. Stereology of Single Objects. *J. Microsc.* **1997**, *186*, 93–107. [CrossRef]
190. Mandarim-de-Lacerda, C.A.; Del-Sol, M. Tips for Studies with Quantitative Morphology (Morphometry and Stereology). *Int. J. Morphol.* **2017**, *35*, 1482–1494. [CrossRef]
191. Peterson, D.A. Stereology. In *Encyclopedia of Movement Disorders*; Kompoliti, K., Metman, L.V., Eds.; Academic Press: Oxford, UK, 2010; pp. 168–170; ISBN 978-0-12-374105-9.

192. Clayton, J.A.; Davis, A.F. Sex/Gender Disparities and Women's Eye Health. *Curr. Eye Res.* **2015**, *40*, 102–109. [CrossRef]
193. Mandarim-de-Lacerda, C.A. Stereological Tools in Biomedical Research. *An. Acad. Bras. Ciênc.* **2003**, *75*, 469–486. [CrossRef] [PubMed]
194. Weibel, E.R. Measuring through the Microscope: Development and Evolution of Stereological Methods. *J. Microsc.* **1989**, *155*, 393–403. [CrossRef]
195. Zetterberg, M. Age-Related Eye Disease and Gender. *Maturitas* **2016**, *83*, 19–26. [CrossRef]
196. Gupta, P.D.; Johar, K.; Nagpal, K.; Vasavada, A.R. Sex Hormone Receptors in the Human Eye. *Surv. Ophthalmol.* **2005**, *50*, 274–284. [CrossRef]
197. Nilsson, S.; Mäkelä, S.; Treuter, E.; Tujague, M.; Thomsen, J.; Andersson, G.; Enmark, E.; Pettersson, K.; Warner, M.; Gustafsson, J.-Å. Mechanisms of Estrogen Action. *Physiol. Rev.* **2001**, *81*, 1535–1565. [CrossRef]
198. Gligorijevic, J.; Krstic, M.; Babic, G. Immunohistochemical Detection of Estrogen and Progesterone Receptors in the Human Lacrimal Gland. *Arch. Biol. Sci.* **2011**, *63*, 319–324. [CrossRef]
199. Spelsberg, H.; Klueppel, M.; Reinhard, T.; Glaeser, M.; Niederacher, D.; Beckmann, M.W.; Sundmacher, R. Detection of Oestrogen Receptors (ER) α and β in Conjunctiva, Lacrimal Gland, and Tarsal Plates. *Eye* **2004**, *18*, 729–733. [CrossRef]
200. Ueno, H.; Ariji, E.; Izumi, M.; Uetani, M.; Hayashi, K.; Nakamura, T. MR imaging of the lacrimal gland: Age-related and gender-dependent changes in size and structure. *Acta Radiol.* **1996**, *37*, 714–719. [CrossRef] [PubMed]
201. Haarsma, L.D.; Ubels, J.L. Patch-clamp recording of K^+ current from lacrimal gland duct cells. *bioRxiv*, **2019**, bioRxiv:670653.
202. Remington, S.; Nelson, D.; Richards, S.; Liu, M.; Sullivan, B.; Sullivan, D. Gender-related differences in gene expression of the lacrimal gland. *Adv. Exp. Med. Biol.* **2002**, *506*, 121–127. [CrossRef]
203. Mani, S.; Mermelstein, P.; Tetel, M.; Anesetti, G. Convergence of Multiple Mechanisms of Steroid Hormone Action. *Horm. Metab. Res.* **2012**, *44*, 569–576. [CrossRef] [PubMed]
204. Handelsman, D.J. Androgen Physiology, Pharmacology, Use and Misuse. In *Endotext*; Feingold, K.R., Anawalt, B., Blackman, M.R., Boyce, A., Chrousos, G., Corpas, E., de Herder, W.W., Dhatariya, K., Dungan, K., Eds.; MDText.com, Inc.: South Dartmouth, MA, USA, 2000.
205. Horstman, A.M.; Dillon, E.L.; Urban, R.J.; Sheffield-Moore, M. The Role of Androgens and Estrogens on Healthy Aging and Longevity. *J. Gerontol. A. Biol. Sci. Med. Sci.* **2012**, *67*, 1140–1152. [CrossRef]
206. Gibson, E.J.; Stapleton, F.; Wolffsohn, J.S.; Golebiowski, B. Local Synthesis of Sex Hormones: Are There Consequences for the Ocular Surface and Dry Eye? *Br. J. Ophthalmol.* **2017**, *101*, 1596–1603. [CrossRef]

International Journal of
Molecular Sciences

MDPI

Review

The Role of Nerve Growth Factor on the Ocular Surface: A Review of the Current Experimental Research and Clinical Practices

Nicolás Kahuam-López, Amir Hosseini, Jennifer Y. M. Ling, Joseph Chiang, Alfonso Iovieno and Sonia N. Yeung *

Department of Ophthalmology and Visual Sciences, University of British Columbia,
Vancouver, BC V5Z 3N9, Canada
* Correspondence: sonia.yeung@ubc.ca

Abstract: The ocular surface is susceptible to a wide spectrum of inflammatory, degenerative, and neurotrophic diseases that can impair vision. The complex pathophysiology and limited therapeutic options associated with these conditions continue to pose significant clinical challenges. Nerve Growth Factor (NGF), a neurotrophin initially recognized for its role in neuronal survival and differentiation, has emerged as a key regulator of ocular surface homeostasis and repair. Beyond its neurotrophic functions, NGF is suggested to influence epithelial proliferation, immune responses, tear secretion, and angiogenesis. Experimental and clinical studies have implicated NGF in both the pathogenesis and potential treatment of various ocular surface diseases, including allergic conjunctivitis, neurotrophic keratopathy (NK), immune-mediated and herpetic keratitis, and dry eye disease (DED), as well as post-surgical corneal wound healing. Notably, recombinant human NGF (rhNGF, cenegermin) has been approved as the first topical biologic therapy for NK. Despite encouraging clinical outcomes, challenges such as high treatment costs, limited long-term data, and potential proangiogenic effects remain. This review consolidates current evidence on the role of NGF in ocular surface health and disease, highlighting its biological mechanisms, clinical applications, and future therapeutic potential.

Keywords: ocular surface; nerve growth factor; cenegermin; corneal wound healing; allergic conjunctivitis; neurotrophic keratopathy; dry eye disease; corneal transplant; refractive surgery; cataract surgery

1. Introduction

Nerve Growth Factor (NGF) is a homodimeric protein initially discovered in the peripheral nervous system and named for its effects on neuron growth and differentiation [1]. Since its discovery, it has been shown to play a role in numerous physiological processes and pathological conditions. On the ocular surface, NGF has been studied in the context of allergic conjunctivitis [2–5], NK [6–12], immune and infectious keratitis [13–16], DED [17–19], corneal transplant [20,21], cataract [22], and refractive surgery [23–25]. This review discusses the current experimental research and clinical practices regarding NGF on the ocular surface.

In the sections that follow, we begin by examining the molecular biology of NGF, including its gene structure, proteolytic processing, and downstream signaling via tyrosine protein kinase receptor-A ($TrkA^{NGFR}$) and p75 pan-NT receptor, named $p75^{NTR}$. These receptors activate pathways that regulate diverse cellular processes such as neuronal survival, apoptosis, calcium homeostasis, inflammation, immune cell recruitment, cell proliferation, and tissue remodeling [26–38]. The ocular expression of NGF receptors is then reviewed, with emphasis on their localization in both neuronal and non-neuronal cells [38–48], supporting NGF's diverse effects.

Building on this foundation, we examine the physiological roles of NGF at the ocular surface, focusing on its contribution to epithelial cell proliferation and differentiation, corneal nerve regeneration, and modulation of local immune responses. To support this, we present ocular-surface-specific in vitro data, demonstrating the effects of exogenous NGF treatment on goblet cell expression and secretion, mucin production and release, conjunctival epithelial cell differentiation [45,49], and corneal epithelial migration and proliferation [36]. We also highlight the upregulation of the $TrkA^{NGFR}$ receptor and matrix metalloproteinase-9 (MMP-9) expression [36,37]. Furthermore, we explore the induction of fibroblastic-keratocyte and conjunctival fibroblast differentiation into myofibroblasts and enhanced migration upon exogenous NGF treatment [48,50].

We then synthesize evidence from animal models and clinical studies evaluating NGF's therapeutic applications in a range of ocular surface diseases. Particular emphasis is placed on NK, a rare but vision-threatening disorder affecting approximately 5 individuals or fewer in 10,000 [51], for which topical rhNGF (cenegermin) remains the only FDA-approved pharmacologic therapy [52]. We also briefly compare NGF therapy with other conventional NK treatment options, such as tear substitutes, amniotic membrane transplantation, neurotization, and autologous serum drops, highlighting why NGF therapy offers great potential as a therapeutic approach to target the underlying neurotrophic deficit.

Lastly, we critically examine the limitations and unresolved questions surrounding NGF-based therapies, including the high cost and limited accessibility of rhNGF, its complex administration schedule, the scarcity of long-term safety and efficacy data, and mechanistic concerns such as the potential proangiogenic effects of NGF in corneal neovascularization [11,53]. We highlight specific knowledge gaps, such as the differential effects of NGF across various cell types and disease contexts, and emphasize the need for further multicenter randomized trials and mechanistic investigations to optimize NGF's clinical utility and expand its approved therapeutic indications.

2. Methods of Literature Search

A comprehensive literature search was performed using PubMed and Embase to identify studies examining the role of NGF in ocular surface diseases.

The PubMed search used the following terms: ("Nerve Growth Factor" or "NGF" or "Cenegermin") combined with ("Cornea" or "Ocular Surface" or "Pterygium Of Conjunctiva And Cornea" or "Pterygium" or "Conjunctiva" or "Dry Eye Syndrome" or "Dry Eye" or "Dry Eye Disease" or "Conjunctivitis Sicca" or "Keratoconjunctivitis Sicca" or "Keratitis Sicca" or "Keratitis" or "Immune Keratitis" or "Herpetic Keratitis" or "Corneal Ulcer" or "Refractive Surgical Procedures" or "Refractive Surgery" or "LASIK" or "Laser-assisted In Situ Keratomileusis" or "PRK" or "Photorefractive Keratectomy" or "SMILE" or "Small Incision Lenticule Extraction" or "Corneal Surgery" or "Corneal Transplantation" or "Corneal Transplant" or "Corneal Neovascularization" or "Corneal Diseases" or "Graft Rejection" or "Graves Ophthalmopathy" or "Thyroid Eye Disease" or "Allergic Conjunctivitis" or "Vernal Keratoconjunctivitis" or "Conjunctivitis" or "Neuralgia" or "Neuropathic Pain").

For Embase, a two-step search was conducted. First, ocular surface and corneal disease terms were searched using the following: ("Cornea" or "Ocular Surface" or "Conjunctiva" or "Pterygium Of Conjunctiva" or "Pterygium Of Cornea" or "Pterygium" or "Dry Eye

Syndrome" or "Dry Eye" or "Dry Eye Disease" or "Conjunctivitis Sicca" or "Keratoconjunctivitis Sicca" or "Keratitis Sicca" or "Keratitis" or "Immune Keratitis" or "Herpetic Keratitis" or "Corneal Ulcer" or "Refractive Surgical Procedures" or "Refractive Surgery" or "LASIK" or "Laser-assisted In Situ Keratomileusis" or "PRK" or "Photorefractive Keratectomy" or "SMILE" or "Small Incision Lenticule Extraction" or "Corneal Surgery" or "Corneal Transplantation" or "Corneal Transplant" or "Graft Rejection" or "Corneal Neovascularization" or "Corneal Diseases" or "Graves Ophthalmopathy" or "Thyroid Eye Disease" or "Allergic Conjunctivitis" or "Vernal Keratoconjunctivitis" or "Conjunctivitis" or "Neuralgia" or "Neuropathic Pain"). These were then combined with NGF-related terms: ("Nerve Growth Factor" or "NGF" or "Cenegermin"). The final search strategy was constructed using the Boolean operator AND to retrieve records containing both sets of terms.

3. Biology of Nerve Growth Factor

NGF is a key neurotrophic factor essential for the development and maintenance of both the central and peripheral nervous systems [54]. It plays a critical role in neuronal repair and apoptosis, which are involved in various neurological disorders [55,56]. NGF is also thought to contribute to several other biological processes, including immune regulation, inflammation, pulmonary hypertension, wound healing, and cancer metastasis [54,56–59]. Furthermore, NGF has several therapeutic applications in neurological, ocular, and skin diseases [13,60–74].

NGF was discovered in 1950 by Rita Levi-Montalcini. It was characterized by its ability to stimulate growth, survival, and differentiation of neurons during development and after injury [38,74]. Since its discovery, NGF has been found to be produced by epithelial cells, fibroblasts/myofibroblasts, endothelial cells, smooth muscle cells, hepatocytes, glial cells, astrocytes, Müller cells, antigen-presenting cells, lymphocytes, granulocytes, mast cells, and eosinophils [75]. The NGF gene is located on the short arm of chromosome 1 at 1p13.2 [74,76–78]. It is initially produced as a 118-amino-acid glycoprotein, formed by the subunits $\alpha 2$, β, and $\gamma 2$, bound by non-covalent bonds. The endoplasmic reticulum synthesizes NGF in its prosomal form (proNGF), which is then folded and transferred to the Golgi apparatus (Figure 1). The majority of active NGF results from the intracellular cleavage of proNGF by the calcium-dependent serine protease of its γ-subunits, exposing the biologically active carboxyl terminus. Some additional proNGF is released by the cells and exists as active NGF after processing by extracellular proteases [54,59].

NGF is part of the neurotrophin family that includes brain-derived neurotrophic factor (BDNF), neurotrophin-3 (NT-3), NT-4/5, and NT-6 [79]. These neurotrophins exert their biological functions through three Trk receptors: NGF binds to the tropomyosin $TrkA^{NGFR}$ tyrosine kinase receptor (termed $p140TrkA^{NGFR}$ or $TrkA^{NGFR}$), BDNF and NT-4 bind to TrkB, and NT-3 binds to TrkC. All neurotrophins also bind with lower affinity to the $p75^{NTR}$ receptor [38,80].

NGF's neurotrophic effects are primarily mediated by the $TrkA^{NGFR}$ receptor, and its secondary effects are mediated by the $p75^{NTR}$ receptor [81,82]. $TrkA^{NGFR}$ consists of a 140 kD molecule that forms a receptor with three domains: an extracellular receptor domain, a single transmembrane helix, and an intracellular tyrosine kinase domain [83]. The extracellular sequence is composed of five additional domains (D1–D5). D5 is an immunoglobulin-like domain responsible for NGF binding [84,85]. $TrkA^{NGFR}$ is extensively expressed in neuronal and non-neuronal tissues, such as immune cells, tumor cells, and stem cells [86,87].

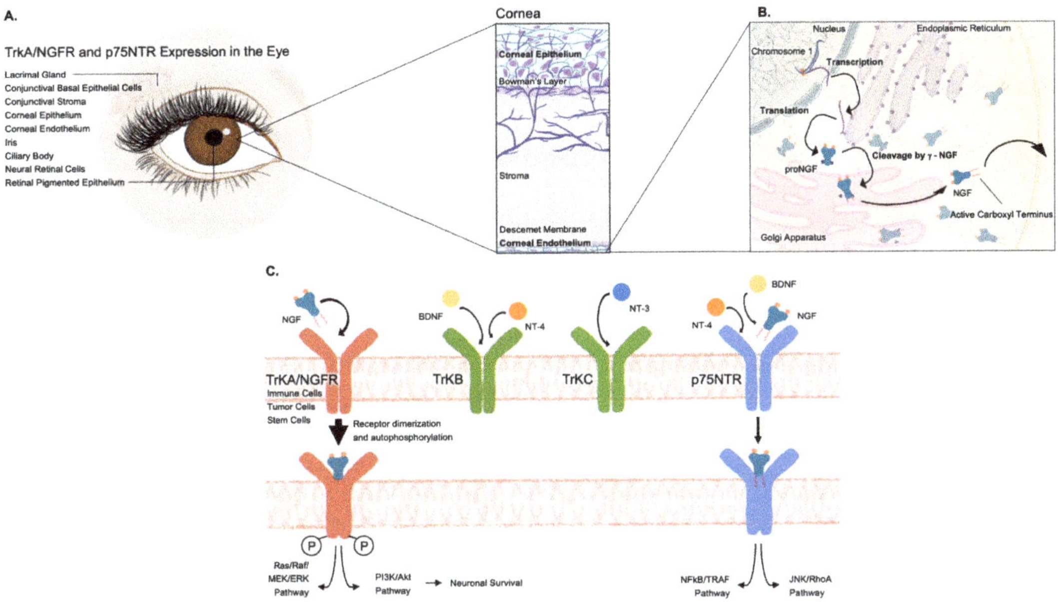

Figure 1. Schematic overview of nerve growth factor in the eye. (**A**) TrkA/NGFR and p75^{NTR} are expressed in the lacrimal gland, conjunctival basal epithelial cells, conjunctival stroma, corneal epithelium, corneal endothelium, iris, ciliary body, neural retinal cells, and retinal pigmented epithelium. (**B**) NGF synthesis and cleavage: the endoplasmic reticulum synthesizes proNGF, which is then folded and transferred to the Golgi apparatus. Intracellular cleavage of proNGF occurs by the calcium-dependent serine protease of its γ-subunits, exposing the biologically active carboxyl terminus. Additional proNGF is released from the cells, and active NGF is formed through the action of extracellular proteases. (**C**) TrkA/NGFR and p75^{NTR} signal transduction pathways: upon NGF binding to TrkA/NGFR, TrkA/NGFR dimerizes and is autophosphorylated at its intracellular domain, resulting in the activation of the Ras–Raf–MEK–ERK and PI3K–AKT signaling pathways. When NGF binds to the receptor p75^{NTR}, it activates the JNK or NFκB signaling pathways, including downstream interactions with RhoA and TRAF proteins.

When NGF binds to TrkA^{NGFR}, TrkA^{NGFR} dimerizes and is autophosphorylated at its intracellular domain, resulting in the activation of signaling pathways rat sarcoma protein (Ras), serine/threonine kinase (Raf), mitogen-activated protein kinase (MEK), extracellular-signal-regulated kinase (ERK), phosphoinositide 3-kinases (PI3K), and protein kinase B (AKT), imperative to neuronal survival [26,79,88,89]. When added exogenously to cultured cells, NGF binding can trigger pro-survival downstream signaling cascades that are critical for regulating neuronal growth, differentiation, and survival [90–94]. Specifically, PI3K/AKT signaling and MEK/ERK signaling suppress apoptosis by inhibiting caspase-3 activation and promote axonal regeneration and synaptic plasticity [90,94,95]. In cultured neurons, NGF also reduces oxidative stress, enhances antioxidant activity, and modulates microglial polarization toward an anti-inflammatory phenotype [90,96].

On the other hand, the union of NGF and p75^{NTR} receptor activates the c-Jun N-terminal kinase (JNK) or nuclear factor kappa B (NFκB) signaling pathways, including downstream interactions with Ras homolog family member A (RhoA) and tumor-necrosis-factor-receptor-associated factor (TRAF) proteins [26,79,88,89]. Binding of NGF to p75^{NTR}, especially in the absence of TrkA^{NGFR}, can trigger apoptotic signaling through the JNK and

NF-κB pathways, thereby underscoring the critical role of cellular context and receptor availability in determining the biological outcomes of NGF signaling [75,90,97].

Both TrkA^{NGFR} and p75^{NTR} are expressed in the basal epithelial cells, goblet cells, fibroblasts, and the stroma of the conjunctiva; limbal epithelial cells; corneal keratocytes and epithelial and endothelial cells; the iris; ciliary body; retinal pigmented epithelium; cells of the neural retina; and the lacrimal gland [39–48,98,99]. Given this, TrkA^{NGFR} and p75^{NTR} expression extends beyond neuronal elements to include resident epithelial, endothelial, stromal, and secretory cells, underscoring NGF's broader role in non-neuronal ocular functions. Moreover, TrkA^{NGFR} and p75^{NTR} have also been detected in skin and lung fibroblasts in vitro [100], providing additional evidence of their non-neuronal expression and activity.

4. The Role of Nerve Growth Factor on the Ocular Surface

The role of TrkA^{NGFR} in ocular surface diseases was first proposed by Lambiase et al. (1998) [39], who examined receptor expression under both normal and pathological conditions. The authors reported elevated levels of TrkA^{NGFR} in patients with vernal keratoconjunctivitis (VKC) and ocular cicatricial pemphigoid (OCP) compared to healthy individuals. In a later study, Micera et al. (2015) [99] further characterized NGF signaling in OCP. OCP conjunctivas showed αSMA-expressing fibroblasts and high NGF levels. Advanced-stage fibroblasts exhibited increased p75^{NTR} and reduced TrkA^{NGFR} expression compared to early-stage cells. NGF exposure reduced αSMA, p75^{NTR}, and cytokine release (TGF-β1, IL-4) in early, but not in advanced, OCP fibroblasts in vitro, suggesting stage-specific differences in NGF responsiveness. Increased receptor expression was also observed in corneal ulcers, suggesting a potential role for TrkA^{NGFR} in corneal epithelial remodeling. Furthermore, TrkA^{NGFR} is expressed in limbal basal epithelial cells in vivo and has been implicated in regulating the differentiation and proliferation of limbal stem cells [43,101]. Together, these findings support a role for NGF in promoting the proliferation and differentiation of limbal epithelial progenitor cells.

Under physiological conditions, NGF is released into the tear film and aqueous humor [41,67] and is suggested to originate from the corneal epithelium, stroma, and endothelial cells, as reported in studies of cadaveric human corneas [69]. Lambiase et al. (2002) [41] demonstrated the presence of NGF and TrkA^{NGFR} in the cornea, iris, ciliary body, and lens of rabbits, with the highest NGF levels found in the iris, suggesting that these molecules may play a role in regenerating sensory and sympathetic nerve fibers [102]. Furthermore, in the cornea, NGF accelerates keratocyte migration, stimulates immunomodulation and healing after injury, induces epithelial cell proliferation and differentiation, and maintains corneal epithelial stem cells [40,103]. Corneal innervation has also been proposed to be NGF-dependent by De Castro et al. (1998) [104], who demonstrated a relationship between NGF and corneal nerve density by analyzing the innervation pattern and response to noxious stimulation in TrkA^{NGFR} knockout mice. They observed reduced corneal nerve density and impaired corneal sensitivity in the knockout group compared to wild-type and heterozygous mice, further supporting the role of NGF in corneal innervation.

Furthermore, in vitro studies demonstrate that NGF exerts its biological effects on corneal epithelial cells, and neurons primarily through high-affinity binding to the TrkA^{NGFR} receptor. This activates key intracellular signaling cascades, particularly the PI3K/AKT and MEK/ERK pathways, which regulate cell survival, proliferation, and differentiation [94,105,106]. In human corneal epithelial cells, NGF stimulation leads to time- and dose-dependent phosphorylation of AKT and ERK, promoting cell cycle progression via upregulation of D-type cyclins and resulting in accelerated growth of these cells [105]. This aligns with broader evidence highlighting the role of PI3K/AKT signaling in supporting corneal epithelial homeostasis and wound healing [107].

In vivo, NGF is endogenously expressed in the murine cornea, with marked upregulation during reinnervation following surgical transection of corneal nerves [108]. Beyond its direct neurotrophic effects, NGF is also suggested to facilitate corneal healing by stimulating the release of pro-neural peptides such as substance P [68,109,110]. Supporting evidence from murine models also reveal that both NGF and glial-cell-line-derived neurotrophic factor (GDNF) are significantly upregulated in regenerating corneal epithelium, correlating with the reappearance of subbasal nerve fibers [111]. Conditioned medium from corneal epithelial cells enriched with NGF and GDNF promotes neurite outgrowth from trigeminal ganglion neurons, characterized by increased elongation and branching. Notably, neutralization of either NGF or GDNF significantly impairs this neuritogenic effect and diminishes corneal nerve regeneration in vivo. Furthermore, diabetic mice exhibit attenuated NGF and GDNF expression in regenerating corneal tissue, which is associated with delayed epithelial and nerve repair. This impairment can be rescued by exogenous supplementation of either growth factor [111]. Finally, functional studies using rats demonstrate that inhibition of endogenous NGF activity through anti-NGF antibodies delays corneal epithelial wound healing, whereas topical administration of exogenous NGF significantly accelerates epithelial closure [40].

NGF has also been suggested to play a role in modulating tear secretion and protecting against the deleterious effects of DED [47,49]. In primary human conjunctival epithelial cells and cell line cultures, NGF induces a dose-dependent increase in goblet cell numbers, promotes the production and storage of mucin-5AC precursor (MUC5AC), and promotes neural innervation and maintenance [49].

Additionally, NGF has been proposed to regulate immune cells infiltrating the cornea and conjunctiva during chronic inflammatory states associated with allergic and autoimmune diseases [39]. Lambiase et al. (1998) [39] demonstrated increased $TrkA^{NGFR}$ expression on eosinophils and T-helper lymphocytes in conjunctival biopsies from patients with VKC. The detection of NGF receptors on immune cells at the ocular surface during inflammatory conditions further supports the proposed role of NGF in modulating inflammatory processes. Finally, NGF may also act as an angiogenic factor under pathological conditions. Ribatti et al. (2009) [112] demonstrated a correlation between microvascular density and NGF/$TrkA^{NGFR}$ expression in endothelial cells of human pterygium. The study proposed that NGF is present and activates $TrkA^{NGFR}$ in pterygium, suggesting its involvement in the angiogenic response characteristic of this condition.

5. Clinical Applications of Nerve Growth Factor on the Ocular Surface

NGF has been extensively studied in both experimental and clinical contexts for its role in ocular surface diseases, including allergic conjunctivitis, NK, immune and infectious keratitis, DED, and corneal transplantation, cataract, and refractive surgeries. This section summarizes the current understanding of NGF as a therapeutic target in these conditions (Table 1).

5.1. Allergic Conjunctivitis

Preliminary experimental evidence suggests that NGF plays an essential role in allergic reactions through its release by neurons, lymphocytes, mast cells, fibroblasts, and smooth muscle cells following antigenic stimulation [113,114]. During allergic conjunctivitis, NGF is released by conjunctival epithelial and immune cells. Upon binding to $TrkA^{NGFR}$ and $p75^{NTR}$, NGF modulates allergic responses via the $p75^{NTR}$/JNK signaling pathway in conjunctival epithelial cells [115]. It is also hypothesized to actively contribute to allergic inflammation by binding to its receptors on eosinophils, mast cells, and T-helper lymphocytes [2–4].

Lambiase et al. (1995, 1997) [3,5] evaluated NGF plasma concentrations in patients with VKC and examined their correlation with plasma levels of substance P, as well as serum levels of eosinophil cationic protein (ECP) and immunoglobulin E. NGF plasma levels were measured, and tarsal and bulbar conjunctival biopsy specimens were collected from both VKC patients and healthy matched controls. The results showed significantly higher plasma concentrations of NGF in VKC patients, which correlated with the number of mast cells in the tarsal and bulbar conjunctiva.

The conjunctival epithelium and NGF may play an active role in ocular allergic inflammation through the $p75^{NTR}$ pathway. Sacchetti et al. (2019) [115] investigated the involvement of $TrkA^{NGFR}$ and $p75^{NTR}$ in patients with allergic rhinoconjunctivitis (ARC) before and after a conjunctival provocation test (CPT) with an allergen. In the quiescent phase, ARC patients exhibited a significant increase in conjunctival $p75^{NTR}$ expression, while NGF and $TrkA^{NGFR}$ were undetectable. Following allergen challenge, patients showed a significant increase in tear NGF levels and upregulation of downstream $p75^{NTR}$ signaling molecules, including JNK/stress-activated protein kinase (SAPK) and p53. These findings suggest an active role for $p75^{NTR}$ in mediating allergic responses on the ocular surface.

5.2. Neurotrophic Keratopathy

Damage to corneal nerves alters the metabolism and survival of the epithelium by depleting the tissue of acetylcholine and substance P, consequently resulting in decreased epithelial mitosis and impaired epithelial healing, which may lead to the development of neurotrophic ulcers [116,117].

Murine NGF purified from submaxillary glands has been used to treat ocular surface diseases such as NK due to herpetic infections, chemical burns, topical anesthetic abuse, and diabetes [66,68]. In 1969, Bocchini and Angeletti [118] described a method for purifying NGF from adult mouse submaxillary glands. Prospective pilot studies later evaluated the effects of intracerebroventricular administration of murine growth factors in patients with Parkinson's and Alzheimer's disease [65,119]. Eriksdotter et al. (1998) [65] and Olson et al. (1991) [119] investigated the administration of murine NGF into the lateral cerebral ventricle and left putamen. The rationale behind these studies was to explore potential therapies that could counteract cholinergic degeneration and/or induce the formation of new cholinergic nerve terminals in Alzheimer's disease, and to support chromaffin cell autografts in patients with severe Parkinson's disease. Although these studies were insufficient to demonstrate the therapeutic intracerebral use of NGF in neurodegenerative diseases, they laid the foundation for future research into NGF's clinical applications.

In 1998, Lambiase et al. [68] evaluated the effect of topical murine NGF in patients with neurotrophic ulcers and observed complete corneal healing in all patients after 10 days to 6 weeks of treatment. Additionally, an observational study by Bonini et al. (2000) [66] evaluated 45 eyes from 43 patients with stage 2 or 3 NK that were unresponsive to artificial tears and therapeutic contact lenses. Patients received murine NGF eye drops at a concentration of 200 µg/mL every two hours (from 6:00 AM to 12:00 AM) for two days, followed by one drop every four hours until complete epithelial healing. Once healed, a lower concentration (100 µg/mL) was administered four times daily for two weeks. Complete corneal healing was achieved in all patients within 2 to 6 weeks of initiating murine NGF treatment. Mild and transient ocular adverse effects (AEs), such as photophobia, burning sensation, and conjunctival hyperemia, were reported, but no systemic AEs occurred during the follow-up period of 16 to 72 months [13,66,120].

Topical rhNGF has also been studied for the treatment of NK. It is the only FDA-approved pharmacologic treatment for NK and the first topical biologic approved in the field of ophthalmology. rhNGF (cenegermin) ophthalmic solution 0.002% received FDA approval in 2018 and is synthesized using recombinant *Escherichia coli* [52].

A case of central NK in Wallenberg syndrome (WS), unresponsive to artificial tears and bandage contact lenses, was treated with rhNGF and reported by Mandarà et al. (2022) [7]. A 47-year-old man with WS, caused by a stroke in the territory of the left vertebrobasilar artery, developed left corneal NK grade 3 of central origin. The patient was treated with topical rhNGF at a concentration of 20 μg/mL, one drop six times daily for eight weeks. The corneal epithelium healed completely, with no recurrence at one-year follow-up. Another case report [8] described an 84-year-old female who developed NK in the context of diabetes mellitus, infectious keratitis, DED, and corneal exposure. She was treated with rhNGF 20 μg/mL, administered six times daily. The epithelial defect began to improve five weeks after initiating treatment and resolved completely after eight weeks.

The long-term clinical efficacy of topical rhNGF, formulated at 20 μg/mL, for the treatment of NK was demonstrated in a retrospective case series from a single center [9]. Eighteen patients with stage 2 or 3 NK were treated with rhNGF six times daily for eight weeks and followed for up to 48 months. All patients achieved complete corneal healing by the end of the treatment period. Three patients experienced recurrence of persistent epithelial defects within 12 months, and one patient experienced recurrence of a corneal ulcer within 36 months. The authors concluded that rhNGF was effective in restoring long-term corneal epithelial stability and highlighted the need for larger, long-term, prospective, controlled trials.

Two randomized controlled trials evaluated the safety and efficacy of rhNGF in patients with NK. Patients were administered 10 or 20 μg/mL rhNGF eye drops six times daily for eight weeks. The rhNGF-treated groups demonstrated both statistically and clinically significant reductions in lesion size and disease progression during treatment [10–12]. The REPARO trial [11,12], a multicenter randomized controlled trial, assessed the use of 10 and 20 μg/mL rhNGF eye drops in patients with stage 2 or 3 NK. The trial confirmed the safety and efficacy of rhNGF in moderate to severe cases. Phase I evaluated safety in 18 patients, while Phase II assessed safety and efficacy in 156 patients. Participants were randomized into three groups: 10 μg/mL rhNGF, 20 μg/mL rhNGF, or vehicle, for an 8-week treatment period. All participants received one eye drop six times daily. At week 8, 43.1% of vehicle-treated patients exhibited less than 0.5 mm of lesion staining compared to 74.5% in the 10 μg/mL rhNGF group and 74.0% in the 20 μg/mL rhNGF group. Another multicenter randomized, vehicle-controlled trial [10] evaluated 20 μg/mL rhNGF in NK patients, using complete healing of persistent epithelial defects or corneal ulcers at 8 weeks as the primary endpoint. Patients received one eye drop six times daily. The study found that 65.2% of patients treated with rhNGF achieved 0 mm of lesion staining with no residual staining compared to only 16.7% of vehicle-treated patients. Additionally, Cheung et al. (2022) [121] conducted a retrospective chart review demonstrating the effectiveness of rhNGF in combination with bandage contact lenses for NK. The study reported a 70% improvement in corneal sensation and complete epithelial healing in 67% of patients with persistent epithelial defects.

NK is infrequent in the pediatric population. Its etiology can be congenital, either as isolated corneal anesthesia or in association with systemic disease, or acquired, resulting from infections, neurological disorders, or the toxicity of topical medications [122]. Several case reports [123–127] and a retrospective case series [53] examined the use of rhNGF in the pediatric population. Papadopoulos et al. (2021) [123] reported the case of a 7-year-old male who developed NK following two years of treatment with antibiotics, steroids, and artificial tears for infectious keratitis. The patient was successfully treated with 20 μg/mL rhNGF eye drops administered six times daily for eight weeks, with no reported AEs. In another case [124], a 3-year-old male developed NK after undergoing surgery for rhabdomyosarcoma of the jaw. Treatment with 20 μg/mL rhNGF eye drops, administered six times daily for eight weeks, resulted in complete corneal epithelial healing within three weeks. A separate case report [127] described a 5-month-old child with congenital corneal anesthesia who developed NK and was treated with 200 μg/mL murine NGF, administered every two hours (from 6:00 AM to 12:00 AM) for two days. This was followed by one drop six times daily until epithelial healing. Once the corneal epithelium was intact, the child received 100 μg/mL murine NGF, administered six times daily for six months. By day 10 of treatment, the mother reported that the child began displaying signs of discomfort upon instillation of the drops, which was postulated to indicate the return of corneal sensation. In a different study, Fausto et al. (2020) [125] reported the case of a 9-year-old patient with pontine tegmental cap dysplasia and bilateral cranial nerve VI and VIII palsies who developed NK and was treated with 20 μg/mL rhNGF, one drop six times daily at two-hour intervals (from 8 AM to 8 PM). After eight weeks of treatment, the authors reported complete epithelial healing and a reduction in corneal opacity and neovascularization. Cochet–Bonnet corneal esthesiometry could not be performed due to the patient's lack of cooperation. No local or systemic AEs were observed. Finally, a retrospective case series [53] involving eight pediatric patients (age range 2 to 18 years) from three tertiary referral institutions treated NK with 20 μg/mL rhNGF. The etiologies of NK included Stickler syndrome (cranial nerve V palsy), surgery for cerebellopontine tumor, cranial nerve V agenesis, trauma (fireworks injury), complex regional pain syndrome, Gómez–López-Hernández syndrome, Stevens–Johnson syndrome, and Herpes Simplex Virus (HSV) keratitis. The authors reported improvement in corneal sensation (Cochet–Bonnet esthesiometry) and Mackie classification staging in 63% of patients. All patients in this series had previously received NK-specific therapies (e.g., tarsorrhaphy, amniotic membrane transplant, autologous serum eye drops). AEs reported during therapy included ocular pain, difficulty sleeping, and continued corneal thinning.

To conclude, rhNGF is unique among current therapies for NK in that it directly targets the underlying pathophysiological deficit: corneal nerve damage. In the meta-analysis by Roumeau et al. (2022) [128], rhNGF achieved complete corneal healing in 75% of patients, comparable to outcomes with autologous serum (92%), amniotic membrane transplantation (AMT, 86%), and corneal neurotization (99%). In contrast, non-specific treatments, such as lubricants, were associated with a markedly lower healing rate of 23%. Surgical and non-surgical treatments demonstrated similar rates of complete healing overall. Notably, only rhNGF and AMT were associated with significant improvements in visual acuity. Moreover, rhNGF demonstrated a relatively short mean time to epithelial healing (24.2 days) compared to 27.6 days for autologous serum, 16.4 days for AMT, and 117 days for neurotization. Vera-Duarte et al. (2024) [129] also emphasized that rhNGF is distinct among therapies for neurotrophic keratopathy due to its ability to restore corneal epithelial integrity while promoting reinnervation, thereby addressing both the epithelial and neural components of the disease, unlike conventional treatments that primarily provide trophic support (e.g., autologous serum, amniotic membrane) or mechanical protection (e.g., artificial tears, bandage contact lenses) without targeting the underlying sensory nerve deficit.

In the case of autologous serum, which can mimic some effects of recombinant NGF therapy through its content of neurotrophic and epithelial-supporting factors such as NGF, epidermal growth factor (EGF), transforming growth factor-beta (TGF-β), insulin-like growth factor-1 (IGF-1), fibronectin, and vitamin A [130–133], its therapeutic benefits are likely multifactorial. Moreover, the concentration of NGF in autologous serum is several orders of magnitude lower than that achieved with pharmacologic formulations like cenegermin [130–132], which are specifically designed to reach effective levels for epithelial healing and corneal nerve regeneration. This difference may account for the greater efficacy of rhNGF in restoring visual acuity, as described above.

5.3. Immune Keratitis

Lambiase et al. (2000) examined the use of murine NGF in patients with autoimmune corneal ulcers and corneal melting unresponsive to immunosuppressive therapy [13]. In the study, four patients with severe corneal melting secondary to immune-related peripheral corneal ulcers received one drop of murine NGF solution (10 μg in 50 μL, equivalent to 200 μg/mL) every two hours (from 6 AM to 12 PM) for two days, followed by six times daily until the ulcer healed. Once complete healing was achieved, the dose was reduced to 5 μg in 50 μL (equivalent to 100 μg/mL), administered four times daily for two weeks. All patients demonstrated complete corneal healing within eight weeks of treatment.

5.4. Herpetic Keratitis

Murine NGF has been proposed as a potential therapy to treat and prevent the recurrence of herpetic keratitis. In a rabbit model, Lambiase et al. (2008) [15] demonstrated that topical administration of murine NGF significantly improved both clinical and laboratory parameters compared to the balanced salt solution (BSS)-treated control group. Notably, the therapeutic effects of NGF were comparable to those of acyclovir, with no significant differences observed between the two treatment groups. In contrast, treatment with neutralizing anti-NGF antibodies worsened disease severity, resulting in fatal HSV encephalitis in two animals. Animals in the study were divided into four groups and treated topically with either NGF, acyclovir, BSS, or neutralizing anti-NGF antibodies. Disease severity was graded using a keratitis scoring system: 0.0 to 0.5 indicated normal or non-specific superficial lesions; 0.6 to 0.9 indicated punctate ulcerations; 1.0 to 1.9 indicated dendritic ulcerations; 2.0 to 2.9 indicated geographic ulcerations or trophic erosions involving less than 50 percent of the cornea; and 3.0 to 3.9 indicated involvement of more than 50 percent of the cornea [14]. A correlation between NGF deficiency and HSV reactivation was also demonstrated in rabbits with latent HSV infection [134]. Although the underlying mechanism remains unclear, the authors suggested that NGF's immunomodulatory effects, such as promoting T and B lymphocyte proliferation and regulating antibody production [135], may contribute to its ability to suppress HSV replication. Supporting its therapeutic potential, a case report [16] describing a 68-year-old HIV-positive male with an acyclovir-resistant herpetic corneal ulcer reported successful treatment with NGF eye drops. NGF was administered at a concentration of 200 μg/mL (10 μg NGF dissolved in 50 μL of 0.9% saline), instilled into the inferior conjunctival fornix every two hours until complete epithelial healing, which was achieved after 23 days. Following ulcer resolution, the drops were continued at the same concentration four times daily for an additional 15 days. No recurrence was observed during one year of follow-up.

Although the molecular mechanisms underlying NGF's protective effects in herpetic keratitis are not yet fully understood, emerging evidence suggests that its therapeutic benefits arise from its immunomodulatory, anti-inflammatory, and neurotrophic properties rather than direct antiviral activity. In addition to the above-mentioned study by Lambiase et al. (2008) [15], recent in vitro studies suggest NGF has the capacity to inhibit Toll-like receptor 3 (TLR3)-mediated inflammatory cascades in human corneal epithelial cells by suppressing NF-κB activation and reducing reactive oxygen species (ROS) production, thereby attenuating the expression of pro-inflammatory cytokines such as IL-6, IL-8, IFN-β, and RANTES [136]. These findings hint at NGF's ability to mitigate virus-induced immunopathology by dampening excessive inflammation through the modulation of innate immune signaling pathways, specifically TLR signaling, which is particularly relevant to HSV pathology. Additional mechanistic insights from diabetic keratopathy models highlight NGF's ability to attenuate hyperglycemia-induced oxidative stress, inflammation, and apoptosis. In vitro and in vivo studies by Park et al. (2016) [137] demonstrated that NGF markedly reduced ROS generation, NF-κB activation, and the expression of IL-1β and TNF-α in corneal epithelial cells cultured under high-glucose conditions. NGF also suppressed the expression of cleaved caspase-3 and BAX, which are key markers of apoptosis, and significantly reversed corneal epithelial damage and inflammatory responses in streptozotocin-induced diabetic rats. These data reinforce the notion that NGF exerts broad cytoprotective effects and suggest possible mechanisms through which it mitigates viral diseases via suppression of inflammatory and apoptotic signaling. Lastly, given that NGF is both produced by and acts upon various immune cell types and is upregulated systemically and locally during inflammation, infection, and stress, it may act as a coactivator of immune responses and contribute to the recruitment, activation, and survival of immune cells, as suggested here [138,139]. Based on this, it is plausible that exogenously administered NGF could similarly modulate immune activity and enhance host responses during immunologic insults.

5.5. Dry Eye Disease

NGF and its receptors are expressed in the lacrimal gland, and NGF has been detected in human tear film [19]. Topical NGF administration has also been shown to stimulate tear secretion in patients with DED [18,25]. Chang et al. (2008) [17] further proposed that NGF may reduce corneal epithelial cell apoptosis and mitigate damage caused by chronic hyperosmolar stress, a hallmark of DED. As previously discussed, NGF may exert cytoprotective effects on the ocular surface through mechanisms relevant to dry eye disease. In vitro, NGF has been shown to reduce TLR3-mediated inflammation and oxidative stress, potentially via NF-κB inhibition and decreased ROS production, leading to lower expression of IL-6, IL-8, and IFN-β [136]. In diabetic keratopathy models, NGF also reduced apoptotic markers and improved epithelial integrity [137]. While not studied directly in DED, these pathways may contribute to epithelial preservation under desiccating stress.

Clinical studies involving human participants [17,140] have also demonstrated a positive correlation between tear NGF levels and dry eye severity. Using enzyme-linked immunoassays, researchers quantified NGF concentrations in tear samples from affected individuals and found correlations with conjunctival hyperemia, fluorescein staining, and OSDI scores greater than 20, thereby supporting the potential utility of NGF as a biomarker for disease severity in DED. A Phase II, prospective, open-label, multiple-dose clinical trial [141] evaluated the safety and efficacy of rhNGF eye drops in 40 patients with DED. This single-center study tested two concentrations of rhNGF eye drop solution (4 μg/mL and 20 μg/mL), administered twice daily in both eyes for 28 days. The outcomes assessed included treatment-emergent AEs; the frequency and severity of DED symptoms, evaluated using the Symptoms Assessment in Dry Eye (SANDE) scale; ocular surface staining assessed with lissamine green using the National Eye Institute scale; tear production measured by Schirmer test type I (without anesthesia); and tear function assessed by tear film break-up time and tear film osmolarity. Both concentrations of rhNGF induced significant improvement in the signs and symptoms of DED; however, improvement in tear film break-up time was observed only in the 20 μg/mL group. These findings suggest that higher concentrations of rhNGF significantly enhance tear production and function.

Interestingly, another Phase II multicenter randomized double-masked vehicle-controlled dose-ranging trial [142] evaluated the safety and efficacy of rhNGF (cenegermin) eye drops at a concentration of 20 μg/mL in 261 patients with moderate to severe DED, including Sjögren's DED. Patients were randomized to receive cenegermin eye drops at a dose of 20 μg/mL either two or three times daily, or vehicle alone, for four weeks, followed by a 12-week follow-up period. Although the primary endpoint of change in Schirmer I score at week 4 was not met, a significantly higher proportion of patients treated with cenegermin achieved clinically meaningful tear production (Schirmer I greater than 10 mm in 5 min) compared to vehicle. Notably, only the group receiving cenegermin three times daily showed sustained and statistically significant improvements in patient-reported symptoms, as measured by the SANDE and (Impact of Dry Eye on Everyday Life) IDEEL questionnaires, throughout the follow-up period. Cenegermin was generally well tolerated, with mild and transient eye pain being the most commonly reported AE. These findings suggest that administering cenegermin 20 μg/mL three times daily may provide greater and longer lasting symptomatic relief in patients with moderate to severe DED.

5.6. Corneal Transplantation

In a preclinical study, Gong et al. (2007) [21] demonstrated that NGF gene therapy may enhance corneal graft survival by modulating immune responses. Using a high-rejection rat model, Lewis rats received corneal grafts from inbred female Dark Agouti donors, which are fully mismatched at major histocompatibility complex (MHC) class I and II loci, resulting in uniform graft rejection. A single local administration of adenovirus-mediated NGF gene transfer one day prior to transplantation significantly prolonged graft survival, preserved endothelial cell density, and suppressed the expression of key pro-inflammatory cytokines, including TNF-α, IFN-γ, IL-12p40, and IL-4, compared to untreated controls. Interestingly, NGF was shown to reduce IL-6 and IL-8 secretion in human corneal epithelial cells in vitro, possibly by modulating NF-κB signaling pathways [136]. While this effect has not been investigated in corneal transplantation models, IL-6 and IL-8 are known to be upregulated in the tear film and aqueous humor following procedures such as endothelial keratoplasty and Descemet's membrane endothelial keratoplasty, where they contribute to postoperative inflammation and increased risk of graft rejection [143–145].

The use of rhNGF in NK following penetrating keratoplasty (PKP) was reported in a case involving a 24-year-old woman who had previously undergone acoustic neuroma surgery [20]. The patient presented with stage 3 NK, which necessitated multilayer amniotic membrane transplantation (AMT) and two PKPs due to recurrence. After the second PKP, 20 μg/mL rhNGF eye drops were administered six times daily for eight weeks, resulting in complete corneal epithelial healing and a stable ocular surface maintained over 12 months of follow-up. Pan et al. (2018) [146] investigated the association between tear NGF levels and corneal subepithelial nerve regeneration following keratoplasty. In this retrospective study, tear samples from 30 eyes of 28 patients undergoing primary keratoplasty were analyzed. NGF concentrations were reduced on postoperative day 1 compared to preoperative levels but showed a progressive increase on days 7, 30, and 90. By day 90, peripheral nerve buds were detected in 80% of the grafts, and their presence significantly correlated with elevated tear NGF levels, suggesting that postoperative upregulation of NGF may contribute to subepithelial nerve regeneration after keratoplasty. Finally, a case study by Gouvea et al. (2021) [147] reported the clinical outcomes of a 75-year-old male with lattice dystrophy and a history of HSV keratitis who developed NK in the right eye two years after undergoing PKP. Following multiple recurrences and failure of NK-specific treatments, including dehydrated amniotic membrane, therapeutic contact lens, and lateral tarsorrhaphy, the patient was started on 20 μg/mL rhNGF eye drops administered six times daily. By week 8, the corneal epithelium had completely healed, and visual acuity (VA) improved from 20/100 to 20/50. The ocular surface remained stable during a six-month follow-up.

5.7. Cataract Surgery

A randomized controlled trial investigated the efficacy of topical murine NGF versus 0.2% hyaluronic acid in promoting corneal wound healing after cataract surgery [22]. The primary objective was to assess whether murine NGF accelerates postoperative epithelial recovery. Patients in the NGF group received 1 drop of 200 μg/mL murine NGF solution (10 μg in 50 μL of 0.9% saline) instilled into the inferior conjunctival fornix every two hours between 6 AM and 12 PM for two weeks, followed by four times daily administration for an additional week. The control group received 0.2% hyaluronic acid on the same schedule. By day 21 postoperatively, anterior segment optical coherence tomography (OCT) revealed complete stromal healing in the NGF-treated group, with no residual injury detectable. In contrast, the control group exhibited persistent incision lines extending from the corneal surface to Descemet's membrane. These findings suggest that topical murine NGF significantly accelerates corneal wound healing following cataract surgery.

NGF may support corneal epithelial repair after cataract surgery by activating PI3K/AKT and MEK/ERK pathways, which are key regulators of epithelial cell survival, proliferation, and migration. As described earlier, NGF stimulation in corneal epithelial cells leads to phosphorylation of AKT and ERK, facilitating cell cycle progression and promoting epithelial regeneration [105]. These findings are consistent with evidence linking PI3K/AKT signaling to corneal wound healing [107] and with studies demonstrating that NGF enhances epithelial cell migration and proliferation [36].

5.8. Refractive Surgery

A trial involving rhesus monkeys evaluated nerve regeneration, as well as NGF mRNA and protein expression, following laser in situ keratomileusis (LASIK) to correct −8.00 diopters of myopia [25]. NGF mRNA expression increased 5.4-fold on day 3, remained elevated at 2-fold above baseline on day 7, and normalized by three months after surgery. NGF protein levels decreased on days 3 and 7 after LASIK but returned to control levels by one month postoperatively. These early changes in NGF mRNA and protein levels correlated with the density of the corneal nerve plexuses. The authors proposed that these alterations may be associated with the initiation of nerve regeneration and the eventual recovery of corneal nerve plexuses. In comparative studies, tear NGF levels are highest following photorefractive keratectomy (PRK), followed by LASIK and small incision lenticule extraction (SMILE) [23,24,148]. Moreover, a positive correlation has been observed between tear NGF levels and the degree of myopia corrected with SMILE [24].

Topical administration of murine NGF following refractive surgery was evaluated by Joo et al. (2004) [149]. In their prospective, double-masked study in rabbits, murine NGF (200 mg in 1 mL of BSS) was applied directly to the exposed stromal bed immediately after photoablation and then to the corneal surface four times daily for three days. Murine NGF treatment was associated with a faster recovery of corneal sensitivity after LASIK compared to the control group. Similarly, Gong et al. (2021) investigated the effects of topical NGF on dry eye following LASIK [150]. In their study, rabbits that underwent LASIK were randomly assigned to one of three treatment groups: 200 μg/mL murine NGF, 0.2% hyaluronate, or normal saline. The authors reported accelerated recovery of subbasal and superficial stromal nerve densities, improved corneal sensitivity, and increased tear film break-up time in the murine NGF group at one and three months postoperatively.

A prospective, nonrandomized, comparative clinical trial by Lee et al. (2005) evaluated tear NGF levels following LASIK and PRK [148]. The study reported an increase in tear NGF levels after both refractive procedures, with a greater elevation observed in the PRK group. Early postoperative NGF levels in tears were associated with reduced postoperative corneal sensation, tear film break-up time, and Schirmer test values. The authors observed lower tear film break-up times at 1, 3, and 6 months in the LASIK group, whereas the PRK group exhibited higher Schirmer test values and improved corneal sensation at 3 and 6 months. The authors hypothesized that the differences observed were due to the higher postoperative NGF levels detected in the PRK group.

Two cases of NK following LASIK treated with rhNGF were reported by Habibi et al. (2021) [151], with both procedures having occurred 20 years prior to presentation. After 8 weeks of treatment, there was a marked improvement in VA, corneal sensitivity, and fluorescein corneal staining. Nonetheless, signs and symptoms recurred in both cases: at 3 months after therapy in the first and 1 month in the second. These findings suggest that a longer duration of treatment may be beneficial for patients with mild chronic manifestations of neurotrophic disease.

5.9. Adverse Events

AEs associated with murine NGF and rhNGF have been reported; however, all were transient [16,22,53,103,120,141,152]. Local AEs include eye pain (affecting 0–63.5%), foreign body sensation (4.3–20%), blurred vision (10.8–16.7%), photophobia (1.9–16.7%), increased lacrimation (0–15%), ocular pruritus (7.7%), eyelid pain (0–10.7%), eye discharge (0–5%), ocular hyperemia (0–4.3%), corneal deposits (0–4.3%), anterior chamber inflammation (4.3%), eye inflammation (4.3%), hyphema (4.3%), keratitis (4.3%), eye paresthesia (4.3%), posterior capsule opacification (4.3%), and corneal neovascularization (0–1.9%). Systemic AEs described in the literature include headache (1.9–25%), rhinitis (0–10%), nasopharyngitis (0–5%), back and neck pain (0–5%), tinnitus (0–5%), and flatulence (0–5%). To date, no serious AEs have been reported with the topical use of NGF on the ocular surface [10,11,141,142,152,153]. Following topical administration, a small proportion of NGF is absorbed by the conjunctiva, peri-orbital tissue, and cornea, with distribution mainly confined to the anterior segment [103]. rhNGF is eliminated through tears and the nasolacrimal duct, with minimal systemic absorption [52]. Notably, murine NGF and rhNGF do not induce the production of circulating NGF antibodies [103,120,152]. The most commonly reported AEs are related to topical application and may, in some cases, reflect corneal reinnervation and sensitivity [103]. A notable limitation in the current body of experimental research is the absence of data on the use of rhNGF in pregnant women [52].

A randomized, double-masked, vehicle-controlled trial [152] evaluated ocular and systemic AEs associated with rhNGF in healthy volunteers. Outcomes measured included blood chemistry, urinalysis, vital signs, electrocardiograms (ECGs), serum NGF antibody levels, ocular and systemic AEs, VA, tear function, intraocular pressure, fundus examination, and ocular symptoms. A few mild and transient ocular AEs related to rhNGF administration were reported, including a transient burning sensation, photophobia, and conjunctival hyperemia. These findings are consistent with those reported by Lambiase et al. (2007) [120] in NK patients treated with murine NGF. It is also noteworthy that a retrospective study in pediatric patients with NK found that 25% of those with pre-existing mild corneal neovascularization exhibited increased conjunctival injection and progression of corneal stromal neovascularization during rhNGF treatment [53]. These findings are consistent with those of Matsuyama et al. (2017) [154], who administered pellets containing murine NGF into 1–2 mm corneal pockets to assess the distribution and characteristics of perivascular nerves in neovascularized tissue using a mouse corneal micropocket model. Immunohistochemistry analysis revealed that NGF promotes the innervation of perivascular nerves, potentially regulating blood flow within neovessels and accelerating the maturation of pre-existing corneal blood vessels.

Table 1. Studies evaluating nerve growth factor as a treatment for ocular surface diseases.

Authors	Study Design	Ocular Surface Disease	No. of Patients (Eyes)	Type of NGF	Treatment Scheme	Outcomes	Follow-Up	Results
Lambiase et al. (1998) [68]	Case series	Neurotrophic keratopathy	12 (14)	Murine NGF	1 drop (200 μg/mL) every 2 h (6–12 AM) for 2 days, then 6 times daily until ulcer healed. 1 drop (100 μg/mL) 4 times daily for 2 weeks post-healing.	Corneal healing.	3 months	All patients had complete resolution of the corneal ulcer after 10 days to 6 weeks of treatment.
Bonini et al. (2000) [66]	Prospective, noncomparative, interventional case series	Neurotrophic keratopathy	43 (45)	Murine NGF	1 drop (200 μg/mL) every 2 h (6–12 AM) for 2 days, then 6 times daily until healed. 1 drop (100 μg/mL) 4 times daily for 2 weeks post-healing.	Size and depth of the ulcer or the epithelial defect, corneal sensitivity, best corrected VA, side effects, and relapse of the disease.	15.8 +/− 11.5 months	Complete resolution of the persistent epithelial defect after 12 days to 6 weeks of treatment in all patients. AE: Hyperemia and ocular and periocular pain.
Tan et al. (2006) [127]	Case report *	Neurotrophic keratopathy	1 (1)	Murine NGF	1 drop (200 μg/mL) every 2 h (6 AM–12 AM) for 2 days, then 6 times daily until healing. 1 drop (100 μg/mL) 6 times daily until a cumulative dose of 3 mg was reached.	Corneal healing.	4 months	Corneal healing at 8 weeks.

Table 1. *Cont.*

Authors	Study Design	Ocular Surface Disease	No. of Patients (Eyes)	Type of NGF	Treatment Scheme	Outcomes	Follow-Up	Results
Bonini et al. (2018) [11,12]	Randomized controlled trial	Neurotrophic keratopathy	Phase I: 18 (18); Phase II: 156 (156)	rhNGF	1 drop (10 µg/mL or 20 µg/mL) 6 times daily for 8 weeks.	Corneal healing, AEs.	56 weeks	At week 8, 74.5% of patients receiving rhNGF 10 µg/mL had less than 0.5 mm of lesion staining compared to 74.0% of those receiving rhNGF 20 µg/mL. During follow-up, 96% of patients remained recurrence-free. AEs were mostly local, mild, and transient.
Pedrotti et al. (2019) [124]	Case report *	Neurotrophic keratopathy	1	rhNGF	1 drop (20 µg/mL) 6 times daily for 8 weeks.	Corneal healing.	21 weeks	Corneal healing at 3 weeks.
Pflugfelder et al. (2020) [10]	Multicenter randomized controlled trial	Neurotrophic keratopathy	48	rhNGF	1 drop (20 µg/mL or vehicle) 6 times daily for 8 weeks.	Corneal healing and sensitivity, changes in VA.	24 weeks	At week 8, 65.2% of patients in the 20 µg/mL rhNGF group achieved 0 mm of lesion staining with no residual staining compared to 16.7% in the control group.

Table 1. *Cont.*

Authors	Study Design	Ocular Surface Disease	No. of Patients (Eyes)	Type of NGF	Treatment Scheme	Outcomes	Follow-Up	Results
Ahuja et al. (2020) [8]	Case report	Neurotrophic keratopathy	1	rhNGF	1 drop (20 μg/mL) 6 times a day for 8 weeks.	Corneal healing.	-	Corneal healing at 8 weeks.
Pocobelli et al. (2020) [20]	Case report	Neurotrophic keratopathy on penetrating keratoplasty	1	rhNGF	1 drop (20 μg/mL) 6 times a day for 8 weeks.	Corneal healing.	12 months	Complete corneal healing was achieved after 5 weeks. NK recurred at week 9. After a second cycle of treatment, no recurrence was observed during follow-up.
Fausto et al. (2020) [125]	Case report *	Neurotrophic keratopathy	1	rhNGF	1 drop (20 μg/mL) 6 times a day for 8 weeks.	Corneal healing.	6 months	Corneal healing was achieved at 8 weeks, with a reduction in corneal opacity and neovascularization.
Mandarà et al. (2022) [7]	Case report	Neurotrophic keratopathy	1	rhNGF	1 drop (20 μg/mL) 6 times a day for 8 weeks.	Corneal healing.	12 months	Corneal healing at 8 weeks.

Table 1. *Cont.*

Authors	Study Design	Ocular Surface Disease	No. of Patients (Eyes)	Type of NGF	Treatment Scheme	Outcomes	Follow-Up	Results
Hatcher et al. (2021) [53]	Retrospective case series *	Neurotrophic keratopathy	8 (9)	rhNGF	1 drop (20 µg/mL) 6 times a day for 8 weeks.	Corneal healing, sensation and scarring, VA, and AEs.	2–13 months	63% experienced clinical improvement with no recurrence in 10 months. AEs: ocular pain, difficulty sleeping, continued corneal thinning, and corneal neovascularization.
Papadopoulos et al. (2021) [123]	Case report *	Neurotrophic keratopathy	1	rhNGF	1 drop (20 µg/mL) 6 times a day for 8 weeks.	Corneal healing.	8 months	Corneal healing was achieved at 8 weeks, with no recurrence during follow-up.
Habibi et al. (2021) [151]	Case series	Neurotrophic keratopathy following LASIK	2 (4)	rhNGF	1 drop (20 µg/mL) 6 times a day for 8 weeks.	Corneal healing, VA, and recurrence.	5 months	Corneal healing and VA improvement at 8 weeks. Recurrence at 1 and 3 months after treatment.
Cheung et al. (2022) [121]	Retrospective chart review	Neurotrophic keratopathy	16 (18)	rhNGF	8 weeks course, drop frequency not specified.	Corneal healing and sensitivity.	3–20 months	Corneal sensation increased from 7% to 79% of eyes. Among patients with a persistent epithelial defect, 67% experienced complete resolution.

Table 1. *Cont.*

Authors	Study Design	Ocular Surface Disease	No. of Patients (Eyes)	Type of NGF	Treatment Scheme	Outcomes	Follow-Up	Results
Bruscolini et al. (2022) [9]	Retrospective chart review	Neurotrophic keratopathy	18	rhNGF	1 drop (20 µg/mL) 6 times daily for 8 weeks.	Corneal healing and sensitivity, VA, and recurrence.	48 months	Corneal healing was observed at 8 weeks, with improvements in corneal sensitivity, VA, and tear production during follow-up. Three cases recurred within 12 months and one case within 36 months.
Hamrah et al. (2024) [153]	Phase IV multicenter, prospective, open-label clinical trial	Neurotrophic Keratopathy (Stage 1)	37	rhNGF	1 drop (20 µg/mL) 6 times daily for 8 weeks.	Corneal epithelial healing (fluorescein staining). Secondary: corneal sensitivity, BCDVA, QoL measures (IDEEL, EQ-5D-5L), Schirmer, TFBUT.	5.5 months	At week 8, 84.8% showed corneal epithelial healing, with 95.2% remaining healed at week 32. Corneal sensitivity improved in 91.2% at week 8 and 82.1% at week 32. Mean BCDVA improved by −0.10 logMAR at week 8. Eye pain (37.8%) was the most common AE, typically mild or moderate.

Table 1. *Cont.*

Authors	Study Design	Ocular Surface Disease	No. of Patients (Eyes)	Type of NGF	Treatment Scheme	Outcomes	Follow-Up	Results
Lambiase et al. (2000) [13]	Case series	Immune corneal ulcer	4 (5)	Murine NGF	1 drop (200 µg/mL) every 2 h (6 AM–12 PM) for 2 days, then 6 times daily until ulcer healed; 1 drop (100 µg/mL) 4 times daily for 2 weeks post-healing.	Corneal healing.	3–12 months	Corneal healing within 8 weeks of treatment.
Cellini et al. (2006) [22]	Randomized controlled trial	Cataract surgery	30 (30)	Murine NGF	NGF group: 1 drop (200 µg/mL) every 2 h (6 AM–12 PM) for 2 weeks, then 4 times daily for 1 week. Hyaluronic acid group: 1 drop (0.2%) every 2 h (6 AM–12 PM) for 2 weeks, then 4 times daily for 1 week.	Corneal thickness at the site of the surgical wound, the endothelial cell count, and the incision line in the stroma (via OCT).	21 days	No significant difference in endothelial cell count. The stromal incision was not visible at day 21 in the NGF group. Corneal thickness at day 21: NGF, 645.2 µm; HA, 704 µm.
Cellini et al. (2007) [16]	Case report	Herpetic keratitis	1	Murine NGF	1 drop (200 µg/mL, 10 µg/50 µL) every 2 h until ulcer healed (23 days), then 4 times daily for 15 additional days.	Corneal healing.	12 months	Corneal healing at 23 days.

Table 1. *Cont.*

Authors	Study Design	Ocular Surface Disease	No. of Patients (Eyes)	Type of NGF	Treatment Scheme	Outcomes	Follow-Up	Results
Ferrari et al. (2014) [152]	Randomized controlled trial	Healthy volunteers	74	rhNGF	Single dose: 1 drop (0.0175 μg, 0.175 μg, or 0.7 μg rhNGF). Single-day dosing: 1 drop (2.1 μg, 6.3 μg, or 18.9 μg total/day) 3 times daily for 1 day. Multiple-day dosing: 1 drop (10.5 μg, 31.5 μg, or 94.5 μg total) 3 times daily for 5 days.	Blood chemistry, urinalyses, vital signs, ECGs, serum NGF antibodies, ocular and systemic AEs, visual acuity, tear function, intraocular pressure, fundus oculi, and ocular symptoms.	10 or 30 days	Treatment did not result in a significant increase in circulating NGF levels, and no antidrug antibodies were detected in serum. There was no detectable clinical evidence of systemic AEs. Ocular AEs were transient and mild in intensity.
Sacchetti et al. (2020) [141]	Phase IIa, prospective, open-label, multiple-dose, clinical trial	Dry eye disease	39 (78)	rhNGF	1 drop (4 μg/mL or 20 μg/mL) twice daily for 28 days.	AE, change in DED symptoms, staining and tear function.	8 weeks	The severity of DED symptoms and ocular surface damage showed significant improvement in both groups, while tear function improved only in the 20 μg/mL group.

Table 1. *Cont.*

Authors	Study Design	Ocular Surface Disease	No. of Patients (Eyes)	Type of NGF	Treatment Scheme	Outcomes	Follow-Up	Results
Wirta et al. (2024) [142]	Phase II, randomized, double-masked, vehicle-controlled, dose-ranging trial	Dry eye disease (including Sjögren's DED)	261 (522)	rhNGF	1 drop (20 µg/mL) two or three times daily for 28 days.	Schirmer I score, SANDE, IDEEL, TFBUT, ocular staining, AE.	12 weeks	Although the primary endpoint (Schirmer I score) was not met, significantly more patients in both rhNGF groups achieved Schirmer >10 mm. Only the three-times-daily group showed sustained symptom improvement. Cenegermin was well tolerated.

* Studies including pediatric patients.

6. Challenges of Nerve Growth Factor as an Ocular Surface Therapy

NGF is a potential therapeutic agent for various ocular surface diseases, particularly those involving epithelial regeneration (e.g., NK), inflammation (e.g., allergic conjunctivitis and immune keratitis), infection (e.g., HSV keratitis), and post-surgical corneal wound healing. NGF exerts downstream effects on neurons, fibroblasts, endothelial and smooth muscle cells, mast cells, eosinophils, and lymphocytes through multiple biochemical pathways. Its ability to modulate this diverse group of cells, each playing a critical role in both physiological and pathological states of the ocular surface, may explain the broad therapeutic applicability of NGF across a range of ocular surface conditions.

The clinical application of NGF in NK is the most extensively studied, with supporting evidence from both randomized controlled trials and basic science research. However, certain reported AEs warrant further investigation to clarify the relationship between topical NGF therapy and their occurrence. Notably, one patient in the 20 μg/mL group of the REPARO trial developed corneal neovascularization [11]. This observation aligns with findings from Hatcher et al. (2021) [53], who reported similar outcomes in a retrospective study involving pediatric patients. The effect of murine NGF and rhNGF on corneal neovascularization remains unclear and requires further evaluation through studies with extended follow-up. Ongoing research into the pathophysiological mechanisms of NGF on the ocular surface may help clarify the potential contribution of NGF to corneal neovascularization in selected cases.

Although NGF is recognized for its neuroprotective properties and its ability to support epithelial healing, its role in ocular surface disease appears to be context dependent. Elevated concentrations of NGF have been reported in the tear film of patients with contact-lens-associated dry eye, Sjögren's syndrome, ocular cicatricial pemphigoid, keratoconjunctivitis sicca, and dry eye following refractive surgery [19,99,131,140,148,155], suggesting that NGF is not consistently deficient across disease states. In such chronic inflammatory conditions, increased NGF levels may contribute to disease persistence by sustaining immune cell activation and inflammation. The occurrence of corneal neovascularization during rhNGF therapy [11,53] also raises concerns about a potential proangiogenic effect in susceptible patients. Finally, while activation of the high-affinity $TrkA^{NGFR}$ receptor is generally associated with beneficial outcomes such as nerve regeneration and epithelial repair through PI3K/Akt and MEK/ERK signaling, unopposed or excessive engagement of the low-affinity $p75^{NTR}$ receptor may initiate proapoptotic and pro-inflammatory cascades via the JNK and NF-κB pathways [75,90,94,97,105–107,156]. Thus, although NGF upregulation may initially aid tissue repair, prolonged or dysregulated signaling may drive nerve dysfunction, chronic inflammation, and tissue remodeling.

The cost-effectiveness and availability of rhNGF are important factors that may pose challenges to its widespread use as a therapy for ocular surface diseases, particularly in publicly funded healthcare systems. The Liverpool Reviews and Implementation Group at the University of Liverpool was commissioned by the National Institute for Health and Care Excellence (NICE) to serve as the evidence review group in evaluating the clinical and cost-effectiveness of cenegermin (rhNGF) for NK. The group found no evidence of long-term benefit, and as a result, it was not possible to establish a reliable estimate of cost-effectiveness [157]. Finally, the administration regimen is complex, requiring eye drops to be instilled up to six times per day over an 8-week treatment period [10,11].

There are several limitations in the current literature on NGF use on the ocular surface. Extrapolating the results to the general population is challenging due to heterogeneous study samples and designs, as well as the limited number of clinical studies focused on specific ocular surface diseases included in this review. Randomized controlled trials evaluating NGF in the context of NK or DED are scarce, and much of the existing data is derived from case reports and small case series. As a result, a substantial portion of the literature consists of studies with low levels of evidence [158]. Inadequate long-term follow-up is another limitation of existing trials. From a clinical perspective, future studies would benefit from incorporating survival analyses (e.g., Kaplan–Meier estimates) to assess recurrence rates in NK patients at 6 to 12 months post-treatment. Future studies, particularly randomized controlled trials, are warranted for a range of conditions in which evidence for NGF use remains limited, such as DED, refractive surgery, and allergic conjunctivitis, among others. Moreover, the role of NGF in these conditions is not yet fully understood. Drug-induced and iatrogenic insults, including chronic use of preservative-containing eye drops, topical anesthetic abuse, and ocular surgery (e.g., cataract, refractive, and corneal transplant surgeries), can also lead to impairments of corneal innervation and epithelial integrity, contributing to DED, NK and various other diseases of the ocular surface [20,66,148,151,159,160]. Given NGF's roles in nerve regeneration, epithelial repair, and stimulation of tear secretion, its therapeutic efficacy in these underexplored contexts warrants further investigation. Although the efficacy of topical NGF has been notable in several studies on NK, further research is needed to guide clinicians in identifying optimal clinical scenarios and appropriate treatment regimens, especially considering that cost remains a barrier to routine use. A more comprehensive understanding of the underlying pathophysiological mechanisms of NGF may facilitate its development as a therapeutic agent for a wider range of ocular surface diseases.

7. Conclusions

NGF has been studied across a range of contexts, from basic science research to non-randomized and randomized clinical trials. In primary human conjunctival epithelial cells and cell line cultures, NGF has been shown to increase goblet cell numbers, enhance mucin precursor production and storage, and support neural innervation and maintenance [49]. Clinically, topical administration of NGF has demonstrated positive outcomes in various ocular surface diseases, with NK being the most extensively studied. Notably, rhNGF is the first FDA-approved topical biologic therapy in the field of ophthalmology, specifically indicated for the treatment of NK. Altogether, NGF is a molecule with notable therapeutic effects on the ocular surface. It regulates tear production and supports the survival and proliferation of epithelial cells, fibroblasts, immune cells, endothelial cells, and corneal sensory nerves. Both experimental and clinical evidence support its role as a potential treatment and biomarker for degenerative and immune-mediated diseases, as well as for post-surgical wound healing of the ocular surface. Addressing the current limitations of NGF-based therapy through well-designed, large-scale, multicenter randomized controlled trials with long-term follow-up across diverse clinical settings may expand its approved indications. Moreover, such efforts may establish rhNGF as a first-line therapy rather than a rescue option for cases unresponsive to conventional treatment.

Author Contributions: Conceptualization—A.I. and S.N.Y.; investigation—N.K.-L., A.H., J.Y.M.L. and J.C.; analysis—N.K.-L., A.H., J.Y.M.L. and J.C.; writing—N.K.-L., A.H., J.Y.M.L. and J.C.; editing—A.I. and S.N.Y.; funding acquisition—A.I. and S.N.Y.; supervision—A.I. and S.N.Y. All authors have read and agreed to the published version of the manuscript.

Funding: This research received no external funding.

Data Availability Statement: No new data were created or analyzed in this study.

Conflicts of Interest: The authors declare no conflicts of interest.

References

1. Aloe, L. Rita Levi-Montalcini and the Discovery of NGF, the First Nerve Cell Growth Factor. *Arch. Ital. Biol.* **2011**, *149*, 175–181. [CrossRef]
2. Dartt, D.A.; Masli, S. Conjunctival Epithelial and Goblet Cell Function in Chronic Inflammation and Ocular Allergic Inflammation. *Curr. Opin. Allergy Clin. Immunol.* **2014**, *14*, 464–470. [CrossRef]
3. Lambiase, A.; Bonini, S.; Micera, A.; Tirassa, P.; Magrini, L.; Bonini, S.; Aloe, L. Increased Plasma Levels of Substance P in Vernal Keratoconjunctivitis. *Investig. Ophthalmol. Vis. Sci.* **1997**, *38*, 2161–2164.
4. Sacchetti, M.; Lambiase, A.; Aronni, S.; Griggi, T.; Ribatti, V.; Bonini, S.; Bonini, S. Hyperosmolar Conjunctival Provocation for the Evaluation of Nonspecific Hyperreactivity in Healthy Patients and Patients with Allergy. *J. Allergy Clin. Immunol.* **2006**, *118*, 872–877. [CrossRef] [PubMed]
5. Lambiase, A.; Bonini, S.; Bonini, S.; Micera, A.; Magrini, L.; Bracci-Laudiero, L.; Aloe, L. Increased Plasma Levels of Nerve Growth Factor in Vernal Keratoconjunctivitis and Relationship to Conjunctival Mast Cells. *Investig. Ophthalmol. Vis. Sci.* **1995**, *36*, 2127–2132.
6. Mantelli, F.; Allegretti, M.; Chao, W.; Filatori, I.; Battigello, P.; Vaja, V.; Goodman, J.; Sinigaglia, F. Phase I/II Randomized, Double-Masked, Vehicle-Controlled Trial of Recombinant Human Nerve Growth Factor (rhNGF) Eye Drops in Stage 2/3 Neurotrophic Keratitis. *Investig. Ophthalmol. Vis. Sci.* **2017**, *58*, 1172.
7. Mandarà, E.; Brocca, D.; Pellegrini, F.; Interlandi, E. Topical Nerve Growth Factor for the Treatment of Neurotrophic Keratopathy Caused by Wallenberg Syndrome. *Cornea* **2022**, *41*, 647–648. [CrossRef]
8. Ahuja, A.S.; Bowden, F.W.; Robben, J.L. A Novel Treatment for Neurotrophic Corneal Ulcer Using Topical Cenegermin (OXERVATE^{TM}) Containing Recombinant Human Nerve Growth Factor. *Cureus* **2020**, *12*, e11724. [CrossRef]
9. Bruscolini, A.; Marenco, M.; Albanese, G.M.; Lambiase, A.; Sacchetti, M. Long-Term Clinical Efficacy of Topical Treatment with Recombinant Human Nerve Growth Factor in Neurotrophic Keratopathy: A Novel Cure for a Rare Degenerative Corneal Disease? *Orphanet J. Rare Dis.* **2022**, *17*, 57. [CrossRef]
10. Pflugfelder, S.C.; Massaro-Giordano, M.; Perez, V.L.; Hamrah, P.; Deng, S.X.; Espandar, L.; Foster, C.S.; Affeldt, J.; Seedor, J.A.; Afshari, N.A.; et al. Topical Recombinant Human Nerve Growth Factor (Cenegermin) for Neurotrophic Keratopathy: A Multicenter Randomized Vehicle-Controlled Pivotal Trial. *Ophthalmology* **2020**, *127*, 14–26. [CrossRef]
11. Bonini, S.; Lambiase, A.; Rama, P.; Sinigaglia, F.; Allegretti, M.; Chao, W.; Mantelli, F.; REPARO Study Group. Phase II Randomized, Double-Masked, Vehicle-Controlled Trial of Recombinant Human Nerve Growth Factor for Neurotrophic Keratitis. *Ophthalmology* **2018**, *125*, 1332–1343. [CrossRef] [PubMed]
12. Bonini, S.; Lambiase, A.; Rama, P.; Filatori, I.; Allegretti, M.; Chao, W.; Mantelli, F.; REPARO Study Group. Phase I Trial of Recombinant Human Nerve Growth Factor for Neurotrophic Keratitis. *Ophthalmology* **2018**, *125*, 1468–1471. [CrossRef] [PubMed]
13. Lambiase, A.; Bonini, S.; Aloe, L.; Rama, P.; Bonini, S. Anti-Inflammatory and Healing Properties of Nerve Growth Factor in Immune Corneal Ulcers with Stromal Melting. *Arch. Ophthalmol.* **2000**, *118*, 1446–1449. [CrossRef]
14. Anand, B.S.; Hill, J.M.; Dey, S.; Maruyama, K.; Bhattacharjee, P.S.; Myles, M.E.; Nashed, Y.E.; Mitra, A.K. In Vivo Antiviral Efficacy of a Dipeptide Acyclovir Prodrug, Val-Val-Acyclovir, against HSV-1 Epithelial and Stromal Keratitis in the Rabbit Eye Model. *Investig. Ophthalmol. Vis. Sci.* **2003**, *44*, 2529–2534. [CrossRef]
15. Lambiase, A.; Coassin, M.; Costa, N.; Lauretti, P.; Micera, A.; Ghinelli, E.; Aloe, L.; Rama, P.; Bonini, S. Topical Treatment with Nerve Growth Factor in an Animal Model of Herpetic Keratitis. *Graefe's Arch. Clin. Exp. Ophthalmol.* **2008**, *246*, 121–127. [CrossRef]
16. Mauro, C.; Pietro, L.; Emilio, C.C. The Use of Nerve Growth Factor in Herpetic Keratitis: A Case Report. *J. Med. Case Rep.* **2007**, *1*, 124. [CrossRef] [PubMed]
17. Chang, E.-J.; Im, Y.S.; Kay, E.P.; Kim, J.Y.; Lee, J.E.; Lee, H.K. The Role of Nerve Growth Factor in Hyperosmolar Stress Induced Apoptosis. *J. Cell. Physiol.* **2008**, *216*, 69–77. [CrossRef]
18. Coassin, M.; Lambiase, A.; Costa, N.; De Gregorio, A.; Sgrulletta, R.; Sacchetti, M.; Aloe, L.; Bonini, S. Efficacy of Topical Nerve Growth Factor Treatment in Dogs Affected by Dry Eye. *Graefe's Arch. Clin. Exp. Ophthalmol.* **2005**, *243*, 151–155. [CrossRef] [PubMed]
19. Lambiase, A.; Micera, A.; Sacchetti, M.; Cortes, M.; Mantelli, F.; Bonini, S. Alterations of Tear Neuromediators in Dry Eye Disease. *Arch. Ophthalmol.* **2011**, *129*, 981–986. [CrossRef]
20. Pocobelli, A.; Komaiha, C.; De Carlo, L.; Pocobelli, G.; Boni, N.; Colabelli Gisoldi, R.A.M. Role of Topical Cenegermin in Management of a Cornea Transplant in a Functionally Monocular Patient with Neurotrophic Keratitis and Facial Nerve Palsy: A Case Report. *Int. Med. Case Rep. J.* **2020**, *13*, 617–621. [CrossRef]
21. Gong, N.; Pleyer, U.; Vogt, K.; Anegon, I.; Flügel, A.; Volk, H.-D.; Ritter, T. Local Overexpression of Nerve Growth Factor in Rat Corneal Transplants Improves Allograft Survival. *Investig. Ophthalmol. Vis. Sci.* **2007**, *48*, 1043–1052. [CrossRef] [PubMed]

22. Cellini, M.; Bendo, E.; Bravetti, G.O.; Campos, E.C. The Use of Nerve Growth Factor in Surgical Wound Healing of the Cornea. *Ophthalmic Res.* **2006**, *38*, 177–181. [CrossRef] [PubMed]
23. Gao, S.; Li, S.; Liu, L.; Wang, Y.; Ding, H.; Li, L.; Zhong, X. Early Changes in Ocular Surface and Tear Inflammatory Mediators after Small-Incision Lenticule Extraction and Femtosecond Laser-Assisted Laser in Situ Keratomileusis. *PLoS ONE* **2014**, *9*, e107370. [CrossRef]
24. Chin, J.Y.; Lin, M.T.-Y.; Lee, I.X.Y.; Mehta, J.S.; Liu, Y.-C. Tear Neuromediator and Corneal Denervation Following SMILE. *J. Refract. Surg.* **2021**, *37*, 516–523. [CrossRef]
25. Chen, L.; Wei, R.H.; Tan, D.T.H.; Beuerman, R.W.; Li, W.; Zhao, S. Nerve Growth Factor Expression and Nerve Regeneration in Monkey Corneas after LASIK. *J. Refract. Surg.* **2014**, *30*, 134–139. [CrossRef] [PubMed]
26. Chao, M.V. Neurotrophins and Their Receptors: A Convergence Point for Many Signalling Pathways. *Nat. Rev. Neurosci.* **2003**, *4*, 299–309. [CrossRef]
27. Kaplan, D.R.; Miller, F.D. Neurotrophin Signal Transduction in the Nervous System. *Curr. Opin. Neurobiol.* **2000**, *10*, 381–391. [CrossRef]
28. Kenchappa, R.S.; Tep, C.; Korade, Z.; Urra, S.; Bronfman, F.C.; Yoon, S.O.; Carter, B.D. P75 Neurotrophin Receptor-Mediated Apoptosis in Sympathetic Neurons Involves a Biphasic Activation of JNK and up-Regulation of Tumor Necrosis Factor-Alpha-Converting Enzyme/ADAM17. *J. Biol. Chem.* **2010**, *285*, 20358–20368. [CrossRef]
29. De Bernardi, M.A.; Rabins, S.J.; Colangelo, A.M.; Brooker, G.; Mocchetti, I. TrkA Mediates the Nerve Growth Factor-Induced Intracellular Calcium Accumulation. *J. Biol. Chem.* **1996**, *271*, 6092–6098. [CrossRef]
30. Ludwiczak, S.; Reinhard, J.; Reinach, P.S.; Li, A.; Oronowicz, J.; Yousf, A.; Kakkassery, V.; Mergler, S. Joint CB1 and NGF Receptor Activation Suppresses TRPM8 Activation in Etoposide-Resistant Retinoblastoma Cells. *Int. J. Mol. Sci.* **2024**, *25*, 1733. [CrossRef]
31. Minnone, G.; De Benedetti, F.; Bracci-Laudiero, L. NGF and Its Receptors in the Regulation of Inflammatory Response. *Int. J. Mol. Sci.* **2017**, *18*, 1028. [CrossRef] [PubMed]
32. Orrenius, S.; Zhivotovsky, B.; Nicotera, P. Regulation of Cell Death: The Calcium–Apoptosis Link. *Nat. Rev. Mol. Cell Biol.* **2003**, *4*, 552–565. [CrossRef]
33. Terracina, S.; Ferraguti, G.; Tarani, L.; Fanfarillo, F.; Tirassa, P.; Ralli, M.; Iannella, G.; Polimeni, A.; Lucarelli, M.; Greco, A.; et al. Nerve Growth Factor and Autoimmune Diseases. *Curr. Issues Mol. Biol.* **2023**, *45*, 8950–8973. [CrossRef]
34. Liu, P.; Li, S.; Tang, L. Nerve Growth Factor: A Potential Therapeutic Target for Lung Diseases. *Int. J. Mol. Sci.* **2021**, *22*, 9112. [CrossRef] [PubMed]
35. Jung, S.I.; Choi, S.H.; Kim, J.-W.; Lim, J.; Rim, Y.A.; Ju, J.H. The Effect of Nerve Growth Factor on Cartilage Fibrosis and Hypertrophy during In Vitro Chondrogenesis Using Induced Pluripotent Stem Cells. *Int. J. Stem Cells* **2025**, *18*, 59–71. [CrossRef] [PubMed]
36. Blanco-Mezquita, T.; Martinez-Garcia, C.; Proença, R.; Zieske, J.D.; Bonini, S.; Lambiase, A.; Merayo-Lloves, J. Nerve Growth Factor Promotes Corneal Epithelial Migration by Enhancing Expression of Matrix Metalloprotease-9. *Investig. Ophthalmol. Vis. Sci.* **2013**, *54*, 3880–3890. [CrossRef]
37. Micera, A.; Lambiase, A.; Stampachiacchiere, B.; Sgrulletta, R.; Normando, E.M.; Bonini, S.; Bonini, S. Nerve Growth Factor Has a Modulatory Role on Human Primary Fibroblast Cultures Derived from Vernal Keratoconjunctivitis-Affected Conjunctiva. *Mol. Vis.* **2007**, *13*, 981–987.
38. Micera, A.; Lambiase, A.; Stampachiacchiere, B.; Bonini, S.; Bonini, S.; Levi-Schaffer, F. Nerve Growth Factor and Tissue Repair Remodeling: TrkA(NGFR) and p75(NTR), Two Receptors One Fate. *Cytokine Growth Factor Rev.* **2007**, *18*, 245–256. [CrossRef]
39. Lambiase, A.; Bonini, S.; Micera, A.; Rama, P.; Bonini, S.; Aloe, L. Expression of Nerve Growth Factor Receptors on the Ocular Surface in Healthy Subjects and during Manifestation of Inflammatory Diseases. *Investig. Ophthalmol. Vis. Sci.* **1998**, *39*, 1272–1275.
40. Lambiase, A.; Manni, L.; Bonini, S.; Rama, P.; Micera, A.; Aloe, L. Nerve Growth Factor Promotes Corneal Healing: Structural, Biochemical, and Molecular Analyses of Rat and Human Corneas. *Investig. Ophthalmol. Vis. Sci.* **2000**, *41*, 1063–1069.
41. Lambiase, A.; Bonini, S.; Manni, L.; Ghinelli, E.; Tirassa, P.; Rama, P.; Aloe, L. Intraocular Production and Release of Nerve Growth Factor after Iridectomy. *Investig. Ophthalmol. Vis. Sci.* **2002**, *43*, 2334–2340.
42. Garcia, T.B.; Hollborn, M.; Bringmann, A. Expression and Signaling of NGF in the Healthy and Injured Retina. *Cytokine Growth Factor Rev.* **2017**, *34*, 43–57. [CrossRef] [PubMed]
43. Qi, H.; Chuang, E.Y.; Yoon, K.-C.; de Paiva, C.S.; Shine, H.D.; Jones, D.B.; Pflugfelder, S.C.; Li, D.-Q. Patterned Expression of Neurotrophic Factors and Receptors in Human Limbal and Corneal Regions. *Mol. Vis.* **2007**, *13*, 1934–1941. [PubMed]
44. You, L.; Kruse, F.E.; Völcker, H.E. Neurotrophic Factors in the Human Cornea. *Investig. Ophthalmol. Vis. Sci.* **2000**, *41*, 692–702.
45. Ríos, J.D.; Ghinelli, E.; Gu, J.; Hodges, R.R.; Dartt, D.A. Role of Neurotrophins and Neurotrophin Receptors in Rat Conjunctival Goblet Cell Secretion and Proliferation. *Investig. Ophthalmol. Vis. Sci.* **2007**, *48*, 1543–1551. [CrossRef]

46. Ghinelli, E.; Johansson, J.; Ríos, J.D.; Chen, L.-L.; Zoukhri, D.; Hodges, R.R.; Dartt, D.A. Presence and Localization of Neurotrophins and Neurotrophin Receptors in Rat Lacrimal Gland. *Investig. Ophthalmol. Vis. Sci.* **2003**, *44*, 3352–3357. [CrossRef]
47. Muzi, S.; Colafrancesco, V.; Sornelli, F.; Mantelli, F.; Lambiase, A.; Aloe, L. Nerve Growth Factor in the Developing and Adult Lacrimal Glands of Rat with and without Inherited Retinitis Pigmentosa. *Cornea* **2010**, *29*, 1163–1168. [CrossRef]
48. Micera, A.; Lambiase, A.; Puxeddu, I.; Aloe, L.; Stampachiacchiere, B.; Levi-Schaffer, F.; Bonini, S.; Bonini, S. Nerve Growth Factor Effect on Human Primary Fibroblastic-Keratocytes: Possible Mechanism during Corneal Healing. *Exp. Eye Res.* **2006**, *83*, 747–757. [CrossRef]
49. Lambiase, A.; Micera, A.; Pellegrini, G.; Merlo, D.; Rama, P.; De Luca, M.; Bonini, S.; Bonini, S. In Vitro Evidence of Nerve Growth Factor Effects on Human Conjunctival Epithelial Cell Differentiation and Mucin Gene Expression. *Investig. Ophthalmol. Vis. Sci.* **2009**, *50*, 4622–4630. [CrossRef]
50. Micera, A.; Puxeddu, I.; Lambiase, A.; Antonelli, A.; Bonini, S.; Bonini, S.; Aloe, L.; Pe'er, J.; Levi-Schaffer, F. The Pro-Fibrogenic Effect of Nerve Growth Factor on Conjunctival Fibroblasts Is Mediated by Transforming Growth Factor-Beta. *Clin. Exp. Allergy* **2005**, *35*, 650–656. [CrossRef]
51. Dua, H.S.; Said, D.G.; Messmer, E.M.; Rolando, M.; Benitez-del-Castillo, J.M.; Hossain, P.N.; Shortt, A.J.; Geerling, G.; Nubile, M.; Figueiredo, F.C.; et al. Neurotrophic Keratopathy. *Prog. Retin. Eye Res.* **2018**, *66*, 107–131. [CrossRef] [PubMed]
52. Adams, B.S.; Patel, A.R. Cenegermin. In *StatPearls*; StatPearls Publishing: Treasure Island, FL, USA, 2025.
53. Hatcher, J.B.; Soifer, M.; Morales, N.G.; Farooq, A.V.; Perez, V.L.; Shieh, C. Aftermarket Effects of Cenegermin for Neurotrophic Keratopathy in Pediatric Patients. *Ocul. Surf.* **2021**, *21*, 52–57. [CrossRef]
54. Sofroniew, M.V.; Howe, C.L.; Mobley, W.C. Nerve Growth Factor Signaling, Neuroprotection, and Neural Repair. *Annu. Rev. Neurosci.* **2001**, *24*, 1217–1281. [CrossRef]
55. Rocco, M.L.; Soligo, M.; Manni, L.; Aloe, L. Nerve Growth Factor: Early Studies and Recent Clinical Trials. *Curr. Neuropharmacol.* **2018**, *16*, 1455–1465. [CrossRef]
56. Aloe, L.; Rocco, M.L.; Balzamino, B.O.; Micera, A. Nerve Growth Factor: Role in Growth, Differentiation and Controlling Cancer Cell Development. *J. Exp. Clin. Cancer Res.* **2016**, *35*, 116. [CrossRef] [PubMed]
57. Rowe, C.W.; Dill, T.; Faulkner, S.; Gedye, C.; Paul, J.W.; Tolosa, J.M.; Jones, M.; King, S.; Smith, R.; Hondermarck, H. The Precursor for Nerve Growth Factor (proNGF) in Thyroid Cancer Lymph Node Metastases: Correlation with Primary Tumour and Pathological Variables. *Int. J. Mol. Sci.* **2019**, *20*, 5924. [CrossRef] [PubMed]
58. Steckiewicz, K.P.; Barcińska, E.; Woźniak, M. Nerve Growth Factor as an Important Possible Component of Novel Therapy for Cancer, Diabetes and Cardiovascular Diseases. *Cell. Mol. Biol.* **2018**, *64*, 16–23. [CrossRef]
59. Liu, Z.; Wu, H.; Huang, S. Role of NGF and Its Receptors in Wound Healing (Review). *Exp. Ther. Med.* **2021**, *21*, 599. [CrossRef]
60. Kim, D.H.; Gutin, P.H.; Noble, L.J.; Nathan, D.; Yu, J.S.; Nockels, R.P. Treatment with Genetically Engineered Fibroblasts Producing NGF or BDNF Can Accelerate Recovery from Traumatic Spinal Cord Injury in the Adult Rat. *Neuroreport* **1996**, *7*, 2221–2225. [CrossRef]
61. Holtzman, D.M.; Sheldon, R.A.; Jaffe, W.; Cheng, Y.; Ferriero, D.M. Nerve Growth Factor Protects the Neonatal Brain against Hypoxic-Ischemic Injury. *Ann. Neurol.* **1996**, *39*, 114–122. [CrossRef]
62. Apfel, S.C.; Schwartz, S.; Adornato, B.T.; Freeman, R.; Biton, V.; Rendell, M.; Vinik, A.; Giuliani, M.; Stevens, J.C.; Barbano, R.; et al. Efficacy and Safety of Recombinant Human Nerve Growth Factor in Patients with Diabetic Polyneuropathy: A Randomized Controlled Trial. rhNGF Clinical Investigator Group. *JAMA* **2000**, *284*, 2215–2221. [CrossRef] [PubMed]
63. Carmignoto, G.; Maffei, L.; Candeo, P.; Canella, R.; Comelli, C. Effect of NGF on the Survival of Rat Retinal Ganglion Cells Following Optic Nerve Section. *J. Neurosci.* **1989**, *9*, 1263–1272. [CrossRef]
64. Chaturvedi, R.K.; Shukla, S.; Seth, K.; Agrawal, A.K. Nerve Growth Factor Increases Survival of Dopaminergic Graft, Rescue Nigral Dopaminergic Neurons and Restores Functional Deficits in Rat Model of Parkinson's Disease. *Neurosci. Lett.* **2006**, *398*, 44–49. [CrossRef] [PubMed]
65. Eriksdotter Jönhagen, M.; Nordberg, A.; Amberla, K.; Bäckman, L.; Ebendal, T.; Meyerson, B.; Olson, L.; Seiger, Å.; Shigeta, M.; Theodorsson, E.; et al. Intracerebroventricular Infusion of Nerve Growth Factor in Three Patients with Alzheimer's Disease. *Dement. Geriatr. Cogn. Disord.* **1998**, *9*, 246–257. [CrossRef]
66. Bonini, S.; Lambiase, A.; Rama, P.; Caprioglio, G.; Aloe, L. Topical Treatment with Nerve Growth Factor for Neurotrophic Keratitis. *Ophthalmology* **2000**, *107*, 1347–1351; discussion 1351–1352. [CrossRef]
67. Lambiase, A.; Centofanti, M.; Micera, A.; Manni, G.L.; Mattei, E.; De Gregorio, A.; de Feo, G.; Bucci, M.G.; Aloe, L. Nerve Growth Factor (NGF) Reduces and NGF Antibody Exacerbates Retinal Damage Induced in Rabbit by Experimental Ocular Hypertension. *Graefe's Arch. Clin. Exp. Ophthalmol.* **1997**, *235*, 780–785. [CrossRef]
68. Lambiase, A.; Rama, P.; Bonini, S.; Caprioglio, G.; Aloe, L. Topical Treatment with Nerve Growth Factor for Corneal Neurotrophic Ulcers. *N. Engl. J. Med.* **1998**, *338*, 1174–1180. [CrossRef] [PubMed]

69. Lambiase, A.; Sacchetti, M.; Bonini, S. Nerve Growth Factor Therapy for Corneal Disease. *Curr. Opin. Ophthalmol.* **2012**, *23*, 296–302. [CrossRef]
70. Landi, F.; Aloe, L.; Russo, A.; Cesari, M.; Onder, G.; Bonini, S.; Carbonin, P.U.; Bernabei, R. Topical Treatment of Pressure Ulcers with Nerve Growth Factor: A Randomized Clinical Trial. *Ann. Intern. Med.* **2003**, *139*, 635–641. [CrossRef]
71. McArthur, J.C.; Yiannoutsos, C.; Simpson, D.M.; Adornato, B.T.; Singer, E.J.; Hollander, H.; Marra, C.; Rubin, M.; Cohen, B.A.; Tucker, T.; et al. A Phase II Trial of Nerve Growth Factor for Sensory Neuropathy Associated with HIV Infection. AIDS Clinical Trials Group Team 291. *Neurology* **2000**, *54*, 1080–1088. [CrossRef]
72. Siliprandi, R.; Canella, R.; Carmignoto, G. Nerve Growth Factor Promotes Functional Recovery of Retinal Ganglion Cells after Ischemia. *Investig. Ophthalmol. Vis. Sci.* **1993**, *34*, 3232–3245.
73. Tuveri, M.; Generini, S.; Matucci-Cerinic, M.; Aloe, L. NGF, a Useful Tool in the Treatment of Chronic Vasculitic Ulcers in Rheumatoid Arthritis. *Lancet* **2000**, *356*, 1739–1740. [CrossRef]
74. Levi-Montalcini, R. The Nerve Growth Factor 35 Years Later. *Science* **1987**, *237*, 1154–1162. [CrossRef]
75. Aloe, L.; Rocco, M.L.; Balzamino, B.O.; Micera, A. Nerve Growth Factor: A Focus on Neuroscience and Therapy. *Curr. Neuropharmacol.* **2015**, *13*, 294–303. [CrossRef] [PubMed]
76. Levi-Montalcini, R.; Hamburger, V. Selective Growth Stimulating Effects of Mouse Sarcoma on the Sensory and Sympathetic Nervous System of the Chick Embryo. *J. Exp. Zool.* **1951**, *116*, 321–361. [CrossRef] [PubMed]
77. Varon, S.; Nomura, J.; Shooter, E.M. The Isolation of the Mouse Nerve Growth Factor Protein in a High Molecular Weight Form. *Biochemistry* **1967**, *6*, 2202–2209. [CrossRef] [PubMed]
78. Smith, A.P.; Varon, S.; Shooter, E.M. Multiple Forms of the Nerve Growth Factor Protein and Its Subunits. *Biochemistry* **1968**, *7*, 3259–3268. [CrossRef]
79. Chao, M.V.; Rajagopal, R.; Lee, F.S. Neurotrophin Signalling in Health and Disease. *Clin. Sci.* **2006**, *110*, 167–173. [CrossRef]
80. Lei, L.; Parada, L.F. Transcriptional Regulation of Trk Family Neurotrophin Receptors. *Cell. Mol. Life Sci.* **2007**, *64*, 522–532. [CrossRef]
81. Kaplan, D.R.; Hempstead, B.L.; Martin-Zanca, D.; Chao, M.V.; Parada, L.F. The Trk Proto-Oncogene Product: A Signal Transducing Receptor for Nerve Growth Factor. *Science* **1991**, *252*, 554–558. [CrossRef]
82. Johnson, D.; Lanahan, A.; Buck, C.R.; Sehgal, A.; Morgan, C.; Mercer, E.; Bothwell, M.; Chao, M. Expression and Structure of the Human NGF Receptor. *Cell* **1986**, *47*, 545–554. [CrossRef] [PubMed]
83. Barbacid, M. Structural and Functional Properties of the TRK Family of Neurotrophin Receptors. *Ann. N. Y. Acad. Sci.* **1995**, *766*, 442–458. [CrossRef]
84. Wiesmann, C.; Ultsch, M.H.; Bass, S.H.; de Vos, A.M. Crystal Structure of Nerve Growth Factor in Complex with the Ligand-Binding Domain of the TrkA Receptor. *Nature* **1999**, *401*, 184–188. [CrossRef] [PubMed]
85. Urfer, R.; Tsoulfas, P.; O'Connell, L.; Hongo, J.A.; Zhao, W.; Presta, L.G. High Resolution Mapping of the Binding Site of TrkA for Nerve Growth Factor and TrkC for Neurotrophin-3 on the Second Immunoglobulin-like Domain of the Trk Receptors. *J. Biol. Chem.* **1998**, *273*, 5829–5840. [CrossRef] [PubMed]
86. Zhang, M.; Zhang, Y.; Ding, J.; Li, X.; Zang, C.; Yin, S.; Ma, J.; Wang, Y.; Cao, Y. The Role of TrkA in the Promoting Wounding-Healing Effect of CD271 on Epidermal Stem Cells. *Arch. Dermatol. Res.* **2018**, *310*, 737–750. [CrossRef]
87. Zheng, M.-G.; Sui, W.-Y.; He, Z.-D.; Liu, Y.; Huang, Y.-L.; Mu, S.-H.; Xu, X.-Z.; Zhang, J.-S.; Qu, J.-L.; Zhang, J.; et al. TrkA Regulates the Regenerative Capacity of Bone Marrow Stromal Stem Cells in Nerve Grafts. *Neural Regen. Res.* **2019**, *14*, 1765–1771. [CrossRef]
88. Troullinaki, M.; Alexaki, V.-I.; Mitroulis, I.; Witt, A.; Klotzsche-von Ameln, A.; Chung, K.-J.; Chavakis, T.; Economopoulou, M. Nerve Growth Factor Regulates Endothelial Cell Survival and Pathological Retinal Angiogenesis. *J. Cell. Mol. Med.* **2019**, *23*, 2362–2371. [CrossRef]
89. Bibel, M.; Barde, Y.A. Neurotrophins: Key Regulators of Cell Fate and Cell Shape in the Vertebrate Nervous System. *Genes Dev.* **2000**, *14*, 2919–2937. [CrossRef]
90. Gu, C.-L.; Zhang, L.; Zhu, Y.; Bao, T.-Y.; Zhu, Y.-T.; Chen, Y.-T.; Pang, H.-Q. Exploring the Cellular and Molecular Basis of Nerve Growth Factor in Cerebral Ischemia Recovery. *Neuroscience* **2025**, *566*, 190–197. [CrossRef]
91. Turney, S.G.; Ahmed, M.; Chandrasekar, I.; Wysolmerski, R.B.; Goeckeler, Z.M.; Rioux, R.M.; Whitesides, G.M.; Bridgman, P.C. Nerve Growth Factor Stimulates Axon Outgrowth through Negative Regulation of Growth Cone Actomyosin Restraint of Microtubule Advance. *Mol. Biol. Cell* **2016**, *27*, 500–517. [CrossRef]
92. Yoon, S.O.; Casaccia-Bonnefil, P.; Carter, B.; Chao, M.V. Competitive Signaling between TrkA and P75 Nerve Growth Factor Receptors Determines Cell Survival. *J. Neurosci.* **1998**, *18*, 3273–3281. [CrossRef] [PubMed]
93. Huang, E.J.; Reichardt, L.F. Trk Receptors: Roles in Neuronal Signal Transduction. *Annu. Rev. Biochem.* **2003**, *72*, 609–642. [CrossRef]

94. Pierchala, B.A.; Ahrens, R.C.; Paden, A.J.; Johnson, E.M. Nerve Growth Factor Promotes the Survival of Sympathetic Neurons through the Cooperative Function of the Protein Kinase C and Phosphatidylinositol 3-Kinase Pathways. *J. Biol. Chem.* **2004**, *279*, 27986–27993. [CrossRef]
95. Mnich, K.; Carleton, L.A.; Kavanagh, E.T.; Doyle, K.M.; Samali, A.; Gorman, A.M. Nerve Growth Factor-Mediated Inhibition of Apoptosis Post-Caspase Activation Is Due to Removal of Active Caspase-3 in a Lysosome-Dependent Manner. *Cell Death Dis.* **2014**, *5*, e1202. [CrossRef]
96. Kirkland, R.A.; Saavedra, G.M.; Franklin, J.L. Rapid Activation of Antioxidant Defenses by Nerve Growth Factor Suppresses Reactive Oxygen Species during Neuronal Apoptosis: Evidence for a Role in Cytochrome c Redistribution. *J. Neurosci.* **2007**, *27*, 11315–11326. [CrossRef] [PubMed]
97. Kuner, P.; Hertel, C. NGF Induces Apoptosis in a Human Neuroblastoma Cell Line Expressing the Neurotrophin Receptor p75NTR. *J. Neurosci. Res.* **1998**, *54*, 465–474. [CrossRef]
98. Qi, H.; Li, D.-Q.; Shine, H.D.; Chen, Z.; Yoon, K.-C.; Jones, D.B.; Pflugfelder, S.C. Nerve Growth Factor and Its Receptor TrkA Serve as Potential Markers for Human Corneal Epithelial Progenitor Cells. *Exp Eye Res.* **2008**, *86*, 34–40. [CrossRef]
99. Micera, A.; Stampachiacchiere, B.; Di Zazzo, A.; Sgrulletta, R.; Cortes, M.; Normando, E.M.; Lambiase, A.; Bonini, S. NGF Modulates trkANGFR/p75NTR in αSMA-Expressing Conjunctival Fibroblasts from Human Ocular Cicatricial Pemphigoid (OCP). *PLoS ONE* **2015**, *10*, e0142737. [CrossRef]
100. Micera, A.; Vigneti, E.; Pickholtz, D.; Reich, R.; Pappo, O.; Bonini, S.; Maquart, F.X.; Aloe, L.; Levi-Schaffer, F. Nerve Growth Factor Displays Stimulatory Effects on Human Skin and Lung Fibroblasts, Demonstrating a Direct Role for This Factor in Tissue Repair. *Proc. Natl. Acad. Sci. USA* **2001**, *98*, 6162–6167. [CrossRef]
101. Li, W.; Sun, X.; Wang, Z.; Li, R.; Li, L. The Effect of Nerve Growth Factor on Differentiation of Corneal Limbal Epithelial Cells to Conjunctival Goblet Cells in Vitro. *Mol. Vis.* **2010**, *16*, 2739–2744.
102. Ebendal, T.; Olson, L.; Seiger, A.; Hedlund, K.O. Nerve Growth Factors in the Rat Iris. *Nature* **1980**, *286*, 25–28. [CrossRef]
103. Deeks, E.D.; Lamb, Y.N. Cenegermin: A Review in Neurotrophic Keratitis. *Drugs* **2020**, *80*, 489–494. [CrossRef]
104. De Castro, F.; Silos-Santiago, I.; De Armentia, M.L.; Barbacid, M.; Belmonte, C. Corneal Innervation and Sensitivity to Noxious Stimuli in *Trk* A Knockout Mice. *Eur. J. Neurosci.* **1998**, *10*, 146–152. [CrossRef] [PubMed]
105. Hong, J.; Qian, T.; Le, Q.; Sun, X.; Wu, J.; Chen, J.; Yu, X.; Xu, J. NGF Promotes Cell Cycle Progression by Regulating D-Type Cyclins via PI3K/Akt and MAPK/Erk Activation in Human Corneal Epithelial Cells. *Mol. Vis.* **2012**, *18*, 758–764. [PubMed]
106. Huang, E.J.; Reichardt, L.F. Neurotrophins: Roles in Neuronal Development and Function. *Annu. Rev. Neurosci.* **2001**, *24*, 677–736. [CrossRef] [PubMed]
107. Chen, K.; Li, Y.; Zhang, X.; Ullah, R.; Tong, J.; Shen, Y. The Role of the PI3K/AKT Signalling Pathway in the Corneal Epithelium: Recent Updates. *Cell Death Dis.* **2022**, *13*, 513. [CrossRef]
108. Chaudhary, S.; Namavari, A.; Yco, L.; Chang, J.-H.; Sonawane, S.; Khanolkar, V.; Sarkar, J.; Jain, S. Neurotrophins and Nerve Regeneration-Associated Genes Are Expressed in the Cornea After Lamellar Flap Surgery. *Cornea* **2012**, *31*, 1460–1467. [CrossRef]
109. Donnerer, J.; Schuligoi, R.; Stein, C. Increased Content and Transport of Substance P and Calcitonin Gene-Related Peptide in Sensory Nerves Innervating Inflamed Tissue: Evidence for a Regulatory Function of Nerve Growth Factor in Vivo. *Neuroscience* **1992**, *49*, 693–698. [CrossRef]
110. Shaheen, B.S.; Bakir, M.; Jain, S. Corneal Nerves in Health and Disease. *Surv. Ophthalmol.* **2014**, *59*, 263–285. [CrossRef]
111. Di, G.; Qi, X.; Zhao, X.; Zhang, S.; Danielson, P.; Zhou, Q. Corneal Epithelium-Derived Neurotrophic Factors Promote Nerve Regeneration. *Investig. Ophthalmol. Vis. Sci.* **2017**, *58*, 4695. [CrossRef]
112. Ribatti, D.; Nico, B.; Perra, M.T.; Maxia, C.; Piras, F.; Murtas, D.; Crivellato, E.; Sirigu, P. Correlation between NGF/TrkA and Microvascular Density in Human Pterygium. *Int. J. Exp. Pathol.* **2009**, *90*, 615–620. [CrossRef] [PubMed]
113. Lambiase, A.; Bracci-Laudiero, L.; Bonini, S.; Bonini, S.; Starace, G.; D'Elios, M.M.; De Carli, M.; Aloe, L. Human CD4+ T Cell Clones Produce and Release Nerve Growth Factor and Express High-Affinity Nerve Growth Factor Receptors. *J. Allergy Clin. Immunol.* **1997**, *100*, 408–414. [CrossRef]
114. Freund-Michel, V.; Frossard, N. The Nerve Growth Factor and Its Receptors in Airway Inflammatory Diseases. *Pharmacol. Ther.* **2008**, *117*, 52–76. [CrossRef]
115. Sacchetti, M.; Segatto, M.; Bruscolini, A.; Abicca, I.; Cavaliere, C.; Lambiase, A. Changes of NGF Pathway in Allergic Rhinoconjunctivitis: A Conjunctival Allergen Challenge Study. *Allergy* **2019**, *74*, 605–607. [CrossRef]
116. Semeraro, F.; Forbice, E.; Romano, V.; Angi, M.; Romano, M.R.; Filippelli, M.E.; Di Iorio, R.; Costagliola, C. Neurotrophic Keratitis. *Ophthalmologica* **2014**, *231*, 191–197. [CrossRef]
117. Cavanagh, H.D.; Colley, A.M. The Molecular Basis of Neurotrophic Keratitis. *Acta Ophthalmol.* **1989**, *192*, 115–134. [CrossRef]
118. Bocchini, V.; Angeletti, P.U. The Nerve Growth Factor: Purification as a 30,000-Molecular-Weight Protein. *Proc. Natl. Acad. Sci. USA* **1969**, *64*, 787–794. [CrossRef] [PubMed]

119. Olson, L.; Backlund, E.O.; Ebendal, T.; Freedman, R.; Hamberger, B.; Hansson, P.; Hoffer, B.; Lindblom, U.; Meyerson, B.; Strömberg, I. Intraputaminal Infusion of Nerve Growth Factor to Support Adrenal Medullary Autografts in Parkinson's Disease. One-Year Follow-up of First Clinical Trial. *Arch. Neurol.* **1991**, *48*, 373–381. [CrossRef] [PubMed]
120. Lambiase, A.; Coassin, M.; Sposato, V.; Micera, A.; Sacchetti, M.; Bonini, S.; Aloe, L. NGF Topical Application in Patients with Corneal Ulcer Does Not Generate Circulating NGF Antibodies. *Pharmacol. Res.* **2007**, *56*, 65–69. [CrossRef]
121. Cheung, A.Y.; Shah, A.P.; Pierson, K.L.; Denny, M.R.; Nordlund, M.L.; Holland, E.J. Use of Cenegermin in the Presence of Bandage Contact Lenses. *Cornea* **2022**, *41*, 78–82. [CrossRef]
122. Mantelli, F.; Nardella, C.; Tiberi, E.; Sacchetti, M.; Bruscolini, A.; Lambiase, A. Congenital Corneal Anesthesia and Neurotrophic Keratitis: Diagnosis and Management. *Biomed. Res. Int.* **2015**, *2015*, 805876. [CrossRef]
123. Papadopoulos, K.; Besgen, V.; Sekundo, W. Successful Treatment of a Pediatric Neurotrophic Keratopathy with Cenegermin. *Cornea* **2021**, *40*, 516–518. [CrossRef] [PubMed]
124. Pedrotti, E.; Bonetto, J.; Cozzini, T.; Fasolo, A.; Marchini, G. Cenegermin in Pediatric Neurotrophic Keratopathy. *Cornea* **2019**, *38*, 1450–1452. [CrossRef] [PubMed]
125. Fausto, R.; Ceccuzzi, R.; Micheletti, E.; Clerici, R.; Riva, I.; Katsanos, A.; Oddone, F.; Quaranta, L. A Case Report of Pediatric Neurotrophic Keratopathy in Pontine Tegmental Cap Dysplasia Treated with Cenegermin Eye Drops. *Medicine* **2020**, *99*, e20816. [CrossRef] [PubMed]
126. Leto, M.G.; Toro, M.E.; Indemini, P.E.; Fruttero, C.; Denina, M.; Dalmazzo, C.; Sannia, A.; Vaiano, A.S. Pediatric Use of Recombinant Human Nerve Growth Factor 20 Mg/mL Eye Drops (Cenegermin) for Bilateral Neurotrophic Keratopathy in Congenital Corneal Anesthesia. *Cornea* **2021**, *40*, 228–231. [CrossRef]
127. Tan, M.H.; Bryars, J.; Moore, J. Use of Nerve Growth Factor to Treat Congenital Neurotrophic Corneal Ulceration. *Cornea* **2006**, *25*, 352–355. [CrossRef]
128. Roumeau, S.; Dutheil, F.; Sapin, V.; Baker, J.S.; Watson, S.L.; Pereira, B.; Chiambaretta, F.; Navel, V. Efficacy of Treatments for Neurotrophic Keratopathy: A Systematic Review and Meta-Analysis. *Graefe's Arch. Clin. Exp. Ophthalmol.* **2022**, *260*, 2623–2637. [CrossRef]
129. Vera-Duarte, G.R.; Jimenez-Collado, D.; Kahuam-López, N.; Ramirez-Miranda, A.; Graue-Hernandez, E.O.; Navas, A.; Rosenblatt, M.I. Neurotrophic Keratopathy: General Features and New Therapies. *Surv. Ophthalmol.* **2024**, *69*, 789–804. [CrossRef]
130. Anitua, E.; Muruzabal, F.; Tayebba, A.; Riestra, A.; Perez, V.L.; Merayo-Lloves, J.; Orive, G. Autologous Serum and Plasma Rich in Growth Factors in Ophthalmology: Preclinical and Clinical Studies. *Acta Ophthalmol.* **2015**, *93*, e605–e614. [CrossRef]
131. Kanu, L.N.; Ciolino, J.B. Nerve Growth Factor as an Ocular Therapy: Applications, Challenges, and Future Directions. *Semin. Ophthalmol.* **2021**, *36*, 224–231. [CrossRef]
132. Matsumoto, Y.; Dogru, M.; Goto, E.; Ohashi, Y.; Kojima, T.; Ishida, R.; Tsubota, K. Autologous Serum Application in the Treatment of Neurotrophic Keratopathy. *Ophthalmology* **2004**, *111*, 1115–1120. [CrossRef]
133. Geerling, G.; Maclennan, S.; Hartwig, D. Autologous Serum Eye Drops for Ocular Surface Disorders. *Br. J. Ophthalmol.* **2004**, *88*, 1467–1474. [CrossRef]
134. Hill, J.M.; Garza, H.H.; Helmy, M.F.; Cook, S.D.; Osborne, P.A.; Johnson, E.M.; Thompson, H.W.; Green, L.C.; O'Callaghan, R.J.; Gebhardt, B.M. Nerve Growth Factor Antibody Stimulates Reactivation of Ocular Herpes Simplex Virus Type 1 in Latently Infected Rabbits. *J. Neurovirol.* **1997**, *3*, 206–211. [CrossRef]
135. Otten, U.; Ehrhard, P.; Peck, R. Nerve Growth Factor Induces Growth and Differentiation of Human B Lymphocytes. *Proc. Natl. Acad. Sci. USA* **1989**, *86*, 10059–10063. [CrossRef] [PubMed]
136. Chen, H.; Zhang, J.; Dai, Y.; Xu, J. Nerve Growth Factor Inhibits TLR3-Induced Inflammatory Cascades in Human Corneal Epithelial Cells. *J. Inflamm.* **2019**, *16*, 27. [CrossRef] [PubMed]
137. Park, J.H.; Kang, S.-S.; Kim, J.Y.; Tchah, H. Nerve Growth Factor Attenuates Apoptosis and Inflammation in the Diabetic Cornea. *Investig. Ophthalmol. Vis. Sci.* **2016**, *57*, 6767–6775. [CrossRef] [PubMed]
138. Aloe, L.; Bracci-Laudiero, L.; Bonini, S.; Manni, L. The Expanding Role of Nerve Growth Factor: From Neurotrophic Activity to Immunologic Diseases. *Allergy* **1997**, *52*, 883–894. [CrossRef]
139. Aloe, L.; Simone, M.D.; Properzi, F. Nerve Growth Factor: A Neurotrophin with Activity on Cells of the Immune System. *Microsc. Res. Tech.* **1999**, *45*, 285–291. [CrossRef]
140. Liu, Q.; McDermott, A.M.; Miller, W.L. Elevated Nerve Growth Factor in Dry Eye Associated with Established Contact Lens Wear. *Eye Contact Lens* **2009**, *35*, 232–237. [CrossRef]
141. Sacchetti, M.; Lambiase, A.; Schmidl, D.; Schmetterer, L.; Ferrari, M.; Mantelli, F.; Allegretti, M.; Garhoefer, G. Effect of Recombinant Human Nerve Growth Factor Eye Drops in Patients with Dry Eye: A Phase IIa, Open Label, Multiple-Dose Study. *Br. J. Ophthalmol.* **2020**, *104*, 127–135. [CrossRef]

142. Wirta, D.; Lipsky, W.; Toyos, M.; Martel, J.; Goosey, J.; Verachtert, A.; El-Harazi, S.; Karpecki, P.; Allegretti, M.; Goisis, G.; et al. Recombinant Human Nerve Growth Factor (Cenegermin) for Moderate-to-Severe Dry Eye: Phase II, Randomized, Vehicle-Controlled, Dose-Ranging Trial. *BMC Ophthalmol.* **2024**, *24*, 290. [CrossRef] [PubMed]
143. Yawata, N.; Awate, S.; Liu, Y.-C.; Yuan, S.; Woon, K.; Siak, J.; Kawano, Y.-I.; Sonoda, K.-H.; Mehta, J.S.; Yawata, M. Kinetics of Tear Fluid Proteins after Endothelial Keratoplasty and Predictive Factors for Recovery from Corneal Haze. *J. Clin. Med.* **2019**, *9*, 63. [CrossRef] [PubMed]
144. Hayashi, T.; Takahashi, H.; Inoda, S.; Shimizu, T.; Kobayashi, A.; Kawashima, H.; Yamaguchi, T.; Yamagami, S. Aqueous Humour Cytokine Profiles after Descemet's Membrane Endothelial Keratoplasty. *Sci. Rep.* **2021**, *11*, 17064. [CrossRef] [PubMed]
145. Kodati, S.; Chauhan, S.K.; Chen, Y.; Emami-Naeini, P.; Omoto, M.; Dohlman, T.H.; Stevenson, W.; Amouzegar, A.; Tummala, G.; Saban, D.R.; et al. Interleukin-6 Neutralization Prolongs Corneal Allograft Survival. *Curr. Trends Immunol.* **2018**, *19*, 105–113.
146. Pan, Y.; Liu, F.; Qi, X.; Hu, Y.; Xu, F.; Jia, H. Nerve Growth Factor Changes and Corneal Nerve Repair after Keratoplasty. *Optom. Vis. Sci.* **2018**, *95*, 27–31. [CrossRef]
147. Gouvea, L.; Penatti, R.; Rocha, K.M. Neurotrophic Keratitis after Penetrating Keratoplasty for Lattice Dystrophy. *Am. J. Ophthalmol. Case Rep.* **2021**, *22*, 101058. [CrossRef]
148. Lee, H.K.; Lee, K.S.; Kim, H.C.; Lee, S.H.; Kim, E.K. Nerve Growth Factor Concentration and Implications in Photorefractive Keratectomy vs. Laser in Situ Keratomileusis. *Am. J. Ophthalmol.* **2005**, *139*, 965–971. [CrossRef]
149. Joo, M.-J.; Yuhan, K.R.; Hyon, J.Y.; Lai, H.; Hose, S.; Sinha, D.; O'Brien, T.P. The Effect of Nerve Growth Factor on Corneal Sensitivity after Laser in Situ Keratomileusis. *Arch. Ophthalmol.* **2004**, *122*, 1338–1341. [CrossRef]
150. Gong, Q.; Zhang, S.; Jiang, L.; Lin, M.; Xu, Z.; Yu, Y.; Wang, Q.; Lu, F.; Hu, L. The Effect of Nerve Growth Factor on Corneal Nerve Regeneration and Dry Eye after LASIK. *Exp. Eye Res.* **2021**, *203*, 108428. [CrossRef]
151. Habibi, R.N.; Lee, M.D. Treatment of Dry Eye from Laser-Assisted In Situ Keratomileusis with Recombinant Human Nerve Growth Factor (Cenegermin). *Cornea* **2021**, *40*, 1059–1061. [CrossRef]
152. Ferrari, M.P.; Mantelli, F.; Sacchetti, M.; Antonangeli, M.I.; Cattani, F.; D'Anniballe, G.; Sinigaglia, F.; Ruffini, P.A.; Lambiase, A. Safety and Pharmacokinetics of Escalating Doses of Human Recombinant Nerve Growth Factor Eye Drops in a Double-Masked, Randomized Clinical Trial. *BioDrugs* **2014**, *28*, 275–283. [CrossRef] [PubMed]
153. Hamrah, P.; Massaro-Giordano, M.; Schanzlin, D.; Holland, E.; Berdy, G.; Goisis, G.; Pasedis, G.; Mantelli, F. Phase IV Multicenter, Prospective, Open-Label Clinical Trial of Cenegermin (rhNGF) for Stage 1 Neurotrophic Keratopathy (DEFENDO). *Ophthalmol. Ther.* **2024**, *13*, 553–570. [CrossRef]
154. Matsuyama, A.; Takatori, S.; Sone, Y.; Ochi, E.; Goda, M.; Zamami, Y.; Hashikawa-Hobara, N.; Kitamura, Y.; Kawasaki, H. Effect of Nerve Growth Factor on Innervation of Perivascular Nerves in Neovasculatures of Mouse Cornea. *Biol. Pharm. Bull.* **2017**, *40*, 396–401. [CrossRef] [PubMed]
155. Lee, H.K.; Ryu, I.H.; Seo, K.Y.; Hong, S.; Kim, H.C.; Kim, E.K. Topical 0.1% Prednisolone Lowers Nerve Growth Factor Expression in Keratoconjunctivitis Sicca Patients. *Ophthalmology* **2006**, *113*, 198–205. [CrossRef] [PubMed]
156. Ibáñez, C.F.; Simi, A. P75 Neurotrophin Receptor Signaling in Nervous System Injury and Degeneration: Paradox and Opportunity. *Trends Neurosci.* **2012**, *35*, 431–440. [CrossRef]
157. Fleeman, N.; Mahon, J.; Nevitt, S.; Duarte, R.; Boland, A.; Kotas, E.; Dundar, Y.; McEntee, J.; Ahmad, S. Cenegermin for Treating Neurotrophic Keratitis: An Evidence Review Group Perspective of a NICE Single Technology Appraisal. *Pharmacoecon. Open* **2019**, *3*, 453–461. [CrossRef]
158. Carter, M.J. Evidence-Based Medicine: An Overview of Key Concepts. *Ostomy Wound Manag.* **2010**, *56*, 68–85.
159. Baudouin, C.; Labbé, A.; Liang, H.; Pauly, A.; Brignole-Baudouin, F. Preservatives in Eyedrops: The Good, the Bad and the Ugly. *Prog. Retin. Eye Res.* **2010**, *29*, 312–334. [CrossRef]
160. Bandeira, F.; Yusoff, N.Z.; Yam, G.H.-F.; Mehta, J.S. Corneal Re-Innervation Following Refractive Surgery Treatments. *Neural Regen. Res.* **2019**, *14*, 557–565. [CrossRef]

International Journal of
Molecular Sciences

Review

Safety and Efficacy of Diquafosol Compared to Artificial Tears for the Treatment of Dry Eye: A Systematic Review and Meta-Analysis

José Gerardo Serrano-Robles [1,2], Ana Karen Pérez-Vázquez [2], Guillermo Raul Vera-Duarte [1], Alejandro Navas [1], Arturo Ramirez-Miranda [1], Enrique O. Graue-Hernandez [1] and Nicolás Kahuam-López [1,2,*]

1 Instituto de Oftalmologia Fundacion Conde de Valenciana IAP, Mexico City 11520, Mexico; gerardoserranorobles@gmail.com (J.G.S.-R.)
2 Centro de Investigación en Ciencias de La Salud Anáhuac (CICSA), Facultad de Ciencias de La Salud, Universidad Anáhuac México, Campus Norte, Mexico City 52786, Mexico
* Correspondence: nkahuam@gmail.com

Abstract: Dry eye disease (DED) is a prevalent and disabling condition. Artificial tears are commonly used but often inadequate for moderate-to-severe cases. Secretagogues such as pilocarpine, cevimeline, and diquafosol offer potential alternatives, though their comparative effectiveness remains unclear. To evaluate the safety and efficacy of these secretagogues versus artificial tears in adults with DED, we searched CENTRAL, PubMed, Scopus, LILACS, ClinicalTrials.gov, and WHO ICTRP without language restrictions. Randomized controlled trials (RCTs) comparing secretagogues to artificial tears were eligible. Data extraction and synthesis were conducted using Covidence and the Cochrane RoB 2 tool, and 19 RCTs (n = 2697) were included. Fifteen were analyzed quantitatively; however, only eight trials evaluating diquafosol were suitable for meta-analysis, as data for pilocarpine and cevimeline were insufficient for quantitative synthesis. GRADE was used to assess evidence certainty. PROSPERO registration: CRD42020218407. Diquafosol significantly improved rose bengal staining at 4 weeks and OSDI scores and TBUT in post-cataract patients at 4 and 12 weeks. However, it increased mild adverse events (RR, 1.81; 95% CI, 1.15–2.84). Evidence for pilocarpine and cevimeline was limited. Diquafosol 3% shows greater efficacy than artificial tears in post-cataract DED but with more side effects. Further research is needed for other secretagogues.

Keywords: systematic review; meta-analysis; secretagogues; artificial tears; dry eye; diquafosol

1. Introduction

Dry eye disease (DED) affects the ocular surface and is a leading cause of ophthalmological consultations [1,2]. The symptoms vary, ranging from a foreign body sensation to severe pain [3,4], disrupting daily activities, which can have a negative impact on the quality of life of patients. The Tear Film & Ocular Surface Society (TFOS) Dry Eye Workshop II (DEWS-II) defines DED as a multifactorial disease of the ocular surface characterized by a loss of homeostasis of the tear film accompanied by ocular symptoms, in which tear film instability and hyperosmolarity, ocular surface inflammation and damage, and neurosensory abnormalities play etiological roles [5]. It is estimated that the prevalence ranges from 5 to 35%, with female predominance and a maximum peak at age 60, where the prevalence reaches 70% with a more significant trend for the Asian population [3,4,6,7]. Different conditions that affect one or more components of the tear film or the glands that produce its components have the potential to cause the disease [4]. Tear hyperosmolarity is considered to be the trigger of a cascade of signaling events within corneal epithelial cells, leading to the release of inflammatory mediators and proteases [3].

The management of DED is complex due to its multifactorial etiology [8–10]. The treatment aims to restore homeostasis to the ocular surface and tear film, breaking the vicious cycle of the disease. Medical therapies for DED include tear replacement, anti-inflammatory medications, tear film retention, stimulation, and environmental modifications [11]. Topical treatment with artificial tears (ATs) is widely used in patients with dry eyes and can alleviate the signs and symptoms of patients with DED [12]. However, ATs alone may be insufficient to improve symptoms in some patients. In recent years, a scheme has been proposed for the treatment of DED [13], with artificial tears being the mainstay of treatment. While the use of secretagogues is suggested as part of the treatment for patients with moderate to severe degrees of the disease [14,15].

Various pharmacological agents with a secretagogue effect can stimulate watery secretion, mucus secretion, or both. Topical diquafosol eye drops have been favorably evaluated in several studies [6,16,17]. This agent can stimulate watery and mucous secretion in both animals and humans. It is also possible for the oral administration of cholinergic agonists, particularly pilocarpine and cevimeline, to treat severe DED. They have FDA-approved indications for the treatment of dry mouth associated with Sjögren's syndrome (SS) [18]. Pilocarpine and cevimeline exert their therapeutic effect primarily through stimulation of muscarinic receptors on the lacrimal glands, enhancing aqueous tear secretion [19–21]. Although both are broadly classified as cholinergic agonists, their action is mainly mediated via muscarinic pathways, particularly the M3 subtype. Pilocarpine has broader activity across muscarinic receptors, while cevimeline shows greater selectivity for M3, which may result in more targeted glandular stimulation and fewer systemic effects. In contrast, diquafosol is a selective $P2Y_2$ purinergic receptor agonist that promotes tear secretion through a distinct mechanism [22,23]. By activating $P2Y_2$ receptors on the ocular surface epithelium, diquafosol stimulates chloride ion transport and mucin secretion from goblet cells, thereby contributing to both aqueous volume and tear film stability. Its local, non-cholinergic action may offer a more favorable tolerability profile and broader effects on the ocular surface environment compared to muscarinic agonists. Recent preclinical studies also suggest that formulations based on nanocarriers, such as gabapentin-loaded ceria nanoparticles combined with mucoadhesive polymers, can enhance ocular retention and promote not only tear secretion but also corneal nerve preservation and epithelial regeneration. In a rabbit model of dry eye, Yang et al. demonstrated that this approach significantly alleviated dry eye symptoms by increasing mucin-binding efficiency, prolonging ocular surface residence time, and exerting antioxidant and neuroprotective effects [24].

The objective of the current systematic review and meta-analysis is to determine the safety and efficacy of pilocarpine, cevimeline, and diquafosol compared to artificial tears for treating dry eye. However, due to limited data, only diquafosol was included in the quantitative synthesis, while the evidence for pilocarpine and cevimeline was assessed qualitatively.

2. Methods

2.1. Protocol and Registration

The review was registered on PROSPERO (registration number CRD42020218407) and was reported following the Preferred Reporting Items for Systematic Reviews and

Meta-analyses (PRISMA) statement standard guidelines [25]. The methodology established in the published protocol [26] was followed during the systematic review.

2.2. Eligibility Criteria

We included randomized controlled trials in which the study population comprised adults aged 18 years or older with a clinical diagnosis of dry eye disease, including subtypes such as aqueous tear deficiency, Sjögren's syndrome, or keratoconjunctivitis sicca. During the full-text review, we verified that the eligibility criteria of each trial met this specification, and when available, we reviewed the corresponding trial registry to confirm this information. Eligible interventions included treatment with pilocarpine, cevimeline, or diquafosol. The comparator was artificial tears. Studies were primarily conducted in outpatient settings, as dry eye disease does not typically require inpatient management. We imposed no restrictions based on language or publication status.

2.3. Databases and Information Sources

RCTs were searched in CENTRAL, PubMed, Scopus, LILACS, ClinicalTrials.gov, WHO, and ICTRP without language or date restrictions. Reference lists of included studies were also reviewed for additional trials.

2.4. Search Methods

A highly sensitive Cochrane strategy was used to identify RCTs, supplemented by the PRESS guideline [27,28]. Full search strategies for each database are available in Supplementary Materials S1.

2.5. Study Eligibility Criteria

Two reviewers (GSR and AKP) independently performed a study assessment following a standardized approach. Any reviewer disagreement was settled by discussion or consulting a third review author if required (NKL). We followed the criteria of inclusion, exclusion, and elimination established in the published protocol [26].

2.6. Outcome Measures

Evaluated changes in dry eye signs (TBUT, rose bengal and fluorescein staining, Schirmer test) and quality of life (VRQoL or OSDI). Adverse events (e.g., irritation, pain, conjunctivitis) were also assessed. Data from all reported time points were extracted, and a stratified analysis was performed using trials with matching time points.

2.7. Shared Time Points and Outcomes

Information regarding shared outcomes and evaluated time points across studies is available in the Supplementary Material. This includes a detailed summary of randomized controlled trials comparing diquafosol, with and without a history of cataract surgery, as well as the specific time points assessed in each study, even in cases where outcomes were comparable but time points differed.

2.8. Data Collection and Analysis

Study selection was independently performed by two reviewers using Covidence [29], with disagreements resolved by a third author. Titles and abstracts were screened, followed by full-text assessment of potentially relevant studies. Reasons for exclusions were recorded, and the selection process was presented in a PRISMA diagram (Figure 1).

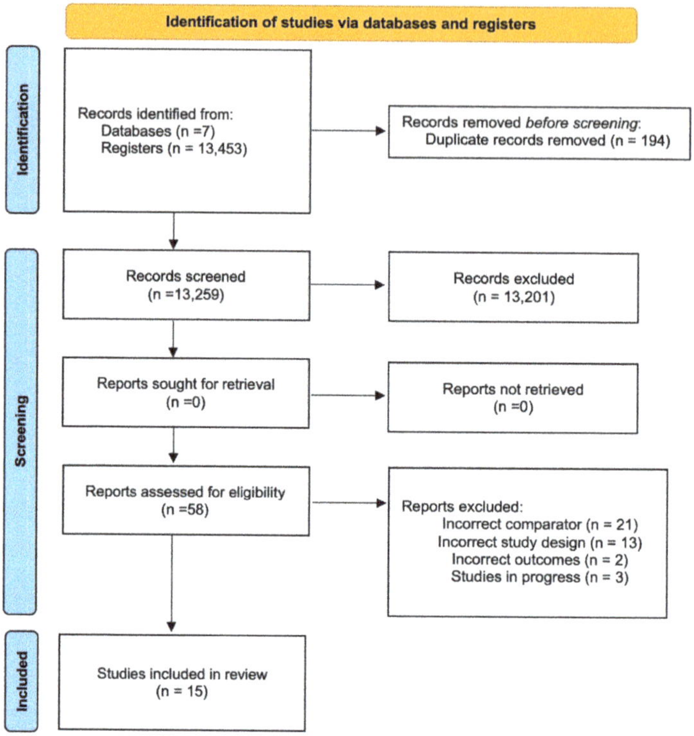

Figure 1. PRISMA flowchart summarizing study selection for the systematic review and meta-analysis.

2.9. Risk of Bias Assessment

The Risk of Bias 2 (RoB 2) tool from the Cochrane Collaboration was used to evaluate bias across key domains. Two reviewers independently assessed each study, classifying risk as "low, high," or "unclear." Discrepancies were resolved by a third reviewer.

2.10. Statistical Analysis

Meta-analyses were conducted using RevMan 5.3. Mean differences (MD) with 95% confidence intervals were calculated for continuous outcomes, and relative risks were used for dichotomous outcomes. Heterogeneity was assessed via forest plots, Chi-square test, and I^2 statistic, following Cochrane guidelines. WebPlotDigitizer was used when outcome data were only available in graphical format.

3. Results

3.1. Literature Search

From 13,453 records, 194 duplicates were removed, and 13,259 titles/abstracts were screened. A total of 58 articles underwent full-text review; 39 were excluded for reasons including incorrect comparator (21), study design (13), outcomes (2), or ongoing status (3). One pilocarpine trial was excluded from meta-analysis due to being a single study. Three cevimeline trials were identified, but none were included in the meta-analysis due to lack of shared outcomes or design heterogeneity. Ultimately, 19 studies were included in the qualitative synthesis and 15 in the meta-analysis. Full study selection details are presented in Figure 1.

Risk-of-Bias Assessment

Supplementary Materials S2 presents bias risk summaries for the trials included in this review. In the comparison between Diquafosol and artificial tears, it is noted that four clinical trials exhibited low bias risk, while four raised some concerns. Potential bias sources were identified across all domains except the outcome selection domain, indicating a 50% overall low bias risk and 50% of trials with some source of concern.

A detailed visual summary of the qualitative synthesis is provided in the Supplementary Material (Supplementary Materials S2).

3.2. Interventions

3.2.1. Diquafosol 3% vs. Artificial Tears

All included trials compared Diquafosol 3% with artificial tears. Some focused on post-cataract patients and were analyzed separately due to their specific clinical context. Most were conducted in outpatient ophthalmology settings. Only studies reporting identical outcomes at the same time points were included in the quantitative synthesis.

Several trials assessed TBUT at 2 weeks [30–32] and 4 weeks [30–33] post-treatment. Fluorescein staining was evaluated at 2 [30–34] and 4 weeks [30–34], while rose bengal staining was reported at 2 [30,32,34] and 4 weeks [30,32–34].

3.2.2. Diquafosol 3% in Post-Cataract Patients

Two trials reported OSDI scores at 1, 4, and 12 weeks post-surgery [16,35]. TBUT was assessed at 1 [16,35], 4 [16,35–39], and 12 weeks [16,35,38]. Four studies reported STT results across 1, 4, and 12 weeks [16,35,36,38], with Jun et al. [38] focusing on 4 and 12 weeks, and Inoue et al. [36] only at 4 weeks. Fluorescein staining was reported at 4 [36–38] and 12 weeks [16,38].

3.2.3. Pilocarpine vs. Artificial Tears

One RCT by Tsifetaki et al. [40] evaluated pilocarpine in 85 subjects randomized to receive pilocarpine, artificial tears, or punctal occlusion. Outcomes included rose bengal and fluorescein staining over 12 weeks. Due to being a single study, it was excluded from meta-analysis.

3.2.4. Cevimeline Trials

Three RCTs evaluated cevimeline in Sjögren's patients. Petrone et al. [41] included 197 subjects; only the 30 mg TID group was analyzed, with STT measured over 12 weeks. Ono et al. [18] evaluated TBUT, STT, and staining at 2 and 4 weeks. Leung et al. [42] conducted a crossover trial with a 4-week washout, but extractable outcomes were unavailable. Quantitative synthesis was not feasible due to heterogeneous endpoints, though all studies reported favorable effects.

3.3. Effects of Interventions

3.3.1. Diquafosol 3% vs. Artificial Tears

TBUT is a continuous quantitative outcome measured in seconds. Thus, an MD analysis with a random-effects model was employed, calculating a 95% confidence interval (CI). Four clinical trials evaluated the effect after two weeks of treatment [30–33]. The combined data from all trials resulted in 342 subjects assigned to the Diquafosol 3% treatment and 346 subjects to artificial tears (MD, −0.05, 95% CI, −0.39 to 0.29; Figure 2). Similarly, four trials assessed the effect after four weeks of treatment [30–33]. The combined data from all trials resulted in 379 subjects assigned to the Diquafosol 3% treatment and 389 subjects to artificial tears (MD, 0.15 with 95% CI, −0.49 to 0.79; Figure 2). In both cases, the p-value was greater than 0.05, indicating no statistically significant difference between using Diquafosol 3% and artificial tears for this outcome.

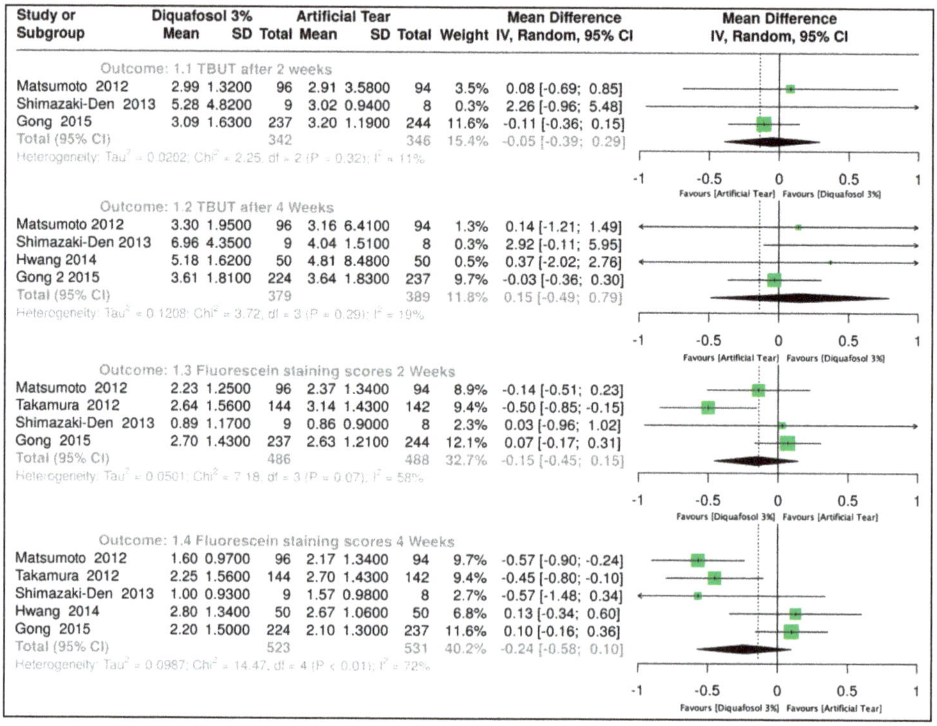

Figure 2. Forest plot comparing 3% diquafosol versus artificial tears for tear breakup time (TBUT) and corneal fluorescein staining. Results are presented as mean differences with 95% confidence intervals (CIs), based on data from studies by Matsumoto et al. [30], Shimazaki-Den et al. [31], Gong et al. [32], Hwang et al. [33], and Takamura et al. [34].

Fluorescein stain score was assessed by MD analysis with a random-effects model employed, with 95% CI. Four clinical trials evaluated the effect of Diquafosol 3% versus artificial tears after two weeks of treatment [30–32,34]. The combined data from all trials resulted in 486 subjects assigned to Diquafosol 3% and 488 subjects assigned to artificial tears treatment (MD, −0.15, 95% CI, −0.45 to 0.15; Figure 2). Five trials assessed the effect of Diquafosol 3% versus artificial tears after four weeks of treatment [30–34]. The combined data from all trials resulted in 523 subjects assigned to Diquafosol 3% and 531 subjects assigned to artificial tears treatment, yielding an MD of −0.24, 95% CI, −0.58 to 0.10 (Figure 2). In both cases, the p-value was greater than 0.05, indicating no statistically significant difference between using Diquafosol 3% and artificial tears for this outcome.

3.3.2. Diquafosol 3% vs. Artificial Tears After Cataract Surgery

OSDI outcome was assessed by MD analysis with a random-effects model performed for this outcome. Two clinical trials [16,35] evaluated the effect of Diquafosol 3% versus artificial tears in subjects post-cataract surgery after one week of treatment. The combined data from these trials resulted in 80 subjects assigned to Diquafosol 3% and 77 subjects assigned to the artificial tears treatment (yielding MD, 4.23, 95% CI, −9.02 to 17.48; Figure 3).

Both trials assessed the outcome at four and twelve weeks of treatment, resulting in MD, −3.97.95% CI, −6.47 to −1.47 and −4.20, 95% CI, −8.29 to −0.11, respectively (Figure 3). In the one-week comparison, there was no difference between the use of Diquafosol 3% and artificial tears in subjects post-cataract surgery ($p > 0.05$). However, in the four-week and twelve-week comparisons, the results were, respectively, Z = 3.12, p-value of 0.002, and Z = 2.01, p-value of 0.04, showing a better response in the Diquafosol 3% group.

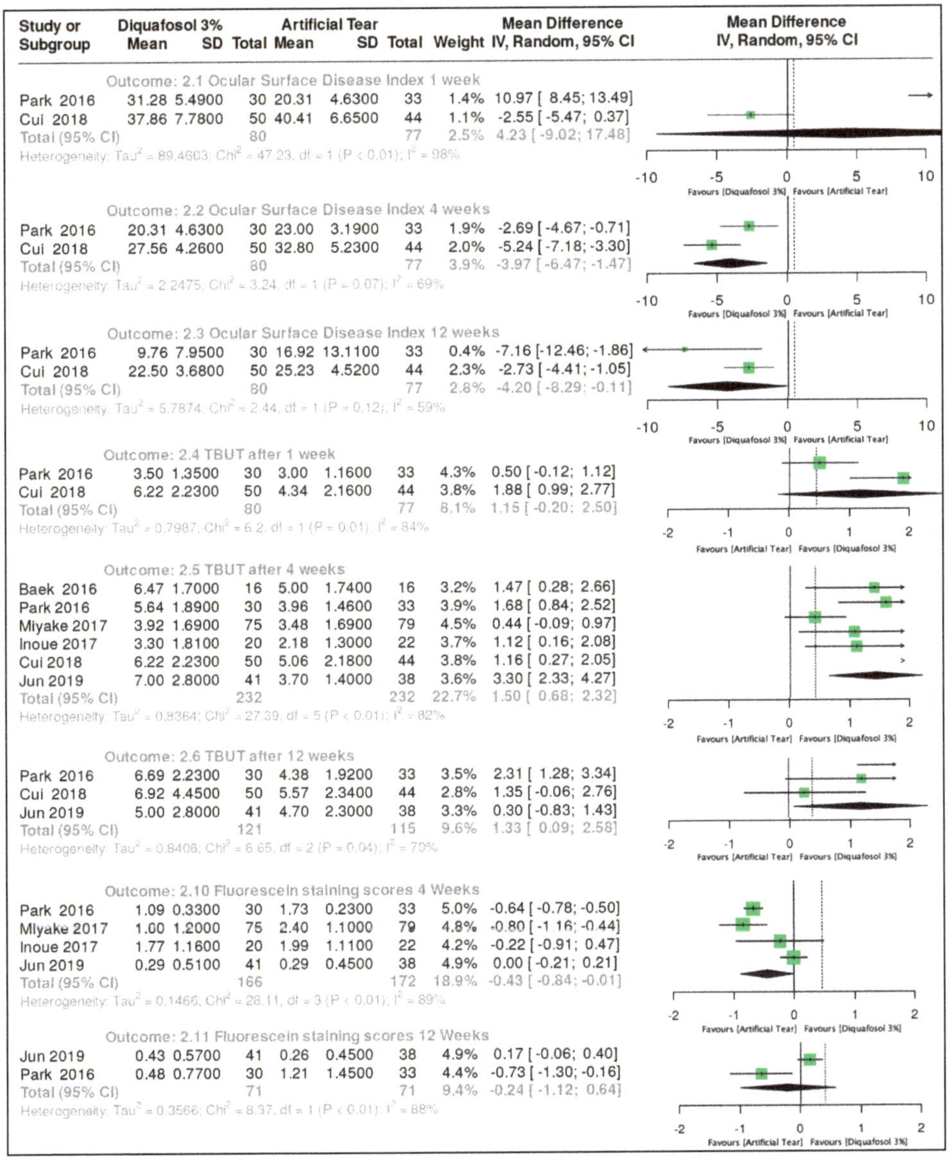

Figure 3. Forest plot comparing 3% diquafosol versus artificial tears in post-cataract surgery patients, evaluating Ocular Surface Disease Index (OSDI), tear breakup time (TBUT), and corneal staining. Results are shown as mean differences with 95% confidence intervals (CIs), based on studies by Park et al. [16], Cui et al. [35], Baek et al. [39], Miyake et al. [37], Inoue et al. [36], and Jun et al. [38].

TBUT is a continuous quantitative outcome; thus, MD analysis with a random-effects model was utilized, 95% CI. Two clinical trials [16,35] evaluated the effect of Diquafosol 3% versus artificial tears in subjects post-cataract surgery after one week of treatment. The combined data from these trials resulted in 80 subjects assigned to Diquafosol 3% and 77 subjects assigned to the artificial tears treatment, yielding MD 1.15, 95% CI, −0.20 to 2.50 (Figure 3). It was also possible to compare this outcome at four weeks of treatment since six clinical trials reported the outcome [16,35–39]. The combined data from these trials resulted in 232 subjects assigned to Diquafosol 3% and 232 subjects assigned to the artificial tears treatment, yielding MD 1.50, 95% CI, 0.68 to 2.32 (Figure 3). A prediction interval was also calculated for this outcome, with 95% of the data falling between −0.18 and 3.18.

The outcome was also evaluated at 12 weeks in three studies [16,35,38]. Combined data from these trials resulted in 121 subjects assigned to Diquafosol 3% and 115 subjects assigned to the artificial tears treatment, yielding an MD of 1.33, 95% CI, 0.09 to 2.58 ($p > 0.05$), in the 1-week comparison (Figure 3). However, in the 4-week and 12-week comparisons, the results were, respectively, $Z = 3.58$, p-value of 0.0003 and $Z = 2.10$, p-value of 0.04, showing a better response in the Diquafosol 3% group.

Fluorescein stain score is a continuous quantitative outcome; hence, MD analysis with a random-effects model was used. Four clinical trials evaluated the effect of Diquafosol 3% versus artificial tears in subjects post-cataract surgery after one week of treatment [16,36–38]. The combined data from these trials resulted in 166 subjects assigned to Diquafosol 3% and 172 subjects assigned to the artificial tears treatment, yielding an MD −0.43 with a 95% CI, −0.84 to −0.01 (Figure 3). It was also possible to compare this outcome at twelve weeks of treatment since two clinical trials reported the outcome [16,38]. The combined data from these trials resulted in 71 subjects assigned to Diquafosol 3% and 71 subjects assigned to the artificial tears treatment, yielding an MD of −0.24 with a 95% CI, −1.12 to 0.64 (Figure 3). The $Z = 2.01$, p-value 0.04 in the 4-week comparison, showing a better response in the Diquafosol 3% group. However, in the 12-week comparison, the p-value was 0.59, indicating no statistically significant difference between the use of Diquafosol 3% and artificial tears in subjects post-cataract surgery at this time point.

3.4. Safety Outcomes

Diquafosol 3% vs. Artificial Tears

Ocular Secretion: Two trials [32,34] reported ocular secretion. Pooled data showed a higher risk in the Diquafosol 3% group (RR = 9.77; 95% CI: 1.83–52.16; $I^2 = 0\%$; Figure 4).

Ocular Irritation: Four trials [30,32–34] reported ocular irritation, with increased risk in the Diquafosol group (RR = 2.48; 95% CI: 1.06–5.78; $I^2 = 33\%$; Figure 4).

Ocular Itching: This was reported in two trials [32,34], with no significant difference between groups (RR = 1.30; 95% CI: 0.49–3.47; $I^2 = 0\%$; Figure 4).

Ocular Pain: This was also reported in two trials [32,34], showing no significant difference (RR = 1.56; 95% CI: 0.52–4.68; $I^2 = 0\%$; Figure 4).

Nasopharyngitis: This was reported by Matsumoto et al. [30] (RR = 0.88; 95% CI: 0.37–2.07). Only one trial reported this outcome, so I^2 was not estimated (Figure 4).

Conjunctivitis: This was reported by Takamura et al. [34] (RR = 1.99; 95% CI: 0.18–21.66). I^2 could not be calculated (Figure 4).

Foreign Body Sensation: Takamura et al. [34] reported this event with higher risk in the artificial tears group (RR = 3.97; 95% CI: 0.08–4.10; Figure 4).

Blepharitis: This was also reported by Takamura et al. [34], favoring Diquafosol (RR = 0.20; 95% CI: 0.01–4.10; Figure 4).

Meta-Analytic Result: Overall, Diquafosol 3% was associated with a higher risk of adverse events (RR = 1.81; 95% CI: 1.15–2.84; Figure 4).

Study or Subgroup	Diquafosol 3% Events	Diquafosol 3% Total	Artificial Tear Events	Artificial Tear Total	Weight	Risk Ratio MH, Random, 95% CI
subgroup = Eye discharge						
Gong 2015	10	246	1	251	4.4%	10.20 [1.32; 79.11]
Takamura 2012	4	144	0	143	2.3%	8.94 [0.49; 164.49]
Total (95% CI)		**390**		**394**	**6.7%**	**9.77 [1.83; 52.16]**
Heterogeneity: $Tau^2 = 0$; $Chi^2 = 0.2$, df = 1 ($P = 0.6553$); $I^2 = 0\%$						
subgroup = Eye irritation						
Gong 2015	7	246	4	251	10.8%	1.79 [0.53; 6.02]
Hwang 2014	4	50	4	50	9.4%	1.00 [0.26; 3.78]
Matsumoto 2012	13	96	3	94	10.7%	4.24 [1.25; 14.41]
Takamura 2012	9	144	1	143	4.4%	8.94 [1.15; 69.63]
Total (95% CI)		**536**		**538**	**35.3%**	**2.48 [1.06; 5.78]**
Heterogeneity: $Tau^2 = 0.2437$; $Chi^2 = 4.45$, df = 3 ($P = 0.2165$); $I^2 = 32.6\%$						
subgroup = Eye pruritus						
Gong 2015	7	246	5	251	12.0%	1.43 [0.46; 4.44]
Takamura 2012	2	144	2	143	4.9%	0.99 [0.14; 6.95]
Total (95% CI)		**390**		**394**	**16.9%**	**1.30 [0.49; 3.47]**
Heterogeneity: $Tau^2 = 0$; $Chi^2 = 0.1$, df = 1 ($P = 0.7517$); $I^2 = 0\%$						
subgroup = Eye pain						
Matsumoto 2012	6	96	4	94	10.6%	1.47 [0.43; 5.04]
Takamura 2012	2	144	1	143	3.3%	1.99 [0.18; 21.66]
Total (95% CI)		**240**		**237**	**13.9%**	**1.56 [0.52; 4.68]**
Heterogeneity: $Tau^2 = 0$; $Chi^2 = 0.05$, df = 1 ($P = 0.8258$); $I^2 = 0\%$						
subgroup = Nasopharyngitis						
Matsumoto 2012	9	96	10	94	17.8%	0.88 [0.37; 2.07]
subgroup = Conjunctivitis						
Takamura 2012	2	144	1	143	3.3%	1.99 [0.18; 21.66]
subgroup = Foreign body sensation						
Takamura 2012	4	144	1	143	4.0%	3.97 [0.45; 35.11]
subgroup = Blepharitis						
Takamura 2012	0	144	2	143	2.1%	0.20 [0.01; 4.10]
Total (95% CI)		**2084**		**2086**	**100.0%**	**1.81 [1.15; 2.85]**

Heterogeneity: $Tau^2 = 0.1087$; $Chi^2 = 15.31$, df = 13 ($P = 0.2885$); $I^2 = 15.1\%$
Test for overall effect: $Z = 2.57$ ($P = 0.0101$)
Test for subgroup differences: $Chi^2 = 10.03$, df = 7 ($P = 0.1867$)

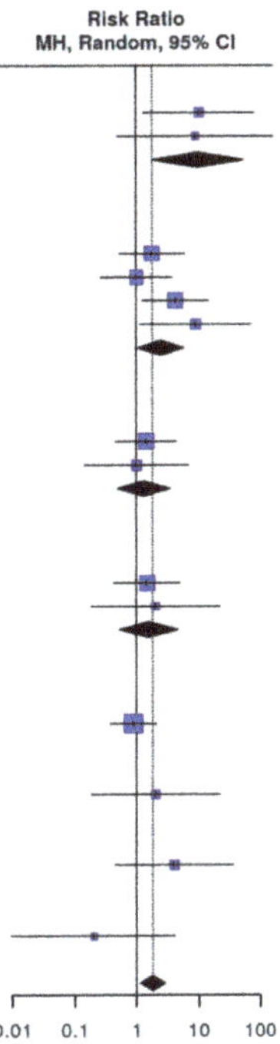

Figure 4. Forest plot comparing the incidence of adverse events between 3% diquafosol and artificial tears. Results are reported as risk ratios with 95% confidence intervals (CIs), based on data from Gong et al. [32], Takamura et al. [34], Hwang et al. [33], and Matsumoto et al. [30].

4. Discussion

This systematic review included only clinical trials assessing the safety and efficacy of pilocarpine, cevimeline, and diquafosol versus artificial tears for dry eye treatment. For pilocarpine (Tsifetak et al. [40]) and cevimeline (three trials: [18,41,42]), quantitative synthesis was not feasible due to a lack of shared outcomes or aligned time points; thus, only qualitative analysis was performed.

Eight clinical trials comparing Diquafosol to artificial tears were identified. A stratified analysis included only studies reporting the same outcomes at the same time points. For TBUT at 2 and 4 weeks, four trials [30–33] involving 768 participants (379 Diquafosol and 389 artificial tears) found no statistically significant difference. For fluorescein staining, four trials [30–32,34] at 2 weeks (n = 974) and five trials [30–34] at 4 weeks (n = 1054) also showed no significant difference.

In post-cataract surgery patients, seven trials were included. Two trials [16,35] assessed OSDI in 157 patients; no difference was found at week 1, but Diquafosol was significantly superior at weeks 4 and 12 (MDs −3.97 and −4.20; $I^2 < 70\%$, high certainty, Table 1). For TBUT, six trials [16,35–39] with 464 subjects showed a significant benefit at 4 weeks (MD 1.5), with moderate certainty.

Table 1. Summary (GRADE) for the comparison of Diquafosol 3% vs. artificial tears in dry eye disease.

Comparison Diquafosol 3% vs. Artificial Tears								
Certainty Assessment					**No. of Patients**		**Effect Size**	**Certainty**
No Studies	**Study Design**	**Risk of Bias**	**Inconsistency**	**Imprecision**	**[Diquafosol 3%]**	**[Artificial Tear]**	**Absolute (95% CI)**	
Tear Film Breakup Time after two weeks of treatment								
3	Randomized trials	Not serious	Not serious	Serious [a]	342	346	MD 0.05 (0.39–0.29)	⊕⊕⊕○ Moderate
Tear Film Breakup Time after four weeks of treatment								
4	Randomized trials	Not serious	Not serious	Serious [a]	379	389	MD 0.15 (0.49–0.79)	⊕⊕⊕○ Moderate
Fluorescein staining score two weeks of treatment								
4	Randomized trials	Not serious	Serious [b]	Serious [a]	486	488	MD 0.15 (0.45–0.15)	⊕⊕○○ Low
Fluorescein staining score four weeks of treatment								
5	Randomized trials	Not serious	Serious [b]	Serious [a]	523	531	MD 0.24 (0.58–0.1)	⊕⊕○○ Low
Comparison Diquafosol 3% vs. Artificial Tears in post-cataract surgery subjects								
Ocular Surface Disease Index after one week of treatment.								
2	Randomized trials	Not serious	Serious [c]	Serious [d]	80	77	MD 4.23 (9.02–17.48)	⊕⊕○○ Low
Ocular Surface Disease Index after four weeks of treatment.								
2	Randomized trials	Not serious	Not serious	Not serious	80	77	MD 3.97 (6.47–1.47)	⊕⊕⊕○ Moderate
Ocular Surface Disease Index after twelve weeks of treatment.								
2	Randomized trials	Not serious	Not serious	Not serious	80	77	MD 4.2 (8.29–0.11)	⊕⊕⊕○ Moderate
Tear Film Breakup Time after one week of treatment.								
2	Randomized trials	Not serious	Serious [e]	Serious [e]	80	77	MD 1.15 (0.2–2.5)	⊕⊕○○ Low
Tear Film Breakup Time after four weeks of treatment.								
6	Randomized trials	Serious [c]	Not serious	Not serious	232	232	MD 1.5 (0.68–2.32)	⊕⊕⊕○ Moderate
Tear Film Breakup Time after twelve weeks of treatment.								
3	Randomized trials	Not serious	Serious [c]	Serious [e]	121	115	MD 1.33 (0.09–2.58)	⊕⊕○○ Low
Fluorescein staining after four weeks of treatment.								
4	Randomized trials	Serious [e]	Serious [e]	Serious [b]	166	172	MD 0.43 (0.84–0.01)	⊕○○○ Very low
Fluorescein staining after four weeks of treatment.								
2	Randomized trials	Not serious	Serious [e]	Serious [b]	71	71	MD 0.24 (1.12–0.64)	⊕⊕○○ Low

Adverse Effects of the Comparison Diquafosol 3% vs. Artificial Tears									
Certainty Assessment					No. of Patients		Effect Size		Certainty
No Studies	Study Design	Inconsistency	Imprecision	Other Considerations	[Diquafosol 3%]	[Artificial Tear]	Relative (95% CI)	Absolute (95% CI)	
Adverse event: Ocular discharge									
2	Randomized trials	Not serious	Serious [a]	Strong association	14/390 (3.6%)	1/394 (0.3%)	RR 9.77 (1.83–52.16)	22 more per 1000 (from 2 more to 130 more)	⊕⊕⊕○ Moderate
Adverse event: Eye Irritation									
4	Randomized trials	Serious [c]	Serious [a]	Strong association	33/536 (6.2%)	12/538 (2.2%)	RR 2.48 (1.06–5.78)	33 more per 1000 (from 1 more to 107 more)	⊕⊕⊕○ Moderate
Adverse event: Ocular itching									
2	Randomized trials	Not serious	Serious [a]	None	9/390 (2.3%)	7/394 (1.8%)	RR 1.30 (0.49–3.47)	5 more per 1000 (from 9 less to 44 more)	⊕⊕⊕○ Moderate

Table 1. *Cont.*

Adverse event: Eye pain									
2	Randomized trials	Not serious	Serious [a]	None	8/240 (3.3%)	5/237 (2.1%)	RR 1.56 (0.52–4.68)	12 more per 1000 (from 10 less to 78 more)	⊕⊕⊕○ Moderate
Adverse event: Conjunctivitis									
1	Randomized trials	Not serious	Serious [a]	None	2/144 (1.4%)	1/143 (0.7%)	RR 1.99 (0.18–21.66)	7 more per 1000 (from 6 less to 144 more)	⊕⊕⊕○ Moderate
Adverse event: Foreign body sensation									
1	Randomized trials	Not serious	Serious [a]	None	4/144 (2.8%)	1/143 (0.7%)	RR 3.97 (0.45–5.11)	7 more per 1000 (from 6 less to 144 more)	⊕⊕⊕○ Moderate
Adverse event: Blepharitis									
1	Randomized trials	Not serious	Serious [a]	None	0/144 (0.0%)	2/143 (1.4%)	RR 0.20 (0.01–4.10)	11 less per 1000 (from 14 less to 43 more)	⊕⊕⊕○ Moderate

CI: confidence interval; MD: mean difference; RR: relative risk. [a] Some trials reported information on this outcome in graphic form, so data extraction software was used, with the possibility of introducing variation. [b] Although all clinical trials used the same method to score this outcome, the perception of each rater may influence the scoring of the reported results. [c] Conflicting evidence reported in clinical trials; [d] inaccurate evidence; [e] some clinical trials included in this comparison had a high risk of bias. Moderate certainty: the estimated effect is probably close to the true effect, although a meaningful difference cannot be ruled out. Low certainty: confidence in the estimate is limited, and the actual effect could differ significantly. Very low certainty: there is minimal confidence in the estimate; the true effect is likely to be markedly different.

Table 1 summarizes adverse effects. Diquafosol 3% was associated with a higher incidence of symptoms such as discharge, irritation, itching, and conjunctivitis. The evidence indicated a significantly increased risk, with moderate certainty despite some imprecision.

4.1. Quality of the Evidence

Only randomized clinical trials were included. Risk of bias was independently assessed using Cochrane's RoB 2 tool, covering five domains: randomization, intervention deviations, missing data, outcome measurement, and selective reporting.

For Diquafosol vs. artificial tears, four studies were rated low risk [30,43–45], while four had moderate risk [31–34], primarily due to randomization and measurement issues. Among post-cataract trials, three were low risk [35,38,46] and three moderate risk [16,39,45]; Inoue et al. [36] was rated high risk due to incomplete data.

Regarding evidence certainty, two outcomes had moderate certainty and four had low certainty in the Diquafosol–artificial tears comparison, mainly downgraded for reliance on graphical data and subjective endpoints. In post-cataract studies, two outcomes had high certainty, one moderate certainty, six low certainty, and one very low certainty, affected by inconsistency, imprecision, and graphical-only reporting, particularly for fluorescein staining. Despite standardized grading, subjectivity in rose bengal scoring may have influenced results. For adverse events, one outcome had high certainty and four had moderate certainty. Ocular secretion was upgraded to high due to strong and consistent effects (RR > 2.0 or <0.5) across studies.

Although a previous meta-analysis by Liu et al. [47] addressed the effects of 3% diquafosol in dry eye disease, our study differs in several important aspects. We conducted a broader and more sensitive literature search, included a larger number of randomized controlled trials, and focused specifically on comparisons with artificial tears. Our review also considered other topical secretagogues such as pilocarpine and cevimeline; while meta-analysis was not feasible for these agents, the search strategy retrieved relevant studies that were narratively reviewed. In addition, we performed a subgroup analysis in post-cataract surgery patients and assessed methodological quality using Cochrane RoB 2.0 and GRADE criteria. For adverse events, one outcome had high and four had moderate certainty; notably, ocular secretion was upgraded to high due to strong and consistent effects (RR > 2.0 or <0.5) across studies. The protocol was prospectively registered and published, ensuring methodological transparency. Xinyu Zhao et al. [48] also conducted a prior meta-analysis on diquafosol in post-cataract patients, reporting favorable outcomes; however, their review lacked protocol registration, risk of bias assessment, and a defined search strategy, which limits its reliability. Nevertheless, their findings are consistent with ours.

This is the first systematic review specifically evaluating 3% Diquafosol vs. artificial tears, showing greater benefits in post-cataract patients likely due to enhanced action in surgically altered ocular surfaces, compared to its tear-like function in non-surgical eyes. A major limitation was the absence of data on tear osmolarity or vision-related quality of life (VR-QoL), despite being pre-specified outcomes. Inconsistent follow-up time points across trials also reduced comparability, limiting both the quantity and certainty of the evidence. Furthermore, the composition of artificial tears varied across the included trials. Some studies used carboxymethylcellulose-based formulations, others used sodium hyaluronate at different concentrations, and several did not specify the exact components of the comparator. These differences may have influenced tear film retention time, osmolarity, and surface coverage, introducing variability in the comparator group and potentially affecting treatment outcomes. We now highlight this formulation heterogeneity as a limitation that may reduce the internal consistency of the control arm. Future trials should clearly specify and, where possible, standardize the artificial tear formulation to improve comparability across studies.

4.2. Overall Completeness and Applicability of Evidence

The clinical trials included in this systematic review were not substantially heterogeneous in terms of population or interventions. However, the available evidence was insufficient to comprehensively address all predefined objectives of the review. Key patient-centered outcomes, such as vision-related quality of life (VRQoL) and tear osmolarity, were not reported in the included studies. Additionally, relevant measures such as intraoperative or postoperative discomfort, treatment adherence, and long-term safety were either inconsistently reported or entirely absent. For pilocarpine and cevimeline, the effects of different doses on both efficacy and adverse events were not systematically explored. Moreover, the potential differences in effectiveness and tolerability between systemic (oral) and topical ophthalmic administration remain unclear, as direct comparisons are lacking. Considering that dry eye disease is driven by tear hyperosmolarity and ocular surface inflammation, future studies and meta-analyses should also incorporate relevant biological markers, such as tear osmolarity, inflammatory cytokine levels, or matrix metalloproteinase activity, to better understand the mechanisms and therapeutic effects of secretagogues. Importantly, dry eye disease encompasses multiple clinical subtypes, including aqueous-deficient and evaporative forms, which may respond differently to treatment. A more granular classification of patients according to disease subtype is needed to accurately assess treatment efficacy and to guide personalized therapy. These limitations restrict the clinical applicability of the current findings and underscore the need for more comprehensive, stratified, and standardized outcome reporting in future randomized trials.

5. Conclusions

Based on the findings of this systematic review and meta-analysis, 3% diquafosol demonstrated superiority over artificial tears in improving rose bengal staining after four weeks of treatment. In post-cataract surgery patients, diquafosol was also superior in improving OSDI and TBUT at four and twelve weeks, and STT at one, four, and twelve weeks. Additionally, fewer adverse effects were reported with diquafosol in some trials. These benefits were supported by moderate- to high-certainty evidence in postoperative populations, suggesting that diquafosol may be considered a more effective treatment option than artificial tears in this subgroup. However, in other populations with dry eye disease, findings were inconsistent and based on low- to very low-certainty evidence, limiting generalizability. Regarding pilocarpine and cevimeline, the current evidence is insufficient to support clinical recommendations due to heterogeneity, limited trial data, and lack of shared outcomes. Therefore, clinical decisions should be made on a case-by-case basis, considering patient characteristics and disease subtype, with diquafosol reserved for specific contexts where evidence supports its use.

Implications for Research

There is a clear need for further well-designed randomized controlled trials evaluating the safety and efficacy of secretagogues in diverse dry eye populations. Future studies should focus on the following:

- Compare treatment outcomes across clinically distinct subtypes of dry eye disease (e.g., aqueous-deficient vs. evaporative);
- Assess the dose–response relationships and adverse event profiles of pilocarpine and cevimeline;
- Investigate potential differences in efficacy and tolerability between systemic (oral) and topical administration routes;
- Incorporate relevant biological indicators (e.g., tear osmolarity, inflammatory cytokines, MMP-9) to better understand mechanisms of action;
- Include validated patient-centered outcomes such as vision-related quality of life and standardized symptom questionnaires;
- Prospectively register protocols and follow predefined methods and outcomes;
- Clearly describe randomization, allocation concealment, and masking procedures;
- Document handling of missing data and perform intention-to-treat analyses;
- Evaluate outcomes at standardized time points (e.g., 4, 12, and 24 weeks);
- Report adverse events in a stratified and comprehensive manner.

Finally, future trials should adopt a more granular classification of participants according to dry eye subtype and disease severity. This stratification, along with improved methodological consistency, will enhance the applicability of findings and inform evidence-based, personalized treatment strategies in dry eye disease.

Supplementary Materials: The following supporting information can be downloaded at: https://www.mdpi.com/article/10.3390/ijms26178113/s1.

Author Contributions: Conceptualization, J.G.S.-R., N.K.-L. and A.N.; methodology, J.G.S.-R., N.K.-L. and A.N.; software, J.G.S.-R.; validation, J.G.S.-R., N.K.-L. and A.K.P.-V.; formal analysis, J.G.S.-R.; investigation, J.G.S.-R. and E.O.G.-H.; resources, J.G.S.-R., A.R.-M. and G.R.V.-D.; data curation, J.G.S.-R. and A.K.P.-V.; writing—original draft preparation, J.G.S.-R. and N.K.-L.; writing—review and editing, J.G.S.-R., A.K.P.-V., E.O.G.-H., A.R.-M., G.R.V.-D. and A.N.; visualization, J.G.S.-R.; supervision, J.G.S.-R., N.K.-L. and G.R.V.-D.; project administration, J.G.S.-R. and N.K.-L.; funding acquisition, J.G.S.-R. and N.K.-L. All review authors contributed to the production of the protocol. J.G.S.-R. and N.K.-L. led the writing of the protocol; A.K.P.-V., E.O.G.-H., A.R.-M., G.R.V.-D. and A.N. provided critical feedback and editorial input throughout the process. All authors have read and agreed to the published version of the manuscript.

Funding: This research received no external funding. The article processing charge (APC) was covered by the authors themselves.

Institutional Review Board Statement: The study was conducted in accordance with the Declaration of Helsinki and was approved by the Research Committee of the Facultad de Ciencias de la Salud, Universidad Anáhuac México (protocol code 202081, approved on 28 January 2021). As this was a systematic review and meta-analysis based exclusively on previously published data, no new data involving human participants or animals were collected, and informed consent was therefore not required. The study was prospectively registered in the International Prospective Register of Systematic Reviews (PROSPERO) under the registration number CRD42020218407 approved 8 December 2020.

Informed Consent Statement: Not applicable.

Data Availability Statement: All data supporting the findings of this study are available in the Supplementary Materials provided with the manuscript. No new primary data were generated during this systematic review and meta-analysis, as all analyses are based on data extracted from previously published studies.

Conflicts of Interest: The authors declare no conflicts of interest.

References

1. Sheppard, J.; Lee, B.S.; Periman, L.M. Dry eye disease: Identification and therapeutic strategies for primary care clinicians and clinical specialists. *Ann. Med.* **2022**, *55*, 241–252. [CrossRef]
2. Bradley, J.L.; Stillman, I.Ö.; Pivneva, I.; Guerin, A.; Evans, A.M.; Dana, R. Dry eye disease ranking among common reasons for seeking eye care in a large US claims database. *Clin. Ophthalmol.* **2019**, *13*, 225–232. [CrossRef]
3. Nichols, K.K. The International Workshop on Meibomian Gland Dysfunction: Introduction. *Investig. Opthalmology Vis. Sci.* **2011**, *52*, 1917–1921. [CrossRef] [PubMed]
4. Clayton, J.A.; Longo, D.L. Dry Eye. *N. Engl. J. Med.* **2018**, *378*, 2212–2223. [CrossRef] [PubMed]
5. Craig, J.P.; Nichols, K.K.; Akpek, E.K.; Caffery, B.; Dua, H.S.; Joo, C.-K.; Liu, Z.; Nelson, J.D.; Nichols, J.J.; Tsubota, K.; et al. TFOS DEWS II Definition and Classification Report. *Ocul. Surf.* **2017**, *15*, 276–283. [CrossRef] [PubMed]
6. Dana, R.; Bradley, J.L.; Guerin, A.; Pivneva, I.; Stillman, I.Ö.; Evans, A.M.; Schaumberg, D.A. Estimated Prevalence and Incidence of Dry Eye Disease Based on Coding Analysis of a Large, All-age United States Health Care System. *Arch. Ophthalmol.* **2019**, *202*, 47–54. [CrossRef]
7. Nelson, J.D.; Shimazaki, J.; Benitez-Del-Castillo, J.M.; Craig, J.P.; McCulley, J.P.; Den, S.; Foulks, G.N. The International Workshop on Meibomian Gland Dysfunction: Report of the Definition and Classification Subcommittee. *Investig. Opthalmology Vis. Sci.* **2011**, *52*, 1930–1937. [CrossRef]
8. Şimşek, C.; Doğru, M.; Kojima, T.; Tsubota, K. Current Management and Treatment of Dry Eye Disease. *Turk. J. Ophthalmol.* **2018**, *48*, 309–313. [CrossRef]
9. Huang, D.; Li, Z. Multidimensional immunotherapy for dry eye disease: Current status and future directions. *Front. Ophthalmol.* **2024**, *4*, 1449283. [CrossRef]
10. Aragona, P.; Giannaccare, G.; Mencucci, R.; Rubino, P.; Cantera, E.; Rolando, M. Modern approach to the treatment of dry eye, a complex multifactorial disease: A P.I.C.A.S.S.O. board review. *Br. J. Ophthalmol.* **2021**, *105*, 446–453. [CrossRef] [PubMed] [PubMed Central]
11. Lee, B.S.; Kabat, A.G.; Bacharach, J.; Karpecki, P.; Luchs, J. Managing Dry Eye Disease and Facilitating Realistic Patient Expectations: A Review and Appraisal of Current Therapies. *Clin. Ophthalmol.* **2020**, *14*, 119–126. [CrossRef] [PubMed]
12. Mohamed, H.B.; El-Hamid, B.N.A.; Fathalla, D.; Fouad, E.A. Current trends in pharmaceutical treatment of dry eye disease: A review. *Eur. J. Pharm. Sci.* **2022**, *175*, 106206. [CrossRef] [PubMed]

13. Rauz, S.; Koay, S.-Y.; Foot, B.; Kaye, S.B.; Figueiredo, F.; Burdon, M.A.; Dancey, E.; Chandrasekar, A.; Lomas, R. The Royal College of Ophthalmologists guidelines on serum eye drops for the treatment of severe ocular surface disease: Full report. *Eye* **2017**, eye2017209. [CrossRef] [PubMed]
14. Donthineni, P.R.; Doctor, M.B.; Shanbhag, S.; Kate, A.; Galor, A.; Djalilian, A.R.; Singh, S.; Basu, S. Aqueous-deficient dry eye disease: Preferred practice pattern guidelines on clinical approach, diagnosis, and management. *Indian J. Ophthalmol.* **2023**, *71*, 1332–1347. [CrossRef]
15. Gupta, P.K.; Toyos, R.; Sheppard, J.D.; Toyos, M.; Mah, F.S.; Bird, B.; Theriot, P.; Higgins, D. Tolerability of Current Treatments for Dry Eye Disease: A Review of Approved and Investigational Therapies. *Clin. Ophthalmol.* **2024**, *18*, 2283–2302. [CrossRef]
16. Park, D.H.; Chung, J.K.; Seo, D.R.; Lee, S.J. Clinical Effects and Safety of 3% Diquafosol Ophthalmic Solution for Patients with Dry Eye After Cataract Surgery: A Randomized Controlled Trial. *Arch. Ophthalmol.* **2016**, *163*, 122–131.e2. [CrossRef]
17. Shimazaki, J.; Seika, D.; Saga, M.; Fukagawa, K.; Sakata, M.; Iwasaki, M.; Okano, T. A Prospective, Randomized Trial of Two Mucin Secretogogues for the Treatment of Dry Eye Syndrome in Office Workers. *Sci. Rep.* **2017**, *7*, 15210. [CrossRef]
18. Ono, M.; Takamura, E.; Shinozaki, K.; Tsumura, T.; Hamano, T.; Yagi, Y.; Tsubota, K. Therapeutic effect of cevimeline on dry eye in patients with Sjögren's syndrome: A randomized, double-blind clinical study. *Arch. Ophthalmol.* **2004**, *138*, 6–17. [CrossRef]
19. Singer, M.C.; Marchal, F.; Angelos, P.; Bernet, V.; Boucai, L.; Buchholzer, S.; Burkey, B.; Eisele, D.; Erkul, E.; Faure, F.; et al. Salivary and lacrimal dysfunction after radioactive iodine for differentiated thyroid cancer: American Head and Neck Society Endocrine Surgery Section and Salivary Gland Section joint multidisciplinary clinical consensus statement of otolaryngology, ophthalmology, nuclear medicine and endocrinology. *Head Neck* **2020**, *42*, 3446–3459. [CrossRef]
20. Dartt, D.A. Neural regulation of lacrimal gland secretory processes: Relevance in dry eye diseases. *Prog. Retin. Eye Res.* **2009**, *28*, 155–177. [CrossRef]
21. Nguyen, D.H.; Vadlamudi, V.; Toshida, H.; Beuerman, R.W. Loss of parasympathetic innervation leads to sustained expression of pro-inflammatory genes in the rat lacrimal gland. *Auton. Neurosci.* **2006**, *124*, 81–89. [CrossRef] [PubMed]
22. Dota, A.; Sakamoto, A.; Nagano, T.; Murakami, T.; Matsugi, T. Effect of Diquafosol Ophthalmic Solution on Airflow-Induced Ocular Surface Disorder in Diabetic Rats. *Clin. Ophthalmol.* **2020**, *14*, 1019–1024. [CrossRef]
23. Ohashi, Y.; Munesue, M.; Shimazaki, J.; Takamura, E.; Yokoi, N.; Watanabe, H.; Nomura, A.; Shimada, F. Long-Term Safety and Effectiveness of Diquafosol for the Treatment of Dry Eye in a Real-World Setting: A Prospective Observational Study. *Adv. Ther.* **2019**, *37*, 707–717. [CrossRef]
24. Yang, C.-J.; Anand, A.; Huang, C.-C.; Lai, J.-Y. Unveiling the Power of Gabapentin-Loaded Nanoceria with Multiple Therapeutic Capabilities for the Treatment of Dry Eye Disease. *ACS Nano* **2023**, *17*, 25118–25135. [CrossRef]
25. Page, M.J.; McKenzie, J.E.; Bossuyt, P.M.; Boutron, I.; Hoffmann, T.C.; Mulrow, C.D.; Shamseer, L.; Tetzlaff, J.M.; Akl, E.A.; Brennan, S.E.; et al. The PRISMA 2020 statement: An updated guideline for reporting systematic reviews. *BMJ* **2021**, *372*, n71. [CrossRef]
26. Serrano-Robles, J.G.; Vázquez, A.K.P.; Navas, A.; Graue-Hernandez, E.O.; Ramirez-Miranda, A.; Kahuam-López, N. Safety and efficacy of pilocarpine, cevimeline, and diquafosol compared to artificial tears for the treatment of dry eye: Protocol for a systematic review. *Syst. Rev.* **2022**, *11*, 105. [CrossRef]
27. McGowan, J.; Sampson, M.; Salzwedel, D.M.; Cogo, E.; Foerster, V.; Lefebvre, C. PRESS Peer Review of Electronic Search Strategies: 2015 Guideline Statement. *J. Clin. Epidemiol.* **2016**, *75*, 40–46. [CrossRef]
28. Rethlefsen, M.L.; Kirtley, S.; Waffenschmidt, S.; Ayala, A.P.; Moher, D.; Page, M.J.; Koffel, J.B.; PRISMA-S Group. PRISMA-S: An extension to the PRISMA Statement for Reporting Literature Searches in Systematic Reviews. *Syst. Rev.* **2021**, *10*, 39. [CrossRef] [PubMed]
29. Covidence. Melbourne: Veritas Health Innovation. Covidence Systematic Review Software [Internet]. 28 June 2022. Available online: https://www.covidence.org/ (accessed on 13 October 2021).
30. Matsumoto, Y.; Ohashi, Y.; Watanabe, H.; Tsubota, K. Efficacy and Safety of Diquafosol Ophthalmic Solution in Patients with Dry Eye Syndrome: A Japanese Phase 2 Clinical Trial. *Ophthalmology* **2012**, *119*, 1954–1960. [CrossRef] [PubMed]
31. Shimazaki-Den, S.; Iseda, H.; Dogru, M.; Shimazaki, J. Effects of Diquafosol Sodium Eye Drops on Tear Film Stability in Short BUT Type of Dry Eye. *Cornea* **2013**, *32*, 1120–1125. [CrossRef] [PubMed]
32. Gong, L.; Sun, X.; Ma, Z.; Wang, Q.; Xu, X.; Chen, X.; Shao, Y.; Yao, K.; Tang, L.; Gu, Y.; et al. A randomised, parallel-group comparison study of diquafosol ophthalmic solution in patients with dry eye in China and Singapore. *Br. J. Ophthalmol.* **2015**, *99*, 903–908. [CrossRef]
33. Hwang, H.S.; Sung, Y.-M.; Lee, W.S.; Kim, E.C. Additive Effect of Preservative-free Sodium Hyaluronate 0.1% in Treatment of Dry Eye Syndrome with Diquafosol 3% Eye Drops. *Cornea* **2014**, *33*, 935–941. [CrossRef]
34. Takamura, E.; Tsubota, K.; Watanabe, H.; Ohashi, Y. A randomised, double-masked comparison study of diquafosol versus sodium hyaluronate ophthalmic solutions in dry eye patients. *Br. J. Ophthalmol.* **2012**, *96*, 1310–1315. [CrossRef] [PubMed]

35. Cui, L.; Li, Y.; Lee, H.S.; Yang, J.M.; Choi, W.; Yoon, K.C. Effect of diquafosol tetrasodium 3% on the conjunctival surface and clinical findings after cataract surgery in patients with dry eye. *Int. Ophthalmol.* **2017**, *38*, 2021–2030. [CrossRef]
36. Inoue, Y.; Ochi, S. Effects of 3% diquafosol sodium ophthalmic solution on higher-order aberrations in patients diagnosed with dry eye after cataract surgery. *Clin. Ophthalmol.* **2016**, *11*, 87–93. [CrossRef]
37. Miyake, K.; Yokoi, N. Influence on ocular surface after cataract surgery and effect of topical diquafosol on postoperative dry eye: A multicenter prospective randomized study. *Clin. Ophthalmol.* **2017**, *11*, 529–540. [CrossRef]
38. Jun, I.; Choi, S.; Lee, G.Y.; Choi, Y.J.; Lee, H.K.; Kim, E.K.; Seo, K.Y.; Kim, T.-I. Effects of Preservative-free 3% Diquafosol in Patients with Pre-existing Dry Eye Disease after Cataract Surgery: A Randomized Clinical Trial. *Sci. Rep.* **2019**, *9*, 12659. [CrossRef]
39. Baek, J.; Doh, S.H.; Chung, S.K. The Effect of Topical Diquafosol Tetrasodium 3% on Dry Eye After Cataract Surgery. *Curr. Eye Res.* **2016**, *41*, 1281–1285. [CrossRef]
40. Tsifetaki, N.; Kitsos, G.; Paschides, C.A.; Alamanos, Y.; Eftaxias, V.; Voulgari, P.V.; Psilas, K.; Drosos, A.A. Oral pilocarpine for the treatment of ocular symptoms in patients with Sjögren's syndrome: A randomised 12 week controlled study. *Ann. Rheum. Dis.* **2003**, *62*, 1204–1207. [CrossRef] [PubMed]
41. Petrone, D.; Condemi, J.J.; Fife, R.; Gluck, O.; Cohen, S.; Dalgin, P. A double-blind, randomized, placebo-controlled study of cevimeline in Sjögren's syndrome patients with xerostomia and keratoconjunctivitis sicca. *Arthritis Rheum.* **2002**, *46*, 748–754. [CrossRef] [PubMed]
42. Leung, K.C.M.; McMillan, A.S.; Wong, M.C.M.; Leung, W.K.; Mok, M.Y.; Lau, C.S. The efficacy of cevimeline hydrochloride in the treatment of xerostomia in Sjögren's syndrome in southern Chinese patients: A randomised double-blind, placebo-controlled crossover study. *Clin. Rheumatol.* **2007**, *27*, 429–436. [CrossRef]
43. Kaido, M.; Kawashima, M.; Shigeno, Y.; Yamada, Y.; Tsubota, K. Randomized Controlled Study to Investigate the Effect of Topical Diquafosol Tetrasodium on Corneal Sensitivity in Short Tear Break-Up Time Dry Eye. *Adv. Ther.* **2018**, *35*, 697–706. [CrossRef]
44. Fukuoka, S.; Arita, R. Tear film lipid layer increase after diquafosol instillation in dry eye patients with meibomian gland dysfunction: A randomized clinical study. *Sci. Rep.* **2019**, *9*, 9091. [CrossRef]
45. Miyake, H.; Kawano, Y.; Tanaka, H.; Iwata, A.; Imanaka, T.; Nakamura, M. Tear volume estimation using a modified Schirmer test: A randomized, multicenter, double-blind trial comparing 3% diquafosol ophthalmic solution and artificial tears in dry eye patients. *Clin. Ophthalmol.* **2016**, *10*, 879–886. [CrossRef]
46. Kim, S.; Shin, J.; Lee, J.E. A randomised, prospective study of the effects of 3% diquafosol on ocular surface following cataract surgery. *Sci. Rep.* **2021**, *11*, 9124. [CrossRef] [PubMed]
47. Liu, Y.; Qian, Y.; Li, M.; Shi, Y.; Liu, L.; Sun, L.; Ye, H.; Zou, J. Combination Therapy with Diquafosol Sodium and Sodium Hyaluronate in Eyes with Dry Eye Disease After Small Incision Lenticule Extraction. *Vivo* **2023**, *37*, 2829–2834. [CrossRef] [PubMed]
48. Zhao, X.; Xia, S.; Chen, Y. Comparison of the efficacy between topical diquafosol and artificial tears in the treatment of dry eye following cataract surgery. *Medicine* **2017**, *96*, e8174. [CrossRef] [PubMed]

International Journal of
Molecular Sciences

MDPI

Review

Translating Biomarker Discovery: From Bench to Bedside in Dry Eye Disease

Jeremy Jones [1], Kyla Frenia [2], Julia Gelman [1], Maria Beatty [1], Melody Zhou [3], Levin Ma [3], Sean Pieramici [4], Noah Eger [5], Deepinder Dhaliwal [6], Leanne T. Labriola [1,*] and Kunhong Xiao [3,7,8,*]

1 Pittsburgh Research Institute, Sewickley, PA 15143, USA; jeremy@pghtrials.com (J.J.); gelmanjulia2@gmail.com (J.G.); maria@pghtrials.com (M.B.)
2 Department of Bioengineering, Swanson School of Engineering, University of Pittsburgh, Pittsburgh, PA 15260, USA; frenia@innsightech.com
3 Department of Biomedical Engineering, College of Engineering, Carnegie Mellon University, Pittsburgh, PA 15213, USA; melody.z9690@gmail.com (M.Z.); llmar1000000@gmail.com (L.M.)
4 Southwestern PA Eye Center, Corneal Services, Washington, PA 15301, USA; spieramici@gmail.com
5 Eger Eye Group, Optometry, Coraopolis, PA 15108, USA; noahod@verizon.net
6 University of Pittsburgh Medical Center, Corneal Services, Pittsburgh, PA 15260, USA; dhaliwaldk@upmc.edu
7 Center for Proteomics & Artificial Intelligence, Allegheny Health Network Cancer Institute, Pittsburgh, PA 15212, USA
8 Center for Clinical Mass Spectrometry, Allegheny Health Network Cancer Institute, Pittsburgh, PA 15212, USA
* Correspondence: labriola@pghtrials.com (L.T.L.); kxiao2@andrew.cmu.edu (K.X.); Tel.: +1-412-641-4160 (L.T.L.); +1-412-592-6549 (K.X.)

Abstract: Dry Eye Disease (DED) is a complex, multifaceted ocular disease characterized by tear film instability and inflammation. It can sometimes be elusive to identify the type of DED in patients, given the overlapping symptoms with other conditions like allergies and the multitude of stimuli that might trigger DED onset. There is also difficulty due to limitations on the diagnostic testing available to clinicians, as poor reliability and a lack of standardization plague accurate diagnoses. Identified biomarkers can help identify DED pathophysiology and category, and these include molecular biomarkers like matrix metalloproteinase-9 (MMP-9), cytokines, lactotransferrin, and lacritin, as well as functional biomarkers such as tear osmolarity. Diagnostic tools, such as the InflammaDry and I-Pen Tear Osmolarity System, also now allow for point-of-care measurement of select biomarkers, including MMP-9 and osmolarity. Nonetheless, there remains a critical need for additional, reliable, and accurate diagnostic devices to better aid in the diagnosis and management of DED. This review uniquely combines a review on the current understanding of various biomarkers with an overview of the emerging technologies available to healthcare providers, aiding in better-informed diagnosis and treatment of DED.

Keywords: dry; diagnostics; eye; inflammation; lactoferrin; matrix metalloproteinase-9; osmolarity; osmometry

1. Introduction

Dry Eye Disease (DED) is a prevalent ocular condition characterized by tear film instability and ocular surface inflammation, ultimately leading to cellular damage, discomfort, and visual disturbances [1]. The tear film, comprising an aqueous, lipid, and mucin layer, is essential to ocular surface health and visual acuity. Tear film instability can arise via several mechanisms, including reduced tear production, excessive tear evaporation, and changes in mucin secretion [2]. Often, individuals experiencing tear film instability experience a mixture of underlying etiologies. Contributors to tear film instability include systemic conditions (e.g., autoimmune disorders), environmental factors (e.g., digital eye strain, air pollution), lifestyle choices (e.g., poor nutrition, contact lens use), and geographic influences (e.g., low humidity, high altitude) [1]. Due to the multifaceted nature of DED, diagnosis remains challenging, especially because DED symptoms often overlap with other ocular conditions and can vary in clinical presentations. Molecular biomarkers have emerged as a reliable and objective metric for the diagnosis and screening of DED. These markers also provide new insights into inflammatory pathways, lacrimal gland dysfunction, and tear film dynamics. This review synthesizes current knowledge on DED molecular biomarkers, focusing on their role in advancing mechanistic understanding. An improved understanding of DED-relevant biomarkers and how to best use the tools currently available to quantify these biomarkers will aid in advancing more accurate diagnosis of DED in patients, leading to treatment specific to DED subtype and improved outcomes in the future.

2. Pathophysiology of DED

DED is complex, often driven by a combination of underlying mechanisms. Often, tear instability presents as the central initiating event, beginning with a breakdown in tear film. This is caused either by a decrease in tear secretion, common in aqueous-deficient DED, or by an increase in tear evaporation, more common in evaporative DED. Once the tear film is compromised, the remaining tear fluid is more concentrated with salts and other solutes, leading to a state of hyperosmolarity. The resulting damage to the ocular surface initiates a self-perpetuating cycle of inflammation, which makes symptoms worse over time and prevents the disease from resolving without intervention [2–7]. The initial stress and damage to the ocular surface epithelial cells leads to the production and release of pro-inflammatory cytokines and matrix metalloproteinases, most notably including matrix metalloproteinase-9 (MMP-9), which compromises the integrity of the corneal epithelium (Figure 1) [5]. This inflammatory cascade is part of a normal bodily inflammatory response, but the chronic presence of these cytokines results in further ocular surface damage and worsens the tear film's state of dysregulation. The chronic inflammation not only impacts the ocular surface but concurrently impairs the lacrimal glands as well, leading to reduced tear production. It also damages the meibomian glands, which alters lipid composition and further increases tear evaporation. This further destabilizes the tear film and reinforces the inflammatory environment of the ocular surface [6]. Neurosensory abnormalities resulting from this inflammation, such as impairment of corneal nerve function and increased nociceptive signaling, can further lead to significant patient discomfort [7]. This complex interplay among tear film instability, immune activation, and neurosensory feedback forms a vicious cycle that sustains the chronic nature of DED. Understanding these interrelated mechanisms is essential for identifying targeted biomarkers and developing more effective, personalized therapeutic strategies for DED.

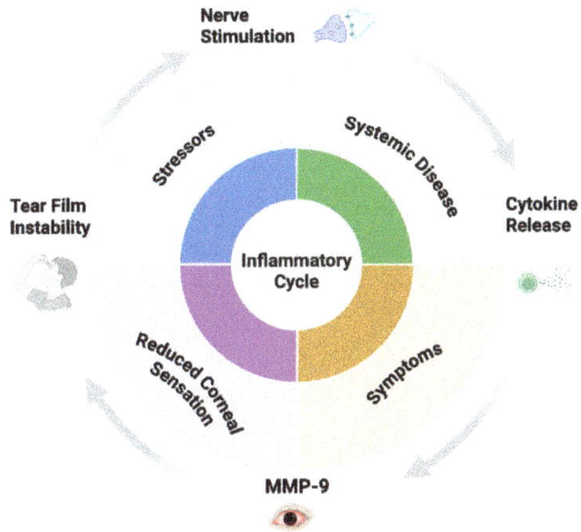

Figure 1. Pathophysiology of DED. This figure illustrates the pathological mechanisms underlying the inflammatory cycle of DED, emphasizing key contributors such as tear film instability, environmental or cellular stress, and systemic conditions. The cycle initiates with tear film instability, which induces ocular surface stress and nerve stimulation, leading to the release of pro-inflammatory cytokines and the activation of an inflammatory response. Elevated levels of MMP-9 further amplify this response by compromising corneal integrity, thereby perpetuating the cycle of inflammation and ocular surface damage. This schematic was developed by the authors' own concept.

3. Molecular Biomarkers of DED

Biomarkers play an emerging role in improving the diagnosis, subtyping, and management of DED, a condition that typically presents with indistinct symptoms and overlapping clinical features. Traditional diagnostic methods, such as Schirmer's test or tear break-up time, are limited by variability and lack of sensitivity, emphasizing the need for objective molecular markers [8–10]. In recent years, a diverse array of candidate biomarkers—including small molecules, proteins, and lipids—have been identified in the tear film (Table 1) [11–18]. Each marker offers unique insights into the underlying pathophysiology of DED, reflecting inflammation, glandular dysfunction, tear composition, or neurosensory abnormalities. Identification of these markers has elucidated the underlying mechanisms of DED, including key processes such as the recruitment of cytotoxic T cells and CD4+ T-helper cells, activation of antigen-presenting cells, and release of inflammatory mediators such as MMP-9, Tumor Necrosis Factor alpha (TNF-α), Interleukin-1 (IL-1), and Interleukin-6 (IL-6) [2,5,19–22]. These markers contribute to ocular surface damage and disease chronicity, making them prime candidates for both diagnostic and therapeutic applications. The following sections provide an overview of key biomarker categories and their clinical relevance, with particular emphasis on MMP-9 and other inflammation-related markers closely associated with DED.

3.1. Inflammatory Markers

Inflammation is a key process that perpetuates DED and contributes to many of the symptoms of discomfort experienced by patients daily. The hyperosmolarity that initiates DED, along with mechanical trauma to the cornea due to reduced lubrication of the ocular surface, both trigger and sustain inflammation. This inflammatory response can further exacerbate DED by damaging the ocular surface and lacrimal glands, leading to a chronic state of injury that continuously stimulates immune and inflammatory pathways. Because inflammation is a primary driver of DED progression, inflammatory proteins are often strong biomarkers of disease. These markers frequently correlate with clinical signs, patient-reported symptoms, and disease severity.

3.1.1. Matrix Metalloproteinases and MMP-9

MMP-9 is the most well-known of the molecular biomarkers for DED, having been successfully translated to clinical use through the InflammaDry™ device (QuidelOrtho, San Diego, CA, USA) [23–26]. As a zinc-dependent endopeptidase, MMP-9 degrades extracellular matrix components, including corneal epithelial tight junction proteins, leading to barrier disruption and accelerated epithelial cell shedding [24]. Elevated MMP-9 levels in tears are strongly correlated with DED severity, shorter tear break-up times, and compromised corneal integrity [27]. Prior clinical studies have supported the implication of MMP-9 in DED patients. One study recruited forty-six patients with newly diagnosed DED and 18 control subjects. They collected 1 microliter of unstimulated tear fluid from each patient and analyzed them for MMP-9 levels. The study found that MMP-9 was significantly higher in DED patients than in the control patients, and the MMP-9 levels even showed to be significantly correlated to DED patients in this study [28]. Mechanistically, MMP-9 is upregulated by pro-inflammatory cytokines like Interleukin-1β (IL-1β) and TNF-α, which are released by activated immune cells, including cytotoxic T cells and CD4+ T-helper cells [19]. This creates an inflammatory feedback loop that exacerbates tissue damage. Due to MMP-9's responsiveness to inflammatory stimuli and its direct impact on ocular surface health, MMP-9 serves as a valuable biomarker for investigating DED pathophysiology and guiding targeted therapeutic strategies.

MMP-9 is also considered an objective biomarker for DED and is correlated with ocular surface integrity [24,29–31]. An increased concentration of MMP-9 is typically associated with a shorter tear break-up time, which serves as a measure of tear film stability. This information is especially useful in clinical settings, as a reduced tear break-up time is reflective of an unstable tear film, making it difficult for patients to maintain visual clarity and comfort. Thus, MMP-9 serves as a meaningful marker of inflammation, ocular surface integrity, and functional tear film deficiency in DED. Other matrix metalloproteinases (MPPs) have also been identified as candidate biomarkers of DED, including MMP-2 and MMP-3, although these are less established.

3.1.2. Cytokines and Chemokines

Cellular communication within the immune system is crucial for coordinating a proper response to pathogens and injury. This communication is mediated by a diverse family of small proteins called cytokines, which act as signaling molecules to regulate the behavior of immune cells. Chemokines are a subset of cytokines that play a specific role in guiding the migration of these cells to sites of inflammation or infection. Cytokines and chemokines both play a significant role in recruiting immune cells to the ocular surface in DED, contributing to the perpetuation of inflammation and corneal damage in DED.

IL-1β is a key pro-inflammatory cytokine involved in ocular surface inflammation, particularly in DED [32,33]. It is primarily produced by activated innate immune cells as an inactive prohormone and can be enzymatically cleaved intracellularly or extracellularly to become active. Extracellular cleavage can be performed by a variety of enzymes, most notably including MMP-9, suggesting IL-1β may play a significant role in the self-perpetuating inflammatory cycle that characterizes DED. IL-1β is widely considered a master regulator of both local and systemic inflammation, playing a pivotal role in the development and progression of acute and chronic inflammation. Although it is present in healthy tear fluid, it exists predominantly in its inactive form. Some studies have shown

IL-1β to be present at higher levels in DED tear fluid compared to healthy tear fluid. IL-1β could pose potential as a biomarker for DED, especially considering its role in regulating inflammatory events and association with MMP-9.

Interleukin-6 (IL-6) is a pleiotropic cytokine also involved in DED, possessing both pro- and anti-inflammatory characteristics. IL-6 is consistently found at significantly elevated concentrations in the tears of patients diagnosed with DED when compared to healthy control individuals [34]. This consistent elevation underscores its potential as a key indicator of disease presence and activity. On the ocular surface, IL-6 is largely produced by corneal epithelial cells in response to DED-like triggers such as hyperosmolarity [21]. Interestingly, IL-6 also plays a significant role in initiating the differentiation of T-helper 17 (Th17) cells, which are known to be critical players in chronic inflammatory diseases and disease relapse [35]. Thus, IL-6 is a strong candidate as a target for therapeutic intervention and as a biomarker, given its potential role in the pathogenesis of DED and elevation in DED tear samples.

TNF-α, a pleiotropic cytokine involved in numerous inflammatory responses, has been found to be elevated in the tear film and ocular surface tissues of patients with DED. Its upregulation contributes to the chronic inflammation characteristic of the disease, affecting both the ocular surface and lacrimal glands [36]. However, while TNF-α plays a critical role in DED pathogenesis and is associated with disease severity, it is not a disease-specific biomarker due to its overlap with broader systemic inflammatory processes, limiting its diagnostic specificity.

Similarly, IgE also plays a significant role in ocular surface inflammation [37,38]. The inflammatory environment brought about by IgE-mediated reactions can compromise the epithelial barrier function. When the epithelial barrier is damaged, increased tear evaporation occurs and irritation persists. Evidently, DED symptoms worsen because of the activity of IgE. While increased IgE levels in tear fluid are not directly associated with DED, they are closely linked to a comorbid condition, allergic conjunctivitis. The symptoms of these two conditions are nearly identical, making it difficult to determine whether ocular surface irritation and dryness are present due to disease or allergic reactions. Simultaneously, researchers are investigating whether an underlying allergy component exists in DED. Moreover, IgE, though elevated in tear fluid during allergic conjunctivitis—a condition often overlapping with DED—primarily reflects allergic comorbidity rather than direct DED pathophysiology, necessitating contextual interpretation to avoid misdiagnosis.

Table 1. Key Biomarkers for DED.

Biomarker	Role	Clinical Relevance	Reference
1. Protein Biomarkers			
MMP-9	Degrades extracellular matrix; upregulated during inflammation	Elevated in DED; used in point-of-care test (InflammaDry); marker of ocular surface inflammation	[23–27,29–31]
Lactoferrin	Iron-binding glycoprotein with antimicrobial and anti-inflammatory properties	Decreased in aqueous-deficient DED; indicates lacrimal gland dysfunction	[39–42]
Lacritin	Tear glycoprotein that promotes epithelial cell survival, autophagy, and secretion	Deficient in aqueous-deficient DED; shown to restore tear secretion and corneal integrity in preclinical models	[43–47]
Lysozyme	Antimicrobial enzyme secreted by lacrimal glands	Reduced levels suggest impaired tear secretion	[48–52]
Lipocalin-1	Stabilizes the tear film lipid layer	Altered levels associated with tear film instability	[43,53–56]

Table 1. *Cont.*

Biomarker	Role	Clinical Relevance	Reference
MUC5AC	Secreted gel-forming mucin from conjunctival goblet cells	Decreased in DED, especially in mucin-deficient or Sjögren's syndrome cases	[57–67]
HLA-DR	Major histocompatibility complex class II molecule	Upregulated in conjunctival epithelial cells; marker of immune activation	[68–72]
2. Cytokines and Chemokines			
IL-1β, IL-6, TNF-α	Pro-inflammatory cytokines	Elevated levels in tears of DED patients; drive ocular surface inflammation	[22,73–81]
IL-8 (CXCL8)	Neutrophil chemoattractant	Reflects active inflammation and epithelial damage	[5,17,75,82–84]
IFN-γ	Activates immune response, especially Th1-mediated	Linked to goblet cell loss and mucin downregulation	[17,75,82,84,85]
CCL5 (RANTES)	Recruits T cells	Found in increased levels in tears and conjunctiva of DED patients	[5,86,87]
3. Lipid Biomarkers			
Meibum Lipids (e.g., wax esters, cholesterol esters)	Maintain tear film stability and reduce evaporation	Altered composition in Meibomian Gland Dysfunction (MGD) contributes to evaporative DED	[88–94]
Phospholipids, sphingolipids	Inflammatory signaling molecules	Lipidomics has revealed dysregulated lipid profiles in DED associated with inflammation	[95–102]
4. Metabolites and Small Molecules			
Lactate, Urea	Indicators of metabolic stress	Elevated levels found in tear fluid of DED patients	[103–105]
Glutamate, Glutamine	Linked to oxidative stress and inflammation	Altered profiles can distinguish DED subtypes	[106–109]
Reactive oxygen species (ROS)	Oxidative stress marker	Associated with cellular damage in DED pathogenesis	[110–113]
5. Nucleic Acid Biomarkers (Genomic/Epigenomic)			
MicroRNAs (e.g., miR-146a, miR-155)	Post-transcriptional gene regulation of inflammation	Dysregulated in tears and conjunctiva; potential non-invasive biomarkers for DED diagnosis and subtype stratification	[114–119]
HLA gene polymorphisms	Immune response genes	Certain variants associated with Sjögren's syndrome and autoimmune-related DED	[120–123]
6. Functional and Imaging Biomarkers			
Tear Osmolarity	Measures tear solute concentration	Elevated (>308 mOsm/L) in DED; reproducible marker for severity	[124–129]
Corneal Sensitivity	Assesses corneal nerve function and ocular surface integrity	Reduced in DED; associated with neurosensory abnormalities and disease severity	[130–133]
Tear Break-Up Time (TBUT/NITBUT)	Measures tear film stability	Decreased in DED, especially in evaporative forms	[134–138]
Meibography	Visualizes meibomian gland structure	Gland dropout seen in MGD-related DED	[139–142]
In vivo confocal microscopy (IVCM)	Assesses corneal nerves and immune cells	Reveals corneal nerve loss or dendritic cell activation in DED	[143–148]

3.2. *Lacrimal Gland Protein Markers*

Differential expression of lacrimal gland-derived proteins, which reflect alterations in tear fluid synthesis and secretion, is also commonly reported as a marker of DED. These proteins may indicate dysfunction or damage to the lacrimal glands, a hallmark of certain DED subtypes, particularly aqueous-deficient DED. Changes in expression levels can signal impaired tear production, glandular inflammation, or structural degeneration, all of which contribute to tear film instability and ocular surface stress. As such, lacrimal gland proteins serve not only as potential biomarkers of disease but also as indicators of underlying pathophysiological mechanisms driving DED progression.

3.2.1. Lactoferrin

Lactoferrin (LTF or LF), also known as lactotransferrin, is an 80 kDa multifunctional glycoprotein. It is one of the most abundant proteins in tear fluid and is a key biomarker for diagnosing DED [40,41]. In the tear film, lactoferrin plays a crucial role in maintaining ocular surface health through its antimicrobial, anti-inflammatory, and antioxidant properties. A marked reduction in tear lactoferrin levels is commonly seen in patients with DED, particularly in the aqueous-deficient subtype caused by lacrimal gland dysfunction. This decline correlates with reduced tear production and increased ocular surface damage. Measuring lactoferrin levels provides a non-invasive and reliable method to differentiate between types of DED, such as Sjögren's syndrome-associated DED or other non-Sjögren's variants [39]. Emerging diagnostic technologies, such as photo-detection devices and microfluidic assays, have enhanced precision and accessibility in lactoferrin measurement, facilitating more personalized treatment strategies. These advancements underscore lactoferrin's value as a diagnostic and prognostic biomarker for DED, facilitating targeted therapies to mitigate inflammation and restore tear film homeostasis.

3.2.2. Lysosome

Lysozyme (LYZ) is a glycoside hydrolase that plays a critical antimicrobial role in the tear film, helping to protect the ocular surface from bacterial invasion [42]. Like lactoferrin, it is produced by the lacrimal gland and secreted into the aqueous layer of the tear film, contributing to the innate immune defense of the ocular surface. In the context of DED, decreased concentrations of lysozyme are commonly associated with aqueous-deficient subtypes and may indicate underlying lacrimal gland dysfunction [44–46]. Because of its high abundance in healthy tear fluid and its sensitivity to changes in glandular output, lysozyme has been proposed as a useful biomarker for assessing tear film integrity and lacrimal gland health. When evaluated alongside other tear proteins such as lactoferrin and lipocalin-1, lysozyme can contribute to a more comprehensive characterization of the ocular surface environment and aid in the stratification of DED subtypes. Moreover, changes in lysozyme levels over time may provide insight into disease progression or response to therapeutic intervention.

3.3. *Lipids*

The lipid layer of the tear film plays a crucial role in maintaining ocular homeostasis, primarily by reducing the rate of tear evaporation and preserving tear film stability. Secreted predominantly by the meibomian glands, this outermost layer forms a barrier that minimizes fluid loss from the aqueous layer beneath it. Disruption or deficiency of the lipid layer, as seen in meibomian gland dysfunction (MGD), leads to increased tear evaporation, tear film instability, and hyperosmolar stress—key drivers of evaporative DED. Consequently, alterations in the composition or integrity of the lipid layer are both contributors to disease pathogenesis and potential targets for biomarker discovery and therapeutic intervention.

3.3.1. Omega-6 and Omega-3 Fatty Acids

The Omega-6 to Omega-3 fatty acid ratio reflects the balance of pro-inflammatory and anti-inflammatory lipid precursors in the tear film. Omega-6 polyunsaturated fatty acids (PUFAs), such as arachidonic acid (AA), give rise to inflammatory mediators, while Omega-3 PUFAs, like DHA and EPA, are precursors to pro-resolving, anti-inflammatory molecules [149,150]. This ratio is influenced by systemic diet and local lipid metabolism on the ocular surface, impacting the overall inflammatory milieu of the tear film. In the context of DED, an elevated Omega-6 to Omega-3 ratio is frequently observed, indicative of a pro-inflammatory state that perpetuates the cycle of ocular surface damage and tear film instability. Due to its direct link to inflammation, this ratio has been proposed as a valuable biomarker for assessing the inflammatory component of DED and for monitoring the efficacy of anti-inflammatory treatments. When evaluated in conjunction with other tear film components, the Omega-6 to Omega-3 ratio can contribute to a more nuanced understanding of DED pathophysiology and help guide personalized therapeutic strategies. Moreover, shifts in this ratio over time may provide insight into disease progression or response to interventions targeting inflammation. A recent extension study to the Dry Eye Assessment and Management (DREAM) trial sought to find if discontinuation of Omega-3 supplementation in patients previously given Omega-3 as part of the main DREAM study would yield different outcomes in symptoms and discomfort. 22 patients were randomized to Omega-3 supplements and 21 were given a placebo. The results of the study showed that there was no significant difference in symptom outcomes in the group continuing to take the supplement and the group that discontinued it [151]. This study calls into question the significance that Omega-3 fatty acid supplementation has on improving DED. The study is limited by the small cohort size, however, and further research needs to be done to fully evaluate the impact Omega-3 fatty acids may have in DED.

3.3.2. O-acyl-ω-hydroxy Fatty Acids (OAHFAs)

O-acyl-ω-hydroxy fatty acids (OAHFAs) are a unique class of lipids critical for the structural integrity and function of the tear film lipid layer (TFLL) [99,152]. Produced primarily by the meibomian glands, these specialized lipids contribute significantly to the outermost layer of the tear film, forming a stable barrier that retards evaporation of the underlying aqueous layer. In the context of DED, particularly evaporative subtypes stemming from meibomian gland dysfunction (MGD), decreased concentrations of OAHFAs are commonly associated with increased tear film evaporation and instability. Because of their direct role in maintaining the TFLL's barrier function and their sensitivity to changes in meibomian gland health, OAHFAs have been proposed as useful biomarkers for assessing evaporative dry eye and meibomian gland function. When evaluated alongside other tear film lipids and structural components, OAHFAs can contribute to a more comprehensive characterization of the tear film's evaporative resistance and aid in the stratification of DED subtypes. Changes in OAHFA levels over time may also provide important insights into disease progression or response to therapeutic interventions targeting MGD.

3.3.3. Diesters (DiEs)

Diesters (DiEs), specifically Type I and Type II Diesters, are prominent components of the tear film lipid layer (TFLL), playing a crucial role in its physical properties and stability [153,154]. These complex lipids are synthesized by the meibomian glands and are essential for forming a uniform and stable lipid monolayer on the aqueous tear surface, which is vital for preventing rapid tear evaporation and ensuring smooth blinking. In the context of DED, particularly in cases linked to meibomian gland dysfunction (MGD), qualitative and quantitative alterations in diester profiles are frequently observed, contributing to tear film instability and increased evaporation. Because of their significant contribution to the TFLL's structure and function and their sensitivity to meibomian gland health, diesters have been proposed as valuable biomarkers for assessing tear film quality and meibomian gland function in DED. When evaluated in conjunction with other tear film lipids like OAHFAs and meibomian gland expression, diester analysis can contribute to a more comprehensive characterization of the tear film's evaporative properties and aid in the diagnosis and subtyping of DED.

3.4. MicroRNAs (miRNAs)

miRNAs are small non-coding RNAs that regulate gene expression and have recently emerged as pivotal biomarkers in DED pathogenesis [117,155]. Research led by Pflugfelder at Baylor College of Medicine, in conjunction with insights from the 2024 TFOS sessions, has elucidated the role of miRNAs in DED's inflammatory processes. Specific miRNAs, such as miR-204, are upregulated in the conjunctival epithelium and tear film of DED patients, modulating inflammatory pathways by targeting receptors like Toll-like receptors (TLRs) and the TNFR superfamily. These miRNAs regulate the expression of pro-inflammatory cytokines, including IL-1β, TNF-α, and Interferon gamma (IFN-γ), which exacerbate ocular surface inflammation and lacrimal gland dysfunction. Advanced molecular techniques, such as quantitative PCR and RNA sequencing, have been instrumental in identifying these miRNA expression profiles, providing a deeper understanding of DED's molecular mechanisms.

4. From Biomarkers to Clinical Diagnosis

Multiple devices are commercially available for rapid, in-clinic use that measure a variety of DED biomarkers and measurements (Table 2). These include a device for MMP-9 measurement (InflammaDry, QuidelOrtho, San Diego, CA, USA), and tear osmolarity measurements (I-Pen, I-MED Pharma, Montreal, QC, Canada, and ScoutPro, Bausch & Lomb, Laval, QC, Canada), esthesiometry (Brill corneal esthesiometer, Brill Engines, Barcelona, Spain), and others. Currently, these devices are typically used in the same patients to gather additional data in patients suspected to have DED, yet they do not have the standalone sensitivity to classify the disease etiology (Figure 2).

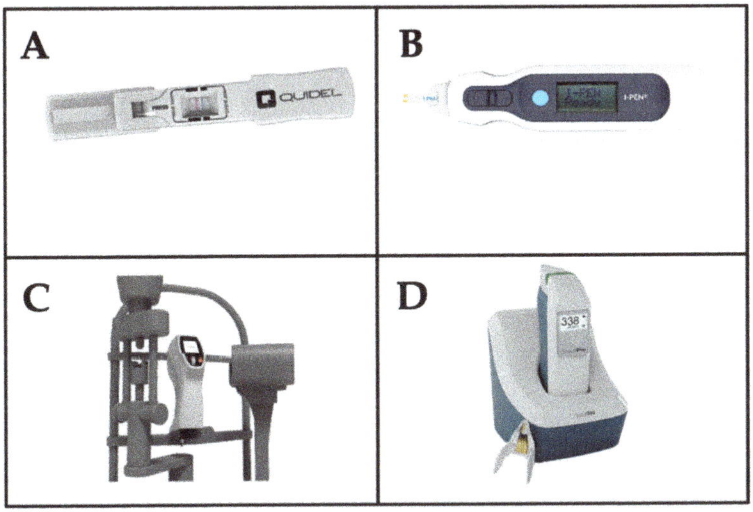

Figure 2. Diagnostic Devices for DED. This figure presents an overview of four distinct medical devices utilized in ophthalmic and diagnostic applications, including (**A**) InflammaDry (MMP-9 detection), (**B**) I-Pen (tear osmolarity), (**C**) Brill Esthesiometer (corneal sensitivity), and (**D**) ScoutPro (tear osmolarity). These tools represent a range of technological innovations aimed at enhancing the accuracy and efficiency of medical assessments in research and clinical settings. Together, these devices provide clinicians with accessible and objective tools for identifying and monitoring biomarkers associated with DED.

4.1. Tools for MMP-9 Measurement

The only device currently available to clinicians for MMP-9 measurement is the InflammaDry device. InflammaDry is a point-of-care diagnostic approach designed to detect the inflammatory biomarker MMP-9 in tears for DED. MMP-9 is the most recognizable molecular biomarker for DED. Recent TFOS discussions emphasized MMP-9's key role in corneal epithelial abnormalities, noting its utility in differentiating DED subtypes due to its association with evaporative DED and MGD [156].

In the clinic, InflammaDry provides a non-invasive method of confirming the presence of ocular surface inflammation and uses lateral flow to detect the concentration of MMP-9 expression. A positive result of two lines means that the MMP-9 concentration is greater than 40 ng/mL. A negative result of only one line indicates an MMP-9 concentration is less than 40 ng/mL [25,26,157,158].

A randomized control trial of 206 patients was performed to assess the specificity and sensitivity of InflammaDry [159]. 143 of the patients presented with the signs and symptoms of DED in clinic, and the other 63 patients were healthy controls. The results showed that InflammaDry had an 85% sensitivity rate (121 of 143 DED patients) and a specificity of 94% (59 of 63 healthy patients). A follow up clinical study sponsored by the company confirmed this finding, citing an 87% sensitivity rate and 97% specificity rate.

While the InflammaDry device has high specificity and sensitivity rates, it can be limited in its role in diagnosing DED. Its ability to measure MMP-9 levels is not a standalone tool; other measurements and observations are often required to confirm a DED diagnosis. MMP-9 levels are known to be elevated as a result of ocular conditions besides DED, highlighting the need for additional data collection when diagnosing. It also does not provide a quantifiable level of MMP-9 concentration in tear film, only giving a positive or negative result based on if the concentration level relative to 40 ng/mL. This is a clinical limitation, as some patients with milder DED may yield MMP-9 levels below the detectable threshold on the InflammaDry. Additionally, monitoring treatment response may be limited here too, as the MMP-9 level cannot be directly measured and tracked. More nuance in MMP-9 levels may be required, especially in low-level or mild dry eye.

Overall, the InflammaDry device can be a reliable tool for aiding in-clinic diagnosis of DED. While limited in standalone diagnostic ability, the device fills a need for accurate measurement of MMP-9 for patients at risk of DED.

4.2. Tools for Tear Osmolarity Measurement

Tear film osmolarity, integrally linked to lacrimal gland function, plays a crucial role in maintaining ocular surface health [128,129]. Osmolarity, which refers to the concentration of dissolved particles in the tear film, is meticulously regulated under normal conditions. Tear osmolarity reflects the balance of electrolytes, water, and proteins in the tear film, regulated by lacrimal gland secretion. In DED, dysfunction of the lacrimal gland can lead to hyperosmolarity, often because of reduced aqueous production or excessive evaporation [126]. This hyperosmolarity damages the ocular surface epithelium and triggers inflammatory cascades [160]. These changes further exacerbate the symptoms of DED, creating a self-perpetuating cycle of ocular surface damage and inflammation. Given that elevated osmolarity is a hallmark of DED, measurement of tear osmolarity can provide insights into lacrimal gland dysfunction and tear film dynamics and has emerged as a valuable diagnostic tool for DED. Additionally, understanding and targeting tear film osmolarity could potentially lead to more effective treatments for DED, aiming to restore the delicate osmotic balance necessary for optimal ocular surface health.

One common device used in clinics for tear osmolarity measurement is the I-Pen tear osmolarity system. The I-Pen system offers a rapid, handheld method of measuring tear film osmolarity to aid in diagnosing DED in patients. The device uses a single-use sensor probe that is gently placed on the lower eyelid's inner surface for approximately two seconds to generate the result. The rapid test displays results immediately in mOsm/L. It requires no anesthesia or sample collection and can be easily performed by trained clinical staff. The I-Pen is very portable and delivers results rapidly, making it a convenient tool for in-clinic use. Comparatively, other similar devices like the Wescor or TearLab are somewhat less portable. Primarily, the differences between these devices are in the collection and analysis methods and in the accuracy of reported results based on prior studies.

A clinical study published in 2021 evaluated the efficacy of the I-Pen in comparison to other standard diagnostic methods. 65 patients were enrolled in the study, with 32 patients presenting with DED pathology and 33 patients presenting with no DED symptoms. Using the osmolarity cutoff of 318 mOsm/L, the study revealed a 90.9% sensitivity and a 90.6% specificity for identifying DED [161]. However, a 2017 in vitro study compared the performance of the I-Med Pharma I-Pen, Wescor 5520 Vapro Pressure Osmometer, and TearLab Osmolarity System, and found that the I-Pen was neither accurate nor precise, especially compared to the other two devices. The study used solutions of known osmolarity to evaluate each device. The Wescor and TearLab devices had correlation coefficient values of $r^2 = 0.98$ and $r^2 = 0.96$, respectively, while the I-Pen had a value of $r^2 = 0.03$. Additionally, its coefficients of variation (CVs) were notably high, ranging from 6.1% to 6.4%. This performance contrasts sharply with the Wescor device (CV = 1.0–1.6%) and the TearLab system (CV = 1.2–2.3%), further supporting a lack of accuracy and precision in the I-Pen device.

Another common device for tear osmolarity measurement is the ScoutPro tear osmolarity system. The ScoutPro is an advanced diagnostic tool designed to quantify tear film osmolarity, a critical biomarker in the pathophysiology of DED. Elevated tear film osmolarity is recognized as a central etiology of DED and is known to correlate with DED severity. The ScoutPro's automated, rapid assay delivers quantitative osmolarity results in milliosmoles per liter (mOsm/L), aiding clinicians in diagnosing DED and objectively assessing disease progression. The system utilizes a test card with a microfluidic channel to collect a tiny tear sample (50 nanoliters) using passive capillary action. Gold electrodes embedded in the channel then measure the electrical impedance of the tear fluid, which is used to calculate and display the osmolarity result. While tear osmolarity may not differentiate DED subtypes, its ability to classify DED severity with accuracy makes it invaluable for diagnosis, including 71% specificity and 64% sensitivity for the device according to a clinical study of 140 patients from Trukera Medical. By targeting this fundamental biomarker, the device facilitates early diagnosis and personalized treatment strategies to mitigate the inflammatory feedback loop in DED [162,163]. A crucial limitation to this device is that it does not aid in diagnosing DED subtype, as it only measures tear osmolarity. This device needs to be used with other metrics and data to effectively determine the most optimal method of treatment for each individual patient.

While tear osmolarity is lauded as a strong biomarker for DED detection and severity assessment, it is important to acknowledge its limitations. Notably, osmolarity testing alone cannot differentiate between the two primary categories of DED: aqueous-deficient dry eye and evaporative dry eye. While it excels at identifying the presence and overall severity of DED, it is insufficient for determining the specific underlying etiology or for guiding subtype-targeted therapies. Consequently, tear osmolarity measurement should always be utilized alongside other clinical evaluation methods. This highlights the necessity of a comprehensive diagnostic approach, where osmolarity provides a crucial objective measure within a broader assessment framework.

Table 2. Summary of common diagnostic devices and their utility for DED.

Device	Primary Function	Biomarkers/Parameters Measured	Role in DED Diagnosis
InflammaDry	Immunoassay for inflammation detection	MMP-9	Detects elevated MMP-9 levels (>40 ng/mL). High sensitivity and specificity for rapid, in-clinic diagnosis [152].
I-Pen	Tear osmolarity system	Tear osmolarity	Measures osmolarity using electrical impedance of the tear fluid of the palpebral conjunctiva [127,128]
Brill	Esthesiometry	Corneal sensitivity	Quantifies corneal sensitivity to aid in early detection of corneal dysesthesia and monitoring of treatment efficacy [129].
ScoutPro	Tear osmolarity system	Tear osmolarity	Measures osmolarity using microfluidics to collect a tiny tear sample for measurement of electrical impedance of the tear fluid, which is used to calculate the osmolarity result with accuracy [162,163]
Corneal Topography	Maps corneal surface to detect irregularities	Corneal surface irregularities, tear film instability	Identifies corneal changes due to tear film instability, enhancing diagnostic precision for DED related ocular surface damage
Anterior Segment OCT	High-resolution imaging of anterior chamber structures	Tear film thickness, corneal epithelium, meibomian gland structure	Visualizes alterations in tear film and glands, correlating with DED severity and aiding in diagnosis
KOWA DR-1a Interferometer	Analyzes tear film lipid layer dynamics	Lipid layer thickness, tear film stability	Assesses evaporative DED by evaluating lipid layer dynamics, providing insights into tear film instability [164].

4.3. Corneal Esthesiometry

Corneal esthesiometry is used to measure the sensitivity of the corneal nerves by applying a controlled stimulus to the corneal surface. The patient's involuntary reflex, such as a blink, or subjective response to the stimulus is used to quantify the nerve's responsiveness. The information gathered from this test helps clinicians in differentiating DED from other ocular surface diseases, assessing DED disease severity based on the observed reduction in corneal sensitivity, and in guiding treatment decisions based on the observed nerve function in individual patients.

The current, most widely used method of measuring corneal sensitivity is with the Cochet-Bonnet Esthesiometer. It is largely considered the gold standard for contact-based esthesiometry and has been long in use by clinicians. The device consists of a handle and a retractable, fine nylon monofilament. The Cochet-Bonnet is used to determine the minimum force of the filament required for a patient to feel a sensation on their cornea. When the patient blinks or reacts to the filament, the length is recorded as the objective measurement for corneal sensitivity. The main benefits of this device are the simplicity, low cost, and portability. It provides a quick and direct measure of nerve function without requiring specialized equipment. However, some limitations exist with this device, as well. Its invasive, contact-based method can cause patient discomfort, induce a reflexive blink, and may potentially lead to a corneal abrasion. The results can also be subjective, as it is easily influenced by the operator's technique and the patient's subjective response, making it less objective and reproducible than non-contact devices.

The other device available to clinicians for measuring corneal sensitivity is the Brill Corneal Esthesiometer. This is a novel, non-invasive, handheld device that uses controlled air pulses to measure corneal sensitivity [130]. By measuring a patient's response to brief corneal stimulation, corneal sensitivity test provides valuable insight into the integrity of corneal nerves and their interaction with the ocular surface [130]. Unlike traditional contact-based esthesiometers, like the Cochet-Bonnet, the Brill esthesiometer employs controlled air pulses to stimulate the cornea, ranging from 2 to 10 mbar across five intensity levels, ensuring precise and reproducible measurements [132]. This non-contact approach minimizes patient discomfort and eliminates the risk of corneal abrasion, making it suitable for use in infectious corneal pathologies. Corneal sensitivity, mediated by the ophthalmic branch of the trigeminal nerve, is often compromised in DED and other conditions like neurotrophic keratopathy, reflecting underlying nerve dysfunction [133]. Corneal sensitivity testing provides valuable insights into the integrity of the corneal nerves, which is essential for diagnosing and managing DED and other ocular surface disorders. The Brill esthesiometer is particularly useful for early detection of DED, monitoring treatment efficacy over time, and providing objective sensitivity data that complements other diagnostic findings. Studies have shown good agreement with the Cochet-Bonnet esthesiometer in healthy and DED patients, though values are not interchangeable, underscoring its role as a complementary diagnostic tool [131]. Additionally, the Brill esthesiometer carries a higher cost and more limited availability in comparison to the Cochet-Bonnet esthesiometer. Additionally, the measurement of corneal sensitivity is not a standalone diagnostic value, as increased sensitivity could be a feature of the different subtypes of DED and even other conditions that impact the ocular surface. Overall, by providing objective data on corneal nerve function, however, the Brill esthesiometer supports tailored therapeutic interventions and improves the management of ocular surface disorders.

4.4. Other Imaging Tools

Advancements in biomarker detection technologies are enhancing our ability to study DED's molecular mechanisms. In ophthalmology, instruments like corneal topography and optical coherence tomography (OCT) are widely used and reliable for assessing DED-related changes. Corneal topography maps the corneal surface to detect irregularities caused by tear film instability, while anterior segment OCT provides high-resolution imaging of the tear film, corneal epithelium, and meibomian glands, revealing structural alterations linked to DED. These imaging modalities enhance diagnosis. The KOWA DR-1α interferometer uses white light illumination to analyze tear film lipid layer dynamics, providing insights into tear film instability. It has a relatively high sensitivity and specificity for diagnosing dry eye, particularly when measuring non-invasive tear break-up time. It is typically used as a complementary device in clinic to help diagnose DED type [164].

4.5. Unmet Needs

The gap between biomarker discovery and clinical translation in DED remains a critical challenge, driven by the complexity of translating molecular insights into practical diagnostic tools. While biomarkers like MMP-9, TNF-α, and lactotransferrin have contributed to our understanding of DED's inflammatory and cellular mechanisms, the integration of some of them into routine clinical practice is hindered by technical, logistical, and economic barriers. MMP-9 has largely broken through these barriers, becoming a strong DED biomarker that is accessible for in-clinic use. However, despite a strong understanding of TNF-α and its role in DED, assessment of it requires more development to become widely adopted in clinical assessment procedures. Similarly, lactrotransferrin has a strong research basis for its relevance in DED but lacks a rapid and reliable method of assessment. Variability in biomarker expression across DED subtypes and patient demographics further complicates the development of standardized assays. This review of current findings demonstrates a need for a device that can reliably test more biomarkers, providing clinicians with a more comprehensive tool for diagnosis of DED.

5. Current Treatment Methods and Limitations

The DEWS TFOS III Report outlines current treatments for dry eye based on the etiologies of the disease. The first line of treatment for all types of DED symptoms is typically artificial tears. Artificial tears, however, provide only temporary relief and do not treat the underlying cause of the DED itself. For evaporative DED, eyelid treatment for blepharitis and lid hygiene are effective. These include warm compresses, lid hygiene, and in-office procedures such as thermal pulsation or Intense Pulsed Light (IPL), which can unblock the glands and improve lipid quality in the tears. Recent advancements in lipid-based artificial tears also directly target the tear film's oily layer, and use of perfluorohexyloctane ophthalmic solution has been shown to help in patients living with evaporative DED. However, the at-home and in-office procedures are limited by efficacy and are not a cure for the disease, meaning repeated treatments are required to maintain relief. The in-office treatments can often be expensive, especially for multiple treatment rounds. Additionally, while the lipid-based tears are more effective at restoring some of the tear film's lipid layer, it still lacks the ability to resolve the underlying meibomian gland dysfunction that is responsible for the DED in the first place. For aqueous deficient DED, the goal is to increase tear production and conserve existing tears. Treatments include preservative-free artificial tears, prescription anti-inflammatory eye drops (e.g., cyclosporine, lifitegrast) to stimulate tear production, and punctal plugs to block tear drainage and keep tears on the ocular surface for a longer period. While effective in many cases, cyclosporine and lifitegrast are slow acting and can sometimes be uncomfortable for patients to use, leading to poor patient adherence. Punctal plugs are limited by epiphora in certain cases and can cause irritation and foreign body sensation in rare cases. New treatments on the horizon include reproxalap, a reactive aldehyde species that has been shown to reduce inflammation associated with DED by a recent randomized, double-masked, vehicle-controlled dry eye chamber trial of 132 patients from Aldeyra Therapeutics [165,166]. Reproxalap was well tolerated and significantly reduced DED symptoms in patients compared to a vehicle control. Another new, recently FDA-approved treatment is acoltremon, which is a TRPM8 thermoreceptor agonist that has been shown in the COMET studies to be safe and effective in treating DED. These treatments and many others in development may improve efficacy and outcomes in future patients suffering from DED.

6. Future Directions

Future advancements in DED diagnosis hinge on the integration of multi-omics approaches, artificial intelligence (AI), and point-of-care devices to enhance precision and accessibility. Emerging technologies, such as exosome profiling and microRNA sequencing, are promising in identifying novel biomarkers that capture the heterogeneity of DED subtypes, potentially enabling personalized treatment strategies. However, significant roadblocks persist, including high costs and limited availability of advanced diagnostic tools in resource-constrained settings, hindering global adoption. For integration of multi-omics into point-of-care diagnostics to be made more feasible, development needs to be done to lower the cost and increase the availability for more widespread use in clinics. Given the extent of sample collection required and high cost, multi-omics remains largely unfeasible at this present moment. Alternatively, AI-driven diagnostic platforms could analyze complex biomarker datasets alongside imaging modalities like corneal topography and OCT, improving diagnostic accuracy and predicting disease progression. It could aid in interpretation of imaging and potentially predict disease progression. However, the challenges of regulatory approval and data privacy remain, and integrating this technology into resource-limited settings could be challenging given high costs and current limited technical support. Standardization of biomarker assays across diverse populations remains challenging due to variability in environmental, genetic, and lifestyle factors. Additionally, the need for large-scale clinical validation studies slows the translation of novel biomarkers into routine clinical practice, necessitating collaborative efforts to establish universal diagnostic criteria and affordable technologies.

Exosomes have emerged as a promising marker for DED, offering potential benefits in both early detection and monitoring of the condition. These nano-sized extracellular vesicles, particularly those found in tear fluid, have shown remarkable potential in identifying DED-specific biomarkers. When analyzed in large scale clinical trials using advanced techniques such as proteomics and RNA sequencing, exosomes from tear samples can reveal distinct molecular signatures associated with various stages and subtypes of DED [167]. Studies have demonstrated significant differences in exosome profiles between healthy individuals and those with DED, including variations in protein content and microRNA expression. Mechanistically, these exosomes can provide valuable insights into the underlying pathological processes of DED, such as inflammation and lacrimal gland dysfunction. Furthermore, exosomes play a crucial role in intercellular communication within the ocular surface ecosystem, making them excellent candidates for monitoring disease progression and treatment response in DED patients.

7. Conclusions

DED arises from a complex interplay of inflammation, tear film dysfunction, and cellular responses. Molecular biomarkers such as MMP-9, TNF-α, lactotransferrin, tear osmolarity, exosomes, and miRNAs provide critical insights into the molecular mechanisms underlying the disease. The integration of advanced diagnostic tools, including the KOWA DR-1α interferometer, InflammaDry, ScoutPro, and Brill esthesiometer, with molecular profiling techniques, enables precise diagnosis and monitoring of DED subtypes. These innovations enhance our ability to correlate molecular data with clinical findings, paving the way for personalized therapeutic strategies. By bridging molecular insights with cutting-edge technologies, biomarker-driven research continues to unravel the complexities of DED, fostering global advancements in ocular surface health and driving scientific discoveries toward improved patient outcomes.

Author Contributions: Conceptualization, L.T.L., K.X.; writing—original draft preparation, J.J., J.G., K.F., M.B., M.Z., L.M.; writing—review and editing, J.J., K.F., M.Z., L.M.; supervision, L.T.L., K.X., S.P., N.E., D.D.; project administration, L.T.L., K.X.; funding acquisition, K.X. All authors have read and agreed to the published version of the manuscript.

Funding: This research received no external funding.

Data Availability Statement: No new data were created in the making of this article.

Acknowledgments: We thank the AHNCI Moonshot Biomarker Program and Highmark Health for their support. We also gratefully acknowledge additional support from the Prostate Cancer

Foundation Challenge Award (to K.X., grant number 2023CHAL4223), The Pittsburgh Foundation (to K.X., cc#45126409), and the Claude Worthington Benedum Foundation.

Conflicts of Interest: The authors declare no conflict of interest.

References

1. Wolffsohn, J.S.; Arita, R.; Chalmers, R.; Djalilian, A.; Dogru, M.; Dumbleton, K.; Gupta, P.K.; Karpecki, P.; Lazreg, S.; Pult, H.; et al. TFOS DEWS II Diagnostic Methodology report. *Ocul. Surf.* **2017**, *15*, 539–574. [CrossRef]
2. Pflugfelder, S.C.; de Paiva, C.S. The Pathophysiology of Dry Eye Disease: What We Know and Future Directions for Research. *Ophthalmology* **2017**, *124*, S4–S13. [CrossRef]
3. Messmer, E.M. The pathophysiology, diagnosis, and treatment of dry eye disease. *Dtsch. Arztebl. Int.* **2015**, *112*, 71–81; quiz 82. [CrossRef] [PubMed]
4. Rao, S.K.; Mohan, R.; Gokhale, N.; Matalia, H.; Mehta, P. Inflammation and dry eye disease-where are we? *Int. J. Ophthalmol.* **2022**, *15*, 820–827. [CrossRef]
5. Stevenson, W.; Chauhan, S.K.; Dana, R. Dry eye disease: An immune-mediated ocular surface disorder. *Arch. Ophthalmol.* **2012**, *130*, 90–100. [CrossRef]
6. Baudouin, C.; Messmer, E.M.; Aragona, P.; Geerling, G.; Akova, Y.A.; Benitez-del-Castillo, J.; Boboridis, K.G.; Merayo-Lloves, J.; Rolando, M.; Labetoulle, M. Revisiting the vicious circle of dry eye disease: A focus on the pathophysiology of meibomian gland dysfunction. *Br. J. Ophthalmol.* **2016**, *100*, 300–306. [CrossRef]
7. Messmer, E.M. Pathophysiology of dry eye disease and novel therapeutic targets. *Exp. Eye Res.* **2022**, *217*, 108944. [CrossRef]
8. Savini, G.; Prabhawasat, P.; Kojima, T.; Grueterich, M.; Espana, E.; Goto, E. The challenge of dry eye diagnosis. *Clin. Ophthalmol.* **2008**, *2*, 31–55. [CrossRef] [PubMed]
9. Roy, N.S.; Wei, Y.; Kuklinski, E.; Asbell, P.A. The Growing Need for Validated Biomarkers and Endpoints for Dry Eye Clinical Research. *Investig. Ophthalmol. Vis. Sci.* **2017**, *58*, BIO1–BIO19. [CrossRef] [PubMed]
10. Sullivan, B. Challenges in using signs and symptoms to evaluate new biomarkers of dry eye disease. *Ocul. Surf.* **2014**, *12*, 2–9. [CrossRef]
11. Choi, W.; Lian, C.; Ying, L.; Kim, G.E.; You, I.C.; Park, S.H.; Yoon, K.C. Expression of Lipid Peroxidation Markers in the Tear Film and Ocular Surface of Patients with Non-Sjogren Syndrome: Potential Biomarkers for Dry Eye Disease. *Curr. Eye Res.* **2016**, *41*, 1143–1149. [CrossRef]
12. Pinto-Fraga, J.; Enriquez-de-Salamanca, A.; Calonge, M.; Gonzalez-Garcia, M.J.; Lopez-Miguel, A.; Lopez-de la Rosa, A.; Garcia-Vazquez, C.; Calder, V.; Stern, M.E.; Fernandez, I. Severity, therapeutic, and activity tear biomarkers in dry eye disease: An analysis from a phase III clinical trial. *Ocul. Surf.* **2018**, *16*, 368–376. [CrossRef]
13. Fong, P.Y.; Shih, K.C.; Lam, P.Y.; Chan, T.C.Y.; Jhanji, V.; Tong, L. Role of tear film biomarkers in the diagnosis and management of dry eye disease. *Taiwan J. Ophthalmol.* **2019**, *9*, 150–159. [CrossRef] [PubMed]
14. Khanal, S.; Bai, Y.; Ngo, W.; Nichols, K.K.; Wilson, L.; Barnes, S.; Nichols, J.J. Human Meibum and Tear Film Derived (O-Acyl)-Omega-Hydroxy Fatty Acids as Biomarkers of Tear Film Dynamics in Meibomian Gland Dysfunction and Dry Eye Disease. *Investig. Ophthalmol. Vis. Sci.* **2021**, *62*, 13. [CrossRef] [PubMed]
15. Suarez-Cortes, T.; Merino-Inda, N.; Benitez-Del-Castillo, J.M. Tear and ocular surface disease biomarkers: A diagnostic and clinical perspective for ocular allergies and dry eye disease. *Exp. Eye Res.* **2022**, *221*, 109121. [CrossRef]
16. Byambajav, M.; Collier, A.; Shu, X.; Hagan, S. Tear Fluid Biomarkers and Quality of Life in People with Type 2 Diabetes and Dry Eye Disease. *Metabolites* **2023**, *13*, 733. [CrossRef]
17. Kumar, N.R.; Praveen, M.; Narasimhan, R.; Khamar, P.; D'Souza, S.; Sinha-Roy, A.; Sethu, S.; Shetty, R.; Ghosh, A. Tear biomarkers in dry eye disease: Progress in the last decade. *Indian J. Ophthalmol.* **2023**, *71*, 1190–1202. [CrossRef]
18. Zhao, L.; Zhang, Y.; Duan, H.; Yang, T.; Zhou, Y.; Ma, B.; Chen, Y.; Qi, H. Clinical Characteristics and Tear Film Biomarkers in Patients with Chronic Dry Eye Disease After Femtosecond Laser-Assisted Laser in Situ Keratomileusis. *J. Refract. Surg.* **2023**, *39*, 556–563. [CrossRef]
19. Liu, R.; Gao, C.; Chen, H.; Li, Y.; Jin, Y.; Qi, H. Analysis of Th17-associated cytokines and clinical correlations in patients with dry eye disease. *PLoS ONE* **2017**, *12*, e0173301. [CrossRef] [PubMed]
20. Kaushik, D.; Xu, B.; Kumar, M. Biomarkers in immunology: Their impact on immune function and response. *Adv. Biomark. Sci. Technol.* **2025**, *7*, 95–110. [CrossRef]
21. Chu, L.; Wang, C.; Zhou, H. Inflammation mechanism and anti-inflammatory therapy of dry eye. *Front. Med.* **2024**, *11*, 1307682. [CrossRef] [PubMed]
22. Perez, V.L.; Stern, M.E.; Pflugfelder, S.C. Inflammatory basis for dry eye disease flares. *Exp. Eye Res.* **2020**, *201*, 108294. [CrossRef]

23. Gupta, S.; Shankar, S.; Bhatta, S.; Mishra, A.; Singh, A. Comparison of tear Matrix Metalloproteinase 9 (MMP-9) estimation with Schirmer's test in Ocular Surface Disorders. *Rom. J. Ophthalmol.* **2024**, *68*, 225–232. [CrossRef]
24. Lanza, N.L.; Valenzuela, F.; Perez, V.L.; Galor, A. The Matrix Metalloproteinase 9 Point-of-Care Test in Dry Eye. *Ocul. Surf.* **2016**, *14*, 189–195. [CrossRef]
25. Kang, M.J.; Kim, H.S.; Kim, M.S.; Kim, E.C. The Correlation between Matrix Metalloproteinase-9 Point-of-Care Immunoassay, Tear Film Osmolarity, and Ocular Surface Parameters. *J. Ophthalmol.* **2022**, *2022*, 6132016. [CrossRef]
26. Messmer, E.M.; von Lindenfels, V.; Garbe, A.; Kampik, A. Matrix Metalloproteinase 9 Testing in Dry Eye Disease Using a Commercially Available Point-of-Care Immunoassay. *Ophthalmology* **2016**, *123*, 2300–2308. [CrossRef]
27. Shoari, A.; Kanavi, M.R.; Rasaee, M.J. Inhibition of matrix metalloproteinase-9 for the treatment of dry eye syndrome; a review study. *Exp. Eye Res.* **2021**, *205*, 108523. [CrossRef]
28. Chotikavanich, S.; de Paiva, C.S.; Li, D.Q.; Chen, J.J.; Bian, F.; Farley, W.J.; Pflugfelder, S.C. Production and activity of matrix metalloproteinase-9 on the ocular surface increase in dysfunctional tear syndrome. *Investig. Ophthalmol. Vis. Sci.* **2009**, *50*, 3203–3209. [CrossRef] [PubMed]
29. Jamerson, E.C.; Elhusseiny, A.M.; ElSheikh, R.H.; Eleiwa, T.K.; El Sayed, Y.M. Role of Matrix Metalloproteinase 9 in Ocular Surface Disorders. *Eye Contact Lens* **2020**, *46* (Suppl. 2), S57–S63. [CrossRef] [PubMed]
30. Aragona, P.; Aguennouz, M.; Rania, L.; Postorino, E.; Sommario, M.S.; Roszkowska, A.M.; De Pasquale, M.G.; Pisani, A.; Puzzolo, D. Matrix metalloproteinase 9 and transglutaminase 2 expression at the ocular surface in patients with different forms of dry eye disease. *Ophthalmology* **2015**, *122*, 62–71. [CrossRef]
31. Caban, M.; Owczarek, K.; Lewandowska, U. The Role of Metalloproteinases and Their Tissue Inhibitors on Ocular Diseases: Focusing on Potential Mechanisms. *Int. J. Mol. Sci.* **2022**, *23*, 4256. [CrossRef]
32. Solomon, A.; Dursun, D.; Liu, Z.; Xie, Y.; Macri, A.; Pflugfelder, S.C. Pro- and anti-inflammatory forms of interleukin-1 in the tear fluid and conjunctiva of patients with dry-eye disease. *Investig. Ophthalmol. Vis. Sci.* **2001**, *42*, 2283–2292.
33. Na, K.S.; Mok, J.W.; Kim, J.Y.; Rho, C.R.; Joo, C.K. Correlations between tear cytokines, chemokines, and soluble receptors and clinical severity of dry eye disease. *Investig. Ophthalmol. Vis. Sci.* **2012**, *53*, 5443–5450. [CrossRef]
34. Zhao, C.S.; Chen, Y.; Ying, G.S.; Asbell, P.A.; Dry Eye, A.; Management Study, G. Association of Tear Cytokine Ratios with Symptoms and Signs of Dry Eye Disease: Biomarker Data from the Dry Eye Assessment and Management Study. *Curr. Eye Res.* **2024**, *49*, 16–24. [CrossRef]
35. Shahini, A.; Shahini, A. Role of interleukin-6-mediated inflammation in the pathogenesis of inflammatory bowel disease: Focus on the available therapeutic approaches and gut microbiome. *J. Cell Commun. Signal* **2023**, *17*, 55–74. [CrossRef] [PubMed]
36. Yoon, K.C.; Jeong, I.Y.; Park, Y.G.; Yang, S.Y. Interleukin-6 and tumor necrosis factor-alpha levels in tears of patients with dry eye syndrome. *Cornea* **2007**, *26*, 431–437. [CrossRef] [PubMed]
37. Dermer, H.; Theotoka, D.; Lee, C.J.; Chhadva, P.; Hackam, A.S.; Galor, A.; Kumar, N. Total Tear IgE Levels Correlate with Allergenic and Irritating Environmental Exposures in Individuals with Dry Eye. *J. Clin. Med.* **2019**, *8*, 1627. [CrossRef] [PubMed]
38. Bao, J.; Tian, L.; Meng, Y.; Wu, B.; Wang, J.; He, J.; Shao, Q.; Wang, C.; Jie, Y.; Zhang, L. Total IgE in tears accurately reflects the severity and predicts the prognosis of seasonal allergic conjunctivitis. *Clin. Transl. Allergy* **2022**, *12*, e12139. [CrossRef]
39. Tsai, C.Y.; Hong, C.; Hsu, M.Y.; Lai, T.T.; Huang, C.W.; Lu, C.Y.; Chen, W.L.; Cheng, C.M. Fluorescence-based reagent and spectrum-based optical reader for lactoferrin detection in tears: Differentiating Sjogren's syndrome from non-Sjogren's dry eye syndrome. *Sci. Rep.* **2024**, *14*, 14505. [CrossRef]
40. Zhang, Y.; Lu, C.; Zhang, J. Lactoferrin and Its Detection Methods: A Review. *Nutrients* **2021**, *13*, 2492. [CrossRef]
41. Zhang, Y.; Yan, P.; Tang, H.; Zhang, J. Rapid detection of tear lactoferrin for diagnosis of dry eyes by using fluorescence polarization-based aptasensor. *Sci. Rep.* **2023**, *13*, 15179. [CrossRef]
42. Connell, S.; Kawashima, M.; Nakamura, S.; Imada, T.; Yamamoto, H.; Tsubota, K.; Fukuda, S. Lactoferrin Ameliorates Dry Eye Disease Potentially through Enhancement of Short-Chain Fatty Acid Production by Gut Microbiota in Mice. *Int. J. Mol. Sci.* **2021**, *22*, 12384. [CrossRef]
43. Karnati, R.; Laurie, D.E.; Laurie, G.W. Lacritin and the tear proteome as natural replacement therapy for dry eye. *Exp. Eye Res.* **2013**, *117*, 39–52. [CrossRef] [PubMed]
44. Dias-Teixeira, K.; Horton, X.; McKown, R.; Romano, J.; Laurie, G.W. The Lacritin-Syndecan-1-Heparanase Axis in Dry Eye Disease. *Adv. Exp. Med. Biol.* **2020**, *1221*, 747–757. [CrossRef]
45. Georgiev, G.A.; Gh, M.S.; Romano, J.; Dias Teixeira, K.L.; Struble, C.; Ryan, D.S.; Sia, R.K.; Kitt, J.P.; Harris, J.M.; Hsu, K.L.; et al. Lacritin proteoforms prevent tear film collapse and maintain epithelial homeostasis. *J. Biol. Chem.* **2021**, *296*, 100070. [CrossRef]
46. Vijmasi, T.; Chen, F.Y.; Balasubbu, S.; Gallup, M.; McKown, R.L.; Laurie, G.W.; McNamara, N.A. Topical administration of lacritin is a novel therapy for aqueous-deficient dry eye disease. *Investig. Ophthalmol. Vis. Sci.* **2014**, *55*, 5401–5409. [CrossRef] [PubMed]

47. McKown, R.L.; Wang, N.; Raab, R.W.; Karnati, R.; Zhang, Y.; Williams, P.B.; Laurie, G.W. Lacritin and other new proteins of the lacrimal functional unit. *Exp. Eye Res.* **2009**, *88*, 848–858. [CrossRef]
48. deLuise, V.P.; Tabbara, K.F. Quantitation of tear lysozyme levels in dry-eye disorders. *Arch. Ophthalmol.* **1983**, *101*, 634–635. [CrossRef] [PubMed]
49. Avisar, R.; Menache, R.; Shaked, P.; Rubinstein, J.; Machtey, I.; Savir, H. Lysozyme content of tears in patients with Sjogren's syndrome and rheumatoid arthritis. *Am. J. Ophthalmol.* **1979**, *87*, 148–151. [CrossRef]
50. Jia, Z.; Wei, W.; Tu, K.; Fang, B.; Zhang, M.; Shi, L. Point-of-care monitoring of dry eye disease using lysozyme in tear based on commercial pregnancy test strips. *Sens. Actuators B Chem.* **2023**, *378*, 133179. [CrossRef]
51. Berra, M.; Galperin, G.; Berra, F.; Marquez, M.I.; Mandaradoni, M.; Tau, J.; Berra, A. Tear Lysozyme in Sjogren s syndrome, Meibomian gland dysfunction, and non-dry-eye. *Arq. Bras. Oftalmol.* **2021**, *85*, 103–108. [CrossRef]
52. Lee, D.; Song, S.; Cho, G.; Dalle Ore, L.C.; Malmstadt, N.; Fuwad, A.; Kim, S.M.; Jeon, T.J. Elucidating the Molecular Interactions between Lipids and Lysozyme: Evaporation Resistance and Bacterial Barriers for Dry Eye Disease. *Nano Lett.* **2023**, *23*, 9451–9460. [CrossRef]
53. Yeh, P.T.; Casey, R.; Glasgow, B.J. A novel fluorescent lipid probe for dry eye: Retrieval by tear lipocalin in humans. *Investig. Ophthalmol. Vis. Sci.* **2013**, *54*, 1398–1410. [CrossRef]
54. Gasymov, O.K.; Abduragimov, A.R.; Prasher, P.; Yusifov, T.N.; Glasgow, B.J. Tear lipocalin: Evidence for a scavenging function to remove lipids from the human corneal surface. *Investig. Ophthalmol. Vis. Sci.* **2005**, *46*, 3589–3596. [CrossRef]
55. Yamada, M.; Mochizuki, H.; Kawai, M.; Tsubota, K.; Bryce, T.J. Decreased tear lipocalin concentration in patients with meibomian gland dysfunction. *Br. J. Ophthalmol.* **2005**, *89*, 803–805. [CrossRef]
56. Subbaraman, L.; Mistry, R.; Thangavelu, M.; Jones, L. Quantification of lipocalin-1 in tears and contact lens deposits using a sandwich ELISA technique. *Contact Lens Anterior Eye* **2013**, *36*, e45–e46. [CrossRef]
57. Gipson, I.K.; Hori, Y.; Argueso, P. Character of ocular surface mucins and their alteration in dry eye disease. *Ocul. Surf.* **2004**, *2*, 131–148. [CrossRef] [PubMed]
58. Hori, Y. Secreted Mucins on the Ocular Surface. *Investig. Ophthalmol. Vis. Sci.* **2018**, *59*, DES151–DES156. [CrossRef] [PubMed]
59. Li, G.; Lu, P.; Song, H.; Zheng, Q.; Nan, K. Expression of mucins MUC5AC and MUC19 on the ocular surface in dry eye syndrome model of ovariectomized female rabbits. *Adv. Clin. Exp. Med.* **2019**, *28*, 165–169. [CrossRef] [PubMed]
60. Carrington, S.D.; Goodall, C.; Myerscough, N.; Corfield, A.P. Canine ocular mucins in health and dry eye disease. *Biochem. Soc. Trans.* **1993**, *21*, 484S. [CrossRef]
61. Shamloo, K.; Barbarino, A.; Alfuraih, S.; Sharma, A. Graft Versus Host Disease-Associated Dry Eye: Role of Ocular Surface Mucins and the Effect of Rebamipide, a Mucin Secretagogue. *Investig. Ophthalmol. Vis. Sci.* **2019**, *60*, 4511–4519. [CrossRef]
62. Portal, C.; Gouyer, V.; Gottrand, F.; Desseyn, J.L. Ocular mucins in dry eye disease. *Exp. Eye Res.* **2019**, *186*, 107724. [CrossRef]
63. Floyd, A.M.; Zhou, X.; Evans, C.; Rompala, O.J.; Zhu, L.; Wang, M.; Chen, Y. Mucin deficiency causes functional and structural changes of the ocular surface. *PLoS ONE* **2012**, *7*, e50704. [CrossRef]
64. Aldina, R.; Sujuti, H.; Permatasari, N.; Widodo, M.A. The effects of genistein on estrogen receptor-β, IL-1β levels, and MUC5AC expression in ovariectomized rats with dry eye. *Clin. Nutr. Exp.* **2019**, *27*, 21–28. [CrossRef]
65. Duan, H.; Yang, T.; Zhou, Y.; Ma, B.; Zhao, L.; Chen, J.; Qi, H. Comparison of mucin levels at the ocular surface of visual display terminal users with and without dry eye disease. *BMC Ophthalmol.* **2023**, *23*, 189. [CrossRef] [PubMed]
66. Corrales, R.M.; Narayanan, S.; Fernandez, I.; Mayo, A.; Galarreta, D.J.; Fuentes-Paez, G.; Chaves, F.J.; Herreras, J.M.; Calonge, M. Ocular mucin gene expression levels as biomarkers for the diagnosis of dry eye syndrome. *Investig. Ophthalmol. Vis. Sci.* **2011**, *52*, 8363–8369. [CrossRef]
67. Xu, K.; Liu, X.N.; Zhang, H.B.; Zhu, X.P.; Zhang, X.J. Tear film instability is associated with weakened colocalization between occludin and MUC5AC in scopolamine-induced dry eye disease (DED) rats. *Int. Ophthalmol.* **2023**, *43*, 463–473. [CrossRef] [PubMed]
68. Blautain, B.; Rabut, G.; Dupas, B.; Riancho, L.; Liang, H.; Luzu, J.; Labbe, A.; Garrigue, J.S.; Brignole-Baudouin, F.; Baudouin, C.; et al. Multimodal Approach in Dry Eye Disease Combining In Vivo Confocal Microscopy and HLA-DR Expression. *Transl. Vis. Sci. Technol.* **2024**, *13*, 39. [CrossRef] [PubMed]
69. Roy, N.S.; Wei, Y.; Yu, Y.; Ying, G.S.; Kuklinski, E.; Barry, B.; Maguire, M.G.; Dana, R.; Brightwell-Arnold, M.; Asbell, P.A.; et al. Conjunctival HLA-DR Expression and Its Association with Symptoms and Signs in the DREAM Study. *Transl. Vis. Sci. Technol.* **2019**, *8*, 31. [CrossRef]
70. Epstein, S.P.; Gadaria-Rathod, N.; Wei, Y.; Maguire, M.G.; Asbell, P.A. HLA-DR expression as a biomarker of inflammation for multicenter clinical trials of ocular surface disease. *Exp. Eye Res.* **2013**, *111*, 95–104. [CrossRef]

71. Roy, N.S.; Yu, Y.; Ying, G.S.; Maguire, M.G.; Asbell, P.A.; Group, D.S. Effect of Omega-3 on HLA-DR Expression by Conjunctival Cells and Tear Cytokine Concentrations in the Dry Eye Assessment and Management Study. *Eye Contact Lens* **2022**, *48*, 384–390. [CrossRef]
72. Fernandez, K.B.; Epstein, S.P.; Raynor, G.S.; Sheyman, A.T.; Massingale, M.L.; Dentone, P.G.; Landegger, L.D.; Asbell, P.A. Modulation of HLA-DR in dry eye patients following 30 days of treatment with a lubricant eyedrop solution. *Clin. Ophthalmol.* **2015**, *9*, 1137–1145. [CrossRef]
73. Wu, J.; Li, G.J.; Niu, J.; Wen, F.; Han, L. Analyze interleukin-1beta, interleukin-6, and tumor necrosis factor-alpha levels in dry eye and the therapeutic effect of cyclosporine A. *World J. Clin. Cases* **2024**, *12*, 5665–5672. [CrossRef] [PubMed]
74. Mrugacz, M.; Ostrowska, L.; Bryl, A.; Szulc, A.; Zelazowska-Rutkowska, B.; Mrugacz, G. Pro-inflammatory cytokines associated with clinical severity of dry eye disease of patients with depression. *Adv. Med. Sci.* **2017**, *62*, 338–344. [CrossRef]
75. Wu, X.; Chen, X.; Ma, Y.; Lin, X.; Yu, X.; He, S.; Luo, C.; Xu, W. Analysis of tear inflammatory molecules and clinical correlations in evaporative dry eye disease caused by meibomian gland dysfunction. *Int. Ophthalmol.* **2020**, *40*, 3049–3058. [CrossRef]
76. Massingale, M.L.; Li, X.; Vallabhajosyula, M.; Chen, D.; Wei, Y.; Asbell, P.A. Analysis of inflammatory cytokines in the tears of dry eye patients. *Cornea* **2009**, *28*, 1023–1027. [CrossRef] [PubMed]
77. Bang, S.P.; Yeon, C.Y.; Adhikari, N.; Neupane, S.; Kim, H.; Lee, D.C.; Son, M.J.; Lee, H.G.; Kim, J.Y.; Jun, J.H. Cyclosporine A eyedrops with self-nanoemulsifying drug delivery systems have improved physicochemical properties and efficacy against dry eye disease in a murine dry eye model. *PLoS ONE* **2019**, *14*, e0224805. [CrossRef]
78. Sun, X.; Zhang, J.; Li, X.; Li, Y.; Zhao, X.; Sun, X.; Li, Y. Fenofibrate inhibits activation of cGAS-STING pathway by alleviating mitochondrial damage to attenuate inflammatory response in diabetic dry eye. *Free Radic. Biol. Med.* **2025**, *235*, 364–378. [CrossRef]
79. Simmons, K.T.; Xiao, Y.; Pflugfelder, S.C.; de Paiva, C.S. Inflammatory Response to Lipopolysaccharide on the Ocular Surface in a Murine Dry Eye Model. *Investig. Ophthalmol. Vis. Sci.* **2016**, *57*, 2443–2451. [CrossRef] [PubMed]
80. Yamaguchi, T. Inflammatory Response in Dry Eye. *Investig. Ophthalmol. Vis. Sci.* **2018**, *59*, DES192–DES199. [CrossRef]
81. Yu, L.; Yu, C.; Dong, H.; Mu, Y.; Zhang, R.; Zhang, Q.; Liang, W.; Li, W.; Wang, X.; Zhang, L. Recent Developments About the Pathogenesis of Dry Eye Disease: Based on Immune Inflammatory Mechanisms. *Front. Pharmacol.* **2021**, *12*, 732887. [CrossRef]
82. Blanco-Vazquez, M.; Vazquez, A.; Fernandez, I.; Novo-Diez, A.; Martinez-Plaza, E.; Garcia-Vazquez, C.; Gonzalez-Garcia, M.J.; Sobas, E.M.; Calonge, M.; Enriquez-de-Salamanca, A. Inflammation-related molecules in tears of patients with chronic ocular pain and dry eye disease. *Exp. Eye Res.* **2022**, *219*, 109057. [CrossRef]
83. Bruscolini, A.; Lambiase, A.; Segatto, M.; La Cava, M.; Nebbioso, M.; Sacchetti, M. Evaluation of IL8 pathway on the ocular surface: New insights in patients with ocular mucous membrane pemphigoid. *Acta Ophthalmol.* **2020**, *98*, e173–e177. [CrossRef]
84. Galvez, B.G.; Martinez-Perez, C.; Villa-Collar, C.; Alvarez-Peregrina, C.; Sanchez-Tena, M.A. Influence of Cytokines on Inflammatory Eye Diseases: A Citation Network Study. *J. Clin. Med.* **2022**, *11*, 661. [CrossRef]
85. Lopez-Miguel, A.; Teson, M.; Martin-Montanez, V.; Enriquez-de-Salamanca, A.; Stern, M.E.; Gonzalez-Garcia, M.J.; Calonge, M. Clinical and Molecular Inflammatory Response in Sjogren Syndrome-Associated Dry Eye Patients Under Desiccating Stress. *Am. J. Ophthalmol.* **2016**, *161*, 133–141.e2. [CrossRef]
86. Lam, H.; Bleiden, L.; de Paiva, C.S.; Farley, W.; Stern, M.E.; Pflugfelder, S.C. Tear cytokine profiles in dysfunctional tear syndrome. *Am. J. Ophthalmol.* **2009**, *147*, 198–205.e1. [CrossRef]
87. El Annan, J.; Goyal, S.; Zhang, Q.; Freeman, G.J.; Sharpe, A.H.; Dana, R. Regulation of T-cell chemotaxis by programmed death-ligand 1 (PD-L1) in dry eye-associated corneal inflammation. *Investig. Ophthalmol. Vis. Sci.* **2010**, *51*, 3418–3423. [CrossRef] [PubMed]
88. Nagar, S.; Ajouz, L.; Nichols, K.K.; Kumar, S.; Zhao, C.; Naidoo, K.K.; Robinson, M.R.; Borchman, D. Relationship Between Human Meibum Lipid Composition and the Severity of Meibomian Gland Dysfunction: A Spectroscopic Analysis. *Investig. Ophthalmol. Vis. Sci.* **2023**, *64*, 22. [CrossRef] [PubMed]
89. Asiedu, K. Candidate Molecular Compounds as Potential Indicators for Meibomian Gland Dysfunction. *Front. Med.* **2022**, *9*, 873538. [CrossRef]
90. Zhao, H.; Wu, S.N.; Shao, Y.; Xiao, D.; Tang, L.Y.; Cheng, Z.; Peng, J. Lipidomics Profiles Revealed Alterations in Patients with Meibomian Gland Dysfunction After Exposure to Intense Pulsed Light. *Front. Neurol.* **2022**, *13*, 827544. [CrossRef] [PubMed]
91. Lam, S.M.; Tong, L.; Yong, S.S.; Li, B.; Chaurasia, S.S.; Shui, G.; Wenk, M.R. Meibum lipid composition in Asians with dry eye disease. *PLoS ONE* **2011**, *6*, e24339. [CrossRef]
92. Nguyen, A.; Naidoo, K.K.; Ajouz, L.; Xu, X.; Zhao, C.; Robinson, M.R.; Borchman, D. Changes in Human Meibum Lipid Composition Related to the Presence and Severity of Meibomian Gland Dysfunction. *J. Ocul. Pharmacol. Ther.* **2024**, *40*, 562–570. [CrossRef]

93. Garcia-Queiruga, J.; Pena-Verdeal, H.; Sabucedo-Villamarin, B.; Paz-Tarrio, M.; Guitian-Fernandez, E.; Garcia-Resua, C.; Yebra-Pimentel, E.; Giraldez, M.J. Meibum Lipidomic Analysis in Evaporative Dry Eye Subjects. *Int. J. Mol. Sci.* **2024**, *25*, 4782. [CrossRef] [PubMed]
94. Sheppard, J.D.; Nichols, K.K. Dry Eye Disease Associated with Meibomian Gland Dysfunction: Focus on Tear Film Characteristics and the Therapeutic Landscape. *Ophthalmol. Ther.* **2023**, *12*, 1397–1418. [CrossRef]
95. Mondal, K.; Mandal, N. Role of Bioactive Sphingolipids in Inflammation and Eye Diseases. *Adv. Exp. Med. Biol.* **2019**, *1161*, 149–167. [CrossRef] [PubMed]
96. Paranjpe, V.; Galor, A.; Grambergs, R.; Mandal, N. The role of sphingolipids in meibomian gland dysfunction and ocular surface inflammation. *Ocul. Surf.* **2022**, *26*, 100–110. [CrossRef]
97. Ham, B.M.; Cole, R.B.; Jacob, J.T. Identification and comparison of the polar phospholipids in normal and dry eye rabbit tears by MALDI-TOF mass spectrometry. *Investig. Ophthalmol. Vis. Sci.* **2006**, *47*, 3330–3338. [CrossRef] [PubMed]
98. Borchman, D. Lipid conformational order and the etiology of cataract and dry eye. *J. Lipid Res.* **2021**, *62*, 100039. [CrossRef]
99. Miyamoto, M.; Sassa, T.; Sawai, M.; Kihara, A. Lipid polarity gradient formed by omega-hydroxy lipids in tear film prevents dry eye disease. *Elife* **2020**, *9*, e53582. [CrossRef]
100. Wan, X.; Zhang, Y.; Zhang, K.; Mou, Y.; Jin, X.; Huang, X. The alterations of ocular surface metabolism and the related immunity inflammation in dry eye. *Adv. Ophthalmol. Pract. Res.* **2025**, *5*, 1–12. [CrossRef]
101. Jantti, J.; Viitaja, T.; Sevon, J.; Lajunen, T.; Raitanen, J.E.; Schlegel, C.; Viljanen, M.; Paananen, R.O.; Moilanen, J.; Ruponen, M.; et al. Early-Stage Development of an Anti-Evaporative Liposomal Formulation for the Potential Treatment of Dry Eyes. *ACS Pharmacol. Transl. Sci.* **2023**, *6*, 1518–1530. [CrossRef] [PubMed]
102. Nishiwaki-Dantas, M.C.; de Freitas, D.; Fornazari, D.; Dos Santos, M.S.; Wakamatsu, T.H.; Barquilha, C.N.; Ferrer, M.T.; Holzhausen, H.C.N.; Alves, M. Phospholipid Nanoemulsion-Based Ocular Lubricant for the Treatment of Dry Eye Subtypes: A Multicenter and Prospective Study. *Ophthalmol. Ther.* **2024**, *13*, 3203–3213. [CrossRef] [PubMed]
103. Singh, S.; Hammer, C.M.; Paulsen, F. Urea and ocular surface: Synthesis, secretion and its role in tear film homeostasis. *Ocul. Surf.* **2023**, *27*, 41–47. [CrossRef]
104. Chai, P.; Zhao, F.; Jia, R.; Zhou, X.; Fan, X. Lactate/lactylation in ocular development and diseases. *Trends Mol. Med.* **2024**. [CrossRef]
105. Mondal, H.; Kim, H.J.; Mohanto, N.; Jee, J.P. A Review on Dry Eye Disease Treatment: Recent Progress, Diagnostics, and Future Perspectives. *Pharmaceutics* **2023**, *15*, 990. [CrossRef]
106. Chen, X.; Zhang, C.; Peng, F.; Wu, L.; Zhuo, D.; Wang, L.; Zhang, M.; Li, Z.; Tian, L.; Jie, Y.; et al. Identification of glutamine as a potential therapeutic target in dry eye disease. *Signal Transduct. Target. Ther.* **2025**, *10*, 27. [CrossRef]
107. Galbis-Estrada, C.; Pinazo-Duran, M.D.; Martinez-Castillo, S.; Morales, J.M.; Monleon, D.; Zanon-Moreno, V. A metabolomic approach to dry eye disorders. The role of oral supplements with antioxidants and omega 3 fatty acids. *Mol. Vis.* **2015**, *21*, 555–567.
108. Jiang, Y.; Yang, C.; Zheng, Y.; Liu, Y.; Chen, Y. A Set of Global Metabolomic Biomarker Candidates to Predict the Risk of Dry Eye Disease. *Front. Cell Dev. Biol.* **2020**, *8*, 344. [CrossRef]
109. Yazdani, M.; Elgstoen, K.B.P.; Rootwelt, H.; Shahdadfar, A.; Utheim, O.A.; Utheim, T.P. Tear Metabolomics in Dry Eye Disease: A Review. *Int. J. Mol. Sci.* **2019**, *20*, 3755. [CrossRef]
110. Seen, S.; Tong, L. Dry eye disease and oxidative stress. *Acta Ophthalmol.* **2018**, *96*, e412–e420. [CrossRef] [PubMed]
111. Dogru, M.; Kojima, T.; Simsek, C.; Tsubota, K. Potential Role of Oxidative Stress in Ocular Surface Inflammation and Dry Eye Disease. *Investig. Ophthalmol. Vis. Sci.* **2018**, *59*, DES163–DES168. [CrossRef]
112. Bu, J.; Liu, Y.; Zhang, R.; Lin, S.; Zhuang, J.; Sun, L.; Zhang, L.; He, H.; Zong, R.; Wu, Y.; et al. Potential New Target for Dry Eye Disease-Oxidative Stress. *Antioxidants* **2024**, *13*, 422. [CrossRef]
113. Ouyang, W.; Yan, D.; Hu, J.; Liu, Z. Multifaceted mitochondrial as a novel therapeutic target in dry eye: Insights and interventions. *Cell Death Discov.* **2024**, *10*, 398. [CrossRef] [PubMed]
114. Shi, H.; Zheng, L.Y.; Zhang, P.; Yu, C.Q. miR-146a and miR-155 expression in PBMCs from patients with Sjogren's syndrome. *J. Oral Pathol. Med.* **2014**, *43*, 792–797. [CrossRef] [PubMed]
115. Zilahi, E.; Tarr, T.; Papp, G.; Griger, Z.; Sipka, S.; Zeher, M. Increased microRNA-146a/b, TRAF6 gene and decreased IRAK1 gene expressions in the peripheral mononuclear cells of patients with Sjogren's syndrome. *Immunol. Lett.* **2012**, *141*, 165–168. [CrossRef]
116. Sun, H.Y.; Lv, A.K.; Yao, H. Relationship of miRNA-146a to primary Sjogren's syndrome and to systemic lupus erythematosus: A meta-analysis. *Rheumatol. Int.* **2017**, *37*, 1311–1316. [CrossRef]
117. Wei, Y.; Li, N.; Zhao, L.; Yang, C.; Ma, B.; Li, X.; Wei, R.; Nian, H. MicroRNAs and Autoimmune-Mediated Eye Diseases. *Front. Cell Dev. Biol.* **2020**, *8*, 818. [CrossRef] [PubMed]

118. Benavides-Aguilar, J.A.; Morales-Rodriguez, J.I.; Ambriz-Gonzalez, H.; Ruiz-Manriquez, L.M.; Banerjee, A.; Pathak, S.; Duttaroy, A.K.; Paul, S. The regulatory role of microRNAs in common eye diseases: A brief review. *Front. Genet.* **2023**, *14*, 1152110. [CrossRef]
119. Rassi, D.M.; De Paiva, C.S.; Dias, L.C.; Modulo, C.M.; Adriano, L.; Fantucci, M.Z.; Rocha, E.M. Review: MicroRNAS in ocular surface and dry eye diseases. *Ocul. Surf.* **2017**, *15*, 660–669. [CrossRef]
120. Kessal, K.; Liang, H.; Rabut, G.; Daull, P.; Garrigue, J.S.; Docquier, M.; Melik Parsadaniantz, S.; Baudouin, C.; Brignole-Baudouin, F. Conjunctival Inflammatory Gene Expression Profiling in Dry Eye Disease: Correlations with HLA-DRA and HLA-DRB1. *Front. Immunol.* **2018**, *9*, 2271. [CrossRef]
121. Brignole-Baudouin, F.; Riancho, L.; Ismail, D.; Deniaud, M.; Amrane, M.; Baudouin, C. Correlation Between the Inflammatory Marker HLA-DR and Signs and Symptoms in Moderate to Severe Dry Eye Disease. *Investig. Ophthalmol. Vis. Sci.* **2017**, *58*, 2438–2448. [CrossRef] [PubMed]
122. Paik, B.; Tong, L. Polymorphisms in Lymphotoxin-Alpha as the "Missing Link" in Prognosticating Favourable Response to Omega-3 Supplementation for Dry Eye Disease: A Narrative Review. *Int. J. Mol. Sci.* **2023**, *24*, 4236. [CrossRef]
123. Roshandel, D.; Semnani, F.; Rayati Damavandi, A.; Masoudi, A.; Baradaran-Rafii, A.; Watson, S.L.; Morgan, W.H.; McLenachan, S. Genetic predisposition to ocular surface disorders and opportunities for gene-based therapies. *Ocul. Surf.* **2023**, *29*, 150–165. [CrossRef]
124. Kim, W.; Woo, I.H.; Eom, Y.; Song, J.S. Short-term changes in tear osmolarity after instillation of different osmolarity eye drops in patients with dry eye. *Sci. Rep.* **2023**, *13*, 11012. [CrossRef]
125. Baudouin, C.; Aragona, P.; Messmer, E.M.; Tomlinson, A.; Calonge, M.; Boboridis, K.G.; Akova, Y.A.; Geerling, G.; Labetoulle, M.; Rolando, M. Role of hyperosmolarity in the pathogenesis and management of dry eye disease: Proceedings of the OCEAN group meeting. *Ocul. Surf.* **2013**, *11*, 246–258. [CrossRef]
126. Lemp, M.A.; Bron, A.J.; Baudouin, C.; Benitez Del Castillo, J.M.; Geffen, D.; Tauber, J.; Foulks, G.N.; Pepose, J.S.; Sullivan, B.D. Tear osmolarity in the diagnosis and management of dry eye disease. *Am. J. Ophthalmol.* **2011**, *151*, 792–798.e1. [CrossRef]
127. Tashbayev, B.; Utheim, T.P.; Utheim, O.A.; Raeder, S.; Jensen, J.L.; Yazdani, M.; Lagali, N.; Vitelli, V.; Dartt, D.A.; Chen, X. Utility of Tear Osmolarity Measurement in Diagnosis of Dry Eye Disease. *Sci. Rep.* **2020**, *10*, 5542. [CrossRef]
128. Tomlinson, A.; Khanal, S.; Ramaesh, K.; Diaper, C.; McFadyen, A. Tear film osmolarity: Determination of a referent for dry eye diagnosis. *Investig. Ophthalmol. Vis. Sci.* **2006**, *47*, 4309–4315. [CrossRef]
129. Suzuki, M.; Massingale, M.L.; Ye, F.; Godbold, J.; Elfassy, T.; Vallabhajosyula, M.; Asbell, P.A. Tear osmolarity as a biomarker for dry eye disease severity. *Investig. Ophthalmol. Vis. Sci.* **2010**, *51*, 4557–4561. [CrossRef] [PubMed]
130. Galor, A.; Lighthizer, N. Corneal Sensitivity Testing Procedure for Ophthalmologic and Optometric Patients. *J. Vis. Exp.* **2024**, *210*, e66597. [CrossRef] [PubMed]
131. Merayo-Lloves, J.; Gomez Martin, C.; Lozano-Sanroma, J.; Renedo Laguna, C. Assessment and safety of the new esthesiometer BRILL: Comparison with the Cochet-Bonnet Esthesiometer. *Eur. J. Ophthalmol.* **2024**, *34*, 1036–1045. [CrossRef] [PubMed]
132. Ruiz-Lozano, R.E.; Quiroga-Garza, M.E.; Ramos-DÁVila, E.M.; PantaleÓN-GarcÍA, J.; Khodor, A.L.I.; Komai, S.; Rodriguez-Gutierrez, L.A.; Ma, S.; Mousa, H.M.; Mattes, R.; et al. Comparative Evaluation of the Corneal Sensitivity Thresholds between the Novel Non-Contact and Cochet-Bonnet Esthesiometers. *Am. J. Ophthalmol.* **2025**, *271*, 407–416. [CrossRef]
133. Vazquez, A.; Blanco-Vazquez, M.; Martinez-Plaza, E.; Sobas, E.M.; Gonzalez-Garcia, M.J.; Lopez-Miguel, A.; Ortega, E.; Enriquez-de-Salamanca, A.; Calonge, M. Corneal Sensory Changes and Nerve Plexus Abnormalities in Chronic Neuropathic Ocular Pain and Dry Eye Postrefractive Surgery. *Am. J. Ophthalmol.* **2025**, *276*, 170–185. [CrossRef]
134. Vidas Pauk, S.; Petricek, I.; Jukic, T.; Popovic-Suic, S.; Tomic, M.; Kalauz, M.; Jandrokovic, S.; Masnec, S. Noninvasive Tear Film Break-up Time Assessment Using Handheld Lipid Layer Examination Instrument. *Acta Clin. Croat.* **2019**, *58*, 63–71. [CrossRef]
135. Tsubota, K. Short Tear Film Breakup Time-Type Dry Eye. *Investig. Ophthalmol. Vis. Sci.* **2018**, *59*, DES64–DES70. [CrossRef] [PubMed]
136. Correa-Sandoval, D.C.; Quintanilla-Treviño, P.M.; Amparo, F.; Garza-Leon, M.A. Noninvasive tear breakup time evaluation with multifunctional topography supports the diagnosis of evaporative dry eye disease. *Pan-Am. J. Ophthalmol.* **2024**, *6*, 80. [CrossRef]
137. Yazdani, M.; Fiskadal, J.; Chen, X.; Utheim, O.A.; Raeder, S.; Vitelli, V.; Utheim, T.P. Tear Film Break-Up Time and Dry Eye Disease Severity in a Large Norwegian Cohort. *J. Clin. Med.* **2021**, *10*, 884. [CrossRef]
138. El Barche, F.Z.; Benyoussef, A.A.; El Habib Daho, M.; Lamard, A.; Quellec, G.; Cochener, B.; Lamard, M. Automated tear film break-up time measurement for dry eye diagnosis using deep learning. *Sci. Rep.* **2024**, *14*, 11723. [CrossRef]
139. Pondelis, N.; Dieckmann, G.M.; Jamali, A.; Kataguiri, P.; Senchyna, M.; Hamrah, P. Infrared meibography allows detection of dimensional changes in meibomian glands following intranasal neurostimulation. *Ocul. Surf.* **2020**, *18*, 511–516. [CrossRef]
140. Palamar, M.; Kiyat, P.; Ertam, I.; Yagci, A. Evaluation of dry eye and meibomian gland dysfunction with meibography in vitiligo. *Eye* **2017**, *31*, 1074–1077. [CrossRef] [PubMed]

141. Wise, R.J.; Sobel, R.K.; Allen, R.C. Meibography: A review of techniques and technologies. *Saudi J. Ophthalmol.* **2012**, *26*, 349–356. [CrossRef]
142. Li, S.; Wang, Y.; Yu, C.; Li, Q.; Chang, P.; Wang, D.; Li, Z.; Zhao, Y.; Zhang, H.; Tang, N.; et al. Unsupervised Learning Based on Meibography Enables Subtyping of Dry Eye Disease and Reveals Ocular Surface Features. *Investig. Ophthalmol. Vis. Sci.* **2023**, *64*, 43. [CrossRef]
143. Alhatem, A.; Cavalcanti, B.; Hamrah, P. In vivo confocal microscopy in dry eye disease and related conditions. *Semin. Ophthalmol.* **2012**, *27*, 138–148. [CrossRef] [PubMed]
144. Aggarwal, S.; Kheirkhah, A.; Cavalcanti, B.M.; Cruzat, A.; Jamali, A.; Hamrah, P. Correlation of corneal immune cell changes with clinical severity in dry eye disease: An in vivo confocal microscopy study. *Ocul. Surf.* **2021**, *19*, 183–189. [CrossRef] [PubMed]
145. Shetty, R.; Dua, H.S.; Tong, L.; Kundu, G.; Khamar, P.; Gorimanipalli, B.; D'Souza, S. Role of in vivo confocal microscopy in dry eye disease and eye pain. *Indian J. Ophthalmol.* **2023**, *71*, 1099–1104. [CrossRef]
146. Sim, R.; Yong, K.; Liu, Y.C.; Tong, L. In Vivo Confocal Microscopy in Different Types of Dry Eye and Meibomian Gland Dysfunction. *J. Clin. Med.* **2022**, *11*, 2349. [CrossRef]
147. He, J.; Ogawa, Y.; Mukai, S.; Saijo-Ban, Y.; Kamoi, M.; Uchino, M.; Yamane, M.; Ozawa, N.; Fukui, M.; Mori, T.; et al. In Vivo Confocal Microscopy Evaluation of Ocular Surface with Graft-Versus-Host Disease-Related Dry Eye Disease. *Sci. Rep.* **2017**, *7*, 10720. [CrossRef] [PubMed]
148. Nicolle, P.; Liang, H.; Reboussin, E.; Rabut, G.; Warcoin, E.; Brignole-Baudouin, F.; Melik-Parsadaniantz, S.; Baudouin, C.; Labbe, A.; Reaux-Le Goazigo, A. Proinflammatory Markers, Chemokines, and Enkephalin in Patients Suffering from Dry Eye Disease. *Int. J. Mol. Sci.* **2018**, *19*, 1221. [CrossRef]
149. Walter, S.D.; Gronert, K.; McClellan, A.L.; Levitt, R.C.; Sarantopoulos, K.D.; Galor, A. omega-3 Tear Film Lipids Correlate with Clinical Measures of Dry Eye. *Investig. Ophthalmol. Vis. Sci.* **2016**, *57*, 2472–2478. [CrossRef]
150. Huang, S.C.; Lei, Y.P.; Hsiao, M.C.; Hsieh, Y.K.; Tang, Q.P.; Chen, C.; Hsu, M.Y. Multicomponent Dietary Supplementation: Impact on Tear Secretion and Ocular Surface Inflammation in Dry Eye Syndrome Patients. *Antioxidants* **2025**, *14*, 103. [CrossRef]
151. Hussain, M.; Shtein, R.M.; Pistilli, M.; Maguire, M.G.; Oydanich, M.; Asbell, P.A.; Group, D.S.R. The Dry Eye Assessment and Management (DREAM) extension study—A randomized clinical trial of withdrawal of supplementation with omega-3 fatty acid in patients with dry eye disease. *Ocul. Surf.* **2020**, *18*, 47–55. [CrossRef]
152. Khanal, S.; Ngo, W.; Nichols, K.K.; Wilson, L.; Barnes, S.; Nichols, J.J. Human meibum and tear film derived (O-acyl)-omega-hydroxy fatty acids in meibomian gland dysfunction. *Ocul. Surf.* **2021**, *21*, 118–128. [CrossRef]
153. Bland, H.C.; Moilanen, J.A.; Ekholm, F.S.; Paananen, R.O. Investigating the Role of Specific Tear Film Lipids Connected to Dry Eye Syndrome: A Study on O-Acyl-omega-hydroxy Fatty Acids and Diesters. *Langmuir* **2019**, *35*, 3545–3552. [CrossRef] [PubMed]
154. Viitaja, T.; Raitanen, J.E.; Moilanen, J.; Paananen, R.O.; Ekholm, F.S. The Properties and Role of O-Acyl-omega-hydroxy Fatty Acids and Type I-St and Type II Diesters in the Tear Film Lipid Layer Revealed by a Combined Chemistry and Biophysics Approach. *J. Org. Chem.* **2021**, *86*, 4965–4976. [CrossRef] [PubMed]
155. Pucker, A.D.; Ngo, W.; Postnikoff, C.K.; Fortinberry, H.; Nichols, J.J. Tear Film miRNAs and Their Association with Human Dry Eye Disease. *Curr. Eye Res.* **2022**, *47*, 1479–1487. [CrossRef]
156. Wolffsohn, J.S.; Benítez-Del-Castillo, J.; Loya-Garcia, D.; Inomata, T.; Iyar, G.; Liang, L.; Pult, H.; Sabater, A.L.; Starr, C.E.; Vehof, J.; et al. TFOS DEWS III Diagnostic Methodology. *Am. J. Ophthalmol.* **2025**, 1–101. [CrossRef]
157. Park, J.Y.; Kim, B.G.; Kim, J.S.; Hwang, J.H. Matrix Metalloproteinase 9 Point-of-Care Immunoassay Result Predicts Response to Topical Cyclosporine Treatment in Dry Eye Disease. *Transl. Vision. Sci. Technol.* **2018**, *7*, 31. [CrossRef] [PubMed]
158. Schargus, M.; Ivanova, S.; Kakkassery, V.; Dick, H.B.; Joachim, S. Correlation of Tear Film Osmolarity and 2 Different MMP-9 Tests with Common Dry Eye Tests in a Cohort of Non-Dry Eye Patients. *Cornea* **2015**, *34*, 739–744. [CrossRef]
159. Sambursky, R.; Davitt, W.F., 3rd; Latkany, R.; Tauber, S.; Starr, C.; Friedberg, M.; Dirks, M.S.; McDonald, M. Sensitivity and specificity of a point-of-care matrix metalloproteinase 9 immunoassay for diagnosing inflammation related to dry eye. *JAMA Ophthalmol.* **2013**, *131*, 24–28. [CrossRef]
160. Bron, A.J.; Willshire, C. Tear Osmolarity in the Diagnosis of Systemic Dehydration and Dry Eye Disease. *Diagnostics* **2021**, *11*, 387. [CrossRef]
161. Park, J.; Choi, Y.; Han, G.; Shin, E.; Han, J.; Chung, T.Y.; Lim, D.H. Evaluation of tear osmolarity measured by I-Pen osmolarity system in patients with dry eye. *Sci. Rep.* **2021**, *11*, 7726. [CrossRef] [PubMed]
162. Greiner, J.V.; Ying, G.S.; Pistilli, M.; Maguire, M.G.; Asbell, P.A.; Dry Eye, A.; Management Study Research, G. Association of Tear Osmolarity with Signs and Symptoms of Dry Eye Disease in the Dry Eye Assessment and Management (DREAM) Study. *Investig. Ophthalmol. Vis. Sci.* **2023**, *64*, 5. [CrossRef]
163. Harrell, C.R.; Feulner, L.; Djonov, V.; Pavlovic, D.; Volarevic, V. The Molecular Mechanisms Responsible for Tear Hyperosmolarity-Induced Pathological Changes in the Eyes of Dry Eye Disease Patients. *Cells* **2023**, *12*, 2755. [CrossRef]

164. Pflugfelder, S.; Nakhleh, L.; Kikukawa, Y.; Tanaka, S.; Kosugi, T. Non-Invasive Tear Break-Up Detection with the Kowa DR-1alpha and Its Relationship to Dry Eye Clinical Severity. *Int. J. Mol. Sci.* **2022**, *23*, 14774. [CrossRef] [PubMed]
165. Aldeyra Therapeutics, Inc. *Reproxalap: Our Novel Small Molecule Drug Candidate for Dry Eye*; Aldeyra Therapeutics, Inc.: Lexington, MA, USA, 2024.
166. Aldeyra Therapeutics, Inc. Aldeyra Therapeutics achieves primary endpoint in phase 3 dry eye disease clinical trial of reproxalap. *Business Wire*, 8 August 2024.
167. Hu, L.; Zhang, T.; Ma, H.; Pan, Y.; Wang, S.; Liu, X.; Dai, X.; Zheng, Y.; Lee, L.P.; Liu, F. Discovering the Secret of Diseases by Incorporated Tear Exosomes Analysis via Rapid-Isolation System: iTEARS. *ACS Nano* **2022**, *16*, 11720–11732. [CrossRef] [PubMed]

International Journal of
Molecular Sciences

MDPI

Article

Effects of Exposure of PHMG-p, a Humidifier Disinfectant Component, on Eye Dryness: A Study on a Rat Model Based on ^{1}H-NMR Metabolomics

Jung Dae Lee [1,2], Hyang Yeon Kim [1,2], Soo Bean Oh [3], Hyeyoon Goo [3], Kyong Jin Cho [3], Gi-Wook Hwang [4], Suhkmann Kim [5] and Kyu-Bong Kim [1,2,*]

1 College of Pharmacy, Dankook University, Cheonan 31116, Republic of Korea; ljd0734@nate.com (J.D.L.); festivalkim@gmail.com (H.Y.K.)
2 Center for Human Risk Assessment, Dankook University, Cheonan 31116, Republic of Korea
3 College of Medicine, Dankook University, Cheonan 31116, Republic of Korea; ohsu9212@naver.com (S.B.O.); ghy1204@hanmail.net (H.G.); perfectcure@dankook.ac.kr (K.J.C.)
4 Division of Environmental and Health Sciences, Faculty of Pharmaceutical Sciences, Tohoku Medical and Pharmaceutical University, Sendai 981-8558, Japan; hwang@tohoku-mpu.ac.jp
5 Department of Chemistry, Center for Proteome Biophysics, and Chemistry Institute for Functional Materials, Pusan National University, Busan 46241, Republic of Korea; suhkmann@pusan.ac.kr
* Correspondence: kyubong@dankook.ac.kr

Abstract: Polyhexamethylene guanidine phosphate (PHMG-p), a widely used disinfectant component in household humidifiers, has been implicated in various health issues, including pulmonary toxicity. Many people use humidifiers to improve dry eye disease (DED). The current study was performed to elucidate the effect of PHMG-p on eye dryness in a rat model using metabolomics. Male Sprague Dawley rats were exposed to PHMG-p (0.1% and 0.3%) following a previously established DED induction model using scopolamine hydrobromide and desiccation stress. Ocular surface damage was assessed using corneal fluorescein staining, tear volume measurement, and tear break-up time (TBUT). Plasma and urine samples were analyzed using ^{1}H-NMR-based metabolomics to identify metabolic alterations associated with PHMG-P-p exposure and DED pathogenesis. PHMG-p exposure exacerbated DED symptoms, as evidenced by a significant reduction in tear volume, shorter TBUT, and increased corneal damage compared to the control group. Metabolomic profiling identified distinct metabolic changes in PHMG-p-exposed groups, including alterations in glutamate, glycine, citrate, and succinate metabolism. These metabolic changes correlated with increased levels of inflammatory cytokines such as IL-1β, IL-6, and TNF-α in the corneal and lacrimal gland tissues. Our findings suggest that PHMG-p exposure contributes to DED pathophysiology by inducing metabolic disturbances and inflammatory responses in the ocular surface. This study highlights the need for further investigation into the potential risks of PHMG-p exposure on ocular health and provides novel insights into the metabolic underpinnings of DED.

Keywords: PHMG-p; eye dryness; NMR; metabolomics; biomarker

1. Introduction

Dry eye disease (DED), also known as dry eye syndrome or keratoconjunctivitis sicca, is a multifactorial and chronic ocular condition characterized by a loss of tear film homeostasis [1]. It affects the ocular surface and is associated with symptoms such as burning, itching, heaviness, eye fatigue, dryness, facial flushing, and blurred vision. DED occurs when the eyes fail to maintain an adequate tear layer, essential for lubricating and nourishing the ocular surface. This leads to increased osmotic pressure in the tear film, resulting in irritation and inflammation, further exacerbated by the release of pro-inflammatory mediators [2]. With an estimated prevalence of 5–50% globally, DED is one of the most common ophthalmic disorders [3]. DED has a variety of causes and risk factors. Age is a significant contributor, with older individuals being more susceptible. Certain medications, such as antihistamines, antihypertensives, and antidepressants, have been associated with DED development. Autoimmune diseases like Sjögren's syndrome, environmental factors such as low humidity and high airflow, and meibomian gland dysfunction, which affects the lipid layer of the tear film, are also prominent causes [1]. Symptoms include stinging or burning sensations, pressure, a gritty feeling, redness, blurry vision, excessive tearing, and difficulty wearing contact lenses, all of which significantly affect the quality of life [1,4].

DED is typically diagnosed using methods such as ocular surface staining, non-invasive evaluation of tear break-up time (TBUT), and measurement of osmotic pressure [5]. The pathophysiology of DED involves inflammation of the ocular surface and increased osmotic pressure of the tear film, which play critical roles in disease progression [6,7]. Common features include inflammation of the ocular surface and major tear glands. Key inflammatory markers such as human leukocyte antigen-DR (HLA-DR) and interleukin (IL)-1β have been detected in the conjunctiva, contributing to the apoptosis or cytotoxicity of conjunctival epithelial cells [8–11]. Increased tear osmotic pressure has also been linked to the overexpression of pro-inflammatory cytokines, including tumor necrosis factor-alpha (TNF-α), IL-1, and IL-6, perpetuating the inflammatory cascade in DED [12–14].

TNF-α, IL-1β, and IL-6 are central to DED pathogenesis. These cytokines are significantly elevated in the tear film and ocular tissues of DED patients, correlating with disease severity and maintaining the chronic inflammatory state [15,16]. TNF-α and IL-6 interact synergistically, amplifying the inflammatory response and stimulating antigen-presenting cell maturation and T-cell function, which further sustain the inflammatory cycle. Elevated IL-1β levels inhibit neurotransmitter secretion, reducing tear production and exacerbating ocular surface damage [16]. Furthermore, TNF-α is pivotal in orchestrating inflammation, with topical TNF-α blockers shown to suppress inflammation in the cornea and lacrimal glands by reducing IFN-γ, IL-21, and IL-6 expression [15,17].

The therapeutic importance of targeting these cytokines is evident in the effectiveness of anti-inflammatory treatments. For instance, cyclosporine A combined with artificial tears significantly reduces TNF-α, IL-1β, and IL-6 levels, improving clinical outcomes in DED patients [15,16]. These findings highlight the critical role of pro-inflammatory cytokines in the pathogenesis and progression of DED and underscore the potential of targeted therapies in managing this disease.

According to recent data, the number of patients visiting hospitals for DED in the Republic of Korea ranges between 2.3 million and 2.5 million annually. As of 2022, women accounted for 66.5% of the total patients, approximately twice the number of men. By age group, patients in their 60s represented the largest proportion at 19.4%, followed by those in their 50s (19.1%) and 40s (15.1%). These statistics highlight that DED is a highly prevalent condition in the Republic of Korea, particularly among women and middle-aged to elderly individuals [18].

Polyhexamethylene guanidine phosphate (PHMG-p) is a guanidine derivative widely used as a biocidal disinfectant due to its fungicidal and bactericidal properties against Gram-positive and Gram-negative bacteria. In the Republic of Korea, PHMG-p was commonly utilized as a disinfectant in household humidifiers to prevent microbial contamination [19,20]. However, in the Republic of Korea, the use of PHMG-p in household humidifiers led to a public health crisis, prompting investigations into its toxicity and long-term effects [21]. PHMG-p exposure was found to primarily target the respiratory system, causing severe health risks, which has driven extensive research across various fields. Studies on the toxicity of PHMG-p have been conducted in areas such as respiratory health, cytotoxicity, immunology, hematology, histology, and omics [22–28]. Due to its harmful effects, ongoing research continues to elucidate the mechanisms of PHMG-p-induced damage and explore potential therapeutic strategies for affected individuals.

The hypothesis that the increase in DED prevalence might be associated with the use of humidifier disinfectants was supported by several observations: (1) the use of humidifiers was often recommended for the treatment of DED [29], (2) while the prevalence of DED has been steadily increasing before and after the discontinuation of humidifier disinfectants in 2011, there was an unexpected decline in 2013, and (3) women, who were more likely to engage in indoor activities, exhibited a prevalence rate more than twice that of men, who were more exposed to outdoor activities [30]. This is contrary to the expected trend if factors such as yellow dust or fine particulate matter were the primary causes of DED. Therefore, investigating the correlation between humidifier disinfectants and DED is both meaningful and important.

Metabolomics has emerged as a powerful tool in disease diagnosis and treatment, offering valuable insights into pathophysiological mechanisms and potential therapeutic targets [31,32]. By comprehensively characterizing metabolites within biological systems, metabolomics provides a unique perspective on disease processes and treatment outcomes, enabling a deeper understanding of the molecular basis of various conditions [33–35]. In the field of disease diagnosis, metabolomics has demonstrated significant potential across a broad spectrum of applications. One of its most promising contributions is the identification of biomarkers for early detection of diseases such as cancer, diabetes, and cardiovascular disorders, allowing for timely intervention and improved patient outcomes [34,36,37]. Clinically, metabolomics has already been implemented in newborn screening programs, enabling the detection of over 50 inherited metabolic disorders, thereby facilitating early treatment and prevention of severe complications [38,39]. Moreover, its potential in infectious disease diagnosis is gaining recognition, as it may allow for the direct detection of pathogens or the identification of host-response biomarkers specific to particular infections [33,40,41]. In the context of complex diseases, metabolomics has provided novel insights into the metabolic underpinnings of conditions such as diabetes, Alzheimer's disease, atherosclerosis, and cancer, uncovering biomarkers and metabolic pathways previously unrecognized [42–45].

Moreover, many studies have employed metabolomics to identify biomarkers and understand the disease mechanisms of DED. Tear metabolomics has been a focal point of research due to the direct relevance of tear composition to ocular surface health. A cross-sectional study involving 113 participants (85 with DED and 28 controls) analyzed reflex tears using UPLC-Q/TOF-MS/MS, revealing 48 metabolites associated with DED incidence [42]. These metabolites showed variations across age groups and were primarily involved in glucose metabolism, amino acid metabolism, and glutathione metabolism. Furthermore, metabolic changes were correlated with clinical indicators such as the Ocular Surface Disease Index (OSDI) and fluorescein breakup time [42]. Serum metabolomics has also provided valuable insights, as evidenced by a large-scale study involving 2819 subjects from the Twins UK cohort [43]. This study identified 222 serum metabolites and highlighted the critical role of androgen metabolism in DED development, particularly among females [43]. Additionally, combined tear and saliva metabolomics studies have advanced the understanding of evaporative DED, particularly in female patients. Recent research identified 56 metabolites in tears that significantly differed between DED patients and controls, with these metabolites linked to meibum composition, antioxidative properties, and the ocular microbiome [44]. Saliva analysis revealed lower levels of hypotaurine in patients with tear film instability, suggesting a potential link between systemic metabolism and ocular health [44]. Animal model studies have further contributed to the field, with scopolamine-induced DED models used to analyze plasma and urine metabolites [45,46]. These studies aimed to identify potential biomarkers and elucidate metabolic changes associated with DED [45,46]. In therapeutic research, in situ metabolomics using MALDI-MSI has identified potential treatment targets [47]. A study published in Nature (2025) demonstrated increased glutamine levels in the cornea following combined mesenchymal stem cell and thymosin beta-4 therapy. This research identified glutaminase 1 (GLS1) as a potential therapeutic target for DED, paving the way for novel treatment approaches [47].

Therefore, in previous studies, we identified biomarkers of dry eye disease (DED) using ^{1}H-NMR in a rat model [45]. Building on this foundation, we aimed to investigate the correlation between PHMG-p, a component of humidifier disinfectants, and its role in inducing or exacerbating DED.

2. Results

2.1. Corneal Fluorescein Staining and Corneal Damage

On day 13, corneal epithelial damage was assessed using corneal fluorescein staining. Both eyes of each rat in the groups (n = 6) were examined, and representative corneal fluorescein staining images from each group on day 13 after DED induction are shown in Figure 1A. The corneal damage scores were 0.68 ± 0.49 and 1.75 ± 0.75 in the control group and the DED group, respectively. The scores for the PC group, DED + PHMG-p 0.1% group, and DED + PHMG-p 0.3% group were 2.25 ± 0.75, 2.08 ± 0.29, and 2.08 ± 0.34, respectively. Additionally, the PHMG-p 0.1% group and the PHMG-p 0.3% group showed scores of 2.25 ± 0.75 and 1.42 ± 0.34, respectively. The corneal damage scores were significantly higher in all groups compared to the control group (Figure 1B).

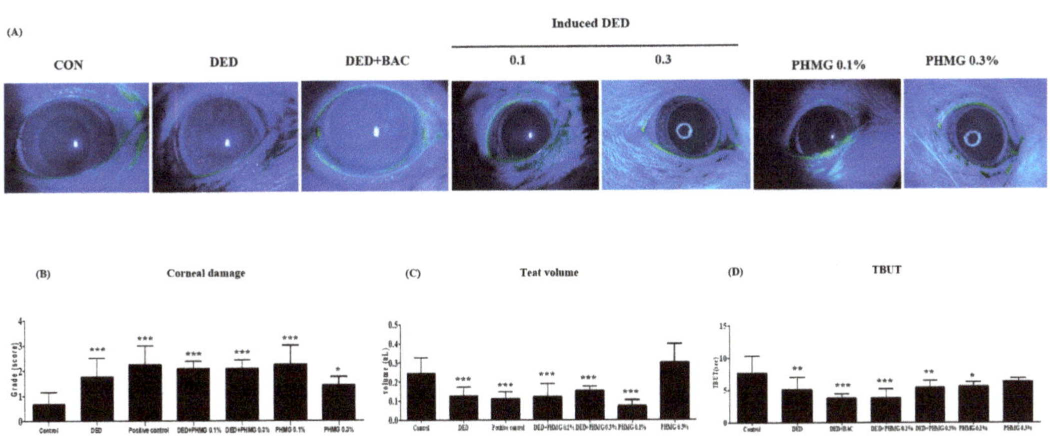

Figure 1. Images of the eyes of rat in the control groups, DED induced group, positive control group and PHMG-p treated groups were photographed with a microscope after 13 day desiccation stress and after the instillation of scopolamine eye drops. (**A**) Corneal fluorescein staining. (**B**) Corneal damage. (**C**) Tear volume. (**D**) Tear break-up time (TBUT). * $p < 0.05$, ** $p < 0.01$, *** $p < 0.001$ compared with the control group.

2.2. Tear Volume

The mean tear volumes across the experimental groups are summarized as follows. In the control group, the tear volume was 0.24 ± 0.08 μL. In the DED group, the tear volume was reduced to 0.13 ± 0.05 μL, confirming a significant decrease in tear production and the successful induction of DED compared to the control group. In the PC group (DED + BAC), treated with benzalkonium chloride (0.1%) after DED induction, the tear volume was further reduced to 0.11 ± 0.04 μL, showing an exacerbation of DED symptoms. The groups treated with 0.1% or 0.3% PHMG-p after DED induction exhibited mean tear volumes of 0.12 ± 0.07 μL and 0.15 ± 0.02 μL, respectively, while the groups treated with PHMG-p (0.1% or 0.3%) alone had mean tear volumes of 0.07 ± 0.03 μL and 0.30 ± 0.10 μL, respectively. All groups, except for the group treated with 0.3% PHMG-p alone, showed significant differences compared to the control group (Figure 1C).

2.3. Tear Break-Up Time (TBUT)

The TBUT results of the control group and the DED group were 7.63 ± 2.64 s and 5.08 ± 1.92 s, respectively, after 13 days of exposure to desiccation stress. The PC group showed a TBUT of 3.79 ± 0.70 s. The groups treated with 0.1% or 0.3% PHMG-p after DED induction had TBUT values of 3.81 ± 1.37 s and 5.40 ± 1.12 s, respectively, while the groups treated with PHMG-p alone had TBUT values of 5.57 ± 0.69 s and 6.32 ± 0.50 s, respectively. Compared to the control group, TBUT was significantly reduced in all groups except for the group treated with only PHMG-p 0.3% (Figure 1D). TBUT was calculated using the mean of three measurements.

2.4. Conjunctival Goblet Cell Counts

The total number of goblet cells in the control group was 89 ± 8.66 cells/mm^2, while in the DED group, the goblet cell count was significantly reduced to 17 ± 13.75 cells/mm^2. The PC group exhibited a further reduction in goblet cell count, with 3 ± 5.20 cells/mm^2. In the DED + PHMG-p 0.1% and DED + PHMG-p 0.3% groups, the goblet cell counts were 0.33 ± 0.58 cells/mm^2 and 38 ± 4.37 cells/mm^2, respectively. The PHMG-p 0.1% group showed a goblet cell count of 3 ± 3.61 cells/mm^2, while the PHMG-p 0.3% group demonstrated 75.5 ± 7.00 cells/mm^2. Compared to the control group, the goblet cell count was significantly reduced in all groups except for the group treated with only PHMG-p 0.3%. Representative histological findings of goblet cell counts in each group are presented in Figure 2.

2.5. Inflammatory Cytokine Concentrations in the Cornea

The expression levels of IL-6, IL-1β, and TNF-α in the corneal tissue were assessed and are shown in Figure 3A. The DED group exhibited a significant increase in all three pro-inflammatory cytokines compared to the control group. The PC group also showed elevated cytokine levels, although the increase was less pronounced compared to the DED group for some markers. In the groups treated with PHMG-p after DED induction, IL-6 and TNF-α levels were significantly elevated in the DED + PHMG-p 0.3% group compared to the control group. IL-1β levels were similarly increased in the DED + PHMG-p 0.3% group, while the DED + PHMG-p 0.1% group exhibited moderately elevated cytokine levels. In the PHMG-p-only groups, IL-6, IL-1β, and TNF-α were slightly increased in the PHMG-p 0.1% group but remained lower than those observed in the DED + PHMG-p groups. The PHMG-p 0.3% only group showed relatively lower cytokine expression levels compared to DED + PHMG-p 0.3%. Representative histological images of IL-1β, IL-6, and TNF-α staining are presented in Figure 3B. Immunohistochemical staining revealed positive immunoreactivity for IL-6, IL-1β, and TNF-α in the DED and DED + PHMG-p groups (indicated by red arrows). These groups exhibited dense chromogenic deposition, suggesting enhanced inflammatory signaling in the corneal tissue. In contrast, weaker or minimal staining was observed in the control and PHMG-p-only groups, indicating relatively low basal cytokine expression. The staining intensity and distribution correspond well with the quantified data shown in Figure 3A, highlighting the pro-inflammatory effects of DED and PHMG-p exposure at the tissue level.

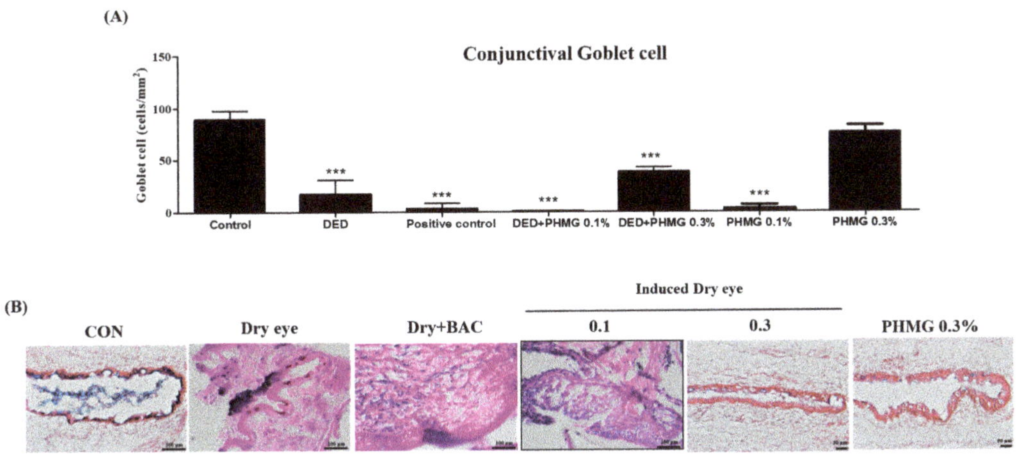

Figure 2. Effect of control groups, DED induced group, positive control group and PHMG-p treated groups on detached conjunctive goblet cell of the rats. (**A**) Quantitative analysis of conjunctive goblet cell density (cells/mm^2) in each group. (**B**) Representative histological image of conjunctive goblet cell. The result of each group are shown as mean ± SD. *** $p < 0.001$ compared with the control group.

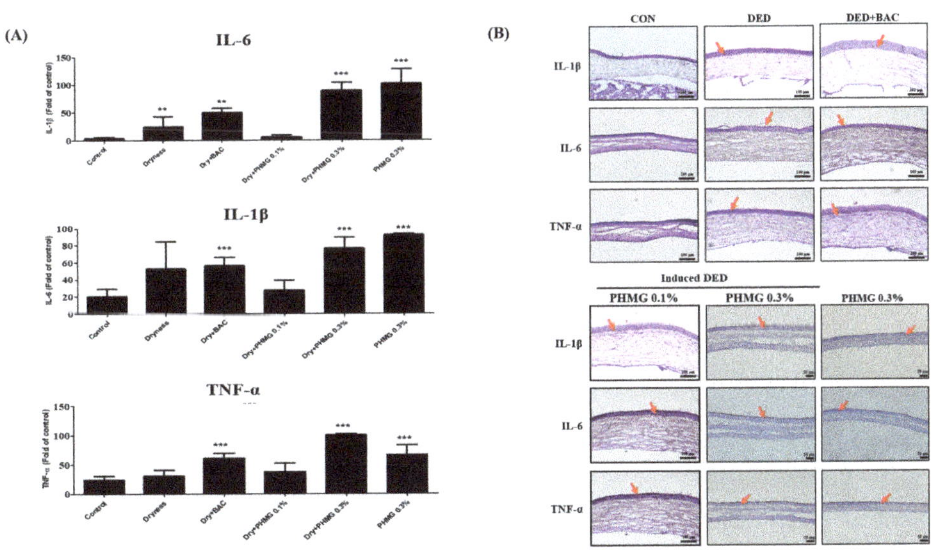

Figure 3. The change of immune index markers in the cornea epithelium of the rats. (**A**) Quantitative analysis of IL-6, IL-1β, and TNF-α expression in the cornea epithelium. (**B**) Representative immunohistochemical images. Values are shown as mean ± SD. ** $p < 0.01$, *** $p < 0.001$ compared with the control group. Red arrows indicate cytokine expression.

2.6. Plasma NMR Profile

NMR spectra for plasma samples of control or treated groups were obtained. The spectral region of δ0.0–10 was segmented into regions of 0.04 ppm width, providing 250 integrated regions in each NMR spectrum for plasma samples. Visual examination of NMR spectra displayed different intensities of several metabolites between groups. The spectral binning data were obtained through NMR analysis of S–D rat plasma samples.

The global profiling data exhibited clear clustering among the control, DED, PC, and PHMG-p-treated groups on the principal component analysis (PCA). Additionally, the orthogonal projections to latent structures discriminant analysis (OPLS-DA) data showed a clear separation of clusters between the groups, as analyzed using the SIMCA-P multivariate analysis program (Figure 4A,B). A total of 41 endogenous metabolites were identified using Chenomx NMR Suite ver. 8.3 (Chenomx Inc., Edmonton, AB, Canada) in plasma samples of control, DED, PC group and PHMG-p-treated groups. The score plots of PCA and OPLS-DA in plasma target profiling demonstrated clearly discriminable clustering between groups. The VIP showed sorting of endogenous metabolites in the order of contribution to the separation of clustering (Figure 5). Significant metabolites were selected according to a VIP value of more than 0.5, which determined meaningfully important metabolites (Figure 5C). In addition, we compared the results with the DED-related metabolites identified in our previous study [44]. In a previous study, the major metabolites associated with DED were identified as 1,3-dimethylurate, 2-hydroxyisobutyrate, alanine, citrate, creatine, glucose, glutamate, lactate, N-nitrosodimethylamine, and succinate. A total of 20 major plasma metabolites were selected in the present study, including 2-hydroxyisobutyrate, 3-hydroxybutyrate, acetate, alanine, arginine, citrate, creatine, glucose, glutamate, glutamine, glycerol, glycine, isoleucine, lactate, leucine, pyruvate, serine, succinate, threonine, and valine. Among them, eight metabolites—2-hydroxyisobutyrate, alanine, citrate, creatine, glucose, glutamate, lactate, and succinate—were identified, which were the same as those reported in the previous study [45]. Figure 6 shows the changes in metabolites for each group.

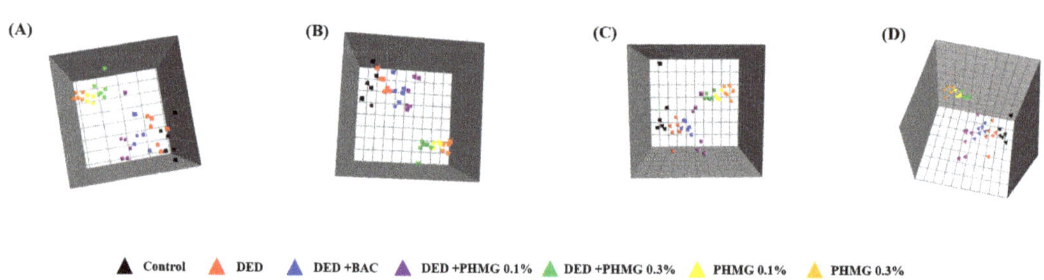

Figure 4. In global profiling, principal component analysis (PCA) ($R^2X = 0.749$, $Q^2 = 0.666$) models (**A**) and orthogonal projections to latent structures-discriminant analysis (OPLS-DA) ($R^2X = 0.738$, $R^2Y = 0.181$, $Q^2 = 0.0871$) models (**B**) results after NMR analysis of control, DED group and PHMG-p treated groups in plasma samples. Global profiling of PCA ($R^2X = 0.883$, $Q^2 = 0.825$) (**C**) and OPLS-DA ($R^2X = 0.882$, $R^2Y = 0.174$, $Q^2 = 0.0955$) (**D**) using NMR data from urine samples. ▲, Control; ▲, DED group; ▲, DED + BAC; ▲, DED + PHMG-p 0.1%; ▲, DED + PHMG-p 0.3%; ▲, PHMG-p 0.1%; ▲, PHMG-p 0.3%.

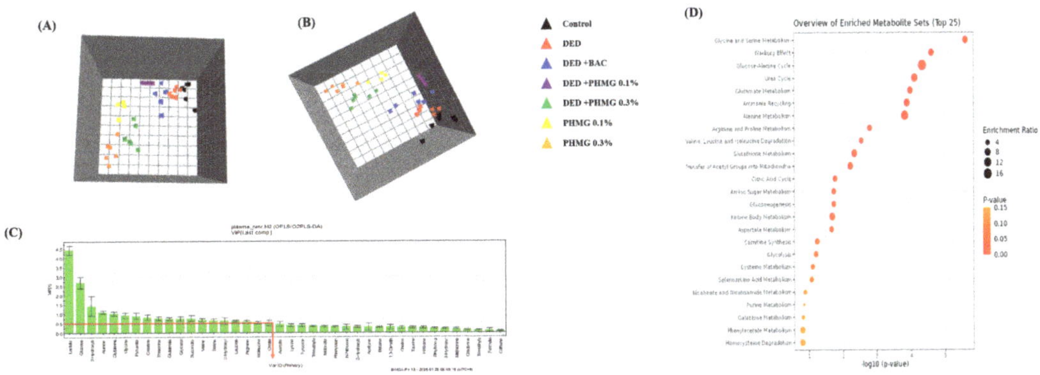

Figure 5. In target profiling, principal component analysis (PCA) ($R^2X = 0.947$, $Q^2 = 0.816$) models (**A**) and orthogonal projections to latent structures-discriminant analysis (OPLS-DA) ($R^2X = 0.991$, $R^2Y = 0.585$, $Q^2 = 0.109$) models (**B**) results after NMR analysis of control and DED group in plasma sample. Variable importance plot (VIP) (**C**) shows the major urine metabolites that contributed to separate the clusters. Metabolites set enrichment overview in plasma samples (**D**). ▲, Control; ▲, DED group; ▲, DED + BAC; ▲, DED + PHMG-p 0.1%; ▲, DED + PHMG-p 0.3%; ▲, PHMG-p 0.1%; ▲, PHMG-p 0.3%.

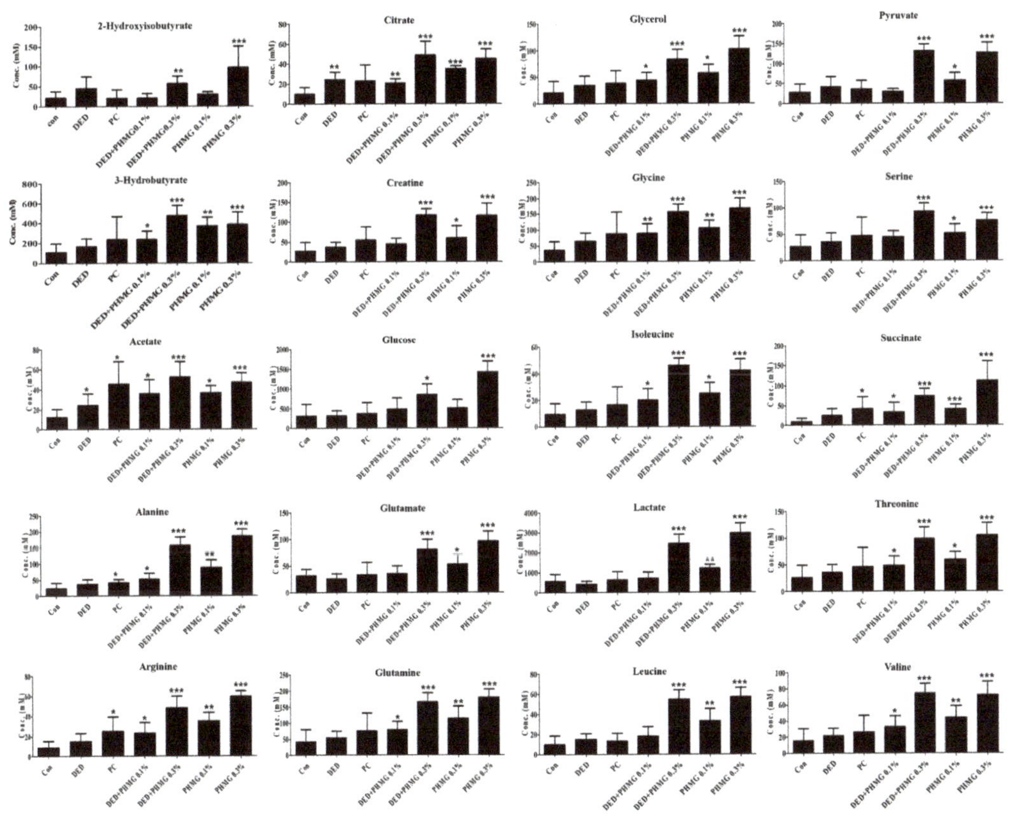

Figure 6. Concentrations of endogenous metabolites in plasma samples for DED induced and PHMG-p treatment to rats. ANOVA test was performed to assess statistical significance compared with control and treatment. Error bars are expressed as S.D. * $p < 0.05$, ** $p < 0.01$, *** $p < 0.001$.

After performing pathway analysis for the selected metabolites using the MetaboAnalyst 6.0 program (http://www.metaboanalyst.ca (accessed on 11 November 2024)) [48], 21 metabolic pathways were predicted in plasma samples. Among these pathways, glycine and serine metabolism, glutamate metabolism, arginine and proline metabolism, glutathione metabolism, the citric acid cycle, amino sugar metabolism, and fatty acid biosynthesis were identified (Table 1). Figure 7 illustrates the expected changes in plasma metabolic pathways in the PHMG-p-treated group after DED induction.

Table 1. Expected pathway based on high-VIP-scored (VIP > 0.5) metabolites in rat plasma using MetaboAnalyst (6.0).

Plasma							
Pathway	**Total**	**Expected**	**Hits**	***p* Value**	**−log(*p*)**	**Holm Adjust**	**FDR**
Glycine and Serine Metabolism	59	1.06	8	2.48×10^{-6}	0.000243	0.000243	0.000243
Glucose-Alanine Cycle	13	0.234	4	4.73×10^{-5}	0.00454	0.00155	0.00155
Urea Cycle	28	0.503	5	7.85×10^{-5}	0.00746	0.00192	0.00192
Glutamate Metabolism	48	0.862	6	0.000106	0.00994	0.00207	0.00207
Ammonia Recycling	31	0.557	5	0.000131	0.0122	0.00211	0.00211
Alanine Metabolism	17	0.305	4	0.000151	0.0139	0.00211	0.00211
Arginine and Proline Metabolism	52	0.934	5	0.00159	0.145	0.0195	0.0195
Valine, Leucine and Isoleucine Degradation	59	1.06	5	0.00283	0.255	0.0308	0.0308
Glutathione Metabolism	20	0.359	3	0.00459	0.409	0.045	0.045
Transfer of Acetyl Groups into Mitochondria	22	0.395	3	0.00606	0.533	0.054	0.054
Citric Acid Cycle	32	0.575	3	0.0174	1	0.133	0.133
Amino Sugar Metabolism	33	0.593	3	0.019	1	0.133	0.133
Gluconeogenesis	33	0.593	3	0.019	1	0.133	0.133
Ketone Body Metabolism	13	0.234	2	0.0212	1	0.136	0.136
Aspartate Metabolism	35	0.629	3	0.0222	1	0.136	0.136
Carnitine Synthesis	22	0.395	2	0.0569	1	0.328	0.328
Glycolysis	23	0.413	2	0.0617	1	0.336	0.336
Cysteine Metabolism	26	0.467	2	0.0768	1	0.396	0.396
Selenoamino Acid Metabolism	27	0.485	2	0.0821	1	0.402	0.402
Nicotinate and Nicotinamide Metabolism	35	0.629	2	0.128	1	0.544	0.544
Fatty Acid Biosynthesis	35	0.629	1	0.476	1	0.992	0.992

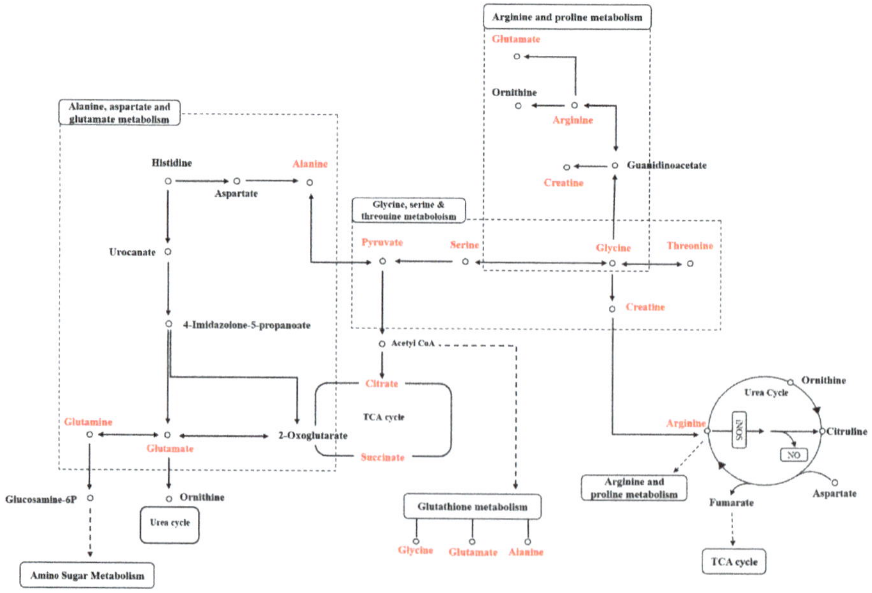

Figure 7. Expected plasma metabolic pathway network of metabolites related to PHMG-p exposure.

2.7. Urinary NMR Profile

NMR spectra for urine samples of control or treated groups were obtained. The spectral region of δ0.0–10 was segmented into regions of 0.04 ppm width, providing 250 integrated regions in each NMR spectrum for urine samples. Visual examination of NMR spectra displayed different intensities of several metabolites between groups.

The global profiling data showed clear separation of clustering among the control, DED, PC, and PHMG-p-treated groups on the par-scale of PCA and OPLS-DA models (Figure 4C,D). A total of 88 endogenous metabolites were identified using Chenomx NMR Suite ver. 8.3 (Chenomx Inc., Edmonton, AL, Canada) in the urine samples of each group. PCA and OPLS-DA score plots in urinary target profiling exhibited clear discrimination of clustering between groups (Figure 8). VIP demonstrated sorting of endogenous metabolites in the order of contribution to separation of clustering. Significant metabolites were selected according to a VIP value of more than 0.5, which determined meaningfully important metabolites (Figure 8C).

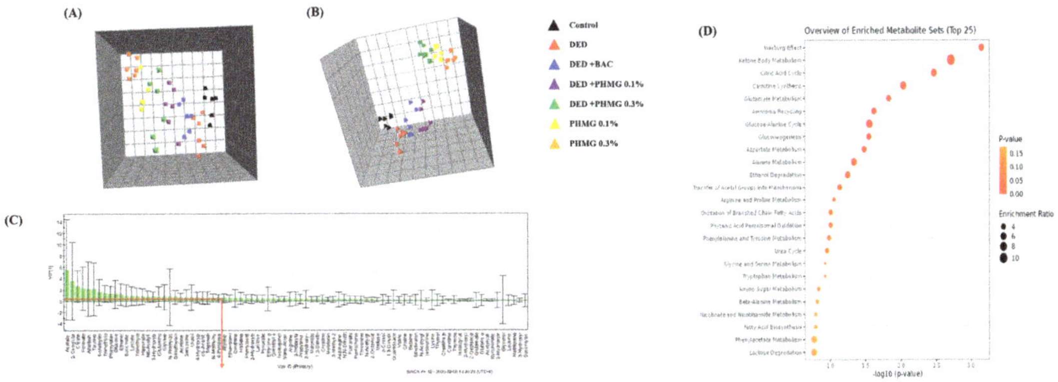

Figure 8. Principal component analysis (PCA) ($R^2X = 0.463$, $Q^2 = 0.0756$) (**A**) model and orthogonal projections to latent structures-discriminant analysis (OPLS-DA) ($R^2X = 0.832$, $R^2Y = 0.586$, $Q^2 = 0.31$) (**B**) in target profiling of urine samples. Variable importance plot (VIP) (**C**) shows the major urine metabolites that contributed to separate the clusters. Metabolites set enrichment overview in urine samples (**D**). ▲, Control; ▲, DED group; ▲, DED+BAC; ▲, DED+PHMG-p 0.1%; ▲, DED+PHMG-p 0.3%; ▲, PHMG-p 0.1%; ▲, PHMG-p 0.3%.

In a previous study, 26 urinary metabolites were screened in the DED group, among which phenylalanine, phenylacetate, pantothenate, glycine, succinate, methanol, valine, propylene glycol, histidine, threonine, lactate, and acetate showed significant differences [45]. In this study, a total of 36 major urinary metabolites were identified, including 1-methylnicotinamide, 2-oxoglutarate, 3-hydroxybutyrate, 4-hydroxyphenylacetate, 4-pyridoxate, acetate, acetone, allantoin, asparagine, cis-aconitate, citrate, dimethylamine, ethanol, ethylene glycol, formate, glucose, glutamine, glycine, hippurate, lactate, lysine, N6-acetyllysine, N-acetylglycine, N-methylhydantoin, N-phenylacetylglycine, ornithine, phenylalanine, propylene glycol, sarcosine, succinate, succinylacetone, taurine, trigonelline, trimethylamine, trimethylamine N-oxide, and uracil. Among them, 12 metabolites were identical to those reported in previous studies: acetate, cis-aconitate, glycine, lactate, N6-acetyllysine, N-methylhydantoin, phenylalanine, propylene glycol, sarcosine, succinate, taurine, and trimethylamine. Figure 9 shows the changes in metabolites for each group.

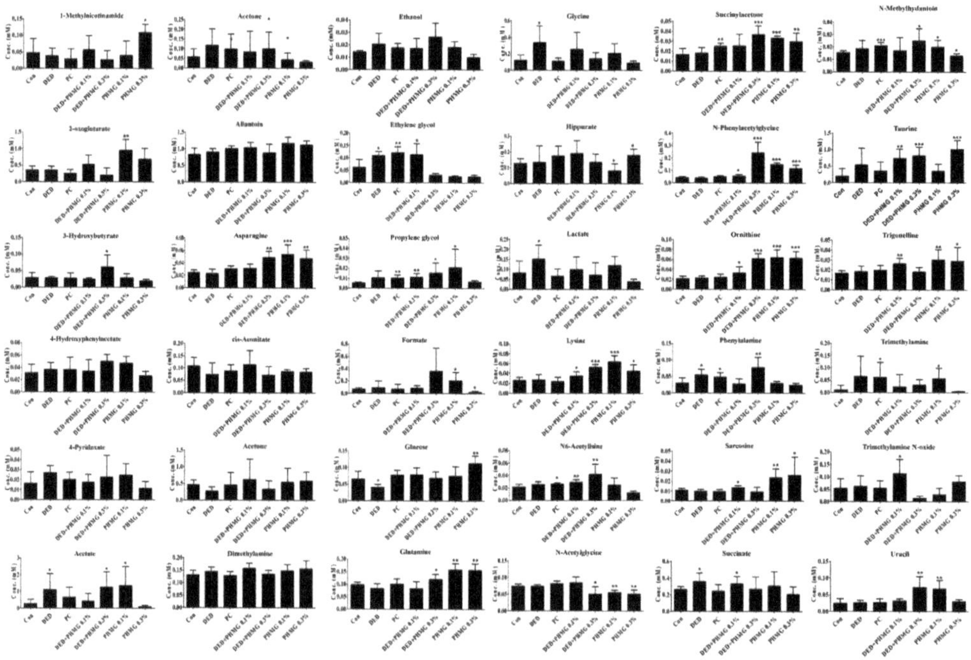

Figure 9. Concentrations of endogenous metabolites in urine samples for DED induced and PHMG-p treatment to rats. ANOVA test was performed to assess statistical significance compared with control and treatment. Error bars are expressed as S.D. * $p < 0.05$, ** $p < 0.01$, *** $p < 0.001$.

Pathway analysis for the selected metabolites in urine samples was also performed in the same manner as for plasma samples, and 26 metabolic pathways were predicted. The predicted metabolic pathways include the citric acid cycle, glutamate metabolism, aspartate metabolism, arginine and proline metabolism, glycine and serine metabolism, amino sugar metabolism, fatty acid biosynthesis, and taurine and hypotaurine metabolism (Table 2). The expected changes in urinary metabolic pathways in the PHMG-p-treated group after DED induction are illustrated in Figure 10.

Table 2. Expected pathway based on high-VIP-scored (VIP > 0.5) metabolites in rat urine using MetaboAnalyst (6.0).

			Urine				
Pathway	**Total**	**Expected**	**Hits**	***p* Value**	**−log(*p*)**	**Holm Adjust**	**FDR**
Ketone Body Metabolism	13	0.272	3	0.00199	0.193	0.0973	0.0973
Citric Acid Cycle	32	0.671	4	0.00351	0.337	0.115	0.115
Carnitine Synthesis	22	0.461	3	0.00946	0.899	0.232	0.232
Glutamate Metabolism	48	1.01	4	0.0152	1	0.298	0.298
Ammonia Recycling	31	0.65	3	0.0245	1	0.354	0.354
Glucose-Alanine Cycle	13	0.272	2	0.0284	1	0.354	0.354
Gluconeogenesis	33	0.692	3	0.0289	1	0.354	0.354
Aspartate Metabolism	35	0.734	3	0.0337	1	0.367	0.367
Alanine Metabolism	17	0.356	2	0.0471	1	0.462	0.462
Ethanol Degradation	19	0.398	2	0.0577	1	0.514	0.514
Transfer of Acetyl Groups into Mitochondria	22	0.461	2	0.0751	1	0.614	0.614
Arginine and Proline Metabolism	52	1.09	3	0.0906	1	0.626	0.626
Oxidation of Branched Chain Fatty Acids	26	0.545	2	0.101	1	0.626	0.626
Phytanic Acid Peroxisomal Oxidation	26	0.545	2	0.101	1	0.626	0.626
Phenylalanine and Tyrosine Metabolism	27	0.566	2	0.107	1	0.626	0.626

Table 2. *Cont.*

Pathway	Total	Expected	Hits	*p* Value	−log(*p*)	Holm Adjust	FDR
		Urine					
Urea Cycle	28	0.587	2	0.114	1	0.626	0.626
Glycine and Serine Metabolism	59	1.24	3	0.121	1	0.626	0.626
Tryptophan Metabolism	59	1.24	3	0.121	1	0.626	0.626
Amino Sugar Metabolism	33	0.692	2	0.15	1	0.683	0.683
Beta-Alanine Metabolism	34	0.713	2	0.157	1	0.683	0.683
Nicotinate and Nicotinamide Metabolism	35	0.734	2	0.165	1	0.683	0.683
Fatty Acid Biosynthesis	35	0.734	2	0.165	1	0.683	0.683
Phenylacetate Metabolism	9	0.189	1	0.174	1	0.683	0.683
Lactose Degradation	9	0.189	1	0.174	1	0.683	0.683
Malate-Aspartate Shuttle	10	0.21	1	0.192	1	0.722	0.722
Taurine and Hypotaurine Metabolism	12	0.251	1	0.226	1	0.762	0.762

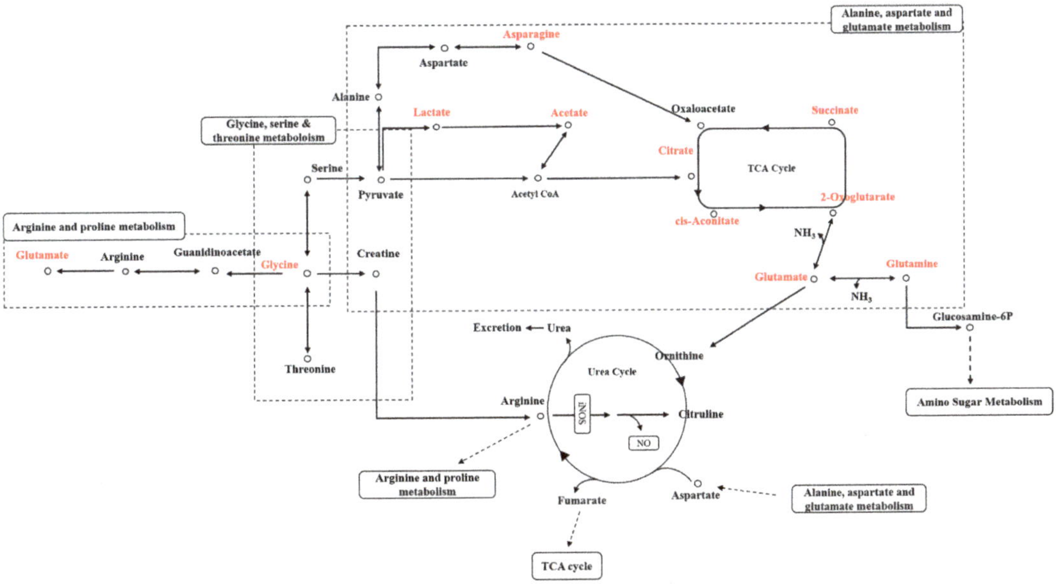

Figure 10. Expected urinary metabolic pathway network of metabolites related to PHMG-p exposure.

3. Discussion

In our previous study, we induced DED in rats and used a metabolomics approach to develop biomarkers and elucidate the mechanisms underlying DED [45,46]. The present study investigated the effects of polyhexamethylene guanidine phosphate (PHMG-p), a humidifier disinfectant component, on DED using a rat model and metabolomic analysis.

Several studies have investigated the ocular effects of polyhexamethylene guanidine (PHMG), highlighting its potential toxicity and concentration-dependent impact on eye health. A study by Lee et al. (2021) examined the role of fibrosis as a manifestation of PHMG toxicity in the eye using Statens Seruminstitut Rabbit Cornea (SIRC) cells [49]. The study demonstrated that PHMG exposure led to an increased expression of fibrosis-related biomarkers, including TGF-β, α-SMA, MMPs, and TIMPs, at both the gene and protein levels. Furthermore, oxidative stress levels were significantly elevated in PHMG-treated cells, supporting the hypothesis that PHMG can induce fibrosis in the cornea. Another study by Park et al. (2019) evaluated the eye irritation potential of PHMG using a reconstructed human cornea-like epithelium model (EpiOcular™) [50]. The results indicated that raw

PHMG materials, with an active ingredient concentration of 26%, were classified under UN GHS Category 1 (serious eye damage) or Category 2 (eye irritation). However, when PHMG solutions were diluted to 0.13% or lower, no significant eye irritation was observed at the tested concentrations. A more recent systematic review by Ivanov et al. (2024) provided a comprehensive assessment of PHMG's toxicity and safety through various exposure routes, including ocular contact [51]. The review concluded that PHMG-p solutions below 0.13% appear to be safe for the human corneal epithelium. However, despite this, even low concentrations of PHMG have been associated with corneal fibrosis, as demonstrated in animal studies. These findings suggest that while diluted PHMG solutions may not cause immediate eye irritation, chronic exposure could still pose a long-term risk to corneal health, particularly through fibrotic changes and oxidative stress-related damage. Although several studies have reported on PHMG and ocular health, no studies have directly investigated its link to DED. Meanwhile, since humidifiers were often recommended for the treatment of DED, this study aimed to explore the potential role of PHMG-p, a component of humidifier disinfectants, in aggravating ocular surface damage and metabolic disorders.

In the present study, changes in conjunctival goblet cell (CGC) density and corneal inflammatory cytokines (IL-6, IL-1β, and TNF-α) were observed, aligning with previous findings. Several studies have investigated the relationship between DED and alterations in CGC numbers, emphasizing their critical role in maintaining tear film stability through mucin secretion. The loss of goblet cells has been strongly implicated in the pathogenesis of DED. Experimental mouse models of DED have demonstrated that DED induction promotes the migration of $CD4^+$ T cells and IFN-γ^+ cells into conjunctival goblet cell zones, leading to progressive goblet cell loss [52]. This immune-mediated response contributes to tear film instability and ocular surface damage commonly observed in DED. More recently, a 2023 study utilized moxifloxacin-based fluorescence microscopy (MBFM) to noninvasively assess goblet cell changes in DED-induced mice [53]. The results revealed a significant reduction in goblet cell density (GCD) and goblet cell area (GCA) in DED mice compared to controls, further supporting the role of goblet cell loss in DED progression [53]. In our study, the number of conjunctival goblet cells (CGCs) was lower in the PHMG-p-treated group after DED induction compared to the DED group, except in the 0.3% PHMG-p only group. These findings confirm that PHMG-p exposure exacerbates DED. Notably, reduction in conjunctival goblet cell (CGC) was not as pronounced in the 0.3% PHMG-p only treated group compared to other groups is likely due to the strong cytotoxicity of high-dose PHMG-p, which may have suppressed immune cell activity. At higher concentrations, intense cytotoxic effects may have inhibited the immune response or induced early cell death, ultimately protecting goblet cells from immune-mediated damage. This finding suggests a concentration-dependent biphasic effect, where lower concentrations of PHMG-p may promote immune activation and inflammatory responses, while higher concentrations may lead to immune suppression and reduced inflammation, resulting in less goblet cell damage.

Additionally, several studies have established a strong association between DED and elevated levels of inflammatory cytokines, particularly IL-1β, IL-6, and TNF-α. These cytokines play a critical role in the pathogenesis and progression of DED, contributing to ocular surface inflammation and tear film instability. Research has consistently shown that IL-1β, IL-6, and TNF-α levels are significantly elevated in the tears and serum of DED patients compared to healthy controls [16,54,55]. Furthermore, a meta-analysis by Roda et al. (2020) confirmed that DED patients exhibit higher levels of these pro-inflammatory cytokines, reinforcing their role in the chronic inflammatory state characteristic of DED [55]. In our study, similar to previous studies, IL-1β, IL-6, and TNF-α levels tended to increase compared to the control group and were further elevated in the PHMG-p only group.

In our previous study, we identified biomarkers of DED through plasma and urinary metabolic profiling [45]. Plasma and urine metabolic profiling provide valuable insights into biochemical processes and have significant applications in research and clinical settings. One of the key advantages of urine metabolic profiling is its non-invasive nature, making sample collection more convenient and patient-friendly [56,57]. Additionally, both plasma and urine contain metabolic signatures from various biochemical pathways, offering a holistic representation of an individual's metabolic status [58]. Another critical advantage of metabolic profiling is its role in biomarker discovery, enabling the identification of potential biomarkers for early disease detection, diagnosis, and prognosis [56,59,60]. Furthermore, urine provides a broader metabolite coverage as it contains end-products from multiple organs, reflecting systemic metabolic changes more comprehensively [56]. Also, urine samples exhibit high stability, making them ideal for metabolomic analysis [61]. By offering a comprehensive and quantitative assessment of metabolic processes, plasma and urine metabolic profiling serve as powerful tools for advancing our understanding of human health, disease mechanisms, and therapeutic monitoring.

In our study, clearer clustering observed in the plasma PCA profile compared to the urinary NMR profile likely reflects inherent differences in biological variability and metabolic dynamics between these two matrices. Plasma provides a more immediate snapshot of systemic metabolic changes, especially in response to acute toxicological stress, such as PHMG-p exposure. In contrast, urine reflects a time-averaged excretory profile that is influenced by hydration status, renal function, and other confounding physiological factors, which may contribute to relatively blurred clustering. Nevertheless, urine remains a valuable biological matrix in metabolomics due to its non-invasive nature, wide metabolite coverage, and ability to capture cumulative metabolic alterations. In our findings, although plasma offered clearer group separation, urinary analysis still yielded meaningful insights—particularly in identifying overlapping pathways such as glutamate, glycine, and citrate metabolism. These complementary features underscore the advantage of integrating both plasma and urine profiles to enhance the overall interpretation of systemic toxicity.

Our findings confirmed that many metabolic pathways were shared between plasma and urinary metabolic profiling, with the following pathways being consistent: alanine metabolism, amino sugar metabolism, ammonia recycling, arginine and proline metabolism, aspartate metabolism, carnitine synthesis, the citric acid cycle, fatty acid biosynthesis, gluconeogenesis, the glucose-alanine cycle, glutamate metabolism, glycine and serine metabolism, ketone body metabolism, nicotinate and nicotinamide metabolism, transfer of acetyl groups into mitochondria, and the urea cycle (Tables 1 and 2). Among these, the metabolic pathways associated with DED include arginine and proline metabolism, the citric acid cycle, glutamate metabolism, and glycine and serine metabolism, among others, which will be discussed in detail below [42,47]. Notably, among the pathways related to dry eye disease, glutathione metabolism was the only one that differed between plasma and urine.

For the plasma and urinary metabolites arginine, glutamate, glutamine, glycine, and pyruvate, their involvement in pathways such as arginine and proline metabolism, glutamate metabolism, glycine and serine metabolism, and the urea cycle has been confirmed. These metabolites show a significant correlation with inflammatory cytokines, including TNF-α, IL-6, and IL-1β. In the current study, glutamine and glutamate was upregulated in PHMG-p treated group in both plasma or urine (Figures 6 and 9). Glutamine plays a vital role in regulating inflammatory responses by supporting lymphocyte proliferation and cytokine production, making it essential for immune homeostasis. Studies have shown that glutamine supplementation reduces pro-inflammatory cytokine levels in the gut mucosa, including IL-1β, IL-6, and TNF-α, suggesting that glutamine availability can modulate immune activation and inflammatory pathways, contributing to a more controlled immune response [62]. In contrast, elevated extracellular glutamate levels have been linked to increased inflammation, particularly through neuroimmune interactions. Inflammatory processes can cause glutamate spillover into the extrasynaptic space, often as a result of glial dysfunction. This excess glutamate further exacerbates immune responses by activating microglial receptors, leading to the release of pro-inflammatory cytokines, such as TNF-α and IL-1β [63]. These findings highlight the dual role of glutamine and glutamate in inflammatory regulation, with glutamine acting as an anti-inflammatory agent, while excessive glutamate contributes to neuroinflammation and cytokine activation. Additionally, glutamate metabolism plays a critical role in inflammation and oxidative stress. Since glutamine can be converted to glutamate, it has been identified as an anti-inflammatory agent by inhibiting the production of reactive oxygen species (ROS), nitric oxide synthase (NOS), inducible nitric oxide synthase (iNOS), and cyclooxygenase-2 (COX-2), all of which are key mediators of inflammation [63]. Furthermore, glutamine suppresses NF-κB activation and inhibits the phosphorylation of STAT1, STAT5, and Akt, leading to reduced levels of TNF-α and IFN-γ [64]. However, at high concentrations, glutamate can induce oxidative stress and apoptosis in cerebral vascular endothelial cells, contributing to neuroinflammation and vascular damage [65]. These findings underscore the complex role of glutamate metabolism in inflammation, balancing both protective and detrimental effects depending on its concentration and metabolic context.

Glycine exhibits a significant anti-inflammatory effect by modulating the production and activity of pro-inflammatory cytokines, particularly TNF-α, IL-6, and IL-1β. Studies have demonstrated that glycine inhibits the production of these cytokines in various cell types and tissues, thereby contributing to the suppression of inflammatory responses [66,67]. This reduction in pro-inflammatory cytokine levels plays a crucial role in mitigating systemic inflammation, highlighting glycine's potential as a therapeutic agent for inflammatory conditions. Beyond its anti-inflammatory properties, glycine is actively involved in glycine and serine metabolism, which is essential for immune regulation and cellular function. One of glycine's key mechanisms in inflammation control is its ability to reduce calcium influx in macrophages, thereby inhibiting the production of toxic free radicals and ultimately reducing oxidative stress and tissue damage [64]. According to our study results, glycine levels were upregulated in all experimental groups compared to the control in plasma, and showed an increasing trend in urine, except in the PHMG-p 0.3% group (Figures 6 and 9). This suggests that glycine levels may have increased in response to suppress the elevation of inflammatory cytokines TNF-α, IL-6, and IL-1β. These findings indicate that glycine and serine metabolism not only regulate inflammatory pathways but also contribute to disease progression in various pathological conditions, including immune-related disorders.

Pyruvate levels were up-regulated in the plasma after DED induction in the high-dose PHMG-p group and in the PHMG-p only group (Figure 6). Pyruvate levels typically increase during inflammation and oxidative stress, representing a metabolic adaptation to cellular stress. This elevation is associated with several protective mechanisms, as pyruvate and lactate contribute to oxidative stress resistance by inducing a mild hormetic increase in reactive oxygen species (ROS). This transient ROS surge activates antioxidant defenses and pro-survival pathways, ultimately enhancing cellular protection [68]. Additionally, pyruvate supplementation has been shown to suppress mitochondrial ROS generation and maintain mitochondrial membrane potential under oxidative stress conditions, highlighting mitochondria as key targets of pyruvate's protective effects [69]. The rise in pyruvate levels during inflammation and oxidative stress may serve a protective function by modulating mitochondrial activity and maintaining redox balance, ultimately supporting cell survival and adaptation [68,69]. These findings suggest that pyruvate plays a critical role in cellular defense mechanisms against oxidative damage. Beyond its role in oxidative stress regulation, pyruvate is a key player in immune cell metabolism. Although not directly part of the TCA cycle, pyruvate serves as a crucial metabolic intermediary that influences immune cell activation and function. In activated immune cells, pyruvate is preferentially converted to lactate rather than entering the TCA cycle, a metabolic shift that supports immune cell activation and proliferation by facilitating glycolytic reprogramming [70]. However, a portion of pyruvate can still enter the TCA cycle to produce citrate, which is then exported to the cytosol to participate in immune-related functions, such as lipid biosynthesis and inflammatory signaling [71].

In our study, arginine levels were increased in plasma across all experimental groups (Figure 6). Arginine plays a crucial role in the urea cycle and nitric oxide (NO) production, making it an essential component in inflammation and oxidative stress regulation [64]. The urea cycle is closely linked to arginine metabolism, as it facilitates nitrogen excretion while also contributing to NO synthesis, which has significant implications for immune function and vascular homeostasis [64]. During inflammatory responses, macrophage M1 polarization promotes the expression of inducible nitric oxide synthase (iNOS), which utilizes arginine to generate NO. This process enhances the antimicrobial and immunomodulatory effects of macrophages while also inhibiting reactive oxygen species (ROS) activity, thereby influencing redox balance and inflammatory signaling [64]. Furthermore, arginine is synthesized from glutamine, glutamate, and proline via the intestinal-renal axis, highlighting its interconnected role in multiple metabolic pathways. Beyond its involvement in NO synthesis, arginine also contributes to creatine biosynthesis and methylation reactions, both of which are critical for maintaining cellular homeostasis and metabolic regulation [72].

The urea cycle is closely linked to inflammatory response, immune regulation, and oxidative stress, playing a critical role in maintaining metabolic and immune homeostasis. Disruptions in the urea cycle, such as urea cycle disorders (UCDs), can lead to hyperammonemia, which negatively affects immune cell function, particularly T cells and macrophages [73]. Additionally, elevated levels of certain amino acids, including glutamine, glycine, and alanine, in UCDs may influence T and B cell activity, further impacting immune function [73]. In our study, glutamine and glycine were increased in both plasma and urine, whereas alanine tended to increase only in plasma (Figures 6 and 9). Beyond its metabolic role, the urea cycle is essential for proper immune responses, particularly in T-cell function. UCDs have been associated with significant immune dysfunctions, including impaired T-cell proliferation [73]. Arginine, a key intermediate in the urea cycle, is critical for T-cell activation and function, and its depletion can lead to increased susceptibility to infections [73].

The citric acid cycle (TCA cycle) plays a fundamental role in cellular metabolism and has significant implications for inflammation, immune responses, and oxidative stress regulation. Beyond its primary function in energy production, key metabolic intermediates such as citrate, succinate, and 2-oxoglutarate act as critical signaling molecules that influence immune cell function and inflammatory processes. In our study, the plasma metabolites associated with the citric acid cycle were citrate, pyruvate, and succinate, while the urinary metabolites included cis-aconitate, citrate, 2-oxoglutarate, and succinate. All plasma metabolites showed an increase, whereas in urine, citrate, 2-oxoglutarate, and succinate exhibited an increasing trend in the PHMG-p treatment groups (Figures 6 and 9). Among these metabolites, citrate has emerged as a key immunometabolite, exerting multiple effects on inflammation and immune regulation. In pro-inflammatory macrophages, citrate accumulation promotes the production of inflammatory mediators, including prostaglandins, nitric oxide (NO), and reactive oxygen species (ROS), which further amplify immune responses [70,74]. Additionally, cytosolic citrate serves as a precursor for acetyl-CoA, which plays a crucial role in histone acetylation and epigenetic regulation, thereby influencing the expression of inflammatory genes [74]. Furthermore, citrate is essential for lipid biosynthesis, a process necessary for membrane expansion in macrophages and dendritic cells, which supports antigen presentation and cytokine production [71]. These findings highlight citrate's dual role as both a metabolic substrate and a regulatory molecule in immune responses. Similarly, succinate accumulation in activated immune cells has profound effects on inflammatory signaling. One of its key functions is stabilizing hypoxia-inducible factor 1α (HIF-1α), which enhances the expression of pro-inflammatory genes, thereby promoting immune activation [75]. Additionally, succinate oxidation by succinate dehydrogenase (SDH) drives mitochondrial ROS production, further amplifying inflammation and immune cell activation [76]. These findings underscore succinate's role as a key regulator of metabolic reprogramming in immune cells. 2-Oxoglutarate also plays a crucial role in immune cell regulation and metabolic sensing. It serves as a co-substrate for demethylases, influencing epigenetic modifications that govern immune cell differentiation and function [77]. Additionally, changes in the isocitrate-to-α-ketoglutarate ratio in pro-inflammatory macrophages serve as metabolic indicators of immune activation [70]. This suggests that 2-oxoglutarate is involved in both cellular adaptation to metabolic stress and the regulation of inflammatory responses. Overall, the Citric Acid Cycle and its intermediates play a critical role in orchestrating immune responses, inflammation, and oxidative stress regulation. These metabolites not only provide energy and biosynthetic precursors, but also function as signaling molecules that mediate metabolic reprogramming in immune cells, further influencing inflammatory and immune regulatory pathways.

Glutathione (GSH) metabolism, which occurs specifically in plasma, involves amino acids such as glycine, glutamate, and alanine and plays a crucial role in regulating inflammation, modulating immune responses, and protecting against oxidative stress. In our study, the levels of glycine, glutamate, and alanine tended to increase in the PHMG-p treatment group (Figures 6 and 9). GSH metabolism plays a critical role in regulating inflammatory responses, immune function, and oxidative stress, serving as a key antioxidant and modulator of immune cell activity. The relationship between GSH and these processes is complex, as it influences cytokine production, cell survival, and redox balance. GSH plays an essential role in modulating pro-inflammatory cytokine production in response to pathogens. Intracellular GSH levels directly regulate the release of cytokines, and GSH depletion has been shown to partially suppress pro-inflammatory responses to certain stimuli, indicating its role in immune activation [78]. Additionally, GSH contributes to cell survival in monocytes exposed to inflammatory stimuli, highlighting its importance in maintaining immune cell function under inflammatory conditions [78]. These findings suggest that GSH is not only a protective antioxidant but also a key regulator of immune homeostasis. Beyond its role in inflammation, GSH is a major cellular antioxidant, crucial for buffering reactive oxygen species (ROS) generated during immune cell activation. By neutralizing ROS, GSH prevents oxidative damage to immune cells and other cellular components, ensuring proper immune function and cellular integrity [79]. These findings underscore the essential role of GSH in controlling oxidative stress and inflammation, making it a potential target for therapeutic interventions in inflammatory and oxidative stress-related diseases.

In conclusion, this study demonstrates that exposure to PHMG-p exacerbates DED by promoting inflammatory responses on the ocular surface. Metabolomic profiling identified distinct metabolic alterations in plasma and urine, particularly in pathways related to glutamate metabolism, glycine and serine metabolism, arginine and proline metabolism, glutathione metabolism, and the citric acid cycle. These metabolic changes correlated with elevated levels of pro-inflammatory cytokines (IL-1β, IL-6, and TNF-α) in corneal and lacrimal gland tissues, reinforcing the role of inflammation in PHMG-p-induced ocular toxicity. Furthermore, glutamate and glycine levels were significantly elevated in both plasma and urine, suggesting their involvement in immune regulation and oxidative stress. The observed increase in pyruvate, succinate, and citrate highlights the role of metabolic reprogramming in inflammatory processes. Notably, arginine levels were elevated in plasma, supporting its role in nitric oxide (NO) production and immune modulation. These findings underscore the potential risks of PHMG-p exposure on ocular health, particularly for individuals using humidifiers in environments prone to DED. Additionally, the metabolomic insights provided in this study contribute to a deeper understanding of DED pathophysiology, offering new perspectives for biomarker discovery and targeted therapeutic strategies.

4. Materials and Methods

4.1. Chemicals

Polyhexamethylene guanidine phosphate (PHMG-p, 25%) was obtained from SK Chemicals (Seoul, Republic of Korea). Scopolamine hydrobromide, 4,4-dimethyl-4-silapentane-1-sulfonic acid (DSS) and 3-(trimethylsilyl)-propionic-2,2,3,3-d4 acid sodium salt (TSP) were obtained from Sigma Aldrich (St. Louis, MO, USA). Sodium azide was purchased from Bio Basic Inc. (Markham, ON, Canada).

4.2. In Vivo Animal Study Design and Experimental Procedures

Forty-two male Sprague Dawley (S-D) rats (7 weeks old, weighing 200–240 g) were purchased from Samtako Co. (Osan, Republic of Korea). The experimental protocol was reviewed and approved by the Institutional Animal Care and Use Committee of Dankook University (IACUC approval number: 2017-035). All animals were acclimatized for one week under controlled environmental conditions: a 12-h light/dark cycle (lights on from 06:00 to 18:00), ambient temperature maintained at 20–24 °C, and relative humidity at 30% ± 5%. During the acclimatization and experimental periods, standard laboratory chow (LabDiet 5L79, Orientbio Inc., Seongnam, Republic of Korea) and tap water were provided ad libitum. The rats were randomly divided into seven groups ($n = 6$ per group). Group 1 served as the untreated control. Groups 2 to 5 were assigned as dry eye disease (DED) induction groups. DED was induced by subcutaneous (SC) injection of scopolamine hydrobromide at a dose of 3 mg/kg (total 12 mg/day), administered four times daily at 9:00, 12:00, 15:00, and 18:00 for 13 consecutive days. In addition to pharmacological induction, animals in these groups were exposed to desiccating environmental stress by housing them in a dry eye chamber for 18 h per day (from 16:00 to 10:00 the following day), followed by 6 h outside the chamber [80–84]. In the positive control (PC) group (Group 3), 0.1% benzalkonium chloride (BAC) in phosphate-buffered saline (PBS) was topically instilled into both eyes once daily at 15:00, with a total of 12 applications per session at 5-min intervals, in addition to scopolamine administration and chamber exposure. Groups 4 and 5 followed the same scopolamine and desiccation regimen as Group 2, but instead received topical PHMG-p at concentrations of 0.1% and 0.3%, respectively, applied using the same method and schedule as BAC in Group 3. Groups 6 and 7 were treated with PHMG-p alone at 0.1% and 0.3%, respectively, following the same topical application schedule and environmental exposure as the other groups. To confirm successful DED induction, diagnostic assessments were conducted on day 8 of scopolamine administration. These included measurement of tear volume, tear film break-up time (TBUT), and microscopic examination of the ocular surface. On day 14, after completion of all treatments, the same diagnostic parameters were evaluated to assess the therapeutic or aggravating effects of the interventions. Final assessments included tear volume, corneal fluorescein staining scores, and TBUT. At the end of the experiment, rats were euthanized for tissue and biofluid collection. Eyeballs were carefully removed for histological evaluation. Urine samples were collected overnight in metabolic cages following the final scopolamine administration. Each urine sample was collected into a glass bottle containing 50 μL of 3% sodium azide. Blood samples were obtained via the abdominal aorta under CO_2 anesthesia using an 18-gauge needle, and centrifuged at 3000× g for 15 min at 4 °C to separate plasma. All urine and plasma samples were stored at −70 °C until further analysis.

4.3. Clinical Evaluation of Animal Models

Tear volume was measured using phenol red-impregnated cotton threads (Zone-Quick, Glendora, CA, USA). The threads were gently placed at the lateral canthus of each eye using fine forceps and removed after 20 s. The wetted length of the thread, which turned red upon contact with tears, was measured under a microscope and expressed in mm [82]. The measured length was converted to tear volume based on the manufacturer's instructions. Tear break-up time (TBUT) was assessed to evaluate tear film stability. A 1% sodium fluorescein solution was instilled into both eyes of non-anesthetized rats, and the time until the appearance of dry spots on the corneal surface after blinking was measured under cobalt blue light. The average of three repeated measurements was recorded as the TBUT. Corneal fluorescein staining was performed to assess epithelial damage. A 5% fluorescein solution was applied to the conjunctival sac, and eyes were examined under a cobalt blue light using a slit-lamp biomicroscope. Corneal damage was scored from 0 to 4 according to the severity of clinical signs, including conjunctival congestion, secretions, conjunctival edema, or edema of the eyelids.

4.4. Histological and Histochemical Analysis

Hematoxylin and eosin (H&E) staining was performed for general morphological evaluation. Whole eyes were surgically excised, fixed in 4% formalin, and embedded in optimal cutting temperature (O.C.T.) compound (Tissue-Tek, Sakura, Tokyo, Japan). Corneal and conjunctival tissues were cryosectioned at a thickness of 5 μm using a cryomicrotome, and stained with H&E. Stained sections were imaged using a virtual microscope system. Periodic acid–Schiff (PAS) staining was conducted to detect goblet cell. Cryosectioned tissues (5 μm) were treated with 0.5% periodic acid (Sigma–Aldrich, Inc, St. Louis, MO, USA, PAS kit.) for 5 min, rinsed with distilled water, and incubated with Schiff's reagent for 30 min at room temperature. After washing under running water for 5 min, the sections were counterstained with hematoxylin for 3 min, dehydrated, cleared, and mounted. Digital images of the stained tissues were obtained using a virtual microscope.

4.5. Immunohistochemistry (IHC)

Tissue slides were fixed in acetone for 15 min and then blocked with 5% bovine serum albumin (BSA) (Albumin, Bioshop Canada Inc., Burlington, ON, Canada) in PBS for 1 h at room temperature. Primary antibodies against IL-1β (Abcam, Cambridge, UK; ab9722), IL-6 (AbPRONTIER, Seoul, Republic of Korea; YF-MA10477), and TNF-α (Abcam, Cambridge,

UK; ab199013), each diluted 1:200 in 5% BSA, were applied and incubated overnight at 4 °C. After three washes in PBS (5 min each), enzyme-conjugated secondary antibodies diluted in 5% BSA were applied for 1 h at room temperature. Following another round of PBS washing, 2.5 mL of 5% BSA containing reagents A and B from the ABC kit (VECTASTAIN Elite ABC HRP Kit, Vector Laboratories, Inc., Burlingame, CA, USA; Cat. No: PK-6100) was added and incubated for 30 min. After washing with PBS for 5 min, a drop of buffer stock solution, a drop of 3,3′-diaminobenzidine (DAB) stock buffer, and 25 μL hydrogen peroxide solution of the DAB Substrate Kit (DAB Peroxidase Substrate, Vector Laboratories, Inc., 30 Ingold Road, Burlingame, CA, USA; Cat. No: SK-4100) were added to 2.5 mL 5% BSA in PBS until a browning reaction appeared. The sections were counterstained with Mayer's hematoxylin (Sigma-Aldrich, Inc, St. Louis, MO, USA) for 30 s and imaged using a virtual microscope.

4.6. ^{1}H NMR-Based Metabolomics Analysis

After thawing the plasma samples at 4 °C, a 350 μL aliquot was transferred into a microcentrifuge tube containing 350 μL of deuterated water (D_2O) solution with 4 mM TSP as an internal standard for chemical shift referencing. Urine samples were also thawed at 4 °C and centrifuged to remove particulates. A 600 μL aliquot of the urine supernatant was added to a microcentrifuge tube containing 70 μL of D_2O solution supplemented with 5 mM DSS and 100 mM imidazole. In addition, 30 μL of 0.42% sodium azide was added to each urine sample to prevent microbial growth. Following vortex mixing, all samples were subjected to ^{1}H-NMR analysis within 48 h. NMR spectra were acquired using a Varian Unity Inova 600 MHz spectrometer (Agilent Technologies, Santa Clara, CA, USA) operating at 26°C, located at Pusan National University (Busan, Republic of Korea). The Carr–Purcell–Meiboom–Gill (CPMG) pulse sequence was applied to attenuate signals from macromolecules and residual water. For urine samples, spectra were acquired using the following parameters: a 16.2 μs 90° pulse width, a 3 s relaxation delay, a 3 s acquisition time, and a total acquisition time of 13 min and 9 s. For plasma samples, the acquisition was performed using a 16.5 μs 90° pulse width, a 3 s relaxation delay, a 3 s acquisition time, and a total acquisition time of 13 min and 20 s. All spectra were acquired with 128 scans and a spectral width of 24,038.5 Hz. Spectral data were processed using the Chenomx NMR Suite software (version 8.3, Chenomx Inc., Edmonton, AB, Canada). The spectral region from δ 0.0 to 10.0 ppm was divided into bins with a width of 0.04 ppm, yielding a total of 250 integrated regions per spectrum. This binning procedure generated a normalized intensity distribution across 250 variables for each spectrum, which was used for subsequent pattern recognition analysis. The water resonance region (δ 4.5–5.0 ppm) was excluded from the analysis to minimize variability associated with differences in water suppression efficiency. Metabolite identification and quantification were also performed using the Chenomx NMR Suite Professional software (version 8.3). TSP (2 mM) and DSS (0.5 mM) were used as the chemical shift and concentration references for plasma and urine samples, respectively.

4.7. Multivariate and Statistical Analysis

All NMR spectral data were exported from the Chenomx NMR Suite Professional software into Microsoft Excel (*.xls) format. The one-dimensional NMR data were then imported into SIMCA-P software (version 12.0, Umetrics Inc., Kinnelon, NJ, USA) for multivariate statistical analysis to explore intrinsic variations in the dataset. Prior to analysis, the data were center-scaled. PCA and OPLS-DA were performed, and the resulting score plots were used to visualize the distribution and clustering of samples across groups. Additionally, VIP values from the OPLS-DA model were used to identify potential biomarkers associated with

PHMG-p exposure in the DED model. For univariate analysis, the means and standard deviations of each metabolite were calculated using Microsoft Excel (version 2019). Quantitative differences in plasma and urinary metabolite concentrations among experimental groups were assessed using ANOVA test in GraphPad Prism (version 5.01, San Diego, CA, USA). A p-value of < 0.05 was considered statistically significant.

Author Contributions: J.D.L. drafted the manuscript; J.D.L., S.B.O. and H.G. performed the animal experiments; J.D.L., S.B.O. and H.G. conducted sample isolation and histopathological evaluation. H.Y.K. performed statistical analyses; S.K. and H.Y.K. analyzed the biological samples using ^{1}H-NMR spectroscopy; K.J.C. and K.-B.K. designed the study; G.-W.H. and K.-B.K. revised and finalized the manuscript. All authors have read and agreed to the published version of the manuscript.

Funding: This work was supported by a National Research Foundation of Republic of Korea (NRF) grant (NRF-2017R1A2B4004758, NRF-2020R1I1A1A01072862 and RS-2024-00463346) funded by the Republic of Korea government (MEST).

Institutional Review Board Statement: Institutional guidelines for the care and use of animals were followed and the experimental protocol was approved by the Institutional Animal Care and Use Committee of Dankook University (IACUC, Approval Date: 12 September 2017, Approval number: 2017-035). All procedures involving animals were in accordance with the ethical standards of the institution or practice at which the studies were conducted.

Conflicts of Interest: The authors have no conflicts of interest to disclose.

Abbreviations

^{1}H-NMR	Proton nuclear magnetic resonance
ANOVA	Analysis of variance
BAC	Benzalkonium chloride
BSA	Bovine serum albumin
COX-2	Cyclooxygenase-2
DED	Dry eye disease
GLS1	Glutaminase 1
GSH	Glutathione
IL-1β	Interleukin-1 beta
IL-6	Interleukin-6
iNOS	Inducible nitric oxide synthase
NO	Nitric oxide
OPLS-DA	Orthogonal projections to latent structures discriminant analysis
OSDI	Ocular Surface Disease Index
PCA	Principal component analysis
PHMG-p	Polyhexamethylene guanidine phosphate.
ROS	Reactive oxygen species
TCA cycle	Citric acid cycle
TNF-α	Tumor necrosis factor-alpha
VIP	Variable importance in projection

References

1. Golden, M.I.; Meyer, J.J.; Zeppieri, M.; Patel, B.C. Dry Eye Syndrome. In *StatPearls [Internet]*; StatPearls Publishing: Treasure Island, FL, USA, 2024. Available online: https://www.ncbi.nlm.nih.gov/books/NBK470411/ (accessed on 21 March 2025).
2. Stern, M.E.; Gao, J.; Siemasko, K.F.; Beuerman, R.W.; Pflugfelder, S.C. The Role of the Lacrimal Functional Unit in the Pathophysiology of Dry Eye. *Exp. Eye Res.* **2004**, *78*, 409–416. [CrossRef]
3. Honavar, S.G. Dry Eye Disease = DED = A Disease Eluding Diagnosis. *Indian J. Ophthalmol.* **2023**, *71*, 1059–1061. [CrossRef]

4. Bravo, C.J.; Martinez, J.A.C.; Gonzalez, P.A. Short-term Health Effects of Tear Agents Chlorobenzylidenemalonitrile and Oleoresin Capsicum During the Civil Riots of Santiago de Chile in 2019–2020. *Toxicol. Res.* **2025**, *41*, 291–301. [CrossRef]
5. Inomata, T.; Iwagami, M.; Hiratsuka, Y.; Fujimoto, K.; Okumura, Y.; Shiang, T.; Murakami, A. Maximum Blink Interval Is Associated with Tear Film Breakup Time: A New Simple, Screening Test for Dry Eye Disease. *Sci. Rep.* **2018**, *8*, 13443. [CrossRef] [PubMed]
6. Research Subcommittee of the International Dry Eye WorkShop. Research in Dry Eye: Report of the Research Subcommittee of the International Dry Eye WorkShop. *Ocul. Surf.* **2007**, *5*, 179–193. [CrossRef] [PubMed]
7. Li, K.; Zhang, C.; Yang, Z.; Wang, Y.; Si, H. Evaluation of a Novel Dry Eye Model Induced by Oral Administration of Finasteride. *Mol. Med. Rep.* **2017**, *16*, 8763–8770. [CrossRef] [PubMed]
8. Brignole, F.; Pisella, P.J.; Goldschild, M.; De Saint Jean, M.; Goguel, A.; Baudouin, C. Flow Cytometric Analysis of Inflammatory Markers in Conjunctival Epithelial Cells of Patients with Dry Eyes. *Investig. Ophthalmol. Vis. Sci.* **2000**, *41*, 1356–1363.
9. Narayanan, S.; Miller, W.L.; McDermott, A.M. Conjunctival Cytokine Expression in Symptomatic Moderate Dry Eye Subjects. *Investig. Ophthalmol. Vis. Sci.* **2006**, *47*, 2445–2450. [CrossRef]
10. Baudouin, C. The Pathology of Dry Eye. *Surv. Ophthalmol.* **2001**, *45*, S211–S220. [CrossRef]
11. Stern, M.E.; Pflugfelder, S.C. Inflammation in Dry Eye. *Ocul. Surf.* **2004**, *2*, 124–130. [CrossRef]
12. Yoon, K.C.; Jeong, I.Y.; Park, Y.G.; Yang, S.Y. Interleukin-6 and Tumor Necrosis Factor-Alpha Levels in Tears of Patients with Dry Eye Syndrome. *Cornea* **2007**, *26*, 431–437. [CrossRef]
13. Li, D.Q.; Chen, Z.; Song, X.J.; Luo, L.; Pflugfelder, S.C. Stimulation of Matrix Metalloproteinases by Hyperosmolarity via a JNK Pathway in Human Corneal Epithelial Cells. *Investig. Ophthalmol. Vis. Sci.* **2004**, *45*, 4302–4311. [CrossRef]
14. Li, D.Q.; Luo, L.; Chen, Z.; Kim, H.S.; Song, X.J.; Pflugfelder, S.C. JNK and ERK MAP Kinases Mediate Induction of IL-1β, TNF-α and IL-8 Following Hyperosmolar Stress in Human Limbal Epithelial Cells. *Exp. Eye Res.* **2006**, *82*, 588–596.
15. Kelagere, Y.; Scholand, K.K.; DeJong, E.N.; Boyd, A.I.; Yu, Z.; Astley, R.A.; Callegan, M.C.; Bowdish, D.M.; Makarenkova, H.P.; de Paiva, C.S. TNF Is a Critical Cytokine in Age-Related Dry Eye Disease. *Ocul. Surf.* **2023**, *30*, 119–128. [CrossRef]
16. Wu, J.; Li, G.J.; Niu, J.; Wen, F.; Han, L. Analyze Interleukin-1β, Interleukin-6, and Tumor Necrosis Factor-Alpha Levels in Dry Eye and the Therapeutic Effect of Cyclosporine A. *World J. Clin. Cases* **2024**, *12*, 5665–5672. [CrossRef] [PubMed]
17. Ji, Y.W.; Byun, Y.J.; Choi, W.; Jeong, E.; Kim, J.S.; Noh, H.; Kim, E.S.; Song, Y.J.; Park, S.K.; Lee, H.K. Neutralization of Ocular Surface TNF-Alpha Reduces Ocular Surface and Lacrimal Gland Inflammation Induced by In Vivo Dry Eye. *Investig. Ophthalmol. Vis. Sci.* **2013**, *54*, 7557–7566. [CrossRef] [PubMed]
18. HIRA (Health Insurance Review and Assessment Service). Information on Statistical Illnesses: Statistics on Diseases. 2025. Available online: https://www.hira.or.kr/ra/stcIlnsInfm/stcIlnsInfmView.do?pgmid=HIRAA030502000000&sortSno=192&utm_source=chatgpt.com (accessed on 21 March 2025).
19. Choi, J.H.; Kim, K. Polyhexamethylene Guanidine Phosphate Enhanced Procoagulant Activity through Oxidative-Stress-Mediated Phosphatidylserine Exposure in Platelets. *Toxics* **2024**, *12*, 50. [CrossRef]
20. Gilbert, P.; Moore, L.E. Cationic Antiseptics: Diversity of Action under a Common Epithet. *J. Appl. Microbiol.* **2005**, *99*, 703–715. [CrossRef]
21. The Special Investigation Commission on Humidifier Disinfectant Disaster and Sewol Ferry Disaster. 2022. Available online: https://socialdisasterscommission.co.kr/ (accessed on 21 March 2025).
22. Park, J.S.; Park, Y.J.; Kim, H.R.; Chung, K.H. Polyhexamethylene Guanidine Phosphate-Induced ROS-Mediated DNA Damage Caused Cell Cycle Arrest and Apoptosis in Lung Epithelial Cells. *J. Toxicol. Sci.* **2019**, *44*, 415–424. [CrossRef]
23. Lee, J.D.; Kim, H.Y.; Kang, K.; Jeong, H.G.; Song, M.K.; Tae, I.H.; Lee, S.H.; Kim, H.R.; Lee, K.; Chae, S.; et al. Integration of Transcriptomics, Proteomics and Metabolomics Identifies Biomarkers for Pulmonary Injury by Polyhexamethylene Guanidine Phosphate (PHMG-P-p), a Humidifier Disinfectant, in Rats. *Arch. Toxicol.* **2020**, *94*, 887–909. [CrossRef]
24. Jeong, M.H.; Jeon, M.S.; Kim, G.E.; Kim, H.R. Polyhexamethylene Guanidine Phosphate Induces Apoptosis through Endoplasmic Reticulum Stress in Lung Epithelial Cells. *Int. J. Mol. Sci.* **2021**, *22*, 1215. [CrossRef] [PubMed]
25. Jeong, S.H.; Lee, H.; Nam, Y.J.; Kang, J.Y.; Lee, H.; Choi, J.Y.; Lee, Y.S.; Kim, J.; Park, Y.H.; Park, S.A.; et al. Longitudinal Long Term Follow-Up Investigation on the Carcinogenic Impact of Polyhexamethylene Guanidine Phosphate in Rat Models. *Sci. Rep.* **2024**, *14*, 7178.
26. Nguyen, H.; Juang, U.; Gwon, S.; Jung, W.; Huang, Q.; Lee, S.; Lee, B.; Kwon, S.H.; Kim, S.-H.; Park, J. Effect of CTMP1 Gene on Pulmonary Fibrosis. *Toxicol. Res.* **2025**, *41*, 235–244. [PubMed]
27. Kang, M.S.; Kim, S.H.; Yang, M.J.; Kim, H.Y.; Kim, I.H.; Kang, J.W.; Choi, H.S.; Jin, S.W.; Park, E.J. Polyhexamethylene Guanidine Phosphate-Induced Necrosis May Be Linked to Pulmonary Fibrosis. *Toxicol. Lett.* **2022**, *362*, 1–16. [CrossRef]
28. Sung, H.J.; Jeong, S.H.; Kang, J.Y.; Kim, C.; Nam, Y.J.; Kim, J.Y.; Choi, J.Y.; Lee, H.J.; Lee, Y.S.; Kim, E.Y.; et al. Hematotoxic Effect of Respiratory Exposure to PHMG-P-p and Its Integrated Genetic Analysis. *Toxics* **2022**, *10*, 694.

29. Wang, M.T.M.; Chan, E.; Ea, L.; Kam, C.; Lu, Y.; Misra, S.L.; Craig, J.P. Randomized Trial of Desktop Humidifier for Dry Eye Relief in Computer Users. *Optom. Vis. Sci.* **2017**, *94*, 1052–1057. [CrossRef]
30. HIRA (Health Insurance Review and Assessment Service). Dry Eye Syndrome' Cannot Be Relieved even in Spring and Summer. 2014. Available online: https://www.hira.or.kr/bbsDummy.do?pgmid=HIRAA020041000100&brdScnBltNo=4&brdBltNo=8709&pageIndex=1 (accessed on 21 March 2025).
31. Kim, H.Y.; Lee, Y.J.; Kim, S.J.; Lee, J.D.; Kim, S.; Ko, M.J.; Kim, J.W.; Shin, C.Y.; Kim, K.B. Metabolomics profiling of valproic acid-induced symptoms resembling autism spectrum disorders using 1H NMR spectral analysis in rat model. *J. Toxicol. Environ. Health A* **2022**, *85*, 1–13.
32. Zhao, Z.; Fan, Y.; Cui, Y.; Yang, L.; Wu, Y.; Yuan, Y.; Zhang, P.; Zhao, R.; Ji, J.; Xu, S.; et al. Integration of serum metabolomics and network pharmacology reveals the immunoenhancing mechanisms of Qishenbuqi capsules. *Toxicol. Res.* **2023**, *12*, 201–215. [CrossRef]
33. Al-Sulaiti, H.; Almaliti, J.; Naman, C.B.; Al Thani, A.A.; Yassine, H.M. Metabolomics approaches for the diagnosis, treatment, and better disease management of viral infections. *Metabolites* **2023**, *13*, 948. [CrossRef]
34. Vo, D.K.; Trinh, K.T.L. Emerging biomarkers in metabolomics: Advancements in precision health and disease diagnosis. *Int. J. Mol. Sci.* **2024**, *25*, 13190. [CrossRef]
35. Pan, S.; Yin, L.; Liu, J.; Tong, J.; Wang, Z.; Zhao, J.; Liu, X.; Chen, Y.; Miao, J.; Zhou, Y.; et al. Metabolomics-driven approaches for identifying therapeutic targets in drug discovery. *MedComm (2020)* **2024**, *5*, e792. [CrossRef] [PubMed]
36. Ghanem, H.Z.; Kadry, M.O.; Abdel-Megeed, R.M.; Abdel-Hamid, A.Z. Metabolomics applications in disease diagnosis, treatment, and drug discovery. *Egypt. Pharm. J.* **2019**, *18*, 290–295. [CrossRef]
37. Rizo-Roca, D.; Henderson, J.D.; Zierath, J.R. Metabolomics in cardiometabolic diseases: Key biomarkers and therapeutic implications for insulin resistance and diabetes. *J. Intern. Med.* **2025**, *297*, 584–607. [CrossRef]
38. Gonzalez-Covarrubias, V.; Martínez-Martínez, E.; Del Bosque-Plata, L. The Potential of Metabolomics in Biomedical Applications. *Metabolites* **2022**, *12*, 194. [CrossRef] [PubMed]
39. Asef, C.K.; Moore, S.G.; Pickens, C.A.; Saavedra-Matiz, C.A.; Orsini, J.J.; Petritis, K.; Gaul, D.A.; Fernández, F.M. Beyond targeted newborn screening: A nontargeted metabolomics workflow to investigate birthweight-metabolome correlations. *Anal. Chem.* **2025**, *97*, 6563–6570. [CrossRef]
40. Hasan, M.R.; Suleiman, M.; Pérez-López, A. Metabolomics in the Diagnosis and Prognosis of COVID-19. *Front. Genet.* **2021**, *12*, 721556. [CrossRef]
41. Rahman, M.; Schellhorn, H.E. Metabolomics of infectious diseases in the era of personalized medicine. *Front. Mol. Biosci.* **2023**, *10*, 1120376. [CrossRef]
42. Jiang, Y.; Yang, C.; Zheng, Y.; Liu, Y.; Chen, Y. A Set of Global Metabolomic Biomarker Candidates to Predict the Risk of Dry Eye Disease. *Front. Cell Dev. Biol.* **2020**, *8*, 344. [CrossRef]
43. Vehof, J.; Hysi, P.G.; Hammond, C.J. A Metabolome-Wide Study of Dry Eye Disease Reveals Serum Androgens as Biomarkers. *Ophthalmology* **2017**, *124*, 505–511. [CrossRef]
44. Fineide, F.A.; Tashbayev, B.; Elgstøen, K.B.P.; Sandås, E.M.; Rootwelt, H.; Hynne, H.; Chen, X.; Ræder, S.; Vehof, J.; Dartt, D.; et al. Tear and Saliva Metabolomics in Evaporative Dry Eye Disease in Females. *Metabolites* **2023**, *13*, 1125. [CrossRef]
45. Lee, J.D.; Kim, H.Y.; Park, J.J.; Oh, S.B.; Goo, H.; Cho, K.J.; Kim, S.; Kim, K.B. Metabolomics approach to biomarkers of dry eye disease using ^{1}H-NMR in rats. *J. Toxicol. Environ. Health A* **2021**, *84*, 313–330.
46. Kim, H.Y.; Lee, J.D.; Kim, H.; Kim, Y.; Park, J.J.; Oh, S.B.; Goo, H.; Cho, K.J.; Kim, K.B. Mass Spectrometry (MS)-Based Metabolomics of Plasma and Urine in Dry Eye Disease (DED)-Induced Rat Model. *J. Toxicol. Environ. Health A* **2025**, *88*, 122–135. [CrossRef] [PubMed]
47. Chen, X.; Zhang, C.; Peng, F.; Wu, L.; Zhuo, D.; Wang, L.; Zhang, M.; Li, Z.; Tian, L.; Jie, Y.; et al. Identification of glutamine as a potential therapeutic target in dry eye disease. *Signal Transduct. Target. Ther.* **2025**, *10*, 27. [CrossRef] [PubMed]
48. Xia, J.; Wishart, D.S. Using MetaboAnalyst 3.0 for comprehensive metabolomics data analysis. *Curr. Protoc. Bioinform.* **2016**, *55*, 14. [CrossRef] [PubMed]
49. Lee, H.; Park, J.; Park, K. Fibrosis as a Result of Polyhexamethylene Guanide Exposure in Cultured Statens Seruminstitut Rabbit Cornea (SIRC) Cells. *Environ. Anal. Health Toxicol.* **2021**, *36*, e2021009.
50. Park, J.Y.; Lee, H.; Park, K. Eye Irritation Tests of Polyhexamethylene Guanidine Phosphate (PHMG) and Chloromethylisothiazolinone/Methylisothiazolinone (CMIT/MIT) Using a Tissue Model of Reconstructed Human Cornea-Like Epithelium. *Environ. Health Toxicol.* **2019**, *34*, e2019004.
51. Ivanov, I.; Kirillova, D.; Erimbetov, K.; Shatalov, D. Toxicity and Safety Analysis of Polyhexamethylene Guanidine: A Comprehensive Systematic Review. *Sci. Pharm.* **2024**, *3*, 153–166. [CrossRef]

52. De Paiva, C.S.; Villarreal, A.L.; Corrales, R.M.; Rahman, H.T.; Chang, V.Y.; Farley, W.J.; Stern, M.E.; Niederkorn, J.Y.; Li, D.Q.; Pflugfelder, S.C. Dry eye-induced conjunctival epithelial squamous metaplasia is modulated by interferon-gamma. *Investig. Ophthalmol. Vis. Sci.* **2007**, *48*, 2553–2560.
53. Kim, J.; Lee, J.; Kim, S.; Yoon, S.H.; Jo, Y.C.; Kim, K.H.; Kim, H.K. Noninvasive Imaging of Conjunctival Goblet Cells as a Method for Diagnosing Dry Eye Disease in an Experimental Mouse Model. *Transl. Vis. Sci. Technol.* **2023**, *12*, 22. [CrossRef]
54. Massingale, M.L.; Li, X.; Vallabhajosyula, M.; Chen, D.; Wei, Y.; Asbell, P.A. Analysis of Inflammatory Cytokines in the Tears of Dry Eye Patients. *Cornea* **2009**, *28*, 1023–1027. [CrossRef]
55. Roda, M.; Corazza, I.; Bacchi Reggiani, M.L.; Pellegrini, M.; Taroni, L.; Giannaccare, G.; Versura, P. Dry Eye Disease and Tear Cytokine Levels—A Meta-Analysis. *Int. J. Mol. Sci.* **2020**, *21*, 3111. [CrossRef]
56. Wang, X.; Zhang, A.; Han, Y.; Wang, P.; Sun, H.; Song, G.; Dong, T.; Yuan, Y.; Yuan, X.; Zhang, M.; et al. Urine Metabolomics Analysis for Biomarker Discovery and Detection of Jaundice Syndrome in Patients with Liver Disease. *Mol. Cell Proteom.* **2012**, *11*, 370–380. [CrossRef] [PubMed]
57. Xu, J.; Chen, Y.; Zhang, R.; He, J.; Song, Y.; Wang, J.; Wang, H.; Wang, L.; Zhan, Q.; Abliz, Z. Global Metabolomics Reveals Potential Urinary Biomarkers of Esophageal Squamous Cell Carcinoma for Diagnosis and Staging. *Sci. Rep.* **2016**, *6*, 35010. [CrossRef]
58. Anesi, A.; Rubert, J.; Oluwagbemigun, K.; Orozco-Ruiz, X.; Nöthlings, U.; Breteler, M.M.B.; Mattivi, F. Metabolic Profiling of Human Plasma and Urine, Targeting Tryptophan, Tyrosine and Branched Chain Amino Acid Pathways. *Metabolites* **2019**, *9*, 261. [CrossRef] [PubMed]
59. Kim, K.; Aronov, P.; Zakharkin, S.O.; Anderson, D.; Perroud, B.; Thompson, I.M.; Weiss, R.H. Urine Metabolomics Analysis for Kidney Cancer Detection and Biomarker Discovery. *Mol. Cell Proteom.* **2009**, *8*, 558–570. [CrossRef]
60. Tohge, T.; Fernie, A.R. Combining Genetic Diversity, Informatics and Metabolomics to Facilitate Annotation of Plant Gene Function. *Nat. Protoc.* **2010**, *5*, 1210–1227. [CrossRef] [PubMed]
61. Wishart, D.S. Metabolomics in humans and other mammals. In *Metabolome Analysis: An Introduction*; Villas-Boas, S.G., Nielsen, J., Smedsgaard, J., Hansen, M.A.E., Roessner-Tunali, U., Eds.; John Wiley and Sons: New York, NY, USA, 2007; pp. 280–296.
62. Cruzat, V.; Macedo Rogero, M.; Keane, K.N.; Curi, R.; Newsholme, P. Glutamine: Metabolism and Immune Function, Supplementation and Clinical Translation. *Nutrients* **2018**, *10*, 1564. [CrossRef]
63. Haroon, E.; Miller, A.H.; Sanacora, G. Inflammation, Glutamate, and Glia: A Trio of Trouble in Mood Disorders. *Neuropsychopharmacology* **2017**, *42*, 193–215. [CrossRef]
64. Zheng, X.; Zhu, Y.; Zhao, Z.; Chu, Y.; Yang, W. The Role of Amino Acid Metabolism in Inflammatory Bowel Disease and Other Inflammatory Diseases. *Front. Immunol.* **2023**, *14*, 1284133. [CrossRef]
65. Parfenova, H.; Basuroy, S.; Bhattacharya, S.; Tcheranova, D.; Qu, Y.; Regan, R.F.; Leffler, C.W. Glutamate Induces Oxidative Stress and Apoptosis in Cerebral Vascular Endothelial Cells: Contributions of HO-1 and HO-2 to Cytoprotection. *Am. J. Physiol. Cell Physiol.* **2006**, *290*, C1399–C1410. [CrossRef]
66. Alarcon-Aguilar, F.J.; Almanza-Perez, J.; Blancas, G.; Angeles, S.; Garcia-Macedo, R.; Roman, R.; Cruz, M. Glycine regulates the production of pro-inflammatory cytokines in lean and monosodium glutamate-obese mice. *Eur. J. Pharmacol.* **2008**, *599*, 152–158.
67. Aguayo-Cerón, K.A.; Sánchez-Muñoz, F.; Gutierrez-Rojas, R.A.; Acevedo-Villavicencio, L.N.; Flores-Zarate, A.V.; Huang, F.; Giacoman-Martinez, A.; Villafaña, S.; Romero-Nava, R. Glycine: The Smallest Anti-Inflammatory Micronutrient. *Int. J. Mol. Sci.* **2023**, *24*, 11236. [CrossRef]
68. Tauffenberger, A.; Fiumelli, H.; Almustafa, S.; Magistretti, P.J. Lactate and Pyruvate Promote Oxidative Stress Resistance Through Hormetic ROS Signaling. *Cell Death Dis.* **2019**, *10*, 653. [CrossRef]
69. Wang, X.; Perez, E.; Liu, R.; Yan, L.J.; Mallet, R.T.; Yang, S.H. Pyruvate Protects Mitochondria from Oxidative Stress in Human Neuroblastoma SK-N-SH Cells. *Brain Res.* **2007**, *1132*, 1–9. [CrossRef] [PubMed]
70. Choi, I.; Son, H.; Baek, J.H. Tricarboxylic Acid (TCA) Cycle Intermediates: Regulators of Immune Responses. *Life* **2021**, *11*, 69. [CrossRef] [PubMed]
71. Williams, N.C.; O'Neill, L.A.J. A Role for the Krebs Cycle Intermediate Citrate in Metabolic Reprogramming in Innate Immunity and Inflammation. *Front. Immunol.* **2018**, *9*, 141. [CrossRef]
72. Wu, G.; Bazer, F.W.; Davis, T.A.; Kim, S.W.; Li, P.; Rhoads, J.M.; Satterfield, M.C.; Smith, S.B.; Spencer, T.E.; Yin, Y. Arginine Metabolism and Nutrition in Growth, Health and Disease. *Amino Acids* **2009**, *37*, 153–168. [CrossRef]
73. Gemici Karaaslan, B.; Kiykim, A.; Burtecene, N.; Gokden, M.; Cansever, M.S.; Hopurcuoglu, D.; Cengiz, G.N.; Topcu, B.; Zubarioğlu, T.; Kiykim, E.; et al. Amino Acid Metabolism and Immune Dysfunction in Urea Cycle Disorders: T and B Cell Perspectives. *J. Inherit. Metab. Dis.* **2025**, *48*, e70009. [CrossRef]
74. Zotta, A.; Zaslona, Z.; O'Neill, L.A. Is Citrate a Critical Signal in Immunity and Inflammation? *J. Cell Signal.* **2020**, *1*, 87–96. [CrossRef]
75. Martínez-Reyes, I.; Chandel, N.S. Mitochondrial TCA Cycle Metabolites Control Physiology and Disease. *Nat. Commun.* **2020**, *11*, 102. [CrossRef]

76. Patil, N.K.; Bohannon, J.K.; Hernandez, A.; Patil, T.K.; Sherwood, E.R. Regulation of Leukocyte Function by Citric Acid Cycle Intermediates. *J. Leukoc. Biol.* **2019**, *106*, 105–117. [CrossRef] [PubMed]
77. Ryan, D.G.; Murphy, M.P.; Frezza, C.; Prag, H.A.; Chouchani, E.T.; O'Neill, L.A.; Mills, E.L. Coupling Krebs Cycle Metabolites to Signalling in Immunity and Cancer. *Nat. Metab.* **2019**, *1*, 16–33. [CrossRef] [PubMed]
78. Ramendra, R.; Mancini, M.; Ayala, J.M.; Tung, L.T.; Isnard, S.; Lin, J.; Routy, J.P.; Nijnik, A.; Langlais, D. Glutathione Metabolism Is a Regulator of the Acute Inflammatory Response of Monocytes to (1→3)-β-D-Glucan. *Front. Immunol.* **2021**, *12*, 694152. [CrossRef] [PubMed]
79. Mak, T.W.; Grusdat, M.; Duncan, G.S.; Dostert, C.; Nonnenmacher, Y.; Cox, M.; Binsfeld, C.; Hao, Z.; Brüstle, A.; Itsumi, M.; et al. Glutathione Primes T Cell Metabolism for Inflammation. *Immunity* **2017**, *46*, 675–689. [CrossRef]
80. Viau, S.; Maire, M.A.; Pasquis, B.; Grégoire, S.; Fourgeux, C.; Acar, N.; Bretillon, L.; Creuzot-Garcher, C.P.; Joffre, C. Time Course of Ocular Surface and Lacrimal Gland Changes in a New Scopolamine-Induced Dry Eye Model. *Graefes Arch. Clin. Exp. Ophthalmol.* **2008**, *246*, 857–867. [CrossRef]
81. Viau, S.; Maire, M.A.; Pasquis, B.; Grégoire, S.; Acar, N.; Bron, A.M.; Bretillon, L.; Creuzot-Garcher, C.P.; Joffre, C. Efficacy of a 2-Month Dietary Supplementation with Polyunsaturated Fatty Acids in Dry Eye Induced by Scopolamine in a Rat Model. *Graefes Arch. Clin. Exp. Ophthalmol.* **2009**, *247*, 1039–1050. [CrossRef]
82. Li, Z.; Choi, W.; Oh, H.J.; Yoon, K.C. Effectiveness of Topical Infliximab in a Mouse Model of Experimental Dry Eye. *Cornea* **2012**, *31* (Suppl. S1), S25–S31. [CrossRef]
83. Li, Z.; Woo, J.M.; Chung, S.W.; Kwon, M.Y.; Choi, J.S.; Oh, H.J.; Yoon, K.C. Therapeutic Effect of Topical Adiponectin in a Mouse Model of Desiccating Stress-Induced Dry Eye. *Investig. Ophthalmol. Vis. Sci.* **2013**, *54*, 155–162. [CrossRef]
84. Yoon, K.C.; Ahn, K.Y.; Choi, W.; Li, Z.; Choi, J.S.; Lee, S.H.; Park, S.H. Tear production and ocular surface changes in experimental dry eye after elimination of desiccating stress. *Investig. Ophthalmol. Vis. Sci.* **2011**, *52*, 7267–7273. [CrossRef]

International Journal of
Molecular Sciences

MDPI

Review

Keratoconjunctivitis Sicca in Sjögren Disease: Diagnostic Challenges and Therapeutic Advances

Muhammad Soyfoo [1,*], Elie Motulsky [2] and Julie Sarrand [1]

[1] Department of Rheumatology, Hôpital Universitaire de Bruxelles (HUB), 1070 Bruxelles, Belgium; julie.sarrand@ulb.be
[2] Department of Ophthalmology, Hôpital Universitaire de Bruxelles (HUB), 1070 Bruxelles, Belgium; elie.motulsky@hubruxelles.be
* Correspondence: msoyfoo@ulb.ac.be

Abstract: Keratoconjunctivitis sicca (KCS), also commonly known as dry eye disease (DED), is one of the most prevalent and crippling features of Sjögren disease (SD), a chronic systemic autoimmune disorder featuring lymphocytic infiltration and progressive impairment of exocrine glands. KCS affects up to 95% of patients with SD and is often the earliest and most persistent manifestation, significantly compromising visual function, ocular comfort, and overall quality of life. Beyond the ocular surface, KCS mirrors a wider spectrum of immune dysregulation and epithelial damage characteristic of the disease, making it a valuable window into the underlying systemic pathology. The pathophysiology of KCS in SD is complex and multifactorial, involving an interplay between autoimmune-mediated lacrimal gland dysfunction, neuroimmune interactions, ocular surface inflammation, and epithelial instability. Tear film instability and epithelial injury result from the aberrant activation of innate and adaptive immunity, involving T and B lymphocytes, pro-inflammatory cytokines, and type I interferon pathways. Despite the clinical significance of KCS, its diagnosis remains challenging, with frequent discrepancies between subjective symptoms and objective findings. Traditional diagnostic tools often lack sensitivity and specificity, prompting the development of novel imaging techniques, tear film biomarkers, and standardized scoring systems. Concurrently, therapeutic strategies have evolved from palliative approaches to immunomodulatory and regenerative treatments, aiming to restore immune homeostasis and epithelial integrity. This review provides a comprehensive update on the pathogenesis, diagnostic landscape, and emerging treatments of KCS in the context of SD.

Keywords: Sjögren's disease; sicca; keratoconjunctivitis; interferon; cytokines

1. Introduction

Sjögren disease (SD) is a chronic systemic autoimmune disorder characterized by lymphoplasmacytic infiltration of exocrine glands, leading to the hallmark sicca symptoms of dry eyes and dry mouth [1,2]. Although its pathophysiology remains incompletely understood, it is thought to involve abnormal lymphocyte activation, pro-inflammatory cytokine secretion, and type I interferon pathway activation [3,4]. With an estimated prevalence of 0.5–1% and a striking female predominance of 9:1, SD ranks among the most common systemic autoimmune diseases [5,6].

Exocrine gland dysfunction is the clinical hallmark of SD, with keratoconjunctivitis sicca (KCS) representing one of its most frequent and debilitating manifestations. Ocular involvement occurs in up to 95% of patients and often constitutes the presenting symptom leading to diagnosis [7–10]. KCS is a multifactorial process in which autoimmune inflammation, altered tear film composition, and impaired ocular surface integrity interact to create a self-perpetuating cycle of dysfunction. Beyond the individual burden, KCS in SD imposes a substantial socioeconomic impact, with annual healthcare costs exceeding 5.9 billion dollars in the United States and quality-of-life reductions comparable to those observed in chronic pain conditions [11,12].

The pathogenesis of SD reflects a complex interplay of genetic and environmental factors. Associations with HLA alleles, particularly HLA-DR3 and HLA-DQ2, support a strong genetic contribution, while viral infections such as Epstein–Barr virus may act as environmental triggers in genetically susceptible individuals [13–15].

Recent advances in ocular surface immunology, tear film biology, and inflammatory mechanisms have reshaped the understanding of KCS in SD. Novel imaging tools now permit in-depth evaluation of the meibomian gland and ocular surface structure, while emerging targeted therapies modulate specific inflammatory pathways. This review summarizes current knowledge of ocular manifestations in SD, highlights diagnostic innovations, and discusses evolving therapeutic strategies, with the goal of providing clinicians and researchers with an updated perspective on the best practices and future directions in KCS management.

2. Pathophysiology of Keratoconjunctivitis Sicca in Sjögren Disease

2.1. Autoimmune Mechanisms and Glandular Dysfunction

The pathophysiology of keratoconjunctivitis sicca (KCS) in Sjögren disease extends beyond simple tear deficiency and reflects a complex autoimmune cascade [16–18]. The process is initiated by infiltration of activated T lymphocytes and other immune cells into the lacrimal glands, producing focal lymphocytic sialadenitis. These infiltrates, composed mainly of $CD4^+$ T-helper cells, B cells, and plasma cells, progressively disrupt acinar and ductal architecture, impairing tear secretion and driving chronic glandular dysfunction [19,20].

The initiating factors in Sjögren disease remain unclear, though molecular mimicry between viral and glandular self-antigens has been implicated [21]. This loss of tolerance favors autoimmune responses against exocrine tissues, with Ro52 and Ro60—major constituents of the Ro/SSA complex—emerging as dominant targets expressed in lacrimal glands [22,23].

The inflammatory process in the lacrimal glands follows a characteristic pattern of progression. Early stages are characterized by periductal lymphocytic infiltration, with preservation of acinar architecture. As the disease progresses, the inflammatory infiltrate expands, forming organized lymphoid structures that may resemble germinal centers [24]. This tertiary lymphoid tissue formation is associated with local production of autoantibodies and pro-inflammatory cytokines [25].

The autoimmune process is characterized by the production of specific autoantibodies, including anti-Ro/SSA and anti-La/Sjögren Syndrome Antigen B (SSB) antibodies, which are present in approximately 60–70% of SD patients [24,26,27]. These antibodies not only serve as diagnostic markers but also contribute directly to tissue damage through complement activation and immune complex formation. Anti-Ro52 antibodies may be particularly important in lacrimal gland dysfunction, as they can interfere with cellular calcium homeostasis and induce apoptosis in acinar cells [28].

In SD, lacrimal gland injury arises from Fas–FasL–induced apoptosis, cytotoxic T-cell activity, and cytokine-mediated inflammation. TNF-α, IL-1β, and IFN-γ sustain a pro-inflammatory niche that perpetuates destruction and hinders repair [29,30].

Type I interferons are central to the pathogenesis of Sjögren disease (SD), with many patients exhibiting an "interferon signature" in their gene expression profiles [31,32]. This activation may be triggered by viral infections or endogenous nucleic acids released from damaged cells. Interferon signaling promotes immune activation, autoantibody production, and tissue injury, thereby representing an attractive therapeutic target [33].

The progression of lacrimal gland dysfunction in SD appears to follow a temporal sequence, in which molecular and cellular alterations precede overt clinical manifestations [34]. Single-cell transcriptomic analyses of murine lacrimal glands have revealed complex changes in epithelial cell populations, including distinct transcriptional alterations in acinar and ductal cells that occur before gross morphological damage becomes evident [35]. Early non-immunologic insults to the glandular microenvironment—such as basement membrane disruption, myoepithelial cell dysfunction, and altered neural innervation—may create a permissive niche for subsequent autoimmune attack [36,37].

Neuroendocrine and hormonal influences further shape disease susceptibility. Dysregulation of the hypothalamic–pituitary–adrenal (HPA) axis, including reduced basal adrenocorticotropic hormone (ACTH) levels and altered cortisol responses, impairs glandular homeostasis in SD patients [38,39]. Androgen deficiency, particularly decreased dehydroepiandrosterone (DHEA) and its sulfate conjugate (DHEA-S), has been linked to reduced structural integrity and secretory activity of lacrimal glands. These hormonal alterations contribute to both glandular dysfunction and immune dysregulation, potentially explaining the strong female predominance and increased susceptibility after menopause [40–43].

At the cellular level, lacrimal gland epithelial cells undergo apoptosis through both intrinsic mitochondrial and extrinsic death receptor pathways, with activation of caspases-3, -8, and -9 leading to progressive acinar cell loss [44,45]. Chronic activation of the unfolded protein response (UPR) in the endoplasmic reticulum, particularly under the influence of IFN-γ, results in sustained cellular stress, misfolded protein accumulation, and eventual cell death [3,46–48]. This failure of adaptive stress responses exacerbates secretory dysfunction and perpetuates ocular surface damage.

2.2. Tear Film Abnormalities and Ocular Surface Changes

The tear film in Sjögren disease (SD) patients shows profound qualitative and quantitative abnormalities that extend beyond simple aqueous deficiency [4,49]. The normal tear film comprises three layers: an outer lipid layer secreted by the meibomian glands, a central aqueous layer produced by the lacrimal glands, and an inner mucin layer derived from conjunctival goblet cells. In SD, dysfunction affects all three layers, creating a complex and multifactorial disturbance of tear film homeostasis [50].

The aqueous layer deficiency, while the most clinically apparent, is accompanied by significant compositional changes. Tear protein concentration increases due to reduced volume, while key protective components such as lactoferrin, lysozyme, and secretory IgA are decreased [51,52]. These alterations compromise antimicrobial defense and disturb osmotic balance at the ocular surface.

Meibomian gland dysfunction (MGD) is also common in SD and contributes to evaporative dry eye that compounds aqueous deficiency [53,54]. Similarly to the lacrimal glands, meibomian glands are affected by inflammatory processes, leading to altered lipid composition and reduced lipid layer stability. The result is increased tear evaporation and further ocular surface desiccation [55].

Finally, mucin layer abnormalities arise from goblet cell loss and altered mucin production [56]. Goblet cell density is markedly reduced in SD, and surviving cells may secrete mucins with altered biochemical properties [57]. These changes diminish tear wettability and weaken the protective barrier function of the ocular surface.

2.3. Inflammatory Cascade and Ocular Surface Damage

The ocular surface in SD becomes a site of chronic inflammation that perpetuates and amplifies the initial autoimmune process [58,59]. Hyperosmolarity resulting from tear deficiency activates inflammatory pathways in the corneal and conjunctival epithelium, leading to the production of inflammatory mediators including matrix metalloproteinases (MMPs), cytokines, and chemokines [60]. Tear film hyperosmolarity (>300 mOsm/L) initiates a complex cascade of inflammatory events that begins with immediate cellular responses to osmotic stress and progresses to sustained inflammatory activation [61,62]. When tear osmolarity exceeds that of epithelial cells, water efflux occurs, causing cell shrinkage and triggering multiple stress-responsive signaling pathways [63,64]. Hyperosmotic stress directly activates the NLRP3 inflammasome complex in corneal and conjunctival epithelial cells, leading to caspase-1 activation and subsequent proteolytic processing of pro-IL-1β and pro-IL-18 into their mature, biologically active forms [65,66]. This process is accompanied by enhanced reactive oxygen species (ROS) generation from damaged mitochondria, which further amplifies inflammasome activation and creates a self-perpetuating cycle of inflammatory mediator release [67,68]. Osmotic stress triggers rapid nuclear translocation of NF-κB, with the degree of translocation directly proportional to tear osmolarity levels [69,70]. Activated NF-κB upregulates transcription of multiple inflammatory genes, including TNF-α, IL-1β, IL-6, and matrix metalloproteinases (MMP-3 and MMP-9), which collectively contribute to epithelial barrier dysfunction and tissue damage [71,72]. The NF-κB pathway also induces expression of adhesion molecules such as ICAM-1 and selectins, facilitating immune cell recruitment to the ocular surface [59,73]. Recent discoveries have highlighted the role of the cGAS-STING pathway in hyperosmolarity-induced inflammation, where oxidized mitochondrial DNA released from stressed cells activates cytosolic DNA sensors, leading to type I interferon production and amplification of inflammatory responses [74,75]. This pathway represents a critical link between cellular stress and innate immune activation in dry eye disease [76].

Hyperosmolarity induces specific changes in epithelial cell function, including disruption of tight junction proteins (particularly occludin and claudin-1), loss of barrier function, and altered mucin production patterns [77,78]. Goblet cells are particularly susceptible to osmotic stress, undergoing apoptosis through ER stress-mediated pathways and showing reduced mucin synthesis even before cell death occurs, contributing to tear film instability [15,79]. The combination of epithelial damage, inflammatory mediator release, and compromised barrier function creates a pathological feedback loop that perpetuates and amplifies the dry eye condition [4,80].

The complement system plays a crucial role in ocular surface damage in SD. Complement activation occurs through both classical and alternative pathways, leading to the formation of membrane attack complexes that directly damage epithelial cells [62,63]. This process is particularly pronounced in areas of epithelial defects, where complement deposition can be demonstrated histologically.

Epithelial cell death occurs through multiple mechanisms, including apoptosis, necrosis, and autophagy [71]. The loss of epithelial cells compromises barrier function, allowing for increased penetration of inflammatory mediators and potential pathogens. This creates a vicious cycle where epithelial damage promotes inflammation, which in turn leads to further epithelial loss [81].

The corneal nerve damage observed in SD patients contributes to both sensory abnormalities and impaired reflex tearing [82,83]. Inflammatory mediators can directly damage corneal nerve fibers, leading to reduced corneal sensitivity and altered blink patterns. This neurogenic component of KCS adds another layer of complexity to the pathophysiology and may explain why some patients experience severe symptoms despite apparently adequate tear production [84] (Figure 1).

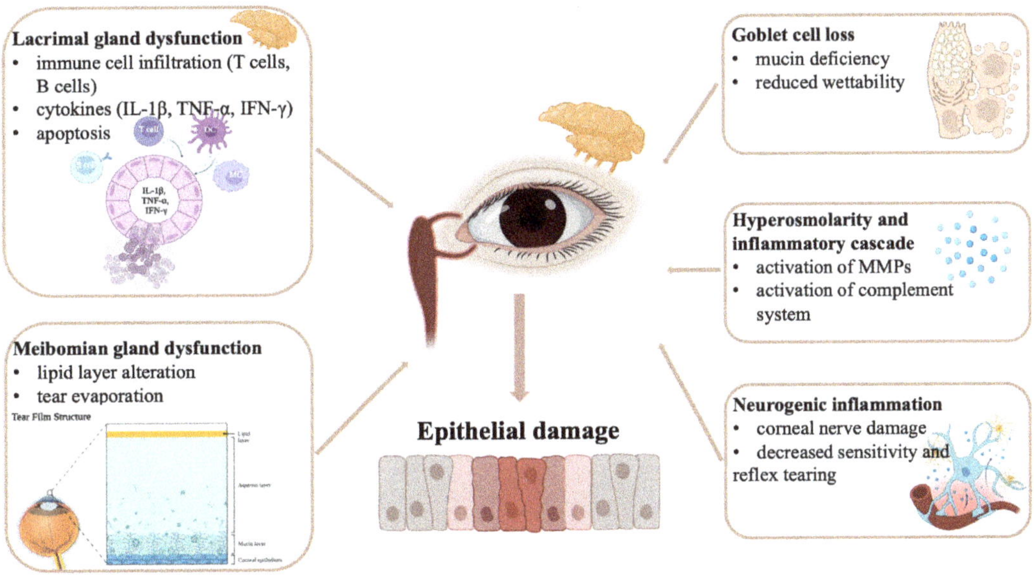

Figure 1. Pathophysiology of keratoconjunctivitis sicca in Sjögren disease. Keratoconjunctivitis sicca arises from lacrimal gland dysfunction, meibomian gland abnormalities, goblet cell loss, and tear film hyperosmolarity. These defects, amplified by immune-mediated inflammation and corneal nerve damage, culminate in chronic ocular surface inflammation and epithelial injury.

3. Diagnostic Challenges in Keratoconjunctivitis Sicca

3.1. Clinical Presentation and Symptom Variability

The diagnosis of KCS in SD presents numerous challenges, beginning with the highly variable and often nonspecific nature of presenting symptoms [7,80]. Patients may report a wide range of ocular complaints, including burning, stinging, foreign body sensation, photophobia, blurred vision, and paradoxical tearing [85,86]. The severity of symptoms does not always correlate with objective findings, making clinical assessment particularly challenging [87,88].

The discordance between symptoms and signs in SD patients is particularly pronounced and represents a unique diagnostic challenge [89,90]. Patients may experience severe discomfort with minimal objective findings, while others may have significant corneal staining with relatively mild symptoms [91]. This phenomenon may be related to altered corneal sensitivity, which is common in SD and can affect both symptom perception and protective reflexes [92,93].

The temporal pattern of symptoms can provide diagnostic clues, with many SD patients experiencing worsening symptoms throughout the day as tear production decreases and environmental factors accumulate [94,95]. Morning symptoms may be relatively mild, while evening discomfort can be severe. However, some patients may experience the opposite pattern, particularly if concurrent MGD is present, as meibomian gland dysfunction may be worse in the morning after prolonged eyelid closure [96].

Symptom triggers are highly individualized but commonly include environmental factors such as air conditioning, wind, low humidity, and visual tasks requiring sustained attention [97,98]. Digital device use has become an increasingly important trigger, as reduced blink rates during screen time can exacerbate tear film instability [99,100]. Understanding these triggers is crucial for both diagnosis and management, as symptom patterns may vary seasonally or with occupational exposures [86].

The psychological impact of chronic KCS cannot be underestimated and adds another layer of complexity to the diagnostic process [12,101]. Many patients experience anxiety, depression, and social isolation related to their ocular symptoms [102,103]. The unpredictable nature of symptom fluctuations can lead to anticipatory anxiety, while the chronic nature of the condition may result in depression and social withdrawal [104]. These psychological factors can influence symptom reporting and may complicate the diagnostic process, particularly when objective findings appear minimal compared to subjective complaints [105].

Sleep disturbances are common in SD patients and may be both a cause and consequence of ocular symptoms [106,107]. Nocturnal lagophthalmos, reduced tear production during sleep, and morning symptoms can create a cycle of poor sleep quality and worsening daytime symptoms. The relationship between sleep and ocular surface health is bidirectional, as poor sleep quality can exacerbate inflammatory processes and reduce pain tolerance [108,109].

3.2. Diagnostic Testing Limitations and Interpretation

Traditional diagnostic tests for KCS, while valuable, have significant limitations when applied to SD patients. The Schirmer test, which measures tear production over a defined time period, can be influenced by reflex tearing, ambient conditions, and patient anxiety [110]. Normal values may be observed in some SD patients, particularly in early disease stages, while abnormal results may occur in patients without systemic autoimmune disease.

Tear break-up time (TBUT) testing provides information about tear film stability but can be affected by factors beyond tear composition, including eyelid abnormalities, surface irregularities, and patient cooperation [111]. The test requires skilled interpretation and may show significant inter-observer variability.

Corneal and conjunctival staining with vital dyes such as fluorescein and lissamine green reveals epithelial damage patterns but may not correlate well with symptom severity [10]. The interpretation of staining patterns requires experience, and mild staining may be overlooked while severe staining may not reflect the full extent of ocular surface compromise.

Tear osmolarity testing has emerged as a valuable diagnostic tool, as hyperosmolarity is a key feature of KCS [64]. However, osmolarity values can fluctuate throughout the day and may be influenced by factors such as recent tear instillation, environmental conditions, and systemic hydration status. Single-point measurements may not capture the full extent of osmotic instability.

3.3. Differential Diagnosis Considerations

The diagnosis of KCS in SD must consider numerous other conditions that can present with similar symptoms and signs. Allergic conjunctivitis, infectious conjunctivitis, and medicamentosa from chronic topical medication use can all mimic aspects of KCS. The presence of concurrent conditions further complicates diagnosis, as many SD patients may have multiple ocular surface disorders simultaneously.

Age-related changes in tear production and composition can overlap with early SD manifestations, making diagnosis particularly challenging in older patients. Hormonal influences, particularly in postmenopausal women, can affect tear production and may confound the assessment of autoimmune-related changes [26].

Medication-induced dry eye from systemic drugs such as antihistamines, antidepressants, and diuretics must be considered in the differential diagnosis. Many SD patients are prescribed medications that can exacerbate ocular surface symptoms, creating a complex interplay between disease-related and medication-related factors.

Contact lens wear can significantly alter ocular surface characteristics and may mask or exacerbate underlying KCS. The assessment of contact lens-wearing SD patients requires careful consideration of lens-related factors and may necessitate a period of lens discontinuation for accurate diagnosis [112].

4. Advanced Diagnostic Approaches

A summary of the diagnostic modalities used in KCS, along with their targets, advantages, and limitations, is presented in Table 1.

Table 1. Diagnostic tools for keratoconjunctivitis sicca in Sjögren Disease.

Test/Tool	Type	Target Parameter	Advantages	Limitations
Schirmer test	Functional	Tear volume	Simple, widely available	Poor specificity, variable reproducibility
TBUT	Functional	Tear film stability	Non-invasive, fast	Operator-dependent
Vital dye staining	Structural	Epithelial integrity	Detects surface damage	Variable correlation with symptoms
Tear osmolarity	Biomarker	Tear composition (osmolarity)	Quantifiable, point-of-care devices	Fluctuates; sensitive to environment
MMP-9 assay (InflammaDry)	Biomarker	Ocular surface inflammation	Fast, POC available	Binary output, not quantifiable
Meibography	Imaging	Meibomian gland morphology	Structural assessment	Limited availability
In vivo confocal microscopy	Imaging	Inflammatory cells, nerve density	High-resolution, detailed	Requires expertise, limited access
Anterior segment OCT	Imaging	Tear meniscus, conjunctiva	Objective, reproducible	Still not routine in many clinics
OSDI/DEQ	Symptom-based	Patient-reported symptom severity	Easy to administer	Subjective, no correlation with signs

Abbreviations: AS-OCT: Anterior Segment Optical Coherence Tomography; DEQ: Dry Eye Questionnaire; IVCM: In Vivo Confocal Microscopy; MMP-9: Matrix Metalloproteinase-9; OSDI: Ocular Surface Disease Index; POC: Point-of-Care; TBUT: Tear Break-Up Time.

4.1. Imaging Technologies and Biomarkers

Recent advances in ocular imaging have revolutionized the diagnostic approach to KCS in SD. Meibography, which provides detailed visualization of meibomian gland structure, has revealed the high prevalence of MGD in SD patients [113]. This non-invasive technique allows for quantitative assessment of gland dropout and morphological changes, providing objective evidence of lipid layer dysfunction. Advanced meibography systems now provide automated calculation of dropout scores using planimetry software to measure the percentage of gland area loss relative to total tarsal area [114,115]. The dropout score correlates directly with functional measures of meibomian gland dysfunction, with scores >30% associated with significant tear film instability and scores >60% indicating severe functional impairment [113,116]. Importantly, upper and lower eyelid dropout patterns differ significantly, with upper lids showing more frequent morphological abnormalities while lower lids demonstrate greater absolute dropout areas [53,117].

Tortuosity index (TI) represents a quantitative measure of meibomian gland shape deviation from normal linear morphology, calculated as the ratio of actual gland path length to the straight-line distance between gland endpoints [118,119]. Normal healthy individuals exhibit TI values < 0.1, while patients with meibomian gland dysfunction show significantly elevated TI values, with each 0.1 increase associated with reduced tear break-up time and increased dry eye symptoms [118,119].

Gland tortuosity often represents the earliest morphological change in meibomian gland dysfunction, preceding visible dropout by months to years, making it a valuable early diagnostic marker [120,121]. The mechanism underlying increased tortuosity involves inflammatory changes in the tarsal plate that alter the mechanical environment of the glands, forcing them to follow tortuous paths as they attempt to maintain their length within a contracting fibrous matrix [122,123]. High tortuosity indices (>0.2) significantly impair meibum expression efficiency during blinking, as the increased path length and multiple directional changes create resistance to flow [124,125].

Modern automated analysis systems provide multiple additional parameters including diameter deformation index (DI), which measures width variations along gland length, and signal index (SI), which reflects gland density and structural integrity based on infrared reflectance patterns [126,127]. These parameters show excellent inter-observer reliability (ICC > 0.8) and provide complementary information to traditional dropout scores, with combined assessment significantly improving diagnostic accuracy for meibomian gland dysfunction [128,129].

Longitudinal studies demonstrate that meibographic parameters predict treatment response, with patients showing high initial tortuosity indices and extensive dropout being less likely to respond to conventional therapies and more likely to require advanced interventions such as intense pulsed light or thermal pulsation treatments [130,131]. The combination of upper eyelid tortuosity and lower eyelid dropout provides the strongest correlation with patient-reported symptoms and objective clinical measures, supporting the importance of comprehensive bilateral assessment in clinical practice [132,133].

Infrared meibography is particularly valuable as it can visualize gland morphology through the eyelid without requiring eyelid eversion. This technique has revealed that meibomian gland dropout in SD patients follows characteristic patterns, with more severe involvement typically seen in the central portions of the eyelids. The correlation between meibography findings and clinical measures of MGD provides valuable insights into the pathophysiology of evaporative dry eye in SD.

In vivo confocal microscopy (IVCM) provides high-resolution visualization of corneal and conjunctival surfaces, allowing assessment of epithelial morphology, inflammatory infiltration, and corneal nerve integrity [134]. In SD, IVCM typically reveals increased dendritic cell density, which reflects active inflammation and may occur before overt clinical progression.

IVCM also reveals characteristic changes in epithelial cell morphology, including increased cell size variability, altered nuclear-to-cytoplasmic ratios, and the presence of inflammatory infiltrates. These changes correlate with disease severity and may serve as biomarkers for treatment response. The technique has also demonstrated reduced corneal nerve fiber density in SD patients, which correlates with decreased corneal sensitivity and may explain the altered pain perception seen in many patients.

Anterior segment optical coherence tomography (AS-OCT) offers high-resolution imaging of the ocular surface and can measure tear meniscus height, providing quantitative assessment of tear volume. This technique is particularly valuable for monitoring treatment response and disease progression over time. Modern AS-OCT systems can also assess conjunctival thickness and identify subclinical inflammatory changes that may not be apparent in clinical examination.

The development of tear film-specific OCT techniques has enabled dynamic assessment of tear film behavior, including measurement of tear film thinning rates and identification of areas of instability. These measurements provide objective correlates of subjective symptoms and can help guide treatment decisions.

Tear film biomarkers have emerged as promising diagnostic tools for KCS in SD, offering objective measures of inflammatory activity and glandular function. Inflammatory markers such as IL-1β, TNF-α, and matrix metalloproteinase-9 (MMP-9) are consistently elevated in SD patients and correlate with disease severity [135]. The development of point-of-care testing devices for MMP-9 has made clinical assessment of tear film inflammation more accessible [115].

Lactoferrin and lysozyme concentrations are typically reduced in SD patients, reflecting impaired lacrimal gland function [113,116]. As these proteins normally provide antimicrobial defense and maintain ocular surface integrity, their deficiency may contribute to the increased susceptibility to ocular surface infections observed in SD [118,119].

Tear osmolarity has also gained prominence as both a diagnostic and monitoring tool [136,137]. With the advent of advanced osmometers requiring only minimal sample volumes, routine clinical implementation has become feasible. Because osmolarity in SD patients fluctuates over time, protocols recommending multiple sequential measurements have been developed to better capture osmotic instability [122,123]. In addition, proteomic and metabolomic profiling of the tear film is revealing novel biomarkers with diagnostic and prognostic value, including proteins involved in inflammation, immune regulation, and tissue repair [124,125]. These approaches not only provide mechanistic insights but also identify potential therapeutic targets [128,129].

4.2. Functional Assessment Techniques

Dynamic assessment of tear film behavior provides insights beyond static measurements [130,131]. High-speed videokeratography can track tear film break-up patterns in real-time, revealing areas of instability and their relationship to symptom patterns [132,133]. This technique provides more detailed information than traditional TBUT testing and can identify subtle abnormalities [134].

Interferometry allows for precise measurement of the tear film lipid layer thickness and can identify patients with MGD-related evaporative dry eye [135,138]. This technique is particularly valuable in SD patients, where both aqueous deficiency and evaporative components may be present simultaneously [139].

Impression cytology enables histological examination of the conjunctival epithelium and can identify inflammatory cells, assess goblet cell density, and evaluate epithelial cell morphology [140,141]. This technique provides objective evidence of ocular surface inflammation and can help differentiate SD-related changes from other causes of KCS [142].

Questionnaire-based assessment tools such as the Ocular Surface Disease Index (OSDI) and Dry Eye Questionnaire (DEQ) provide standardized methods for symptom assessment [143,144]. These tools are particularly valuable for monitoring treatment response and can help identify patients who may benefit from additional interventions [145,146].

5. Current Therapeutic Approaches

A classification of therapeutic strategies for KCS in SD is provided in Table 2.

Table 2. Therapeutic approaches for keratoconjunctivitis sicca in Sjögren Disease.

Treatment Class	Examples	Mechanism of Action	Indication/Utility	Limitations/Notes
Artificial tears	Hyaluronic acid, CMC, lipid-based drops	Tear replacement, lubrication	First-line for all severities	Temporary relief, frequent use needed
Topical corticosteroids	Loteprednol, fluorometholone	Inhibit inflammation	Short-term flare control	Risk of IOP rise, cataract with prolonged use
Topical immunomodulators	Cyclosporine, lifitegrast	T-cell inhibition (calcineurin/LFA-1 pathways)	Chronic inflammation, maintenance therapy	Delayed onset; stinging on instillation
Oral secretagogues	Pilocarpine, cevimeline	Muscarinic receptor agonists	Residual gland function	Cholinergic side effects
Punctal occlusion	Silicone or collagen plugs	Reduces tear drainage	Moderate-to-severe aqueous deficiency	Epiphora, plug extrusion
Biologic therapies	Rituximab, abatacept, tocilizumab	Target B/T cells, cytokines (CD20, CD80/86, IL-6)	Refractory systemic and ocular disease	Off-label; systemic risks; cost
Regenerative therapy	Autologous serum, PRP, stem cells	Growth factors, epithelial healing	Severe epithelial damage, neurotrophic KCS	Access, standardization challenges
Procedural	IPL, scleral lenses	MGD treatment, tear reservoir creation	Severe or refractory cases	Requires expertise; cost

Abbreviations: CMC: Carboxymethylcellulose; IOP: Intraocular Pressure; LFA-1: Lymphocyte Function-Associated Antigen-1; PRP: Platelet-Rich Plasma; NSAID: Nonsteroidal Anti-Inflammatory Drug; MGD: Meibomian Gland Dysfunction; KCS: Keratoconjunctivitis Sicca; SD: Sjögren Disease.

5.1. Artificial Tears and Lubricants

The foundation of KCS management in SD remains the replacement of deficient tear volume and improvement of tear film stability through artificial tears and lubricants. The selection of appropriate formulations requires consideration of tear film abnormalities, symptom patterns, and patient preferences. Modern artificial tears are formulated with various viscosity agents, electrolyte compositions, and osmolarity levels to address different aspects of tear film dysfunction.

The evolution of artificial tear formulations has led to increasingly sophisticated products designed to address specific tear film deficiencies. Hyaluronic acid-based formulations provide excellent mucoadhesive properties and long-lasting relief, while also promoting epithelial healing through interaction with CD44 receptors. These formulations are particularly beneficial for SD patients with significant epithelial damage.

Carboxymethylcellulose (CMC) and hydroxypropyl methylcellulose (HPMC) remain popular viscosity agents, offering good retention time and patient comfort. Newer formulations combining multiple polymers aim to provide both immediate relief and sustained protection. The addition of osmoprotectants such as L-carnitine and erythritol helps protect epithelial cells from osmotic stress.

Preservative-free formulations are strongly preferred for SD patients due to the potential for preservative toxicity in compromised ocular surfaces. Benzalkonium chloride, the most commonly used preservative in ophthalmic preparations, can cause epithelial damage, reduce goblet cell density, and exacerbate inflammatory processes. The development of multi-dose preservative-free systems using alternative preservation technologies has improved patient compliance while maintaining product sterility.

The concentration and type of electrolytes in artificial tears significantly influence their therapeutic effectiveness. Formulations with balanced electrolyte compositions that more closely mimic natural tears may provide superior comfort and healing promotion. The addition of potassium, which is typically depleted in SD patients, may help restore normal cellular function.

Hypotonic formulations may provide benefits for patients with hyperosmolar tears, though the optimal osmolarity for artificial tears remains debated. Some studies suggest that isotonic formulations may be better tolerated initially, while others indicate that slightly hypotonic solutions may help restore normal osmotic balance over time. The choice may need to be individualized based on patient response and tear film characteristics.

The frequency of artificial tear instillation must be individualized based on symptom severity, environmental factors, and tear clearance rates. Many SD patients require hourly or more frequent instillation during symptomatic periods, which can significantly impact quality of life and treatment adherence. The development of longer-lasting formulations using advanced polymer technology and lipid-containing drops has improved patient convenience and potentially enhanced therapeutic efficacy.

Gel formulations and ointments provide longer-lasting relief but may cause temporary vision blurring, making them more suitable for nighttime use. The strategic use of different viscosity products throughout the day, lighter formulations for daytime use and heavier preparations for nighttime, can optimize symptom control while minimizing visual interference.

5.2. Anti-Inflammatory Therapies

Topical corticosteroids may provide rapid symptom relief in keratoconjunctivitis sicca, particularly during acute inflammatory flares. However, their use should be limited to short-term courses given the well-recognized risks of long-term therapy, including glaucoma, cataract formation, and ocular surface complications.

Among steroid-sparing options, topical cyclosporine and lifitegrast have emerged as the mainstays of anti-inflammatory therapy. Cyclosporine, a calcineurin inhibitor, reduces T-lymphocyte activation and inflammatory cytokine production, while lifitegrast, an antagonist of lymphocyte function–associated antigen-1 (LFA-1), interrupts T-cell adhesion and migration. Both agents directly address the underlying autoimmune inflammation, albeit through distinct mechanisms. Clinical trials have demonstrated that cyclosporine 0.05% emulsion, administered twice daily, improves tear production and symptoms, although the onset of action may require several weeks. Lifitegrast, in contrast, has shown improvement in both signs and symptoms within the first few weeks of treatment [147]. This calcineurin inhibitor reduces T-lymphocyte activation and inflammatory cytokine production, addressing the underlying autoimmune process. Clinical trials have demonstrated significant improvements in tear production and symptom relief with twice-daily cyclosporine 0.05% emulsion. The onset of action is typically gradual, requiring several weeks to months for optimal benefit.

Topical lifitegrast, a lymphocyte function-associated antigen-1 (LFA-1) antagonist, represents a novel approach to anti-inflammatory therapy [148,149]. By blocking T-cell activation and migration, lifitegrast interrupts the inflammatory cascade at a different point than cyclosporine. Clinical studies have shown improvements in both signs and symptoms of KCS, with benefits often apparent within the first few weeks of treatment.

The development of newer anti-inflammatory agents continues to expand therapeutic options. Topical corticosteroids with improved safety profiles, such as loteprednol etabonate, may provide anti-inflammatory benefits with reduced systemic absorption and fewer side effects.

5.3. Secretagogues and Tear Stimulants

Oral pilocarpine, a muscarinic agonist, stimulates residual lacrimal gland function and can increase tear production in SD patients with remaining functional glandular tissue [150,151]. The drug is most effective in patients with mild to moderate glandular dysfunction and may provide additional benefits for salivary gland function. Side effects include sweating, nausea, and urinary frequency, which limit its use in some patients.

Cevimeline, another muscarinic agonist, offers similar benefits to pilocarpine but with potentially improved tolerability [150]. The drug has shown efficacy in increasing tear production and reducing symptoms in SD patients, though individual responses vary considerably.

Topical secretagogues are under investigation as potential alternatives to systemic therapy. These agents could theoretically provide localized stimulation of tear production without systemic side effects, though clinical development remains in early stages.

Diquafosol, a P2Y2 receptor agonist, stimulates mucin and fluid secretion from conjunctival epithelial cells and goblet cells. While not available in all markets, this agent has shown promise in clinical trials for improving tear film stability and reducing symptoms.

5.4. Procedural Interventions

Punctal occlusion offers a mechanical strategy for tear conservation and is particularly useful in patients with severe aqueous deficiency [43,152]. Temporary collagen plugs are often placed initially to evaluate benefit before considering permanent silicone plugs. The procedure is generally safe and well tolerated, although potential complications include plug extrusion, infection, and epiphora.

Adjunctive mechanical techniques such as lacrimal gland massage and expression may provide short-term symptom relief by promoting glandular secretion, but their long-term efficacy remains limited.

Intense pulsed light (IPL) therapy has emerged as a novel approach for meibomian gland dysfunction–associated evaporative dry eye in SD. By targeting abnormal periocular vessels, IPL may improve gland function, though additional studies are required to establish standardized treatment protocols.

For patients with severe, refractory keratoconjunctivitis sicca, scleral contact lenses provide a protective fluid reservoir over the cornea, improving ocular surface hydration and reducing symptom burden [153]. Although these devices require specialized fitting and close follow-up, they can substantially enhance quality of life.

6. Emerging Therapeutic Strategies

6.1. Biologic Therapies and Targeted Interventions

The development of biologic therapies represents a paradigm shift in KCS treatment, offering the potential to target specific inflammatory pathways involved in SD pathogenesis.

These treatments address the underlying autoimmune mechanisms rather than merely providing symptomatic relief, potentially offering disease-modifying effects that could slow or halt disease progression.

Rituximab, a monoclonal antibody targeting CD20+ B cells, has shown promise in multiple studies of SD patients, with improvements in both systemic and ocular manifestations [154,155]. Clinical trials have demonstrated improvements in tear production, ocular surface staining, and patient-reported symptoms following rituximab treatment. Yet these benefits are often temporary, necessitating repeated courses. Moreover, the use of rituximab is constrained by its high cost, limited access in many healthcare systems, and the increased risk of infections associated with prolonged B-cell.

The mechanism of action of rituximab in SD extends beyond simple B-cell depletion. The treatment appears to reset the immune system, reducing the production of autoantibodies and pro-inflammatory cytokines. Some patients experience prolonged remissions following treatment, suggesting that rituximab may help restore immune tolerance in certain individuals.

TNF-α inhibitors, including infliximab, etanercept, and adalimumab, have been investigated for SD treatment with mixed results [156,157]. While some studies have shown improvements in systemic symptoms, ocular benefits have been less consistent. The heterogeneity of SD patients and varying degrees of TNF-α involvement may explain these disparate results. Some patients may benefit significantly from TNF-α inhibition, while others show minimal response.

The use of TNF-α inhibitors in SD requires careful patient selection and monitoring. These agents carry risks of serious infections and may exacerbate certain autoimmune conditions. The decision to use TNF-α inhibitors should be based on disease severity, failure of conventional therapy, and careful risk-benefit assessment.

Abatacept, a selective co-stimulation modulator that blocks T-cell activation, has shown promising results in early clinical trials for SD [158]. By interrupting the interaction between CD80/CD86 on antigen-presenting cells and CD28 on T cells, abatacept may help reduce the autoimmune response responsible for glandular destruction. The drug has demonstrated improvements in both glandular function and systemic symptoms in some patients.

The advantage of abatacept lies in its mechanism of action, which targets the fundamental T-cell activation process central to SD pathogenesis. Unlike treatments that target downstream effector molecules, abatacept may address the root cause of autoimmune activation. However, like other biologic therapies, it requires careful monitoring for adverse effects and may not be suitable for all patients.

Interferon-α therapy has demonstrated efficacy in treating systemic manifestations of SD and may have ocular benefits [159]. The treatment appears to modulate immune function and may help restore glandular function in some patients. However, the significant side effect profile of interferon therapy, including flu-like symptoms, depression, and autoimmune complications, limits its use to carefully selected patients with severe disease.

Newer biologic agents targeting other inflammatory pathways are under investigation. Interleukin-6 inhibitors, such as tocilizumab, have shown promise in preliminary studies. IL-6 plays a crucial role in B-cell activation and autoantibody production, making it an attractive therapeutic target. Other potential targets include the BAFF (B-cell activating factor) pathway, which is important for B-cell survival and activation.

The development of biomarkers to predict responses to biologic therapy is an active area of research. Factors such as autoantibody profiles, cytokine levels, and genetic markers may help identify patients most likely to benefit from specific treatments. This personalized approach could improve treatment outcomes while reducing unnecessary exposure to expensive and potentially harmful therapies.

6.2. Regenerative Medicine Approaches

Stem cell therapy represents a promising frontier in KCS treatment, with potential applications for both lacrimal gland regeneration and ocular surface repair. Mesenchymal stem cells (MSCs) derived from various sources, including bone marrow, adipose tissue, and umbilical cord, have shown anti-inflammatory and regenerative properties in preclinical studies. Recent clinical trials have demonstrated the potential of allogeneic stem cell therapy in treating immune-mediated keratoconjunctivitis sicca, with significant improvements in Schirmer test scores observed in canine models of autoimmune dry eye disease [160,161]. The mechanisms underlying stem cell therapeutic effects include paracrine secretion of growth factors, immunomodulatory cytokines, and extracellular vesicles that promote tissue regeneration and reduce local inflammation [162,163].

Advanced tissue engineering approaches are being developed for lacrimal gland reconstruction, including bioengineered organoids that recapitulate the complex three-dimensional architecture of native glands [164,165]. These organoid systems have shown promise in preclinical studies for restoring secretory function and may eventually provide alternatives to conventional medical therapy for patients with severe glandular destruction [166,167].

Autologous serum eye drops have gained popularity as a treatment for severe KCS, providing growth factors, vitamins, and other biological components that may promote epithelial healing [33]. While evidence for efficacy is limited, many patients report subjective improvements, and the treatment is generally well-tolerated.

Platelet-rich plasma (PRP) eye drops represent an evolution of serum therapy, providing concentrated growth factors and cytokines that may enhance healing. Early clinical studies suggest potential benefits, though standardization of preparation methods and treatment protocols remains challenging. Recent advances in PRP preparation techniques have improved standardization, with studies showing that PRP eye drops containing optimal concentrations of platelet-derived growth factor (PDGF) and transforming growth factor-β (TGF-β) provide superior healing outcomes compared to conventional artificial tears [168,169]. The development of autologous plasma-rich in growth factors (PRGF) represents a further refinement of this approach, offering enhanced bioavailability and sustained release of therapeutic factors [170,171].

Tissue engineering approaches for lacrimal gland reconstruction are in early developmental stages. The complex structure and function of the lacrimal gland present significant challenges, but advances in 3D bioprinting and organoid technology may eventually enable gland replacement or augmentation.

6.3. Gene Therapy and Molecular Interventions

Gene therapy approaches for KCS are being investigated, with potential applications including enhancement of tear production, reduction in inflammation, and promotion of epithelial healing [61,172]. Viral vectors could theoretically deliver therapeutic genes to lacrimal glands or ocular surface tissues, providing sustained therapeutic effects [173,174]. Recent advances in adeno-associated virus (AAV) vector technology have improved targeting specificity and reduced immunogenicity, making clinical translation more feasible [175,176].

Epigenetic modulation represents an emerging therapeutic strategy, with studies identifying specific DNA methylation patterns and histone modifications associated with SS pathogenesis [177,178]. Targeting these epigenetic changes through selective inhibitors may offer new approaches to restoring normal gene expression patterns in affected tissues [168].

Antisense oligonucleotides and small interfering RNAs (siRNAs) offer precise methods for modulating gene expression in target tissues. These approaches could potentially reduce inflammatory mediator production or enhance protective factor expression in the ocular surface [179–181].

Nanotechnology applications in KCS treatment include drug delivery systems that can provide sustained release of therapeutic agents and targeted delivery to specific ocular surface tissues. Nanoparticles, liposomes, and other delivery systems may enhance therapeutic efficacy while reducing systemic exposure. Recent developments in nanocarrier systems include thermosensitive hydrogels that provide prolonged drug residence time on the ocular surface, and targeted nanoparticles that can selectively deliver anti-inflammatory agents to activated immune cells [182,183]. These advanced delivery systems show promise for improving treatment outcomes while minimizing side effects [182,184].

7. Future Directions and Research Priorities

7.1. Personalized Medicine Approaches

The heterogeneity of SD patients and their varying responses to treatment highlight the need for personalized medicine approaches that consider individual patient characteristics, disease phenotypes, and molecular profiles [13,185]. This approach represents a fundamental shift from the traditional "one-size-fits-all" treatment paradigm to tailored interventions based on specific patient needs and disease mechanisms [186–188].

Biomarker-guided therapy selection is becoming increasingly important in SD management, with recent advances in tear proteomics and metabolomics enabling identification of patient-specific inflammatory profiles for targeted treatment selection [189–191]. Patients with high levels of specific inflammatory markers may benefit more from anti-inflammatory therapies, while those with evidence of glandular dysfunction may require secretagogues or regenerative approaches [192,193]. The development of point-of-care testing devices for key biomarkers is making personalized treatment selection more feasible in clinical practice [194,195].

Genetic profiling may reveal susceptibility factors and therapeutic targets specific to individual patients. Polymorphisms in genes involved in drug metabolism, such as cytochrome P450 enzymes, could influence optimal dosing of medications like cyclosporine [196,197]. Additionally, genetic variants in inflammatory pathways may predict response to specific anti-inflammatory treatments [198].

Endotypes are one of the most novel concepts emerging in SD research is the recognition of disease *endotypes*—biologically distinct subgroups characterized by different underlying mechanisms [199,200]. This framework moves beyond clinical phenotyping toward mechanism-based stratification. Patients with predominantly inflammatory endotypes may respond preferentially to immunosuppressive therapies, while those with neurogenic or glandular dysfunction endotypes may require alternative interventions [135,201]. Identification of endotype-specific biomarkers could revolutionize therapeutic algorithms, and they represent a key step toward precision medicine in SD [187].

Pharmacogenomics applications in SD are still in early stages but hold promise for optimizing treatment selection and dosing [202]. Genetic variants affecting drug absorption, metabolism, and target receptor expression could influence treatment outcomes [203]. The integration of pharmacogenomic data into clinical decision-making tools could improve treatment efficacy while reducing adverse effects.

Tear film proteomic and metabolomic analyses are providing new insights into disease mechanisms and potential therapeutic targets [204]. These approaches may eventually enable the development of personalized treatment protocols based on individual tear film profiles. The identification of specific metabolic pathways that are dysregulated in individual patients could guide targeted interventions.

Patient-centered outcomes: The refinement of patient-reported outcome measures is essential to capture the heterogeneous impact of SD and treatment response. Personalized symptom profiles, aligned with individual quality-of-life priorities, may further guide therapy and monitoring [205,206].

Systems medicine and AI: Integration of multi-omic data (clinical, genetic, biochemical, and imaging) using artificial intelligence and machine learning is being developed to create predictive models of treatment response and long-term outcomes [207,208]. Recent applications in ophthalmology illustrate this potential: for example, deep learning algorithms applied to in vivo confocal microscopy and optical coherence tomography (OCT) have been shown to accurately classify dry eye severity and detect subtle corneal nerve alterations before clinical symptoms emerge. For instance, a recent deep learning model applied to anterior segment optical coherence tomography (AS-OCT) images demonstrated robust diagnostic performance for dry eye disease, achieving 85% accuracy, 86% sensitivity, and 82% specificity when compared to traditional clinical tests—suggesting that AI can provide fast, objective, and reproducible assessments of tear film abnormalities. Such tools could assist clinicians in delivering more precise, individualized care in SD. Emerging AI techniques are also being applied to in vivo confocal microscopy (IVCM). A novel machine learning algorithm now enables unbiased quantification of corneal nerve features—such as nerve density and dendritic cell infiltration—offering objective biomarkers that correlate with ocular surface inflammation.

Collectively, these advances highlight a paradigm shift toward precision medicine in SD. By integrating biomarkers, genetics, and computational tools, future treatment strategies may be tailored to individual disease mechanisms, with the ultimate goal of improving outcomes while reducing treatment burden.

7.2. Combination Therapy Strategies

The complex pathophysiology of KCS in SD suggests that combination therapies targeting multiple pathways may be more effective than single-agent approaches. Combinations of anti-inflammatory agents, tear replacements, and procedural interventions may provide synergistic benefits. Recent studies have shown that combining topical cyclosporine with punctal occlusion provides superior outcomes compared to either treatment alone.

Network medicine approaches are revealing unexpected therapeutic targets through analysis of protein–protein interaction networks and pathway crosstalk. The integration of traditional Chinese medicine with Western pharmacological approaches has shown promise in clinical trials, suggesting that combination strategies may benefit from both Eastern and Western therapeutic traditions.

Sequential therapy protocols that adapt treatment based on patient response and disease progression may optimize outcomes while minimizing side effects. The development of treatment algorithms incorporating objective measures of treatment response could guide therapy selection and adjustment.

8. Conclusions

Keratoconjunctivitis sicca (KCS) in Sjögren disease represents a complex autoimmune condition that extends far beyond simple tear deficiency. Its multifactorial pathophysiology involves immune, inflammatory, hormonal, and neurogenic mechanisms, making effective management particularly challenging.

Recent advances in diagnostics, including high-resolution imaging and biomarker discovery, are improving early detection and enabling more objective disease monitoring. Therapeutic strategies have evolved from symptomatic tear replacement to targeted anti-inflammatory agents, procedural interventions, and emerging biologic and regenerative therapies, with the potential to modify disease progression rather than simply alleviate symptoms. If validated in larger trials, these innovations could ultimately reshape international treatment guidelines.

Among the most novel concepts highlighted in this review is the recognition of disease endotypes—biologically distinct subgroups of Sjögren disease defined by their underlying mechanisms rather than clinical manifestations. This framework represents a paradigm shift toward mechanism-based classification, offering the potential to refine therapeutic selection, accelerate personalized medicine, and fundamentally alter future treatment algorithms.

Looking ahead, the integration of endotype-specific biomarkers, genetic and pharmacogenomic data, and computational approaches such as artificial intelligence will pave the way toward precision medicine in Sjögren disease. Multidisciplinary collaboration between ophthalmologists, rheumatologists, and other specialists, combined with patient-centered care models, will be essential for translating these scientific advances into improved outcomes and quality of life for patients.

Funding: This research received no external funding.

Conflicts of Interest: The authors declare no conflict of interest.

Abbreviations

AS-OCT	Anterior Segment Optical Coherence Tomography
BAFF	B-cell Activating Factor
CD	Cluster of Differentiation
DED	Dry Eye Disease
DEQ	Dry Eye Questionnaire
HLA	Human Leukocyte Antigen
IFN-γ	Interferon gamma
IFN-I	Type I Interferon
IL-1β	Interleukin-1 beta
IVCM	In Vivo Confocal Microscopy
KCS	Keratoconjunctivitis Sicca
MGD	Meibomian Gland Dysfunction
MMP-9	Matrix Metalloproteinase-9
MSC	Mesenchymal Stem Cell
NSAID	Nonsteroidal Anti-Inflammatory Drug
OSDI	Ocular Surface Disease Index
PRP	Platelet-Rich Plasma
SD	Sjögren's Disease
sIgA	Secretory Immunoglobulin A
SSA/Ro	Sjögren Syndrome Antigen A (Ro)
SSB/La	Sjögren Syndrome Antigen B (La)
SS	Sjögren's Syndrome
TBUT	Tear Break-Up Time
TGF-β	Transforming Growth Factor-beta
TFOS DEWS II	Tear Film and Ocular Surface Society Dry Eye Workshop II
TNF-α	Tumor Necrosis Factor-alpha

References

1. Qin, B.; Wang, J.; Yang, Z.; Yang, M.; Ma, N.; Huang, F.; Zhong, R. Epidemiology of primary Sjogren's syndrome: A systematic review and meta-analysis. *Ann. Rheum. Dis.* **2015**, *74*, 1983–1989. [CrossRef] [PubMed]
2. Ramos-Casals, M.; Brito-Zeron, P.; Siso-Almirall, A.; Bosch, X. Primary Sjogren syndrome. *BMJ* **2012**, *344*, e3821. [CrossRef] [PubMed]
3. Pflugfelder, S.C.; de Paiva, C.S. The Pathophysiology of Dry Eye Disease: What We Know and Future Directions for Research. *Ophthalmology* **2017**, *124*, S4–S13. [CrossRef] [PubMed]
4. Bron, A.J.; de Paiva, C.S.; Chauhan, S.K.; Bonini, S.; Gabison, E.E.; Jain, S.; Knop, E.; Markoulli, M.; Ogawa, Y.; Perez, V.; et al. TFOS DEWS II pathophysiology report. *Ocul. Surf.* **2017**, *15*, 438–510, Erratum in *Ocul. Surf.* **2019**, *17*, 842. [CrossRef]
5. Mavragani, C.P.; Moutsopoulos, H.M. Sjogren's syndrome. *Annu. Rev. Pathol.* **2014**, *9*, 273–285. [CrossRef]
6. Patel, R.; Shahane, A. The epidemiology of Sjogren's syndrome. *Clin. Epidemiol.* **2014**, *6*, 247–255.
7. Stapleton, F.; Alves, M.; Bunya, V.Y.; Jalbert, I.; Lekhanont, K.; Malet, F.; Na, K.-S.; Schaumberg, D.; Uchino, M.; Vehof, J.; et al. TFOS DEWS II Epidemiology Report. *Ocul. Surf.* **2017**, *15*, 334–365. [CrossRef]
8. Galor, A.; Feuer, W.; Lee, D.J.; Florez, H.; Carter, D.; Pouyeh, B.; Prunty, W.J.; Perez, V.L. Prevalence and risk factors of dry eye syndrome in a United States veterans affairs population. *Am. J. Ophthalmol.* **2011**, *152*, 377–384.e2. [CrossRef]
9. Ramos-Casals, M.; Solans, R.; Rosas, J.; Camps, M.T.; Gil, A.; Del Pino-Montes, J.; Calvo-Alen, J.; Jiménez-Alonso, J.; Micó, M.-L.; Beltrán, J.; et al. Primary Sjogren syndrome in Spain: Clinical and immunologic expression in 1010 patients. *Medicine* **2008**, *87*, 210–219. [CrossRef]
10. Akpek, E.K.; Klimava, A.; Thorne, J.E.; Martin, D.; Lekhanont, K.; Ostrovsky, A. Evaluation of patients with dry eye for presence of underlying Sjogren syndrome. *Cornea* **2009**, *28*, 493–497. [CrossRef]
11. Caffery, B.E.; Richter, D.; Simpson, T.; Fonn, D.; Doughty, M.; Gordon, K. CANDEES. The Canadian Dry Eye Epidemiology Study. *Adv. Exp. Med. Biol.* **1998**, *438*, 805–806.
12. Miljanovic, B.; Dana, R.; Sullivan, D.A.; Schaumberg, D.A. Impact of dry eye syndrome on vision-related quality of life. *Am. J. Ophthalmol.* **2007**, *143*, 409–415. [CrossRef] [PubMed]
13. Lessard, C.J.; Li, H.; Adrianto, I.; Ice, J.A.; Rasmussen, A.; Grundahl, K.M.; Kelly, J.A.; Dozmorov, M.G.; Miceli-Richard, C.; Bowman, S.; et al. Variants at multiple loci implicated in both innate and adaptive immune responses are associated with Sjogren's syndrome. *Nat. Genet.* **2013**, *45*, 1284–1292. [CrossRef] [PubMed]
14. Igoe, A.; Scofield, R.H. Autoimmunity and infection in Sjogren's syndrome. *Curr. Opin. Rheumatol.* **2013**, *25*, 480–487. [CrossRef]
15. Baudouin, C.; Messmer, E.M.; Aragona, P.; Geerling, G.; Akova, Y.A.; Benítez-Del-Castillo, J.; Boboridis, K.G.; Merayo-Lloves, J.; Rolando, M.; Labetoulle, M. Revisiting the vicious circle of dry eye disease: A focus on the pathophysiology of meibomian gland dysfunction. *Br. J. Ophthalmol.* **2016**, *100*, 300–306. [CrossRef] [PubMed]
16. Jones, L.; Downie, L.E.; Korb, D.; Benitez-Del-Castillo, J.M.; Dana, R.; Deng, S.X.; Dong, P.N.; Geerling, G.; Hida, R.Y.; Liu, Y.; et al. TFOS DEWS II Management and Therapy Report. *Ocul. Surf.* **2017**, *15*, 575–628. [CrossRef]
17. Manoussakis, M.N.; Boiu, S.; Korkolopoulou, P.; Kapsogeorgou, E.K.; Kavantzas, N.; Ziakas, P.; Patsouris, E.; Moutsopoulos, H.M. Rates of infiltration by macrophages and dendritic cells and expression of interleukin-18 and interleukin-12 in the chronic inflammatory lesions of Sjogren's syndrome: Correlation with certain features of immune hyperactivity and factors associated with high risk of lymphoma development. *Arthritis Rheum.* **2007**, *56*, 3977–3988.
18. Christodoulou, M.I.; Kapsogeorgou, E.K.; Moutsopoulos, H.M. Characteristics of the minor salivary gland infiltrates in Sjogren's syndrome. *J. Autoimmun.* **2010**, *34*, 400–407. [CrossRef]
19. Scofield, R.H.; Farris, A.D.; Horsfall, A.C.; Harley, J.B. Fine specificity of the autoimmune response to the Ro/SSA and La/SSB ribonucleoproteins. *Arthritis Rheum.* **1999**, *42*, 199–209. [CrossRef]
20. Bacman, S.; Berra, A.; Sterin-Borda, L.; Borda, E. Muscarinic acetylcholine receptor antibodies as a new marker of dry eye Sjogren syndrome. *Investig. Opthalmol. Vis. Sci.* **2001**, *42*, 321–327.
21. Peri, Y.; Agmon-Levin, N.; Theodor, E.; Shoenfeld, Y. Sjogren's syndrome, the old and the new. *Best Pract. Res. Clin. Rheumatol.* **2012**, *26*, 105–117. [CrossRef]
22. Wahren-Herlenius, M.; Dorner, T. Immunopathogenic mechanisms of systemic autoimmune disease. *Lancet* **2013**, *382*, 819–831. [CrossRef]
23. Yiannaki, E.E.; Tzioufas, A.G.; Bachmann, M.; Hantoumi, J.; Tsikaris, V.; Sakarellos-Daitsiotis, M.; Sakarellos, C.; Moutsopoulos, H.M. The value of synthetic linear epitope analogues of La/SSB for the detection of autoantibodies to La/SSB; specificity, sensitivity and comparison of methods. *Clin. Exp. Immunol.* **1998**, *112*, 152–158. [CrossRef] [PubMed]
24. Galletti, J.G.; de Paiva, C.S. The ocular surface immune system through the eyes of aging. *Ocul. Surf.* **2021**, *20*, 139–162. [CrossRef]

25. Kroneld, U.; Jonsson, R.; Carlsten, H.; Bremell, T.; Johannessen, A.C.; Tarkowski, A. Expression of the mucosal lymphocyte integrin alphaEbeta7 and its ligand E-cadherin in salivary glands of patients with Sjogren's syndrome. *Scand. J. Rheumatol.* **1998**, *27*, 215–218. [PubMed]
26. Song, Y.; Li, J.; Wu, Y. Evolving understanding of autoimmune mechanisms and new therapeutic strategies of autoimmune disorders. *Signal Transduct. Target. Ther.* **2024**, *9*, 263. [CrossRef] [PubMed]
27. Cusick, M.F.; Libbey, J.E.; Fujinami, R.S. Molecular mimicry as a mechanism of autoimmune disease. *Clin. Rev. Allergy Immunol.* **2012**, *42*, 102–111. [CrossRef]
28. Baer, A.N.; Maynard, J.W.; Shaikh, F.; Magder, L.S.; Petri, M. Secondary Sjogren's syndrome in systemic lupus erythematosus defines a distinct disease subset. *J. Rheumatol.* **2010**, *37*, 1143–1149. [CrossRef]
29. Tsunawaki, S.; Sporn, M.; Ding, A.; Nathan, C. Deactivation of macrophages by transforming growth factor-beta. *Nature* **1988**, *334*, 260–262. [CrossRef]
30. Kapsogeorgou, E.K.; Christodoulou, M.I.; Panagiotakos, D.B.; Paikos, S.; Tassidou, A.; Tzioufas, A.G.; Moutsopoulos, H.M. Minor salivary gland inflammatory lesions in Sjogren syndrome: Do they evolve? *J. Rheumatol.* **2013**, *40*, 1566–1571. [CrossRef]
31. Båve, U.; Nordmark, G.; Lövgren, T.; Rönnelid, J.; Cajander, S.; Eloranta, M.; Alm, G.V.; Rönnblom, L. Activation of the type I interferon system in primary Sjogren's syndrome: A possible etiopathogenic mechanism. *Arthritis Rheum.* **2005**, *52*, 1185–1195. [CrossRef]
32. Gottenberg, J.-E.; Cagnard, N.; Lucchesi, C.; Letourneur, F.; Mistou, S.; Lazure, T.; Jacques, S.; Ba, N.; Ittah, M.; Lepajolec, C.; et al. Activation of IFN pathways and plasmacytoid dendritic cell recruitment in target organs of primary Sjogren's syndrome. *Proc. Natl. Acad. Sci. USA* **2006**, *103*, 2770–2775, Erratum in *Proc. Natl. Acad. Sci. USA* **2006**, *103*, 5242. [CrossRef] [PubMed]
33. Imgenberg-Kreuz, J.; Sandling, J.K.; Almlöf, J.C.; Nordlund, J.; Signér, L.; Norheim, K.B.; Omdal, R.; Rönnblom, L.; Eloranta, M.-L.; Syvänen, A.-C.; et al. Genome-wide DNA methylation analysis in multiple tissues in primary Sjogren's syndrome reveals regulatory effects at interferon-induced genes. *Ann. Rheum. Dis.* **2016**, *75*, 2029–2036. [CrossRef] [PubMed]
34. Delcroix, V.; Mauduit, O.; Lee, H.S.; Ivanova, A.; Umazume, T.; Knox, S.M.; de Paiva, C.S.; Dartt, D.A.; Makarenkova, H.P. The First Transcriptomic Atlas of the Adult Lacrimal Gland Reveals Epithelial Complexity and Identifies Novel Progenitor Cells in Mice. *Cells* **2023**, *12*, 1435. [CrossRef] [PubMed]
35. Bjordal, O.; Norheim, K.B.; Rodahl, E.; Jonsson, R.; Omdal, R. Primary Sjogren's syndrome and the eye. *Surv. Ophthalmol.* **2020**, *65*, 119–132. [CrossRef]
36. Hayashi, T. Dysfunction of lacrimal and salivary glands in Sjogren's syndrome: Nonimmunologic injury in preinflammatory phase and mouse model. *J. Biomed. Biotechnol.* **2011**, *2011*, 407031. [CrossRef]
37. Nguyen, C.Q.; Cha, S.R.; Peck, A.B. Sjogren's syndrome (SjS)-like disease of mice: The importance of B lymphocytes and autoantibodies. *Front. Biosci.* **2007**, *12*, 1767–1789. [CrossRef]
38. Tzioufas, A.G.; Kapsogeorgou, E.K.; Moutsopoulos, H.M. Pathogenesis of Sjogren's syndrome: What we know and what we should learn. *J. Autoimmun.* **2012**, *39*, 4–8. [CrossRef]
39. Hernandez-Molina, G.; Leal-Alegre, G.; Michel-Peregrina, M. The meaning of anti-Ro and anti-La antibodies in primary Sjogren's syndrome. *Autoimmun. Rev.* **2011**, *10*, 123–125. [CrossRef]
40. Baimpa, E.; Dahabreh, I.J.; Voulgarelis, M.; Moutsopoulos, H.M. Hematologic manifestations and predictors of lymphoma development in primary Sjogren syndrome: Clinical and pathophysiologic aspects. *Medicine* **2009**, *88*, 284–293. [CrossRef]
41. Ramos-Casals, M.; Brito-Zerón, P.; Kostov, B.; Sisó-Almirall, A.; Bosch, X.; Buss, D.; Trilla, A.; Stone, J.H.; Khamashta, M.A.; Shoenfeld, Y. Google-driven search for big data in autoimmune geoepidemiology: Analysis of 394,827 patients with systemic autoimmune diseases. *Autoimmun. Rev.* **2015**, *14*, 670–679. [CrossRef] [PubMed]
42. Chivasso, C.; D'Agostino, C.; Parisis, D.; Soyfoo, M.S.; Delporte, C. Involvement of aquaporin 5 in Sjogren's syndrome. *Autoimmun. Rev.* **2023**, *22*, 103268. [CrossRef] [PubMed]
43. Hermida-Prieto, M.; Garcia-Castro, J.; Marinas-Pardo, L. Systemic Treatment of Immune-Mediated Keratoconjunctivitis Sicca with Allogeneic Stem Cells Improves the Schirmer Tear Test Score in a Canine Spontaneous Model of Disease. *J. Clin. Med.* **2021**, *10*, 5981. [CrossRef] [PubMed]
44. Harrell, C.R.; Feulner, L.; Djonov, V.; Pavlovic, D.; Volarevic, V. The Molecular Mechanisms Responsible for Tear Hyperosmolarity-Induced Pathological Changes in the Eyes of Dry Eye Disease Patients. *Cells* **2023**, *12*, 2755. [CrossRef]
45. De Paiva, C.S.; Pflugfelder, S.C. Rationale for anti-inflammatory therapy in dry eye syndrome. *Arq. Bras. Oftalmol.* **2008**, *71* (Suppl. 6), 89–95. [CrossRef]
46. Stern, M.E.; Schaumburg, C.S.; Pflugfelder, S.C. Dry eye as a mucosal autoimmune disease. *Int. Rev. Immunol.* **2013**, *32*, 19–41. [CrossRef]
47. Yoon, S.P.; Yu, Z.; Pflugfelder, S.C.; de Paiva, C.S. Differentially Expressed Tear Proteins in Sjogren's Syndrome Keratoconjunctivitis Sicca. *Transl. Vis. Sci. Technol.* **2023**, *12*, 8. [CrossRef]

48. Carnahan, M.C.; Goldstein, D.A. Ocular complications of topical, peri-ocular, and systemic corticosteroids. *Curr. Opin. Ophthalmol.* **2000**, *11*, 478–483. [CrossRef]
49. Pflugfelder, S.C.; Tseng, S.C.; Sanabria, O.; Kell, H.; Garcia, C.G.; Felix, C.; Feuer, W.; Reis, B.L. Evaluation of subjective assessments and objective diagnostic tests for diagnosing tear-film disorders known to cause ocular irritation. *Cornea* **1998**, *17*, 38–56. [CrossRef]
50. Lemp, M.A.; Crews, L.A.; Bron, A.J.; Foulks, G.N.; Sullivan, B.D. Distribution of aqueous-deficient and evaporative dry eye in a clinic-based patient cohort: A retrospective study. *Cornea* **2012**, *31*, 472–478. [CrossRef]
51. Caffery, B.; Joyce, E.; Boone, A.; Slomovic, A.; Simpson, T.; Jones, L.; Senchyna, M. Tear lipocalin and lysozyme in Sjogren and non-Sjogren dry eye. *Optom. Vis. Sci.* **2008**, *85*, 661–667. [CrossRef]
52. Boukes, R.J.; Boonstra, A.; Breebaart, A.C.; Reits, D.; Glasius, E.; Luyendyk, L.; Kijlstra, A. Analysis of human tear protein profiles using high performance liquid chromatography (HPLC). *Doc. Ophthalmol.* **1987**, *67*, 105–113. [CrossRef] [PubMed]
53. Villani, E.; Beretta, S.; De Capitani, M.; Galimberti, D.; Viola, F.; Ratiglia, R. In vivo confocal microscopy of meibomian glands in Sjogren's syndrome. *Investig. Ophthalmol. Vis. Sci.* **2011**, *52*, 933–939. [CrossRef] [PubMed]
54. Goto, E.; Matsumoto, Y.; Kamoi, M.; Endo, K.; Ishida, R.; Dogru, M.; Kaido, M.; Kojima, T.; Tsubota, K. Tear evaporation rates in Sjogren syndrome and non-Sjogren dry eye patients. *Am. J. Ophthalmol.* **2007**, *144*, 81–85. [CrossRef] [PubMed]
55. Bron, A.J.; Tiffany, J.M.; Gouveia, S.M.; Yokoi, N.; Voon, L.W. Functional aspects of the tear film lipid layer. *Exp. Eye Res.* **2004**, *78*, 347–360. [CrossRef]
56. Pflugfelder, S.C.; Huang, A.J.; Feuer, W.; Chuchovski, P.T.; Pereira, I.C.; Tseng, S.C. Conjunctival cytologic features of primary Sjogren's syndrome. *Ophthalmology* **1990**, *97*, 985–991. [CrossRef]
57. Mathers, W.D.; Stovall, D.; Lane, J.A.; Zimmerman, M.B.; Johnson, S. Menopause and tear function: The influence of prolactin and sex hormones on human tear production. *Cornea* **1998**, *17*, 353–358. [CrossRef]
58. Lam, H.; Bleiden, L.; de Paiva, C.S.; Farley, W.; Stern, M.E.; Pflugfelder, S.C. Tear cytokine profiles in dysfunctional tear syndrome. *Am. J. Ophthalmol.* **2009**, *147*, 198–205.e1. [CrossRef]
59. Stern, M.E.; Gao, J.; Siemasko, K.F.; Beuerman, R.W.; Pflugfelder, S.C. The role of the lacrimal functional unit in the pathophysiology of dry eye. *Exp. Eye Res.* **2004**, *78*, 409–416. [CrossRef]
60. De Paiva, C.S.; Villarreal, A.L.; Corrales, R.M.; Rahman, H.T.; Chang, V.Y.; Farley, W.J.; Stern, M.E.; Niederkorn, J.Y.; Li, D.-Q.; Pflugfelder, S.C. Dry eye-induced conjunctival epithelial squamous metaplasia is modulated by interferon-gamma. *Investig. Ophthalmol. Vis. Sci.* **2007**, *48*, 2553–2560. [CrossRef]
61. Huang, D.; Li, Z. Multidimensional immunotherapy for dry eye disease: Current status and future directions. *Front. Ophthalmol.* **2024**, *4*, 1449283. [CrossRef]
62. Baudouin, C.; Aragona, P.; Messmer, E.M.; Tomlinson, A.; Calonge, M.; Boboridis, K.G.; Akova, Y.A.; Geerling, G.; Labetoulle, M.; Rolando, M. Role of hyperosmolarity in the pathogenesis and management of dry eye disease: Proceedings of the OCEAN group meeting. *Ocul. Surf.* **2013**, *11*, 246–258. [CrossRef]
63. Versura, P.; Profazio, V.; Campos, E.C. Performance of tear osmolarity compared to previous diagnostic tests for dry eye diseases. *Curr. Eye Res.* **2010**, *35*, 553–564. [CrossRef]
64. Lemp, M.A.; Bron, A.J.; Baudouin, C.; del Castillo, J.M.B.; Geffen, D.; Tauber, J.; Foulks, G.N.; Pepose, J.S.; Sullivan, B.D. Tear osmolarity in the diagnosis and management of dry eye disease. *Am. J. Ophthalmol.* **2011**, *151*, 792–798.e1. [CrossRef]
65. Zheng, Q.; Ren, Y.; Reinach, P.S.; Xiao, B.; Lu, H.; Zhu, Y.; Qu, J.; Chen, W. Reactive oxygen species activated NLRP3 inflammasomes initiate inflammation in hyperosmolarity stressed human corneal epithelial cells and environment-induced dry eye patients. *Exp. Eye Res.* **2015**, *134*, 133–140. [CrossRef]
66. Chi, W.; Li, F.; Chen, H.; Wang, Y.; Zhu, Y.; Yang, X.; Zhu, J.; Wu, F.; Ouyang, H.; Ge, J.; et al. Caspase-8 promotes NLRP1/NLRP3 inflammasome activation and IL-1beta production in acute glaucoma. *Proc. Natl. Acad. Sci. USA* **2014**, *111*, 11181–11186. [CrossRef] [PubMed]
67. Bian, F.; Qi, H.; Ma, P.; Zhang, L.; Yoon, K.-C.; Pflugfelder, S.C.; Li, D.-Q. An immunoprotective privilege of corneal epithelial stem cells against Th17 inflammatory stress by producing glial cell-derived neurotrophic factor. *Stem Cells* **2010**, *28*, 2172–2181. [CrossRef] [PubMed]
68. Lee, H.S.; Hattori, T.; Park, E.Y.; Stevenson, W.; Chauhan, S.K.; Dana, R. Expression of toll-like receptor 4 contributes to corneal inflammation in experimental dry eye disease. *Investig. Ophthalmol. Vis. Sci.* **2012**, *53*, 5632–5640. [CrossRef] [PubMed]
69. Luo, L.; Li, D.Q.; Doshi, A.; Farley, W.; Corrales, R.M.; Pflugfelder, S.C. Experimental dry eye stimulates production of inflammatory cytokines and MMP-9 and activates MAPK signaling pathways on the ocular surface. *Investig. Ophthalmol. Vis. Sci.* **2004**, *45*, 4293–4301. [CrossRef]
70. Li, D.Q.; Chen, Z.; Song, X.J.; Luo, L.; Pflugfelder, S.C. Stimulation of matrix metalloproteinases by hyperosmolarity via a JNK pathway in human corneal epithelial cells. *Investig. Ophthalmol. Vis. Sci.* **2004**, *45*, 4302–4311. [CrossRef]

71. Yagci, A.; Gurdal, C. The role and treatment of inflammation in dry eye disease. *Int. Ophthalmol.* **2014**, *34*, 1291–1301. [CrossRef]
72. De Paiva, C.S.; Corrales, R.M.; Villarreal, A.L.; Farley, W.J.; Li, D.-Q.; Stern, M.E.; Pflugfelder, S.C. Corticosteroid and doxycycline suppress MMP-9 and inflammatory cytokine expression, MAPK activation in the corneal epithelium in experimental dry eye. *Exp. Eye Res.* **2006**, *83*, 526–535. [CrossRef] [PubMed]
73. Kunert, K.S.; Tisdale, A.S.; Stern, M.E.; Smith, J.A.; Gipson, I.K. Analysis of topical cyclosporine treatment of patients with dry eye syndrome: Effect on conjunctival lymphocytes. *Arch. Ophthalmol.* **2000**, *118*, 1489–1496. [CrossRef] [PubMed]
74. Gao, J.; Schwalb, T.A.; Addeo, J.V.; Ghosn, C.R.; Stern, M.E. The role of apoptosis in the pathogenesis of canine keratoconjunctivitis sicca: The effect of topical Cyclosporin A therapy. *Cornea* **1998**, *17*, 654–663. [CrossRef] [PubMed]
75. Wang, Y.; Ogawa, Y.; Dogru, M.; Kawai, M.; Tatematsu, Y.; Uchino, M.; Okada, N.; Igarashi, A.; Kujira, A.; Fujishima, H.; et al. Ocular surface and tear functions after topical cyclosporine treatment in dry eye patients with chronic graft-versus-host disease. *Bone Marrow Transplant.* **2008**, *41*, 293–302. [CrossRef]
76. Chauhan, S.K.; El Annan, J.; Ecoiffier, T.; Goyal, S.; Zhang, Q.; Saban, D.R.; Dana, R. Autoimmunity in dry eye is due to resistance of Th17 to Treg suppression. *J. Immunol.* **2009**, *182*, 1247–1252. [CrossRef]
77. Pelegrino, F.S.; Volpe, E.A.; Gandhi, N.B.; Li, D.Q.; Pflugfelder, S.C.; de Paiva, C.S. Deletion of interferon-gamma delays onset and severity of dacryoadenitis in CD25KO mice. *Arthritis Res. Ther.* **2012**, *14*, R234. [CrossRef]
78. Zoukhri, D.; Fix, A.; Alroy, J.; Kublin, C.L. Mechanisms of murine lacrimal gland repair after experimentally induced inflammation. *Investig. Ophthalmol. Vis. Sci.* **2008**, *49*, 4399–4406. [CrossRef]
79. Mantelli, F.; Massaro-Giordano, M.; Macchi, I.; Lambiase, A.; Bonini, S. The cellular mechanisms of dry eye: From pathogenesis to treatment. *J. Cell. Physiol.* **2013**, *228*, 2253–2256. [CrossRef]
80. Craig, J.P.; Nichols, K.K.; Akpek, E.K.; Caffery, B.; Dua, H.S.; Joo, C.-K.; Liu, Z.; Nelson, J.D.; Nichols, J.J.; Tsubota, K.; et al. TFOS DEWS II Definition and Classification Report. *Ocul. Surf.* **2017**, *15*, 276–283. [CrossRef]
81. Benitez-Del-Castillo, J.M.; Acosta, M.C.; Wassfi, M.A.; Diaz-Valle, D.; Gegundez, J.A.; Fernandez, C.; Garcia-SanChez, J. Relation between corneal innervation with confocal microscopy and corneal sensitivity with noncontact esthesiometry in patients with dry eye. *Investig. Ophthalmol. Vis. Sci.* **2007**, *48*, 173–181. [CrossRef] [PubMed]
82. Tuisku, I.S.; Konttinen, Y.T.; Konttinen, L.M.; Tervo, T.M. Alterations in corneal sensitivity and nerve morphology in patients with primary Sjogren's syndrome. *Exp. Eye Res.* **2008**, *86*, 879–885. [CrossRef] [PubMed]
83. Hwang, D.D.; Lee, S.J.; Kim, J.H.; Lee, S.M. The Role of Neuropeptides in Pathogenesis of Dry Dye. *J. Clin. Med.* **2021**, *10*, 4248. [CrossRef] [PubMed]
84. Bourcier, T.; Acosta, M.C.; Borderie, V.; Borra's, F.; Gallar, J.; Bury, T.; Laroche, L.; Belmonte, C. Decreased corneal sensitivity in patients with dry eye. *Investig. Ophthalmol. Vis. Sci.* **2005**, *46*, 2341–2345. [CrossRef]
85. McDonald, M.; Patel, D.A.; Keith, M.S.; Snedecor, S.J. Economic and Humanistic Burden of Dry Eye Disease in Europe, North America, and Asia: A Systematic Literature Review. *Ocul. Surf.* **2016**, *14*, 144–167. [CrossRef]
86. Uchino, M.; Schaumberg, D.A. Dry Eye Disease: Impact on Quality of Life and Vision. *Curr. Ophthalmol. Rep.* **2013**, *1*, 51–57. [CrossRef]
87. Bartlett, J.D.; Keith, M.S.; Sudharshan, L.; Snedecor, S.J. Associations between signs and symptoms of dry eye disease: A systematic review. *Clin. Ophthalmol.* **2015**, *9*, 1719–1730. [CrossRef]
88. McMonnies, C.W. The clinical and experimental significance of blinking behavior. *J. Optom.* **2020**, *13*, 74–80. [CrossRef]
89. Korb, D.R.; Greiner, J.V.; Glonek, T.; Esbah, R.; Finnemore, V.M.; Whalen, A.C. Effect of periocular humidity on the tear film lipid layer. *Cornea* **1996**, *15*, 129–134. [CrossRef]
90. Knop, E.; Knop, N.; Millar, T.; Obata, H.; Sullivan, D.A. The international workshop on meibomian gland dysfunction: Report of the subcommittee on anatomy, physiology, and pathophysiology of the meibomian gland. *Investig. Ophthalmol. Vis. Sci.* **2011**, *52*, 1938–1978. [CrossRef]
91. Sullivan, B.D.; Whitmer, D.; Nichols, K.K.; Tomlinson, A.; Foulks, G.N.; Geerling, G.; Pepose, J.S.; Kosheleff, V.; Porreco, A.; Lemp, M.A. An objective approach to dry eye disease severity. *Investig. Ophthalmol. Vis. Sci.* **2010**, *51*, 6125–6130. [CrossRef]
92. Belmonte, C.; Nichols, J.J.; Cox, S.M.; Brock, J.A.; Begley, C.G.; Bereiter, D.A.; Dartt, D.A.; Galor, A.; Hamrah, P.; Ivanusic, J.J.; et al. TFOS DEWS II pain and sensation report. *Ocul. Surf.* **2017**, *15*, 404–437. [CrossRef]
93. Galor, A.; Levitt, R.C.; Felix, E.R.; Martin, E.R.; Sarantopoulos, C.D. Neuropathic ocular pain: An important yet underevaluated feature of dry eye. *Eye* **2015**, *29*, 301–312. [CrossRef]
94. Nettune, G.R.; Pflugfelder, S.C. Post-LASIK tear dysfunction and dysesthesia. *Ocul. Surf.* **2010**, *8*, 135–145. [CrossRef] [PubMed]
95. Nichols, K.K.; Mitchell, G.L.; Zadnik, K. The repeatability of clinical measurements of dry eye. *Cornea* **2004**, *23*, 272–285. [CrossRef] [PubMed]
96. Willcox, M.D.; Argüeso, P.; Georgiev, G.A.; Holopainen, J.M.; Laurie, G.W.; Millar, T.J.; Papas, E.B.; Rolland, J.P.; Schmidt, T.A.; Stahl, U.; et al. TFOS DEWS II Tear Film Report. *Ocul. Surf.* **2017**, *15*, 366–403. [CrossRef] [PubMed]

97. Wolkoff, P.; Nojgaard, J.K.; Troiano, P.; Piccoli, B. Eye complaints in the office environment: Precorneal tear film integrity influenced by eye blinking efficiency. *Occup. Environ. Med.* **2005**, *62*, 4–12. [CrossRef]
98. Portello, J.K.; Rosenfield, M.; Bababekova, Y.; Estrada, J.M.; Leon, A. Computer-related visual symptoms in office workers. *Ophthalmic Physiol. Opt.* **2012**, *32*, 375–382. [CrossRef]
99. Blehm, C.; Vishnu, S.; Khattak, A.; Mitra, S.; Yee, R.W. Computer vision syndrome: A review. *Surv. Ophthalmol.* **2005**, *50*, 253–262. [CrossRef]
100. Rosenfield, M. Computer vision syndrome: A review of ocular causes and potential treatments. *Ophthalmic Physiol. Opt.* **2011**, *31*, 502–515. [CrossRef]
101. Galor, A.; Feuer, W.; Lee, D.J.; Florez, H.; Faler, A.L.; Zann, K.L.; Perez, V.L. Depression, post-traumatic stress disorder, and dry eye syndrome: A study utilizing the national United States Veterans Affairs administrative database. *Am. J. Ophthalmol.* **2012**, *154*, 340–346.e2. [CrossRef]
102. Labbe, A.; Wang, Y.X.; Jie, Y.; Baudouin, C.; Jonas, J.B.; Xu, L. Dry eye disease, dry eye symptoms and depression: The Beijing Eye Study. *Br. J. Ophthalmol.* **2013**, *97*, 1399–1403. [CrossRef]
103. Fernandez, C.A.; Galor, A.; Arheart, K.L.; Musselman, D.L.; Venincasa, V.D.; Florez, H.J.; Lee, D.J. Dry eye syndrome, posttraumatic stress disorder, and depression in an older male veteran population. *Investig. Ophthalmol. Vis. Sci.* **2013**, *54*, 3666–3672. [CrossRef] [PubMed]
104. Vehof, J.; Kozareva, D.; Hysi, P.G.; Hammond, C.J. Prevalence and risk factors of dry eye disease in a British female cohort. *Br. J. Ophthalmol.* **2014**, *98*, 1712–1717. [CrossRef] [PubMed]
105. Li, M.; Gong, L.; Sun, X.; Chapin, W.J. Anxiety and depression in patients with dry eye syndrome. *Curr. Eye Res.* **2011**, *36*, 1–7. [CrossRef] [PubMed]
106. Ayaki, M.; Kawashima, M.; Negishi, K.; Tsubota, K. High prevalence of sleep and mood disorders in dry eye patients: Survey of 1000 eye clinic visitors. *Neuropsychiatr. Dis. Treat.* **2015**, *11*, 889–894. [CrossRef]
107. Ayaki, M.; Tsubota, K.; Kawashima, M.; Kishimoto, T.; Mimura, M.; Negishi, K. Sleep Disorders are a Prevalent and Serious Comorbidity in Dry Eye. *Investig. Ophthalmol. Vis. Sci.* **2018**, *59*, DES143–DES150. [CrossRef]
108. Srinivasan, S.; Menzies, K.; Sorbara, L.; Jones, L. Infrared imaging of meibomian gland structure using a novel keratograph. *Optom. Vis. Sci.* **2012**, *89*, 788–794. [CrossRef]
109. Tavakoli, M.; Hossain, P.; Malik, R.A. Clinical applications of corneal confocal microscopy. *Clin. Ophthalmol.* **2008**, *2*, 435–445. [CrossRef]
110. Schiffman, R.M.; Christianson, M.D.; Jacobsen, G.; Hirsch, J.D.; Reis, B.L. Reliability and validity of the Ocular Surface Disease Index. *Arch. Ophthalmol.* **2000**, *118*, 615–621. [CrossRef]
111. Begley, C.G.; Chalmers, R.L.; Abetz, L.; Venkataraman, K.; Mertzanis, P.; Caffery, B.A.; Snyder, C.; Edrington, T.; Nelson, D.; Simpson, T. The relationship between habitual patient-reported symptoms and clinical signs among patients with dry eye of varying severity. *Investig. Ophthalmol. Vis. Sci.* **2003**, *44*, 4753–4761. [CrossRef] [PubMed]
112. Markoulli, M.; Kolanu, S. Contact lens wear and dry eyes: Challenges and solutions. *Clin. Optom.* **2017**, *9*, 41–48. [CrossRef] [PubMed]
113. Arita, R.; Itoh, K.; Inoue, K.; Amano, S. Noncontact infrared meibography to document age-related changes of the meibomian glands in a normal population. *Ophthalmology* **2008**, *115*, 911–915. [CrossRef] [PubMed]
114. Wang, M.T.M.; Power, B.; Xue, A.L.; Kim, J.S.; Craig, J.P. Diagnostic performance of qualitative and quantitative methods of meibomian gland dropout evaluation in dry eye disease: An investigator-masked, randomised crossover study. *Cont Lens Anterior Eye* **2025**, *48*, 102324. [CrossRef]
115. Daniel, E.; Maguire, M.G.; Pistilli, M.; Bunya, V.Y.; Massaro-Giordano, G.M.; Smith, E.; Kadakia, P.A.; Asbell, P.A. Grading and baseline characteristics of meibomian glands in meibography images and their clinical associations in the Dry Eye Assessment and Management (DREAM) study. *Ocul. Surf.* **2019**, *17*, 491–501. [CrossRef]
116. Pult, H.; Riede-Pult, B.H. Non-contact meibography: Keep it simple but effective. *Cont Lens Anterior Eye* **2012**, *35*, 77–80. [CrossRef]
117. Gupta, P.K.; Karpecki, P. Comprehensive Assessment of the Meibomian Glands by Meibography: Why the Upper Eyelids Matter. *Cornea* **2025**, *44*, 128–135. [CrossRef]
118. Ban, Y.; Shimazaki-Den, S.; Tsubota, K.; Shimazaki, J. Morphological evaluation of meibomian glands using noncontact infrared meibography. *Ocul. Surf.* **2013**, *11*, 47–53. [CrossRef]
119. Lin, X.; Fu, Y.; Li, L.; Chen, C.; Chen, X.; Mao, Y.; Lian, H.; Yang, W.; Dai, Q. A Novel Quantitative Index of Meibomian Gland Dysfunction, the Meibomian Gland Tortuosity. *Transl. Vis. Sci. Technol.* **2020**, *9*, 34. [CrossRef]
120. Arita, R.; Itoh, K.; Maeda, S.; Maeda, K.; Furuta, A.; Fukuoka, S.; Tomidokoro, A.; Amano, S. Proposed diagnostic criteria for obstructive meibomian gland dysfunction. *Ophthalmology* **2009**, *116*, 2058–2063.e1. [CrossRef]

121. Llorens-Quintana, C.; Rico-Del-Viejo, L.; Syga, P.; Madrid-Costa, D.; Iskander, D.R. A Novel Automated Approach for Infrared-Based Assessment of Meibomian Gland Morphology. *Transl. Vis. Sci. Technol.* **2019**, *8*, 17. [CrossRef]
122. Nichols, J.J.; Berntsen, D.A.; Mitchell, G.L.; Nichols, K.K. An assessment of grading scales for meibography images. *Cornea* **2005**, *24*, 382–388. [CrossRef] [PubMed]
123. Tomlinson, A.; Bron, A.J.; Korb, D.R.; Amano, S.; Paugh, J.R.; Pearce, E.I.; Yee, R.; Yokoi, N.; Arita, R.; Dogru, M. The international workshop on meibomian gland dysfunction: Report of the diagnosis subcommittee. *Investig. Ophthalmol. Vis. Sci.* **2011**, *52*, 2006–2049. [CrossRef] [PubMed]
124. Shimazaki, J.; Sakata, M.; Tsubota, K. Ocular surface changes and discomfort in patients with meibomian gland dysfunction. *Arch. Ophthalmol.* **1995**, *113*, 1266–1270. [CrossRef] [PubMed]
125. Yokoi, N.; Mossa, F.; Tiffany, J.M.; Bron, A.J. Assessment of meibomian gland function in dry eye using meibometry. *Arch. Ophthalmol.* **1999**, *117*, 723–729. [CrossRef]
126. Liu, S.; Richards, S.M.; Lo, K.; Hatton, M.; Fay, A.; Sullivan, D.A. Changes in gene expression in human meibomian gland dysfunction. *Investig. Ophthalmol. Vis. Sci.* **2011**, *52*, 2727–2740. [CrossRef]
127. Nichols, K.K.; Foulks, G.N.; Bron, A.J.; Glasgow, B.J.; Dogru, M.; Tsubota, K.; Lemp, M.A.; Sullivan, D.A. The international workshop on meibomian gland dysfunction: Executive summary. *Investig. Ophthalmol. Vis. Sci.* **2011**, *52*, 1922–1929. [CrossRef]
128. Koh, Y.W.; Celik, T.; Lee, H.K.; Petznick, A.; Tong, L. Detection of meibomian glands and classification of meibography images. *J. Biomed. Opt.* **2012**, *17*, 086008. [CrossRef]
129. Xiao, J.; Adil, M.Y.; Chen, X.; Utheim, Ø.A.; Ræder, S.; Tønseth, K.A.; Lagali, N.S.; Dartt, D.A.; Utheim, T.P. Functional and Morphological Evaluation of Meibomian Glands in the Assessment of Meibomian Gland Dysfunction Subtype and Severity. *Am. J. Ophthalmol.* **2020**, *209*, 160–167. [CrossRef]
130. Özer, H.; Yılmaz, S.; Bozkurt, B.; Tezcan, D.; Yazol, M.; Hakbilen, S.; Topaloğlu, Ö.F.; Durmaz, M.S. Assessment of lacrimal gland involvement in primary Sjogren's syndrome using gray-scale ultrasonography and shear wave elastography. *Eur. Radiol.* **2023**, *33*, 9368–9377. [CrossRef]
131. Zhong, W.; Zhang, H.; Ran, H. Advances in imaging of the lacrimal gland in Sjogren's syndrome: A narrative review. *J. Clin. Ultrasound.* **2024**, *52*, 68–77. [CrossRef]
132. Zhang, M.; Pan, J.; Sheng, J. Systematic review and meta-analysis of the diagnostic performance of lacrimal gland ultrasound elastography in primary Sjogren's syndrome. *Int. Ophthalmol.* **2024**, *44*, 271. [CrossRef]
133. Cornec, D.; Jousse-Joulin, S.; Pers, J.; Marhadour, T.; Cochener, B.; Boisramé-Gastrin, S.; Nowak, E.; Youinou, P.; Saraux, A.; Devauchelle-Pensec, V. Contribution of salivary gland ultrasonography to the diagnosis of Sjogren's syndrome: Toward new diagnostic criteria? *Arthritis Rheum.* **2013**, *65*, 216–225. [CrossRef] [PubMed]
134. Villani, E.; Magnani, F.; Viola, F.; Santaniello, A.; Scorza, R.; Nucci, P.; Ratiglia, R. In vivo confocal evaluation of the ocular surface morpho-functional unit in dry eye. *Optom. Vis. Sci.* **2013**, *90*, 576–586. [CrossRef]
135. Aragona, P.; Aguennouz, M.; Rania, L.; Postorino, E.; Sommario, M.S.; Roszkowska, A.M.; De Pasquale, M.G.; Pisani, A.; Puzzolo, D. Matrix metalloproteinase 9 and transglutaminase 2 expression at the ocular surface in patients with different forms of dry eye disease. *Ophthalmology* **2015**, *122*, 62–71. [CrossRef] [PubMed]
136. Ban, Y.; Ogawa, Y.; Ibrahim, O.M.; Tatematsu, Y.; Kamoi, M.; Uchino, M.; Yaguchi, S.; Dogru, M.; Tsubota, K. Morphologic evaluation of meibomian glands in chronic graft-versus-host disease using in vivo laser confocal microscopy. *Mol. Vis.* **2011**, *17*, 2533–2543. [PubMed]
137. Ibrahim, O.M.; Matsumoto, Y.; Dogru, M.; Adan, E.S.; Wakamatsu, T.H.; Goto, T.; Negishi, K.; Tsubota, K. The efficacy, sensitivity, and specificity of in vivo laser confocal microscopy in the diagnosis of meibomian gland dysfunction. *Ophthalmology* **2010**, *117*, 665–672. [CrossRef]
138. Sambursky, R.; Davitt, W.F., 3rd; Latkany, R.; Tauber, S.; Starr, C.; Friedberg, M.; Dirks, M.S.; McDonald, M. Sensitivity and specificity of a point-of-care matrix metalloproteinase 9 immunoassay for diagnosing inflammation related to dry eye. *JAMA Ophthalmol.* **2013**, *131*, 24–28. [CrossRef]
139. Sall, K.; Stevenson, O.D.; Mundorf, T.K.; Reis, B.L. Two multicenter, randomized studies of the efficacy and safety of cyclosporine ophthalmic emulsion in moderate to severe dry eye disease. CsA Phase 3 Study Group. *Ophthalmology* **2000**, *107*, 631–639. [CrossRef]
140. Tauber, J.; Karpecki, P.; Latkany, R.; Luchs, J.; Martel, J.; Sall, K.; Raychaudhuri, A.; Smith, V.; Semba, C.P.; OPUS-2 Investigators. Lifitegrast Ophthalmic Solution 5.0% versus Placebo for Treatment of Dry Eye Disease: Results of the Randomized Phase III OPUS-2 Study. *Ophthalmology* **2015**, *122*, 2423–2431. [CrossRef]
141. Sheppard, J.D.; Torkildsen, G.L.; Lonsdale, J.D.; D'Ambrosio, F.A., Jr.; McLaurin, E.B.; Eiferman, R.A.; Kennedy, K.S.; Semba, C.P.; OPUS-1 Study Group. Lifitegrast ophthalmic solution 5.0% for treatment of dry eye disease: Results of the OPUS-1 phase 3 study. *Ophthalmology* **2014**, *121*, 475–483. [CrossRef] [PubMed]

142. Vivino, F.B.; Al-Hashimi, I.; Khan, Z.; LeVeque, F.G.; Salisbury, P.L., 3rd; Tran-Johnson, T.K.; Muscoplat, C.C.; Trivedi, M.; Goldlust, B.; Gallagher, S.C. Pilocarpine tablets for the treatment of dry mouth and dry eye symptoms in patients with Sjogren syndrome: A randomized, placebo-controlled, fixed-dose, multicenter trial. P92-01 Study Group. *Arch. Intern. Med.* **1999**, *159*, 174–181. [CrossRef] [PubMed]
143. Petrone, D.; Condemi, J.J.; Fife, R.; Gluck, O.; Cohen, S.; Dalgin, P. A double-blind, randomized, placebo-controlled study of cevimeline in Sjogren's syndrome patients with xerostomia and keratoconjunctivitis sicca. *Arthritis Rheum.* **2002**, *46*, 748–754. [CrossRef] [PubMed]
144. Ervin, A.M.; Law, A.; Pucker, A.D. Punctal occlusion for dry eye syndrome. *Cochrane Database Syst. Rev.* **2017**, *6*, CD006775. [CrossRef]
145. Ervin, A.M.; Wojciechowski, R.; Schein, O. Punctal occlusion for dry eye syndrome. *Cochrane Database Syst. Rev.* **2010**, CD006775. [CrossRef]
146. Rosenthal, P.; Cotter, J.M.; Baum, J. Treatment of persistent corneal epithelial defect with extended wear of a fluid-ventilated gas-permeable scleral contact lens. *Am. J. Ophthalmol.* **2000**, *130*, 33–41. [CrossRef]
147. Meijer, J.M.; Meiners, P.M.; Vissink, A.; Spijkervet, F.K.L.; Abdulahad, W.; Kamminga, N.; Brouwer, E.; Kallenberg, C.G.M.; Bootsma, H. Effectiveness of rituximab treatment in primary Sjogren's syndrome: A randomized, double-blind, placebo-controlled trial. *Arthritis Rheum.* **2010**, *62*, 960–968. [CrossRef]
148. Dass, S.; Bowman, S.J.; Vital, E.M.; Ikeda, K.; Pease, C.T.; Hamburger, J.; Richards, A.; Rauz, S.; Emery, P. Reduction of fatigue in Sjogren syndrome with rituximab: Results of a randomised, double-blind, placebo-controlled pilot study. *Ann. Rheum. Dis.* **2008**, *67*, 1541–1544. [CrossRef]
149. Zandbelt, M.M.; de Wilde, P.; van Damme, P.; Hoyng, C.B.; van de Putte, L.; van den Hoogen, F. Etanercept in the treatment of patients with primary Sjogren's syndrome: A pilot study. *J. Rheumatol.* **2004**, *31*, 96–101.
150. Shiozawa, S.; Tanaka, Y.; Shiozawa, K. Single-blinded controlled trial of low-dose oral IFN-alpha for the treatment of xerostomia in patients with Sjogren's syndrome. *J. Interferon Cytokine Res.* **1998**, *18*, 255–262. [CrossRef]
151. Adler, S.; Korner, M.; Forger, F.; Huscher, D.; Caversaccio, M.D.; Villiger, P.M. Evaluation of histologic, serologic, and clinical changes in response to abatacept treatment of primary Sjogren's syndrome: A pilot study. *Arthritis Care Res.* **2013**, *65*, 1862–1868. [CrossRef] [PubMed]
152. Geerling, G.; Maclennan, S.; Hartwig, D. Autologous serum eye drops for ocular surface disorders. *Br. J. Ophthalmol.* **2004**, *88*, 1467–1474. [CrossRef] [PubMed]
153. Harthan, J.S.; Shorter, E. Therapeutic uses of scleral contact lenses for ocular surface disease: Patient selection and special considerations. *Clin. Optom.* **2018**, *10*, 65–74. [CrossRef] [PubMed]
154. Galipeau, J.; Sensebe, L. Mesenchymal Stromal Cells: Clinical Challenges and Therapeutic Opportunities. *Cell Stem Cell* **2018**, *22*, 824–833. [CrossRef]
155. Squillaro, T.; Peluso, G.; Galderisi, U. Clinical Trials With Mesenchymal Stem Cells: An Update. *Cell Transplant.* **2016**, *25*, 829–848. [CrossRef]
156. Garg, A.; Zhang, X. Lacrimal gland development: From signaling interactions to regenerative medicine. *Dev. Dyn.* **2017**, *246*, 970–980. [CrossRef]
157. Miletich, I. Molecular regulation of ocular gland development. *Semin. Cell Dev. Biol.* **2019**, *91*, 66–74. [CrossRef]
158. Khan, S.; Fitch, S.; Knox, S.; Arora, R. Exocrine gland structure-function relationships. *Development* **2022**, *149*, dev197657. [CrossRef]
159. Clayton, J.A. Dry Eye. *N. Engl. J. Med.* **2018**, *378*, 2212–2223. [CrossRef]
160. Alio, J.L.; Rodriguez, A.E.; Martinez, L.M.; Rio, A.L. Autologous fibrin membrane combined with solid platelet-rich plasma in the management of perforated corneal ulcers: A pilot study. *JAMA Ophthalmol.* **2013**, *131*, 745–751. [CrossRef]
161. Freire, V.; Andollo, N.; Etxebarria, J.; Hernaez-Moya, R.; Duran, J.A.; Morales, M.C. Corneal wound healing promoted by 3 blood derivatives: An in vitro and in vivo comparative study. *Cornea* **2014**, *33*, 614–620. [CrossRef]
162. Anitua, E.; Muruzabal, F.; Tayebba, A.; Riestra, A.; Perez, V.L.; Merayo-Lloves, J.; Orive, G. Autologous serum and plasma rich in growth factors in ophthalmology: Preclinical and clinical studies. *Acta Ophthalmol.* **2015**, *93*, e605-14. [CrossRef]
163. Lopez-Plandolit, S.; Morales, M.C.; Freire, V.; Etxebarria, J.; Duran, J.A. Plasma rich in growth factors as a therapeutic agent for persistent corneal epithelial defects. *Cornea* **2010**, *29*, 843–848. [CrossRef] [PubMed]
164. Zhang, K.; Luo, Z.; Yao, X.; Lu, D.; Hong, T.; Zhu, X.; Chen, M.; Wang, X. Identification of Epigenetic Alteration of the IFI44L Gene in B Cells of Sjogren's Syndrome as a Clinical Biomarker and Molecular Significance. *J. Inflamm. Res.* **2025**, *18*, 2499–2512. [CrossRef] [PubMed]
165. Mu, S.; Wang, W.; Liu, Q.; Ke, N.; Li, H.; Sun, F.; Zhang, J.; Zhu, Z. Autoimmune disease: A view of epigenetics and therapeutic targeting. *Front. Immunol.* **2024**, *15*, 1482728. [CrossRef] [PubMed]

166. Zhou, T.; Chen, D.; Li, Q.; Sun, X.; Song, Y.; Wang, C. Curcumin inhibits inflammatory response and bone loss during experimental periodontitis in rats. *Acta Odontol. Scand.* **2013**, *71*, 349–356. [CrossRef]
167. Ice, J.A.; Li, H.; Adrianto, I.; Lin, P.C.; Kelly, J.A.; Montgomery, C.G.; Lessard, C.J.; Moser, K.L. Genetics of Sjogren's syndrome in the genome-wide association era. *J. Autoimmun.* **2012**, *39*, 57–63. [CrossRef]
168. Konsta, O.D.; Thabet, Y.; Le Dantec, C.; Brooks, W.H.; Tzioufas, A.G.; Pers, J.-O.; Renaudineau, Y. The contribution of epigenetics in Sjogren's Syndrome. *Front. Genet.* **2014**, *5*, 71. [CrossRef]
169. Imgenberg-Kreuz, J.; Almlöf, J.C.; Leonard, D.; Alexsson, A.; Nordmark, G.; Eloranta, M.-L.; Rantapää-Dahlqvist, S.; Bengtsson, A.A.; Jönsen, A.; Padyukov, L.; et al. DNA methylation mapping identifies gene regulatory effects in patients with systemic lupus erythematosus. *Ann. Rheum. Dis.* **2018**, *77*, 736–743. [CrossRef]
170. Charras, A.; Arvaniti, P.; Le Dantec, C.; Dalekos, G.N.; Zachou, K.; Bordron, A.; Renaudineau, Y. JAK Inhibitors and Oxidative Stress Control. *Front. Immunol.* **2019**, *10*, 2814. [CrossRef]
171. Tsokos, G.C.; Lo, M.S.; Costa Reis, P.; Sullivan, K.E. New insights into the immunopathogenesis of systemic lupus erythematosus. *Nat. Rev. Rheumatol.* **2016**, *12*, 716–730. [CrossRef] [PubMed]
172. Alunno, A.; Bistoni, O.; Bartoloni, E.; Caterbi, S.; Bigerna, B.; Tabarrini, A.; Mannucci, R.; Falini, B.; Gerli, R. IL-17-producing CD4-CD8- T cells are expanded in the peripheral blood, infiltrate salivary glands and are resistant to corticosteroids in patients with primary Sjogren's syndrome. *Ann. Rheum. Dis.* **2013**, *72*, 286–292. [CrossRef] [PubMed]
173. Selvam, S.; Thomas, P.B.; Hamm-Alvarez, S.F.; Schechter, J.E.; Stevenson, D.; Mircheff, A.K.; Trousdale, M.D. Current status of gene delivery and gene therapy in lacrimal gland using viral vectors. *Adv. Drug Deliv. Rev.* **2006**, *58*, 1243–1257. [CrossRef] [PubMed]
174. Cholkar, K.; Patel, S.P.; Vadlapudi, A.D.; Mitra, A.K. Novel strategies for anterior segment ocular drug delivery. *J. Ocul. Pharmacol. Ther.* **2013**, *29*, 106–123. [CrossRef]
175. Gaudana, R.; Ananthula, H.K.; Parenky, A.; Mitra, A.K. Ocular drug delivery. *AAPS J.* **2010**, *12*, 348–360. [CrossRef]
176. Brito-Zeron, P.; Baldini, C.; Bootsma, H.; Bowman, S.J.; Jonsson, R.; Mariette, X.; Sivils, K.; Theander, E.; Tzioufas, A.; Ramos-Casals, M. Sjogren syndrome. *Nat. Rev. Dis. Primers* **2016**, *2*, 16047. [CrossRef]
177. Imgenberg-Kreuz, J.; Sandling, J.K.; Nordmark, G. Epigenetic alterations in primary Sjogren's syndrome—An overview. *Clin. Immunol.* **2018**, *196*, 12–20. [CrossRef]
178. Li, P.; Han, M.; Zhao, X.; Ren, G.; Mei, S.; Zhong, C. Abnormal Epigenetic Regulations in the Immunocytes of Sjogren's Syndrome Patients and Therapeutic Potentials. *Cells* **2022**, *11*, 1767. [CrossRef]
179. Moreno-Montanes, J.; Bleau, A.M.; Jimenez, A.I. Tivanisiran, a novel siRNA for the treatment of dry eye disease. *Expert Opin. Investig. Drugs* **2018**, *27*, 421–426. [CrossRef]
180. Xue, K.; MacLaren, R.E. Antisense oligonucleotide therapeutics in clinical trials for the treatment of inherited retinal diseases. *Expert Opin. Investig. Drugs* **2020**, *29*, 1163–1170. [CrossRef]
181. Gupta, A.; Kafetzis, K.N.; Tagalakis, A.D.; Yu-Wai-Man, C. RNA therapeutics in ophthalmology—Translation to clinical trials. *Exp. Eye Res.* **2021**, *205*, 108482. [CrossRef]
182. Ci, Z.; Wang, H.; Luo, J.; Wei, C.; Chen, J.; Wang, D.; Zhou, Y. Application of Nanomaterials Targeting Immune Cells in the Treatment of Chronic Inflammation. *Int. J. Nanomed.* **2024**, *19*, 13925–13946. [CrossRef] [PubMed]
183. Wei, J.; Mu, J.; Tang, Y.; Qin, D.; Duan, J.; Wu, A. Next-generation nanomaterials: Advancing ocular anti-inflammatory drug therapy. *J. Nanobiotechnology* **2023**, *21*, 282. [CrossRef] [PubMed]
184. Wen, Y.; Jia, H.; Mo, Z.; Zheng, K.; Chen, S.; Ding, Y.; Zhang, Y.; Wen, Y.; Xie, Q.; Qiu, J.; et al. Cross-linked thermosensitive nanohydrogels for ocular drug delivery with a prolonged residence time and enhanced bioavailability. *Mater. Sci. Eng. C Mater. Biol. Appl.* **2021**, *119*, 111445. [CrossRef] [PubMed]
185. Jackson, D.C.; Zeng, W.; Wong, C.Y.; Mifsud, E.J.; Williamson, N.A.; Ang, C.-S.; Vingrys, A.J.; Downie, L.E. Tear Interferon-Gamma as a Biomarker for Evaporative Dry Eye Disease. *Investig. Ophthalmol. Vis. Sci.* **2016**, *57*, 4824–4830. [CrossRef]
186. Li, Y.; Zhang, K.; Chen, H.; Sun, F.; Xu, J.; Wu, Z.; Li, P.; Zhang, L.; Du, Y.; Luan, H.; et al. A genome-wide association study in Han Chinese identifies a susceptibility locus for primary Sjogren's syndrome at 7q11.23. *Nat. Genet.* **2013**, *45*, 1361–1365. [CrossRef]
187. Gandolfo, S.; Bombardieri, M.; Pers, J.O.; Mariette, X.; Ciccia, F. Precision medicine in Sjogren's disease. *Lancet Rheumatol.* **2024**, *6*, e636–e647. [CrossRef]
188. Soret, P.; Le Dantec, C.; Desvaux, E.; Foulquier, N.; Chassagnol, B.; Hubert, S.; Jamin, C.; Barturen, G.; Desachy, G.; Devauchelle-Pensec, V.; et al. A new molecular classification to drive precision treatment strategies in primary Sjogren's syndrome. *Nat. Commun.* **2021**, *12*, 3523. [CrossRef]
189. Verstappen, G.M.; van Nimwegen, J.F.; Vissink, A.; Kroese, F.G.M.; Bootsma, H. The value of rituximab treatment in primary Sjogren's syndrome. *Clin. Immunol.* **2017**, *182*, 62–71. [CrossRef]

190. Kuo, M.-T.; Fang, P.-C.; Chao, T.-L.; Chen, A.; Lai, Y.-H.; Huang, Y.-T.; Tseng, C.-Y. Tear Proteomics Approach to Monitoring Sjogren Syndrome or Dry Eye Disease. *Int. J. Mol. Sci.* **2019**, *20*, 1932. [CrossRef]
191. Urbanski, G.; Assad, S.; Chabrun, F.; de la Barca, J.M.C.; Blanchet, O.; Simard, G.; Lenaers, G.; Prunier-Mirebeau, D.; Gohier, P.; Lavigne, C.; et al. Tear metabolomics highlights new potential biomarkers for differentiating between Sjogren's syndrome and other causes of dry eye. *Ocul. Surf.* **2021**, *22*, 110–116. [CrossRef]
192. Retamozo, S.; Gheitasi, H.; Quartuccio, L.; Kostov, B.; Corazza, L.; Bové, A.; Sisó-Almirall, A.; Gandía, M.; Ramos-Casals, M.; De Vita, S.; et al. Cryoglobulinaemic vasculitis at diagnosis predicts mortality in primary Sjogren syndrome: Analysis of 515 patients. *Rheumatology* **2016**, *55*, 1443–1451. [CrossRef]
193. Liu, X.; Wang, H.; Wang, X.; Jiang, X.; Jin, Y.; Han, Y.; Zhang, Z. Identification and verification of inflammatory biomarkers for primary Sjogren's syndrome. *Clin. Rheumatol.* **2024**, *43*, 1335–1352. [CrossRef] [PubMed]
194. Shetty, R.; Khamar, P.; Shirodkar, S.; Sethu, S.; Nair, A.P.; Ghosh, A. Patient stratification using point of care biomarkers in dry eye disease. *Indian J. Ophthalmol.* **2023**, *71*, 1391–1400. [CrossRef] [PubMed]
195. Hagan, S.; Martin, E.; Enriquez-de-Salamanca, A. Tear fluid biomarkers in ocular and systemic disease: Potential use for predictive, preventive and personalised medicine. *EPMA J.* **2016**, *7*, 15. [CrossRef] [PubMed]
196. Mavragani, C.P.; Moutsopoulos, H.M. Sjogren's syndrome: Old and new therapeutic targets. *J. Autoimmun.* **2020**, *110*, 102364. [CrossRef]
197. Zochowska, D.; Wyzgal, J.; Paczek, L. Impact of CYP3A4*1B and CYP3A5*3 polymorphisms on the pharmacokinetics of cyclosporine and sirolimus in renal transplant recipients. *Ann. Transplant.* **2012**, *17*, 36–44.
198. Li, R.-N.; Ou, T.-T.; Lin, C.-H.; Lin, Y.-Z.; Fang, T.-J.; Chen, Y.-J.; Tseng, C.-C.; Sung, W.-Y.; Wu, C.-C.; Yen, J.-H. NLRP3 Gene Polymorphisms in Rheumatoid Arthritis and Primary Sjogren's Syndrome Patients. *Diagnostics* **2023**, *13*, 206. [CrossRef]
199. Pecorelli, L.; Klein, K. Insights into Patient Heterogeneity in Sjogren's Disease. *Int. J. Mol. Sci.* **2025**, *26*, 6367. [CrossRef]
200. Nguyen, Y.; Nocturne, G.; Henry, J.; Ng, W.-F.; Belkhir, R.; Desmoulins, F.; Bergé, E.; Morel, J.; Perdriger, A.; Dernis, E.; et al. Identification of distinct subgroups of Sjogren's disease by cluster analysis based on clinical and biological manifestations: Data from the cross-sectional Paris-Saclay and the prospective ASSESS cohorts. *Lancet Rheumatol.* **2024**, *6*, e216–e225. [CrossRef]
201. Cummins, M.J.; Papas, A.; Kammer, G.M.; Fox, P.C. Treatment of primary Sjogren's syndrome with low-dose human interferon alfa administered by the oromucosal route: Combined phase III results. *Arthritis Rheum.* **2003**, *49*, 585–593. [CrossRef] [PubMed]
202. Li, X.X.; Maitiyaer, M.; Tan, Q.; Huang, W.H.; Liu, Y.; Liu, Z.P.; Wen, Y.Q.; Zheng, Y.; Chen, X.; Chen, R.L.; et al. Emerging biologic frontiers for Sjogren's syndrome: Unveiling novel approaches with emphasis on extra glandular pathology. *Front. Pharmacol.* **2024**, *15*, 1377055. [CrossRef] [PubMed]
203. Anghel, S.A.; Dinu-Pirvu, C.-E.; Costache, M.-A.; Voiculescu, A.M.; Ghica, M.V.; Anuța, V.; Popa, L. Receptor Pharmacogenomics: Deciphering Genetic Influence on Drug Response. *Int. J. Mol. Sci.* **2024**, *25*, 9371. [CrossRef] [PubMed]
204. Plaza-Puche, A.B.; Salerno, L.C.; Versaci, F.; Romero, D.; Alio, J.L. Clinical evaluation of the repeatability of ocular aberrometry obtained with a new pyramid wavefront sensor. *Eur. J. Ophthalmol.* **2019**, *29*, 585–592. [CrossRef]
205. Marvel, J.; Gargon, E.; Howse, C.; Chohan, A.; Mayhew, M.; Kenney, G.; Stone, L.; Fisher, B.A.; Steenackers, M.; Williamson, N.; et al. The Development and Content Validation of the Sjogren's Related Quality of Life Instrument (SRQoL). *Rheumatol. Ther.* **2024**, *11*, 1591–1609. [CrossRef]
206. Unger, J.; Mattsson, M.; Drăgoi, R.G.; Avram, C.; Boström, C.; Buttgereit, F.; Lackner, A.; Witte, T.; Raffeiner, B.; Peichl, P.; et al. The Experiences of Functioning and Health of Patients With Primary Sjogren's Syndrome: A Multicenter Qualitative European Study. *Front. Med.* **2021**, *8*, 770422. [CrossRef]
207. Hopkins, A.L. Network pharmacology: The next paradigm in drug discovery. *Nat. Chem. Biol.* **2008**, *4*, 682–690. [CrossRef]
208. Ren, Y.; Xia, W.; Wu, J.; Yang, Z.; Jiang, Y.; Wen, Y.; Guo, Q.; Gu, J.; Yang, J.; Luo, J.; et al. Artificial intelligence-based prediction of organ involvement in Sjogren's syndrome using labial gland biopsy whole-slide images. *Clin. Rheumatol.* **2025**, *44*, 2919–2927. [CrossRef]

International Journal of
Molecular Sciences

MDPI

Article

Long-Term Clinical and Molecular Changes in Dry Eye Disease and Chronic Ocular Pain

Cristina Valencia-Sandonís [1], Andrés Ángel Calderón-García [1], Marta Blanco-Vázquez [1], Laura Valencia-Nieto [1], Andrea Novo-Diez [1], Amanda Vázquez [1,2], Margarita Calonge [1,3], María J. González-García [1,3,*,†] and Amalia Enríquez-de-Salamanca [1,3,†]

1 Institute of Applied Ophthalmobiology (IOBA), Universidad de Valladolid (UVa), Campus Miguel Delibes, Paseo de Belén 17, 47011 Valladolid, Spain; cristina.valencia@uva.es (C.V.-S.); andresangel.calderon@uva.es (A.Á.C.-G.); marta.blanco.vazquez@uva.es (M.B.-V.); laura.valencia@uva.es (L.V.-N.); andrea.novo@uva.es (A.N.-D.); amanda.vazquez@uva.es (A.V.); mcalonge@uva.es (M.C.); amalia.enriquez-salamanca@uva.es (A.E.-d.-S.)

2 Pain Unit, Alliance of University Hospitals, Health System of Castilla y León, Calle Dulzaina 2, 47012 Valladolid, Spain

3 Biomedical Research Networking Center in Bioengineering, Biomaterials and Nanomedicine (CIBER-BBN), Campus Miguel Delibes, Paseo de Belén 17, 47011 Valladolid, Spain

* Correspondence: mariajesus.gonzalez.garcia@uva.es; Tel.: +34-983-184-191

† These authors contributed equally to this work.

Abstract: Dry eye disease (DED) is a prevalent condition characterized by ocular surface inflammation and pain. This study evaluated the long-term progression of DED by analyzing clinical and molecular status, considering the impact of chronic ocular pain. Patients with DED were evaluated at two visits (V1 and V2) separated by at least two years. Evaluations included validated symptom questionnaires alongside slit-lamp examination, corneal sensitivity testing, and sub-basal nerve plexus analysis. Basal tear samples were collected for multiplex quantification of 20 cytokines and substance P (SP), and conjunctival cells were obtained to analyze 25 genes and 12 microRNAs (miRNA). Based on the presence or absence of chronic ocular pain, patients were then divided into two groups. Patients improved in DED-related symptoms, with no changes observed in ocular surface signs. Corneal dendritic cell density decreased, along with epidermal growth factor (EGF), fractalkine, and monocyte chemoattractant protein (MCP-1) tear levels, whereas interleukin (IL)-10 and SP tear levels increased. Neurotrophic tyrosine kinase, receptor, type *(NTRK)1* gene expression was significantly downregulated, especially in patients without chronic ocular pain. miR-665 expression decreased significantly in DED patients. Monitoring corneal dendritic cells, tear cytokines, and gene/miRNA expression offers promising tools for tracking DED progression. Distinguishing the presence of chronic ocular pain as a separate symptom is crucial to optimizing therapeutic strategies and DED progression.

Keywords: dry eye; chronic ocular pain; tear biomarkers; gene expression; miRNAs expression

1. Introduction

Dry eye disease (DED) is a common, complex, multifactorial, and symptomatic disease that significantly affects patient's quality of life [1]. Its prevalence varies depending on the diagnostic criteria, disease severity, and population characteristics, with estimates ranging from 2.7% in individuals aged 20–29 to over 30% in women above 80 [2,3]. In Spain, a recent population-based survey reported a 12.3% prevalence of clinically diagnosed DED, with a notable proportion of young women (18–29 years old) reporting symptoms [4]. Several risk factors have been associated with DED, including increasing age, female sex, ocular surgeries, prolonged screen exposure, and mental health disorders such as anxiety and depression [2,3]. Given its high prevalence and clinical impact, DED represents a major public health issue and a significant burden on healthcare systems worldwide.

Pain is a fundamental protective mechanism that signals actual or potential tissue damage. In DED, tear film instability and hyperosmolarity activate corneal nociceptors, triggering nociceptive signaling through afferent pathways to the central nervous system. Although initially protective, sustained ocular surface stress promotes the release of inflammatory mediators and structural damage to nerve terminals, resulting in peripheral sensitization. If the noxious stimulus or inflammation persists, central sensitization may develop, amplifying pain responses at the level of the central nervous system [5,6].

Traditionally regarded as a symptom of DED, ocular pain is now increasingly recognized as a distinct closely interconnected clinical entity that may coexist with DED, complicating diagnosis and management [1,6]. These interrelated conditions are often difficult to differentiate, but accurate diagnosis is essential to guide effective treatment. Patients with chronic ocular pain secondary to DED may show poor response to conventional therapies and often require a multimodal approach that includes interventions targeting the nervous system [1,7].

In this context, the identification of biomarkers for diagnosing and monitoring DED and ocular pain is being extensively investigated, supported by the accessibility and minimally invasive nature of tear fluid and conjunctival cell sampling [8,9]. Elevated levels of cytokines and neuropeptides involved in inflammation and/or pain have been detected in the tears of patients with DED. Cytokines such as interleukin (IL)-1 receptor antagonist (Ra), IL-6, IL-8/CXCL8, and matrix metalloproteinase (MMP)-9 have been associated with DED [9–11]. Previous studies have identified an association between the concentration or percentage of detection levels of IL-9 in tears and the development of chronic ocular pain; similarly, associations have been published between ocular surface inflammation and IL-2, IL-8/CXCL8, macrophage inflammatory protein (MIP)-1α/CCL3, and interferon (IFN)-γ [9].

Moreover, the study of gene and microRNA (miRNA) expression related to inflammation and pain expression is emerging as a promising tool in ocular surface disease research. The analysis of conjunctival gene expression has gained attention as a valuable approach for diagnosing and monitoring inflammatory ocular surface diseases [12–14]. miRNAs are short noncoding RNA molecules that regulate gene expression at the post-transcriptional level which have been proposed as very promising biomarkers because of their high stability. Emerging evidence highlights a reciprocal relationship between miRNAs and epigenetic regulation in which miRNAs influence the expression of epigenetic regulators while their own transcription is subject to epigenetic control [15]. Changes in miRNA expression have also been actively investigated in the context of ocular surface inflammation [16–19]. In patients with DED, upregulation of inflammation-related miRNAs has been reported, including miR-127-5p, miR-1273h-3p, miR-1288-5p, miR-130b-5p, miR-139-3p, miR-1910-5p, miR-203b-5p, miR-22-5p, and miR-4632-3p [1,19]. Animal models of Sjögren's syndrome have also demonstrated altered tear miRNA profiles associated with autoimmune-mediated DED [18]. In particular, miRNA-146a-5p acts as a regulator of inflammation in DED by inhibiting target genes such as *IRAK1*, which leads to decreased expression of proinflammatory mediators including IL-6 and tumor necrosis factor (TNF)-α [17].

Thus, the aim of this study was to evaluate the long-term progression of DED by assessing clinical and molecular changes over a minimum follow-up period of two years. Specifically, we analyzed the evolution of symptoms, clinical signs, tear levels of cytokines and neuropeptides related to inflammation and pain, and the expression of genes and miRNAs involved in these pathways. In addition, the DED patients included herein were stratified based on the presence or absence of chronic ocular pain to investigate whether pain influences the long-term trajectory of disease-related biomarkers and clinical outcomes.

2. Results

This study corresponds to the second phase of a longitudinal study that initially included 63 patients at the first visit (V1) [9,20]. At the beginning of the second phase, all participants were invited to return for a follow-up visit (V2), which occurred after a mean interval of 3.82 ± 0.64 (range 2.83–3.92) years from V1. A total of 22 patients attended the V2. The flow of participants through the study is summarized in Figure 1. To address potential selection bias, we additionally compared baseline characteristics between participants who returned at V2 and those who did not (Supplementary Table S1). Of these, 19 (86.4%) were women and 3 (13.6%) were men. The overall mean age at V2 was 61.09 ± 7.95 (range, 43–71) years. Participants reported experiencing DED-related symptoms for a mean duration of 15.76 ± 12.52 (range, 5.33–53.58) years.

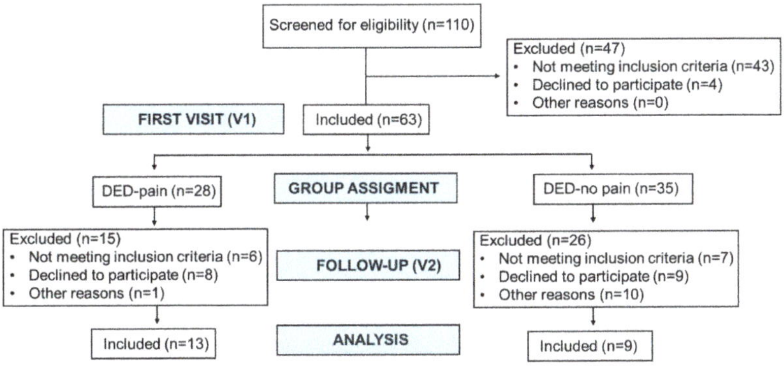

Figure 1. Flow of participants through the study from the first visit (V1) to the follow-up visit (V2).

Patients were subsequently stratified into two groups based on the presence (DED-pain) or absence (DED-no pain) of chronic ocular pain. The DED-pain group included 13 patients, with a mean age of 61.38 ± 8.56 (range, 43–71) years, of whom 11 (84.6%) were women. The DED-no pain group included 9 patients, with a mean age of 60.67 ± 7.45 (range, 49–71) years, including 8 women (88.9%).

2.1. Clinical Evaluation

The treatments used to manage systemic conditions and DED at the time of V1 and V2 are summarized in Table 1. As this was an observational study, data on treatments used between visits were not collected.

Table 2 summarizes the results of symptom questionnaires assessing DED-related symptoms, ocular pain, anxiety, and depression in the entire patient cohort. A significant improvement in DED-related symptoms, as assessed by the Ocular Surface Disease Index (OSDI) questionnaire, was observed, whereas no other significant changes in symptom scores were detected between visits. Importantly, when considering the minimal clinically important difference for OSDI, 15 patients (68.2%) achieved a clinically meaningful improvement in symptoms.

Table 1. Systemic and ocular topical treatments for dry eye disease at V1 and V2.

Systemic Treatments	All (n = 22)			DED-Pain (n = 13)			DED-No Pain (n = 9)		
	V1	V2	*p*-Value	V1	V2	*p*-Value	V1	V2	*p*-Value
Analgesics and NSAIDs	8 (36.4)	3 (13.6)	0.125	6 (46.2)	3 (23.1)	0.375	2 (22.2)	0 (0)	0.500
Antacids	6 (27.3)	5 (22.7)	1.000	4 (30.8)	3 (23.1)	1.000	2 (22.2)	2 (22.2)	1.000
Anticoagulants	2 (9.1)	2 (9.1)	1.000	1 (7.7)	1 (7.7)	1.000	1 (11.1)	1 (11.1)	1.000
Antihypertensives	4 (18.2)	5 (22.7)	1.000	3 (23.1)	3 (23.1)	1.000	1 (11.1)	2 (22.2)	1.000
Asthma treatments	3 (13.6)	3 (13.6)	1.000	3 (23.1)	3 (23.1)	1.000	0 (0)	0 (0)	1.000
Cholesterol-lowering drugs	6 (27.3)	7 (31.8)	1.000	3 (23.1)	4 (30.8)	1.000	3 (33.3)	3 (33.3)	1.000
Neuropsychiatric treatments	3 (13.6)	2 (9.1)	1.000	2 (15.4)	1 (7.7)	1.000	1 (11.1)	1 (11.1)	1.000
Neurological disease treatments	0	1 (4.5)	1.000	2 (15.4)	1 (7.7)	1.000	0 (0)	0 (0)	1.000
Anxiolytics	2 (9.1)	1 (4.5)	1.000	1 (7.7)	0 (0)	1.000	0 (0)	0 (0)	1.000
Antidepressants	2 (9.1)	1 (4.5)	1.000	0 (0)	1 (7.7)	1.000	1 (11.1)	1 (11.1)	1.000
Antiepileptics	1 (4.5)	1 (4.5)	1.000	0 (0)	1 (7.7)	1.000	1 (11.1)	0 (0)	1.000
Other	1 (4.5)	2 (9.1)	1.000	1 (7.7)	0 (0)	1.000	1 (11.1)	1 (11.1)	1.000
Immunosuppressants and corticosteroids	3 (13.6)	0	0.250	2 (15.4)	3 (23.1)	1.000	2 (22.2)	0 (0)	0.500
Hormonal and genitourinary treatments	5 (22.7)	6 (27.3)	1.000	1 (7.7)	0 (0)	1.000	3 (33.3)	3 (33.3)	1.000
Antidiabetic agents	1 (4.5)	0	1.000	3 (23.1)	4 (30.8)	1.000	0 (0)	0 (0)	1.000
Miscellanea	5 (22.7)	6 (27.3)	1.000	3 (23.1)	4 (30.8)	1.000	2 (22.2)	2 (22.2)	1.000
Vitamins and food supplements	4 (18.2)	6 (27.3)	0.500	0 (0)	0 (0)	1.000	1 (11.1)	1 (11.1)	1.000
Muscle relaxants	1 (4.5)	0	1.000	0 (0)	1 (7.7)	1.000	1 (11.1)	1 (11.1)	1.000
Cardiovascular treatments	0	1 (4.5)	1.000	0 (0)	0 (0)	1.000	0 (0)	0 (0)	1.000
Ocular topical treatments	**All (n = 22)**			**DED-Pain (n = 13)**			**DED-No Pain (n = 9)**		
	V1	**V2**	***p*-Value**	**V1**	**V2**	***p*-Value**	**V1**	**V2**	***p*-Value**
Lubricants	15 (68.2)	14 (63.3)	1.000	9 (69.2)	10 (76.9)	1.000	6 (66.7)	4 (44.4)	0.500
Artificial tears	15 (68.2)	14 (63.3)	1.000	9 (69.2)	10 (76.9)	1.000	6 (66.7)	4 (44.4)	0.500
Gels	1 (4.5)	0 (0)	1.000	1 (7.7)	0 (0)	1.000	0 (0)	0 (0)	1.000
Ointments	1 (4.5)	1 (4.5)	1.000	1 (7.7)	1 (7.7)	1.000	0 (0)	0 (0)	1.000
Eyelid hygiene	8 (36.4)	4 (18.2)	0.125	5 (38.5)	2 (15.4)	0.250	3 (33.3)	2 (22.2)	1.000
Punctal plugs	3 (13.6)	2 (9.1)	1.000	2 (15.4)	2 (15.4)	1.000	1 (11.1)	0 (0)	1.000
Blood derivates	3 (13.6)	2 (9.1)	1.000	3 (23.1)	2 (15.4)	1.000	0 (0)	0 (0)	1.000
Corticosteroids	1 (4.5)	2 (9.1)	1.000	1 (7.7)	1 (7.7)	1.000	0 (0)	1 (11.1)	1.000
Cyclosporine	0 (0)	1 (4.5)	1.000	0 (0)	1 (7.7)	1.000	0 (0)	0 (0)	1.000

Data are presented as frequencies n (%). V1: visit 1; V2: visit 2; NSAIDs: nonsteroidal anti-inflammatory drugs.

Table 2. Changes in symptoms between V1 and V2 in the overall cohort (n = 22).

	V1	V2	p-Value
OSDI (0–100)	38.88 ± 19.31	25.09 ± 17.35	**0.002**
mSIDEQ (0–28)	13.68 ± 4.59	13.64 ± 4.69	1.000
Intensity of pain (NRS scale, 0–10)	3.98 ± 3.58	2.89 ± 3.48	0.378
Intensity of pain (WFPRS scale, 0–10)	4.00 ± 3.75	3.11 ± 3.53	0.445
HADS questionnaire (0–42)	8.55 ± 6.04	8.36 ± 4.45	1.000
Anxiety subscale (0–21)	5.82 ± 3.50	5.86 ± 2.96	1.000
Depression subscale (0–21)	2.73 ± 2.83	2.50 ± 2.15	1.000
CDES-Q1			
Better n (%)	-	5 (22.7)	-
Worse n (%)	-	6 (27.3)	-
Same n (%)	-	11 (50.0)	-
CDES-Q2			
Improvement intensity (0–10)	-	7.00 ± 2.32	-
Worsening intensity (0–10)	-	5.33 ± 0.82	-

Data are presented as mean ± standard deviation. V1: visit 1; V2: visit 2. CDES-Q: Change in Dry Eye Symptoms Questionnaire; OSDI: Ocular Surface Disease Index; mSIDEQ: Modified Single Item Dry Eye Questionnaire; NRS: Numerical Rating Scale; WFPRS: Wong–Baker Faces Pain Rating Scale; HADS: Hospital Anxiety and Depression Scale. p-values in bold indicate statistically significant changes from V1 to V2.

Similarly, when stratified by group, patients in the DED-pain group showed a significant reduction in OSDI scores (Table 3). Although a decrease was also observed in the DED-no pain group, it did not reach statistical significance. No other statistically significant changes were observed between visits in either group.

Table 3. Changes in symptoms between V1 and V2 in the subgroups.

	DED-Pain (n = 13)			DED-No Pain (n = 9)		
	V1	V2	p-Value	V1	V2	p-Value
OSDI (0–100)	44.42 ± 21.24	29.37 ± 20.24	**0.021**	30.87 ± 13.42	18.91 ± 10.12	0.336
mSIDEQ (0–28)	16.15 ± 3.91	15.00 ± 4.78	0.442	10.11 ± 2.85	11.67 ± 4.00	0.336
Intensity of pain (NRS scale, 0–10)	6.65 ± 1.84	4.50 ± 3.53	0.189	0.11 ± 0.33	0.56 ± 1.67	0.665
Intensity of pain (WFPRS scale, 0–10)	6.77 ± 2.09	4.96 ± 3.39	0.205	0.00 ± 0.00	0.44 ± 1.33	0.370
HADS questionnaire (0–42)	8.31 ± 4.84	10.00 ± 4.16	0.254	8.89 ± 7.77	6.00 ± 3.91	0.336
Anxiety subscale (0–21)	5.69 ± 3.04	6.85 ± 2.91	0.254	6.00 ± 4.27	4.44 ± 2.55	0.336
Depression subscale (0–21)	2.62 ± 2.33	3.15 ± 2.23	0.442	2.89 ± 3.59	1.56 ± 1.74	0.336
CDES-Q1						
Better n (%)	-	4 (30.8)	-	-	1 (11.1)	-
Worse n (%)	-	4 (30.8)	-	-	2 (22.2)	-
Same n (%)	-	5 (38.5)	-	-	6 (66.7)	-
CDES-Q2						
Improvement intensity (0–10)	-	7.75 ± 1.85	-	-	4.00	-
Worsening intensity (0–10)	-	5.50 ± 0.58	-	-	5.00 ± 1.41	-

Data are presented as mean ± standard deviation. DED: dry eye disease; V1: visit 1; V2: visit 2. CDES-Q: Change in Dry Eye Symptoms Questionnaire; OSDI: Ocular Surface Disease Index; mSIDEQ: Modified Single Item Dry Eye Questionnaire; NRS: Numerical Rating Scale; WFPRS: Wong–Baker Faces Pain Rating Scale; HADS: Hospital Anxiety and Depression Scale. p-values in bold indicate statistically significant changes from V1 to V2.

Regarding ocular surface signs evaluated by slit-lamp biomicroscopy, no significant differences were found between visits in the overall cohort or within subgroups (Table 4).

Corneal sensitivity, assessed with the Belmonte noncontact esthesiometer, remained stable across visits in the entire sample, with no significant changes in mechanical, heat, or cold thresholds. Similarly, contact esthesiometry using the Cochet–Bonnet esthesiometer revealed no differences in sensitivity measurements before or after the application of topical anesthesia. Global Rating of Change scores were also consistent between visits (Table 5). Significant reductions in both total and small dendritic cell density were observed on in vivo confocal microscopy (IVCM), in the total sample analysis (Table 5).

Table 4. Changes in ocular surface signs between V1 and V2 in the overall cohort and in the subgroups.

	All (n = 22)			DED-Pain (n = 13)			DED-No Pain (n = 9)		
	V1	V2	*p*-Value	V1	V2	*p*-Value	V1	V2	*p*-Value
Conjunctival hyperemia (Efron scale, 0–4)	1.00 [2.00–1.00]	2.00 [2.00–1.00]	0.460	1.00 [2.00–1.00]	2.00 [2.00–1.00]	0.579	1.00 [1.00–1.00]	2.00 [2.00–0.50]	0.988
Blepharitis (Efron scale, 0–4)	2.00 [2.25–1.00]	1.00 [2.00–1.00]	0.176	2.00 [2.50–1.00]	1.00 [2.00–1.00]	0.447	2.00 [2.50–1.00]	1.00 [2.00–0.50]	0.405
Nasal LIPCOF (0–3 scales)	2.00 [2.00–1.00]	1.00 [2.00–1.00]	0.127	2.00 [2.50–1.00]	1.00 [2.00–1.00]	0.360	2.00 [2.00–1.00]	1.00 [1.00–0.50]	0.420
Temporal LIPCOF (0–3 scales)	2.00 [2.00–1.00]	1.00 [2.00–1.00]	0.298	2.00 [2.00–1.50]	2.00 [2.00–1.00]	0.360	2.00 [2.00–0.50]	1.00 [2.50–0.50]	0.988
TBUT (seconds)	3.42 ± 1.33	3.50 ± 1.46	0.830	3.64 ± 1.44	3.13 ± 1.24	0.360	3.11 ± 1.16	4.04 ± 1.66	0.639
Corneal staining (Oxford scale, 0–5)	1.27 ± 0.94	0.78 ± 1.02	0.176	1.38 ± 0.96	1.00 ± 1.15	0.360	1.11 ± 0.93	0.44 ± 0.73	0.420
Conjunctival staining (Oxford scale, 0–5)	0.93 ± 0.71	0.59 ± 0.78	0.275	0.92 ± 0.70	0.23 ± 0.39	0.210	0.94 ± 0.77	1.11 ± 0.93	0.988
LWE (0–3 scale)	0.55 ± 0.63	0.82 ± 0.88	0.338	0.58 ± 0.64	1.08 ± 0.93	0.360	0.50 ± 0.66	0.44 ± 0.68	0.988
Meibum quality (0–3 scale)	1.00 [2.00–1.00]	2.00 [2.00–1.00]	0.275	1.00 [2.00–1.00]	2.00 [2.00–1.00]	0.360	2.00 [2.00–1.00]	2.00 [2.00–1.00]	0.988
Meibum Expressibility (0–3 scale)	2.00 [2.00–1.00]	2.00 [2.00–1.75]	0.176	2.00 [2.00–1.00]	2.00 [2.50–1.50]	0.290	2.00 [2.00–0.50]	2.00 [2.00–1.00]	0.988
Schirmer's Test (mm)	10.41 ± 7.56	10.45 ± 9.94	0.350	11.08 ± 7.35	9.92 ± 9.79	0.360	9.44 ± 8.20	11.22 ± 10.69	0.999

Data are presented as mean ± standard deviation or as median [interquartile range]. DED: dry eye disease; V1: visit 1; V2: visit 2; LIPCOF: lid-parallel conjunctival folds: TBUT: tear break-up time; LWE: lid wiper epitheliopathy.

Table 5. Changes in corneal sensitivity and sub-basal nerve plexus between V1 and V2 in the overall cohort (n = 22).

	V1	V2	*p*-Value
Noncontact corneal esthesiometry			
Mechanical threshold (mL/min)	87.28 ± 41.96	114.76 ± 43.77	0.060
Heat threshold (°C)	2.12 ± 1.24	1.16 ± 0.73	0.060
Cold threshold (°C)	−2.23 ± 1.13	−1.31 ± 0.89	0.060
Contact corneal esthesiometry			
Before topical anesthesia (mm)	56.14 ± 7.86	55.68 ± 7.12	0.812
After topical anesthesia (mm)	8.81 ± 16.95	6.90 ± 12.09	0.812
Anesthetic challenge test (GRC scale; −5 to 5)	−1.77 ± 2.35	−1.16 ± 2.22	0.543
Number of nerves (n/mm^2)	46.78 ± 20.87	51.89 ± 23.00	0.792
Nerve density (mm/mm^2)	10,494.99 ± 4564.65	11,610.99 ± 4396.22	0.792
Nerve length (mm/mm^2)	1414.71 ± 335.98	1518.27 ± 266.52	0.685
Density of nerve branch points (n/mm^2)	26.89 ± 26.35	30.87 ± 21.26	0.827
Nerve tortuosity (0–4)	2.70 ± 0.71	2.65 ± 0.73	0.962
Density of microneuromas (n/mm^2)	1.52 ± 2.40	1.99 ± 2.36	0.827
Density of dendritic cells (n/mm^2)	74.05 ± 88.23	25.66 ± 23.79	**0.044**
Small dendritic cells (n/mm^2)	56.82 ± 73.16	16.19 ± 20.17	**0.044**
Large dendritic cells (n/mm^2)	15.81 ± 21.52	8.24 ± 9.65	0.169
Globular cells (n/mm^2)	1.42 ± 2.97	1.23 ± 2.85	0.962
Reflectivity	102.67 ± 11.55	103.44 ± 12.55	0.962

Data are presented as mean ± standard deviation. V1: visit 1; V2: visit 2; GRC: Global Rating of Change. *p*-values in bold indicate statistically significant changes from V1 to V2.

However, when analyzed by group, no statistically significant differences were detected in any of the evaluated parameters (Table 6).

Table 6. Changes in symptoms, ocular surface signs, corneal sensitivity, and sub-basal nerve plexus between V1 and V2 in the subgroups.

	DED-Pain (n = 13)			DED-No Pain (n = 9)		
	V1	V2	*p*-Value	V1	V2	*p*-Value
Noncontact corneal esthesiometry						
Mechanical threshold (mL/min)	91.57 ± 53.68	104.58 ± 38.82	0.915	81.56 ± 19.36	128.33 ± 48.54	0.090
Heat threshold (°C)	2.37 ± 1.20	1.40 ± 0.61	0.246	1.81 ± 1.28	0.87 ± 0.80	0.240
Cold threshold (°C)	−2.07 ± 1.15	−1.29 ± 0.77	0.342	−2.44 ± 1.15	−1.33 ± 1.09	0.240

Table 6. *Cont.*

	DED-Pain (n = 13)			DED-No Pain (n = 9)		
	V1	V2	*p*-Value	V1	V2	*p*-Value
Contact corneal esthesiometry						
Before topical anesthesia (mm)	55.77 ± 8.62	55.77 ± 7.03	0.886	56.67 ± 7.07	55.56 ± 7.68	1.000
After topical anesthesia (mm)	11.67 ± 20.71	9.17 ± 15.50	0.794	5.00 ± 10.00	3.89 ± 4.17	1.000
Anesthetic challenge test (GRC scale; −5 to 5)	−2.31 ± 2.18	−1.50 ± 2.35	0.760	−1.00 ± 2.50	−0.67 ± 2.06	1.000
Number of nerves (n/mm²)	41.99 ± 17.02	53.04 ± 25.64	0.209	53.70 ± 24.85	50.23 ± 19.94	0.844
Nerve density (mm/mm²)	9508.85 ± 4523.93	11,734.28 ± 4538.24	0.209	11,919.40 ± 4486.96	11,432.90 ± 4447.34	0.825
Nerve length (mm/mm²)	1387.18 ± 381.08	1515.77 ± 330.36	0.828	1454.48 ± 274.76	1521.88 ± 150.79	0.825
Density of nerve branch points (n/mm²)	19.79 ± 16.63	33.33 ± 24.03	0.209	37.15 ± 34.75	27.31 ± 17.23	0.825
Nerve tortuosity (0–4)	2.60 ± 0.75	2.77 ± 0.67	0.759	2.83 ± 0.65	2.48 ± 0.82	0.825
Density of microneuromas (n/mm²)	2.08 ± 2.79	1.76 ± 1.87	0.828	0.69 ± 1.47	2.31 ± 3.03	0.825
Density of dendritic cells (n/mm²)	82.53 ± 110.21	20.03 ± 26.47	0.209	61.81 ± 43.91	33.80 ± 17.58	0.600
Small dendritic cells (n/mm²)	64.10 ± 89.76	12.98 ± 23.94	0.209	46.30 ± 41.86	20.83 ± 12.93	0.825
Large dendritic cells (n/mm²)	16.83 ± 25.80	6.57 ± 8.06	0.209	14.35 ± 14.60	10.65 ± 11.67	0.825
Globular cells (n/mm²)	1.60 ± 2.71	0.48 ± 1.25	0.262	1.16 ± 3.47	2.31 ± 4.09	0.825
Reflectivity	99.76 ± 9.01	100.69 ± 14.14	0.759	106.87 ± 13.95	107.41 ± 9.16	0.844

Data are presented as mean ± standard deviation. DED: Dry Eye Disease; V1: visit 1; V2: visit 2; GRC: Global Rating of Change.

2.2. Sample Analysis

2.2.1. Tear Cytokine and Substance P Analysis

Epidermal growth factor (EGF), IL-1Ra, IL-4, IL-8/CXCL8, monocyte chemoattractant protein (MCP)-1/CCL2, MCP-3/CCL7, growth-related oncogene (GRO), and substance P (SP) were detected in at least 90.9% of the subjects at both visits. Fractalkine/CX3CL1, IL-6, IL-10, MIP-1β/CCL4, and regulated on activation, normal T cell expressed and secreted (RANTES)/CCL5 exhibited detection rates ranging from 50 to 100% (Table 7). IL-1β, IL-2, IL-9, IL-17A, IFN-γ, MIP-1α/CCL3, nerve growth factor (NGF), and TNF-α were detected in less than 50% of samples in at least one visit and were therefore analyzed as qualitative variables (detected/undetected).

Table 7. Tear detection rates and concentrations of the 20 analyzed cytokines and substance P at V1 and V2 in the total study population.

	V1		V2		
	Detection Rate (%)	**Concentration (pg/mL)**	**Detection Rate (%)**	**Concentration (pg/mL)**	***p*-Value**
EGF	100	1917.45 ± 894.45 (1520.88–2314.03)	100	845.50 ± 469.99 (637.12–1053.88)	**<0.001** [a]
Fractalkine/CX3CL1	50	1359.33 ± 1871.83 (529.40–2189.25)	100	1061.55 ± 583.81 (802.70–1320.39)	**0.020** [a]
IL-1β	*45.5*	-	*31.8*	-	0.664 [b]
IL-1Ra	100	6846.06 ± 11,331.55 (1821.93–11,870.19)	100	7060.59 ± 8099.22 (3469.60–10,651.58)	0.299 [a]
IL-2	*4.5*	-	63.6	30.02 ± 23.11 (19.77–40.27)	**0.004** [b]
IL-4	90.9	236.72 ± 328.95 (90.87–382.57)	95.5	405.65 ± 328.95 (155.43–655.87)	0.212 [a]
IL-6	63.6	58.38 ± 88.34 (19.17–97.51)	59.1	90.00 ± 128.38 (33.08–146.92)	0.516 [a]
IL-8/CXCL8	100	975.47 ± 3001.24 (−355.20–2306.15)	100	349.35 ± 509.40 (123.50–575.21)	0.971 [a]
IL-9	*9.1*	-	59.1	30.02 ± 23.11 (19.77–40.27)	**0.004** [b]
IL-10	59.1	21.80 ± 26.85 (9.90–33.71)	68.2	87.53 ± 70.83 (56.13–118.94)	0.084 [a]
IL-17A	*0*	-	68.2	45.92 ± 32.01 (31.73–60.12)	**<0.001** [b]

Table 7. *Cont.*

	V1		V2		
	Detection Rate (%)	**Concentration (pg/mL)**	**Detection Rate (%)**	**Concentration (pg/mL)**	***p*-Value**
MCP-1/CCL2	100	801.95 ± 733.80 (476.61–1127.30)	95.5	492.19 ± 363.47 (331.03–653.34)	**0.020** [a]
MCP-3/CCL7	95.5	251.88 ± 138.45 (190.49–313.26)	100	272.22 ± 284.51 (146.07–398.36)	0.930 [a]
TNF-α	59.1	9.25 ± 16.19 (2.07–16.42)	*18.2*	-	**0.024** [b]
IFN-γ	*27.3*	-	59.1	29.54 ± 22.37 (19.62–39.46)	0.087 [b]
GRO	100	6592.32 ± 9261.33 (2486.07–10,698.56)	100	5223.36 ± 4675.23 (3150.48–7296,25)	0.690 [a]
MIP-1α/CCL3	*9.1*	-	*4.5*	-	1.000 [b]
MIP-1β/CCL4	59.1	71.20 ± 268.24 (−47.73–190.13)	59.1	14.26 ± 11.68 (9.08–19.44)	1.000 [a]
NGF	77.3	8.09 ± 8.81 (4.18–11.99)	*36.4*	-	**0.035** [b]
RANTES/CCL5	86.4	82.68 ± 82.67 (46.03–119.34)	68.2	124.84 ± 89.03 (85.36–164.31)	1.000 [a]
SP	100	1172.80 ± 662.72 (862.64–1482.96)	100	4094.55 ± 3155.11 (2617.92–5571.19)	**<0.001** [a]

Detection rates are expressed as percentages, and concentrations are presented as means (95% confidence interval) pg/mL. Molecules with a percentage of detection lower than 50% are in italics. [a] *p*-values correspond to comparisons of concentrations levels between both visits. [b] *p*-values correspond to comparison of detection rates between both visits. V1: visit 1; V2: visit 2; EGF: epidermal growth factor; IL: interleukin; IL-1Ra: interleukin-1 receptor antagonist; MCP: monocyte chemoattractant protein; TNF: tumor necrosis factor; IFN: interferon; GRO: growth related oncogene; MIP: macrophage inflammatory protein; NGF: nerve growth factor; RANTES: regulated on activation normal T cell expressed and secreted; SP: substance P. *p*-values in bold indicate statistically significant changes from V1 to V2.

Quantitative analysis revealed significant decreases in the concentration levels of EGF, fractalkine/CX3CL1, and MCP1/CCL2 at V2 compared with V1, while SP levels significantly increased (Table 7). Among qualitatively analyzed molecules, IL-2, IL-9, and IL-17A showed significantly higher detection percentages at V2, whereas TNF-α and NGF showed significantly lower detection rates.

When patients were stratified into groups, the significant changes observed in the overall cohort were confirmed. In both the DED-pain and DED-no pain groups, EGF levels significantly decreased between visits. Specifically, EGF concentrations declined from 1730.69 ± 893.71 pg/mL at V1 to 935.46 ± 548.38 pg/mL at V2 in the DED-pain group ($p < 0.001$) and from 2187.22 ± 873.73 pg/mL to 715.56 ± 310.81 pg/mL in the DED-no pain group ($p = 0.018$). SP levels significantly increased in both groups: from 1289.75 ± 713.85 pg/mL to 3954.58 ± 3638.18 pg/mL in the DED-pain group ($p = 0.006$) and from 997.38 ± 576.82 pg/mL to 4304.51 ± 2477.08 pg/mL in the DED-no pain group ($p < 0.001$).

2.2.2. Gene Expression Analysis

The expression levels of the 25 analyzed genes, grouped according to their biological function, are shown in Table 8. Among these, only one gene, *NTRK1*, showed a statistically significant downregulation at V2 compared with V1.

In addition, when gene expression was analyzed separately by group, a significant downregulation of *NTRK1* was observed in the DED-no pain group (V1: 9.74 [6.49–12.99] vs. V2: 17.63 [14.75–20.51]; $p = 0.05$). In contrast, no significant differences were detected in the DED-pain group (V1: 11.88 [9.42–14.33] vs. V2: 14.51 [13.36–15.66]; $p= 0.625$). No other significant changes in gene expression were detected between visits in either group.

Table 8. Changes in gene expression between V1 and V2.

Category		Gene	ΔCt V1	ΔCt V2	Fold Change	Fold Regulation	*p*-Value
Modulation of pain responses	Inflammation	*BDKRB1*	11.21 (8.95–13.49)	15.38 (13.09–17.68)	0.06	−18.00	0.125
		IL1A	18.21 (16.38–20.03)	18.13 (16.55–19.71)	1.06	1.06	1.000
		IL2	12.48 (10.74–14.23)	12.88 (12.20–13.56)	0.76	−1.32	1.000
		CALCA	11.62 (9.09–14.15)	14.09 (12.35–15.83)	0.18	−5.54	0.396
		IL6	10.79 (9.24–12.33)	11.39 (9.84–12.95)	0.66	−1.52	0.833
		CCL2	15.96 (13.86–18.05)	16.57 (14.74–18.39)	0.66	−1.52	1.000
		ITGAM	14.74 (12.50–16.98)	13.24 (11.51–14.97)	2.83	2.83	0.605
		TAC1	19.36 (17.82–20.90)	19.17 (17.98–20.35)	1.14	1.14	1.000
		CD200	12.58 (11.45–13.71)	14.76 (12.72–16.80)	0.22	−4.53	0.295
		TACR1	18.89 (16.94–20.84)	19.49 (18.84–20.13)	0.66	−1.52	1.000
		TNF	12.03 (9.84–14.21)	12.14 (10.23–14.05)	0.93	−1.08	1.000
		CX3CR1	10.82 (8.18–13.46)	10.95 (9.85–12.04)	0.91	−1.09	1.000
		IL18	4.68 (3.92–5.44)	4.58 (4.28–4.88)	1.07	1.07	1.000
	Neurotrophins	*BDNF*	7.86 (7.02–8.69)	8.94 (7.55–10.33)	0.47	−2.11	0.295
		NGF	14.79 (12.78–16.81)	15.39 (14.24–16.54)	0.66	−1.52	1.000
		NTRK1	11.21 (9.38–13.04)	15.48 (14.22–16.75)	0.05	−19.29	**0.025**
	Inflammation and neurotransmitters	*PENK1*	12.36 (9.57–15.14)	15.41 (13.05–17.76)	0.12	−8.28	0.295
Conduction of pain	Opioid receptors	*OPRM1*	19.49 (17.93–21.05)	19.85 (19.22–20.48)	0.78	−1.28	1.000
		OPRD1	19.56 (18.00–21.12)	19.85 (19.22–20.48)	0.82	−1.22	1.000
		OPRK1	13.73 (12.00–15.45)	14.25 (13.44–15.06)	0.70	−1.43	1.000
	Ion channels	*TRPV3*	13.74 (12.25–15.23)	16.43 (15.08–17.78)	0.15	−6.45	0.125
		TRPA1	17.90 (16.14–19.66)	19.26 (18.29–20.24)	0.39	−2.57	0.605
		TRPV1	9.28 (8.26–10.30)	8.63 (7.34–9.91)	1.57	1.57	0.675
	Cannabinoid receptors	*CNR2*	12.40 (9.65–15.14)	17.22 (15.15–19.29)	0.04	−28.25	0.125
Synaptic transmission	Eicosanoid metabolism	*PTGS1*	14.37 (12.56–16.19)	14.84 (12.90–16.79)	0.72	−1.39	1.000

Data are expressed as mean ΔCt (cycle threshold (Ct) gene of interest—Ct *GAPDH*) values (95% CI) for each gene. Gene fold change between visits was calculated using the $2^{(-\Delta\Delta Ct)}$ method; when fold-change values were greater than one (upregulation), fold regulation was equal to the fold change; when fold-change values were less than one (downregulation), fold regulation is reported as the negative inverse of the fold change. Note that high values of ΔCt indicate lower gene expression, whereas low ΔCt values indicate higher gene expression. Significant *p*-values are denoted in bold.

2.2.3. miRNA Expression Analysis

Among the 12 miRNAs evaluated, a significant downregulation of miR-665 was observed at V2 compared with V1 (Table 9). However, when miRNA expression was analyzed separately by groups, no significant differences were found between visits.

Table 9. Changes in miRNA expression between V1 and V2.

miRNA	ΔCt V1	ΔCt V2	Fold Change	Fold Regulation	*p*-Value
20a-5p	1.46 (1.05–1.87)	1.50 (1.33–1.66)	0.97	−1.03	0.945
23b-3p	1.69 (2.16–1.22)	1.10 (1.34–0.86)	1.51	1.51	0.203
29a-3p	0.12 (−0.44–0.67)	0.19 (0.11–0.49)	0.95	−1.05	0.868

Table 9. *Cont.*

miRNA	ΔCt V1	ΔCt V2	Fold Change	Fold Regulation	*p*-Value
92b-3p	5.70 (5.25–6.15)	6.05 (5.75–6.34)	0.78	−1.27	0.434
99a-5p	0.72 (1.14–0.29)	0.52 (0.68–0.36)	1.15	1.15	0.595
137-3p	19.33 (18.47–20.19)	18.64 (18.07–19.21)	1.61	1.61	0.252
143-3p	16.43 (14.35–18.51)	16.17 (14.13–18.22)	1.20	1.20	0.945
208a-3p	17.62 (16.53–18.71)	17.80 (16.76–18.84)	0.88	−1.13	0.945
302d-3p	19.50 (18.76–20.25)	18.64 (18.07–19.21)	1.82	1.82	0.203
379-3p	15.52 (13.88–17.16)	17.40 (16.23–18.57)	0.27	−3.68	0.203
543	15.68 (14.75–16.60)	16.58 (15.69–17.47)	0.54	−1.87	0.375
665	5.68 (5.04–6.31)	7.47 (6.89–8.05)	0.29	−3.46	**<0.001**

Data are expressed as estimated mean ΔCt, which was calculated as micro(mi)RNA of interest Ct—housekeeping miRNA Ct, and 95% confidence interval. MiRNA fold change between visits was calculated using the $2^{(-\Delta\Delta Ct)}$ method; when fold-change values were greater than one (upregulation), fold regulation was equal to the fold change; when fold-change values were less than one (downregulation), fold regulation was reported as the negative inverse of the fold change. Note that high values of ΔCt indicate lower miRNA expression, whereas low ΔCt values indicate higher miRNA expression. Significant *p*-values are denoted in bold.

3. Discussion

The overlap between DED-related symptoms and chronic-ocular-pain-related symptoms, combined with the frequent lack of correlation between clinical signs and patient-reported symptoms, significantly complicates early diagnosis and appropriate management of these conditions [21]. This diagnostic challenge underscores the urgent need for reliable biomarkers to improve early identification and monitor the progression of these coexistent and interrelated conditions. Accordingly, this study aimed to evaluate the longitudinal progression of patients with DED both as a whole and stratified by the presence or absence of chronic ocular pain, to better elucidate the impact of persistent pain on disease evolution. To date, and to our knowledge, this is the first study to longitudinally investigate the clinical, molecular, and gene and miRNA expression profiles of these patients.

Our results demonstrated a significant improvement in DED-related symptoms, both in the overall cohort and specifically within the DED-pain group. Ocular surface parameters and corneal sensitivity remained stable between visits, regardless of whether the analysis was conducted on the full sample or stratified by group. At the level of the corneal sub-basal nerve plexus, a significant reduction in total and small dendritic cell density was observed in the whole cohort, although this finding was not maintained when groups were analyzed separately. Changes in EGF and SP concentrations were found both in the total sample and in the group-based analysis. Additionally, alterations in fractalkine/CX3CL1 and MCP-1/CCL2 levels were found in the full cohort. For molecules analyzed qualitatively as detected and nondetected, significant differences were observed in the percentage of detection of IL-2, IL-9, IL-17A, TNF-α and NGF. At the gene and miRNA expression level, *NTRK1* gene expression was downregulated in the overall cohort and in the DED-no pain group, while miR-665 expression was significantly downregulated only in the total sample.

Patients included in this study exhibited a severe degree of DED symptoms at V1. When analyzing the full cohort, a significant improvement was found in DED-related symptoms over time, as measured with the OSDI questionnaire, decreasing from severe to moderate intensity, with 68.2% of patients achieving the minimal clinically important difference for OSDI values. This improvement was also significant within the DED-pain group, with symptoms decreasing from a severe to a moderate level. Although the DED-no pain group did not show statistically significant change, symptom scores also decreased from severe to moderate. While this difference did not reach statistical significance—likely because of the smaller sample size—it may still reflect a clinically meaningful improvement. Patients with chronic ocular pain reported a moderate intensity of pain, and this intensity remained stable throughout the study. Approximately 4 years after their first visit, most patients reported similar symptoms to those experienced at V1, as assessed by the Change in Dry Eye Symptoms Questionnaire (CDES-Q). This outcome may be partly explained by the nature of the questionnaire, which assesses global symptom perception rather than distinguishing between specific complaints such as dryness or pain. In patients with chronic ocular pain, the lack of improvement in pain intensity may have influenced their overall perception of symptom stability, despite the OSDI score improvement found. These results are in line with previous studies showing that individuals with ocular pain tend to report more severe and persistent DED symptoms over time, which is consistent with our findings [22,23]. Furthermore, pain has been consistently identified as one of the most prevalent symptoms in chronic DED [23]. This is particularly relevant since patients exhibiting chronic ocular pain often respond inadequately to first-line topical therapies and may benefit from multimodal treatment strategies targeting the ocular sensory system [24]. In this context, the observed improvement in DED symptoms across the full cohort may reflect a positive response to the standard topical therapies these patients were using. However, the persistence and lack of improvement in ocular pain symptoms may be attributable to the absence of specific treatments targeting ocular pain mechanisms in the DED-pain group. While patients in our sample were treated with standard topical therapies, those with chronic ocular pain may require more advanced treatment options. No changes were observed in the topical or systemic medications that these subjects were receiving. It is important to acknowledge that this was an observational study, and patients were not monitored at our center between the two study visits. During that period, they continued their clinical care at their referring centers, where it can be assumed they received the best available treatment. Nonetheless, our findings highlight that chronic ocular pain, although closely related to DED, is often under-recognized as a specific component within this condition, leading to suboptimal management when not properly identified. This underscores the need to increase awareness of ocular pain mechanisms and promote individualized, multimodal treatment approaches.

No significant changes were found in slit-lamp-based ocular surface signs [24], indicating the stability of these clinical parameters over time. Consistently with our findings, a previous longitudinal study in patients with chronic ocular pain and DED after corneal refractive surgery reported only an improvement in corneal staining, which was not clinically significant, and no other relevant changes in ocular surface signs over time [25].

Similarly, corneal sensitivity showed no significant changes between visits, regardless of the measurement method used or the study group. Alterations in corneal sensitivity are common in DED patients [26–28]. However, the nature of these sensory changes remains controversial because of inconsistent findings in the literature. While some studies have reported corneal hypersensitivity [26], others have documented hyposensitivity when using noncontact esthesiometers to assess corneal sensitivity [27]. These discrepancies have been attributed to differences in measurement techniques, disease severity, and DED subtypes [28]. Despite this variability, there is a consensus that patients with DED exhibit a decreased corneal mechanical sensitivity when assessed using the Cochet–Bonnet esthesiometer [29–31]. Additionally, corneal hypersensitivity has been linked to increased DED-related symptoms and ocular pain [32].

Similarly, sub-basal corneal nerve parameters remained stable between visits, consistently with the absence of differences in corneal sensitivity. Interestingly, a reduction in total corneal dendritic cell density, primarily due to a decrease in the number of small dendritic cells, was observed across all patients. However, stratification by patient groups revealed no significant changes, suggesting that ocular pain does not significantly influence these cellular alterations, which appear to be primarily related to the underlying DED. Since increases in dendritic cell density are generally considered as markers of inflammation or immune activation, the observed reduction may reflect a decrease in immune activity at the ocular surface [28,33]. Previous studies have shown increased dendritic cell density in the central corneas of DED patients compared with healthy controls, particularly those with severe symptoms [34–36]. Although previous studies have associated higher microneuroma density with chronic ocular pain in patients with DED [22,37], no significant differences were observed between visits in our study. These findings underscore the potential utility of IVCM and the study of corneal dendritic cell analysis as valuable biomarkers for monitoring disease progression and inflammatory status in DED patients.

Tear film analysis of the entire cohort revealed significant decreases in the concentrations of EGF, fractalkine/CX3CL1, and MCP-1/CCL2, along with a significant increase in SP levels. Analysis by pain classification indicated that both DED-pain and DED-no pain patients showed reduced EGF and elevated SP concentration.

EGF levels were consistently reduced in the overall sample and in each of the two subgroups. EGF is a key growth factor involved in epithelial cell proliferation and differentiation, as well as wound healing, playing an essential role in maintaining ocular surface integrity [38]. Furthermore, EGF is a cytokine secreted by the lacrimal glands and has been shown to inversely correlate with Schirmer test results [39]. Previous studies have reported reduced EGF levels in tears of DED patients [39,40]. Comparison of our findings with the mean concentrations reported in healthy controls from a previous study conducted by our research group suggests that EGF concentration remained altered over time in this population. In healthy individuals, a mean decrease of approximately 6.3% in tear EGF concentration was observed over a similar follow-up period of time and mean age, likely reflecting physiological aging. In contrast, our cohort exhibited a markedly higher decline of approximately 56% between visits [41], indicating that the observed reduction was unlikely to be solely attributable to normal aging processes. Further research is needed to determine the clinical significance of this sustained decrease.

There was a significant reduction in fractalkine/CX3CL1 in the overall patient analysis. Fractalkine/CX3CL1 is a chemokine critical for neuroimmune communication, acting as a strong chemoattractant for immune cells. Persistent elevation of fractalkine/CX3CL1 has been linked to enhanced neuroinflammation and central sensitization mechanisms involved in chronic pain [42,43]. While our group previously reported increased fractalkine levels in DED patients compared with healthy controls [44], the present study found a decrease in fractalkine concentrations over time, potentially reflecting a reduction in neuroinflammatory activity with time in these patients.

Similarly, a decrease in MCP-1/CCL2 concentration was observed in the overall patient analysis. MCP-1/CCL2, a key chemokine involved in monocyte recruitment to sites of tissue injury or inflammation, is also implicated in pain modulation [45,46]. Prior studies demonstrated that spinal administration of TNF-α induces pain hypersensitivity and upregulates MCP-1, supporting its role in neuroinflammatory sensitization [47]. The decrease observed in this study may indicate a transition from an active neuroinflammatory state to a reduced inflammatory condition.

An increase with time in SP was found in both study groups and in the overall cohort. SP is a neuropeptide expressed by corneal nerves that regulates neuroinflammation and pain pathways [28,48,49]. Increased tear SP levels have been observed in DED patients, with concentrations correlating positively with symptom severity measures such as in OSDI score, photophobia frequency, and blurred vision [50]. However, another recent study found a negative correlation between SP and OSDI scores, which aligns with the reduction in OSDI scores and the increase in SP levels over time found in our study [51]. Also in line with our findings, experimental models of DED in mice have shown that SP expression in ocular surface tissues and trigeminal ganglia increases during the course of DED [52]. Interestingly, DED patients often report symptoms disproportionate to clinical signs [52], a discrepancy especially marked in those with chronic ocular pain, particularly in cases with neuropathic pain component [53]. Increased levels of SP have been shown to impair the function of regulatory T cells, which typically act to suppress effector immune cell activity, thereby sustaining chronic inflammation [49]. Previous research has pointed to SP as a promising target for therapeutic intervention in DED [54,55].

On the other hand, significant differences in the detection percentages of TNF-α, NGF, IL-2, IL-9, and IL-17A were found. The results of the present study showed a decrease in TNF-α detection over time. TNF-α is a well-established key mediator of inflammatory pain and plays a crucial role in chronic inflammatory diseases such as rheumatoid arthritis, where TNF-α inhibitors are widely used as effective treatments. Moreover, TNF-α is recognized as a proinflammatory and pronociceptive cytokine that is rapidly upregulated following tissue injury [56]. Its increased expression has also been reported in DED patients [38]. In our study, the reduction in TNF-α detection over time coincided with improvement in DE-related symptoms. Likewise, the NGF detection rate decreased in V2 compared with V1. NGF is a neurotrophic factor critically involved in the pathophysiology of inflammatory pain and has emerged as a promising therapeutic target for chronic pain management [57]. Additionally, NGF plays an important role in corneal nerve regeneration after corneal surgery [58,59]. In contrast, the detection rates of IL-2, IL-9, and IL-17A increased over time in our cohort, consistently with findings reported in other studies involving patients with DED [38,60]. However, since their percentage of detection was lower than 50%, no further conclusions could be obtained from their concentration.

To gain further insight into the molecular mechanisms underlying ocular surface inflammation and pain and their persistence over time, we examined both gene and miRNA expression profiles in this study. We found a downregulation of the *NTRK1* gene, which encodes for tyrosine kinase receptor (Trk)A, the high-affinity receptor for NGF. Neurotrophins and their corresponding TRKs, encoded by the *NTRK* gene family (*NTRK1*, *NTRK2*, *NTRK3*), are essential for the development and maintenance of both the central and peripheral nervous systems [61]. As the high-affinity NGF receptor, *NTRK1* plays a crucial role in mediating inflammatory and neuropathic pain by sensitizing sensory neurons [62]. Interestingly, when patients were analyzed based on the presence of chronic ocular pain, the downregulation of *NTRK1* was observed only in those without pain, while patients reporting chronic pain showed no significant change in *NTRK1* expression. This finding may suggest a compensatory regulatory mechanism whereby individuals without chronic ocular pain retain or increase TrkA-mediated signaling, possibly contributing to tissue repair or protective neuroimmune modulation. On the other hand, in patients with stablished chronic pain, the lack of TrkA downregulation might be involved in maintenance of pain; actually, several chronic pain states are associated with increased TrkA immunoreactivity and enhanced NGF/TrkA signaling [63–65]. Notably, pharmacological inhibition of the NGF–TrkA pathway is currently under investigation as a therapeutic strategy for various chronic pain syndromes [66], highlighting the clinical relevance of this signaling axis. Regarding miRNA expression analysis, we observed a downregulation of miR-665 across all patient samples. Its upregulation has been previously associated with neuroprotection and modulation of inflammatory responses [67,68], whereas its downregulation has been shown to reduce both pain sensitivity and inflammatory responses in neuropathic pain animal models [69]. To our knowledge, this is the first study reporting miR-665 expression changes in the context of DED, highlighting the novelty of this finding for ocular-surface research. Therefore, miR-665 could represent a promising therapeutic target for the treatment of chronic ocular pain.

This study has some limitations. Because of the study's observational nature, treatments received and disease progression during the intervals between visits were not systematically recorded. As these patients require frequent follow-ups and often attend different centers across various cities, it was unfortunately not possible to access their medical records. Therefore, potential changes in medication that could have influenced the observed symptom improvement and molecular shifts cannot be analyzed. A control group would not be ethically feasible, which prevented monitoring the natural progression of the disease over time. Additionally, the relatively small sample size may limit the generalizability of our findings. Moreover, dividing the sample into subgroups further reduced the statistical power, which may explain the loss of significance observed in some parameters measured. In addition, we cannot completely exclude that the decrease in cytokine detection percentages observed at V2 was influenced by the lower sensitivity of the second assay kit. However, this would not affect cases in which detection percentages increased. Moreover, different customized assay kits were used for V1 and V2 (SPR 1549 and SPR 2141, respectively). Although both were based on the HCYTA-60 K Milliplex Kit, these differences could contribute to variability in detection values between visits. Finally, the stability over time observed in some parameters could reflect either effective long-term management of the ocular surface or that the follow-up period, although relatively long, was still insufficient to detect progressive changes.

Despite the relatively small sample size, the main strength of this study is its long-term longitudinal design, which enables a thorough evaluation of disease progression over time. This approach provides novel evidence of the clinical and molecular changes in patients with DED, with and without chronic ocular pain. By integrating clinical assessments, tear biomarkers, confocal microscopy, and gene and miRNA expression analysis, our findings contribute to a better understanding of the underlying neuroinflammatory mechanisms and highlight potential biomarkers for monitoring disease progression. These results reinforce the importance of differentiating ocular pain as a distinct clinical entity and may guide future research toward more personalized and mechanism-based therapeutic strategies.

4. Materials and Methods

This prospective observational study included patients with DED. Ethical approval was obtained from the East Valladolid Health Area Ethics Committee (Spain), and the study was conducted in accordance with the tenets of the Declaration of Helsinki. All participants provided written informed consent after receiving detailed information about the study objectives.

4.1. Participants and Study Design

Patients with DED attended two visits (V1 and V2) separated by a minimum interval of two years, following the same evaluation protocol. The initial visit was conducted as part of a previous study [9,20], and eligibility for V2 required prior enrollment in that study. The same exclusion criteria were applied at both visits and included: the presence of any ocular surface disease other that DED or chronic ocular pain within the previous 3 months; a history of ocular, periocular, or orbital surgeries; diagnosis of a systemic condition with potential ocular involvement within the previous 3 months; initiation of any systemic therapy that could affect ocular surface health in the last 3 months; initiation of lacrimal punctum occlusion within the previous 3 months; contact lens wear in the 7 days before to the study (for contact lens users); and the use of topical medications or lubricants within 24 and 12 h, respectively, before the study visit.

DED diagnosis was determined based on the presence of DED-related symptoms, defined as an OSDI questionnaire score > 13, along with at least two of the following signs present in both eyes: (1) fluorescein tear break-up time (TBUT) $\leq$ 7 s; (2) corneal fluorescein staining $\geq$ grade 1 (Oxford scale), (3) conjunctival lissamine green staining $\geq$ grade 1 (Oxford scale); or (4) Schirmer test with topical anesthesia $\leq$ 5 mm in 5 min [39,70,71].

Patients were subsequently classified into two groups: those with DED and chronic ocular pain (DED-pain) and those with DED without chronic ocular pain (DED-no pain). Ocular pain was defined as a score of $\geq$2 on both Numerical Rating Scale and Wong–Baker Faces Pain Rating Scale [72]. Pain was considered chronic when it persisted for 3 months or longer [73].

4.2. Clinical Evaluation

All participants underwent assessment after a 20 min period under normal controlled environmental conditions (23 °C, 50% relative humidity, and no localized air flow) in the Controlled Environment Laboratory (CELab) (www.visionrd.com/celab/, accessed on 5 September 2025) [74].

4.2.1. Medical History and Symptom Assessment

A comprehensive medical history was recorded to evaluate both ocular and systemic health and to confirm eligibility based on the exclusion criteria. Participants then completed standardized questionnaires to assess the severity of DED-related symptoms, including the OSDI questionnaire, which categorizes symptom severity as asymptomatic (0–12), mild (13–22), moderate (23–32), or severe (33–100), and the modified Single-Item Dry Eye Questionnaire (mSIDEQ), which evaluates the frequency of symptoms related to DE (score range: 0–28) [75]. In addition to mean changes, the minimal clinically important difference for OSDI was calculated for each participant, defined as 4.5–7.3 points for patients with mild to moderate disease and 7.3–14.3 for those with severe intensity. The proportion of patients achieving an improvement greater than or equal to the thresholds was calculated [76]. The presence and intensity of ocular pain were assessed using the NRS, a scale from 0 to 10 in which scores of 0–1 indicate no pain; 2–4, mild pain; 5–7, moderate pain; and 8–10, severe pain. The Wong–Baker Faces Pain Rating Scale was also administered, using facial expressions to visually represent increasing levels of pain, from 0 (no pain) to 10 (unbearable pain) (https://wongbakerfaces.org/) [72,77,78].

Levels of anxiety and depression were measured with the Hospital Anxiety and Depression Scale, which includes two subscales (anxiety and depression), each scored from 0 to 21, with total scores ranging from 0 to 42. Scores of 0–7 are considered normal; 8–10, borderline; and 11–21, indicative of clinically significant symptoms [79,80].

Finally, changes in ocular pain and DE related symptoms were evaluated using the CDES-Q, consisting of two parts: CDES-Q1, which assesses symptom progression (improved, worsened, or unchanged), and CDES-Q2, which rates the magnitude of change on a scale from 0 to 10 [81].

4.2.2. Tear Sample Collection

Basal tear samples were collected from the external canthus using glass capillary micropipettes (Drummond Scientific Co., Broomall, PA, USA), taking care to avoid inducing reflex tearing. For cytokine quantification, a 1 μL basal tear sample was obtained from one randomly selected eye and diluted at a 1:10 ratio in a cryotube prefilled with 9 μL of chilled Milliplex Cytokine Assay Buffer (Merck Millipore, Burlington, MA, USA). In parallel, a 2 μL sample from the contralateral eye was collected for SP analysis and diluted 1:25 in the appropriate SP assay buffer (Cayman Chemical, Ann Arbor, MI, USA). Throughout the study visit, all tear samples were stored at 4 °C and promptly frozen at −80 °C until biochemical analysis was performed.

4.2.3. Ocular Surface Evaluation

The ocular surface of both eyes was evaluated using a slit lamp (SL-D7, Topcon Corporation, Tokyo, Japan). Bulbar conjunctival hyperemia and blepharitis were evaluated with the Efron scale (range, 0–4) [82]. Lid-parallel conjunctival folds were assessed nasally and temporally and scored on a 0–3 scale [83]. Following the instillation of prewetted sodium fluorescein strips (I-DEW flo, Entod Research Cell UK Ltd., London, UK), TBUT was measured three consecutive times, and the mean value was used for analysis [21]. Two minutes after TBUT measurement, corneal fluorescein staining was graded according to the Oxford grading scale (range, 0–5) [84]. Conjunctival staining was subsequently evaluated using lissamine green strips (I-DEW green, Entod Research Cell UK Ltd., London, UK) and scored with the same scale [84]. Lid wiper epitheliopathy was evaluated using the method described by Korb et al., with scores ranging from 0 to 3, based on the average of horizontal and vertical involvement [85]. Meibomian gland function was assessed by evaluating both meibum quality and expressibility. Digital pressure was applied to the upper and lower eyelid margins. Secretion quality was graded on a 0–3 scale according to Bron et al. [86], and expressibility was evaluated using the 0–3 scale described by Shimazaki et al. [87].

Noncontact esthesiometry was performed using a noncontact Belmonte's gas esthesiometer to determine mechanical and thermal sensitivity thresholds (heat and cold) following protocols previously described by our research group [88]. Additionally, mechanical sensitivity thresholds were assessed using the Cochet–Bonnet contact esthesiometer (Luneau Ophthalmology, Chartres, Paris, France), both before and after instillation of topical anesthetic (1 drop of 0.1% tetracaine and 0.4% oxibuprocaine; Anestésico Doble Colirio, Alcon Cusí, El Masnou, Spain), following standard procedures. Corneal sensitivity threshold was defined as the longest filament length (range, 0–60 mm) that elicited a positive response [70,89]. The anesthetic challenge test was conducted immediately after postanesthetic Cochet–Bonnet esthesiometry. The Global Rating Change (GRC) scale was used to assess changes in symptom intensity, ranging from −5 (complete recovery) to 0 (no change) to +5 (marked worsening) [89].

Basal tear production was assessed with the Schirmer's test with topical anesthesia [70].

Following the instillation of a topical anesthetic, IVCM was conducted bilaterally using the Heidelberg Retina Tomograph III coupled with the Rostock Cornea Module (Heidelberg Engineering GmbH, Heidelberg, Germany). One eye was randomly selected for analysis, and three high-quality (same for V1 and V2), nonoverlapping images of the central subbasal nerve plexus were selected and evaluated. Quantitative analysis was carried out using the ImageJ software, version 1.54g4 along with the NeuronJ plugin (https://imagescience.org/meijering/software/neuronj, accessed on 7 September 2025). The analysis included the following parameters: (1) total number of nerves (n/mm^2), defined as the sum of visible nerve fibers per image; (2) nerve density (mm/mm^2), measured as the cumulative length of all nerves within each frame; (3) average nerve length (mm/mm^2) per image; (4) density of nerve branch points (n/mm^2), referring to the count of nerve bifurcations per image; (5) nerve tortuosity, graded on a 0–4 scale according to the Oliveira-Soto and Efron classification [90]; (6) microneuroma density (n/mm^2), assessed by counting irregularly shaped terminal nerve endings; (7); total dendritic cell density (n/mm^2), corresponding to the number of hyperreflective dendriform structures identified—these were further classified into large (≥25 μm) dendritic cells, small (<25 μm) dendritic cells, and globular immune cells, the latter defined as round-shaped cells lacking dendrites [91,92]; and (8) image reflectivity, quantified as the mean optical density of the sub-basal plexus using the histogram tool in ImageJ. For each metric, the average from three selected images was used in the final analysis. All images from V2 were evaluated by a single trained observer, who was trained using the same protocol as for V1, and all analyses were performed following the same procedures. Excellent interobserver reliability (intraclass correlation coefficient > 0.90 for all nerve parameters except tortuosity, which showed moderate agreement with an intraclass correlation coefficient of 0.63) was previously demonstrated in a previous study in the same patient population [93].

4.2.4. Conjunctival Impression Cytology

Conjunctival impression cytology was performed under topical anesthesia to collect conjunctival cells. A polyethersulfone filter (Supor 200, pore size: 0.20 μm, diameter: 13 mm; Gelman Laboratory, Ann Arbor, MI, USA) was halved and gently applied with light pressure to the upper temporal bulbar conjunctiva, one per eye. The filters were then carefully removed and transferred, one to 350 μL of RLT buffer (Qiagen, Hilden, Germany) containing 1% 2-mercaptoethanol for gene expression analysis and the other to 350 μL of Qiazol buffer for miRNA expression analysis. Samples were stored at −80 °C until further analysis [13].

4.3. Sample Analysis

4.3.1. Tear Analysis

Cytokine concentrations in tear samples were measured using X-MAP technology with two customized multiplexed immunobead-based assays: SPR 1549 (for samples in V1) and SPR 2141 (for samples in V2). These assays utilized the Custom 20-plex Magnetic Human Cytokine Milliplex MAP panels (Millipore, Merck, MA, USA) and were analyzed on a MAGPIX® system (Luminex Corporation, Austin, TX, USA) following the manufacturer's low-volume protocol, which uses 10 μL of either sample or standard per assay, as previously described [44]. A total of 20 cytokines were simultaneously quantified, including EGF, fractalkine/CX3CL1, IL-1β, IL-1Ra, IL-2, IL-4, IL-6, IL-8/CXCL8, IL-9, IL-10, IL-17A, MCP-1/CCL2, MCP-3/CCL7, TNF-α, IFN-γ, GRO, MIP-1α/CCL3, MIP-1β/CCL4, NGF, and RANTES/CCL5. Cytokine concentrations were determined by converting fluorescence readings into cytokine levels (pg/mL) using standard curves. The minimum detectable concentrations, according to the manufacturer's guidelines, were 3.2 pg/mL for EGF, Fractalkine/CX3CL1, IL-1Ra, IL-2, IL-4, IL-8/CXCL8, IL-9, IL-10, IL-17A, MCP-3/CCL7, IFN-γ, GRO, MIP-1α/CCL3, MIP-1β/CCL4, NGF, and RANTES/CCL5; 6.14 pg/mL for IL-6; 6.4 pg/mL for TNF-α; and 9.6 pg/mL for IL-1β and MCP-1/CCL2.

4.3.2. Gene Expression Analysis

The expression of 25 human genes involved in neuropathic and inflammatory pain was analyzed and is listed in Table 10 in alphabetical order. First, RNA was extracted from CIC samples through a commercial kit (RNeasy Micro Kit, Qiagen, Redwood City, CA, USA) and 20 ng of cDNA from each sample was synthesized (iScript cDNA Synthesis kit, BioRad Laboratories Inc., Hercules, CA, USA). Second, gene expression was calculated by real time (RT)-PCR in a 7500 thermocycler (Applied Biosystems, Waltham, MA, USA) using a customized PCR array (BioRad, Hercules, CA, USA), following the manufacturer's instructions. Finally, relative gene expression data were calculated by the Δ cycle threshold (Ct) method using glyceraldehyde-3-phosphate dehydrogenase (*GAPDH*) as housekeeping reference gene [94]. Gene fold change between visits was calculated using the $2^{(-\Delta\Delta Ct)}$ method [95]. Values greater than 1 were considered upregulated, while values lower than 1 were considered downregulated. Fold regulation was calculated to express fold change values in a biologically meaningful way: when fold-change values were greater than one (upregulation), fold regulation was equal to the fold change; when fold-change values were less than one (downregulation), fold regulation was reported as the negative inverse of the fold change.

Table 10. Panel of genes involved in neuropathic and inflammatory pain included in the customized PCR array.

Gene	Description	Gene	Description
BDKRB1	Bradykinin receptor B1	*NTRK1*	Neurotrophic tyrosine kinase, receptor, type 1
BDNF	Brain-derived neurotrophic factor	*OPRD1*	Opioid receptor, delta 1
CALCA	Calcitonin-related polypeptide alpha	*OPRK1*	Opioid receptor, kappa 1
CCL2	Chemokine (C-C motif) ligand 2	*OPRM1*	Opioid receptor, mu 1
CD200	CD200 molecule	*PENK1*	Proenkephalin 1
CNR2	Cannabinoid receptor 2 (macrophage)	*PTGS1*	Prostaglandin-endoperoxide synthase 1 (prostaglandin G/H synthase and cyclooxygenase)
CX3CR1	Chemokine (C-X3-C motif) receptor 1	*TAC1*	Tachykinin, precursor 1
IL18	Interleukin 18	*TACR1*	Tachykinin receptor 1
IL1A	Interleukin 1A	*TNF*	Tumor necrosis factor
IL2	Interleukin 2	*TRPA1*	Transient receptor potential caption channel 1
IL6	Interleukin 6	*TRPV1*	Transient receptor potential cation channel, subfamily V, member 1
ITGAM	Integrin, alpha M (complement component 3 receptor 3 subunit)	*TRPV3*	Transient receptor potential cation channel, subfamily V, member 3
NGF	Nerve growth factor		

4.3.3. MicroRNA Expression Analysis

The expression of 12 human miRNAs (20a-5p; 23b-3p; 29a-3p; 92b-3p; 99a-5p; 137-3p; 143-3p; 208a-3p; 302d-3p; 379-3p; 543; 665) related to pain and inflammation was analyzed. First, miRNA was extracted from CIC samples using a commercial kit (miRNeasy Mini Kit, Qiagen, Hilden, Germany), and 10 ng of cDNA from each sample was synthesized using a commercial kit (miRCURY® LNA® RT Kit, Qiagen). Second, miRNA expression was calculated through real time (RT)-PCR in a 7500 thermocycler (Applied Biosystem) using customized miRNA PCR Panels (Qiagen), following the manufacturer's instructions. Finally, relative miRNA expression data were calculated by the ΔCt method, using hsa-miR-103a-3p as housekeeping reference miRNA, and miRNA fold change between visits was calculated using the $2^{(-\Delta\Delta Ct)}$ method as explained above.

4.4. Statistical Analysis

Statistical analysis was conducted using SPSS software version 26.0 (SPSS Inc., Chicago, IL, USA). Data from both visits were compared. For each patient, one eye was randomly selected and used consistently for the analysis. Quantitative variables were expressed as mean $\pm$ standard deviation; categorical variables, as percentages; and ordinal variables, as median with interquartile range (IQR).

The Shapiro–Wilk test was employed to examine the assumption of normality. When this assumption was met, comparisons between visits in the entire cohort were performed using parametric tests. In contrast, because of the limited number of subjects in each subgroup, nonparametric tests were used to assess within-group changes between visits in the DED-pain and DED-no pain groups.

Specifically, for quantitative variables with a normal distribution, the paired Student's *t*-test was used, after checking homogeneity of variance with Levene's test. For non-normally distributed, ordinal, or qualitative data, the Wilcoxon signed-rank test was applied.

In the analysis of tear molecules, only those with a detection rate $\geq$ 50% were considered for quantitative analysis. Undetected values were imputed using the minimum concentration value of the V1 standard curve, and concentrations were log-transformed (log 2) to normalize the distribution. Molecules detected at rates lower than 50% were not imputed and were analyzed as binary variables (detected vs. undetected) using the McNemar test.

For gene and miRNA expression analysis, nondetected values (Ct > 40) were assigned a value of 40. Gene and miRNA changes between visits were evaluated individually in each patient through the paired Student's *t*-test.

The false discovery rate was controlled using the Benjamini–Hochberg correction method for multiple testing. *p*-values $\leq$ 0.05 were considered statistically significant.

5. Conclusions

This observational study captured the real-life evolution of patients with DED disease, with and without chronic ocular pain, within the context of everyday clinical care. No significant changes were observed in ocular surface clinical signs that could reliably monitor disease progression. However, IVCM revealed a reduction in the density of dendritic cells within the sub-basal nerve plexus, suggesting decreased immune activity or inflammation. Additionally, tear film analysis revealed significant molecular changes, including a decrease in levels of EGF, fractalkine/CX3CL1, and MCP-1/CCL2, alongside an increase in SP concentrations over time. The persistent increase in SP further highlights ongoing neuroimmune dysregulation and pain sensitization. Downregulation of *NTRK1* gene expression, particularly in the DED-no pain group may reflect a protective or compensatory neuroimmune mechanism in less severe stages of the disease. Moreover, the observed downregulation of miR-665 reinforces the presence of molecular adaptations associated with the chronicity of DED.

In conclusion, our findings indicate that although overall DED symptoms may improve with standard therapies, patients experiencing chronic ocular pain show persistent pain severity, underscoring the necessity to consider DED and ocular pain as distinct entities that require individualized, multimodal treatment approaches. These considerations are increasingly recognized in the literature [96].

Supplementary Materials: The following supporting information can be downloaded at: https://www.mdpi.com/article/10.3390/ijms26188918/s1.

Author Contributions: Conceptualization, C.V.-S., A.Á.C.-G., M.B.-V., M.C., A.E.-d.-S. and M.J.G.-G.; methodology, C.V.-S., A.Á.C.-G., M.B.-V., M.C., A.E.-d.-S. and M.J.G.-G.; software, C.V.-S., A.Á.C.-G., M.B.-V. and A.V.; validation, C.V.-S., A.Á.C.-G., M.B.-V. and A.N.-D.; formal analysis, C.V.-S.; investigation, C.V.-S., A.Á.C.-G., M.B.-V., L.V.-N., A.N.-D., A.V. and M.C.; resources, C.V.-S., A.Á.C.-G. and M.B.-V.; data curation, C.V.-S. and M.B.-V.; writing—original draft preparation, C.V.-S.; writing—review and editing, C.V.-S., A.Á.C.-G., M.B.-V., L.V.-N., A.N.-D., A.V., M.C., A.E.-d.-S. and M.J.G.-G.; visualization, C.V.-S., A.E.-d.-S. and M.J.G.-G.; supervision, M.C., A.E.-d.-S. and M.J.G.-G.; project administration, M.C., A.E.-d.-S. and M.J.G.-G.; funding acquisition, M.C., A.E.-d.-S. and M.J.G.-G. All authors have read and agreed to the published version of the manuscript.

Funding: This research was funded by Junta de Castilla y León and the European Social Fund, grant reference EDU/1192/2020 and CLU-2023-1-04; the Ministry of Science, Innovation, and Universities (Government of Spain), AEI/FEDER/UE, grant reference SAF-2016-77080-P and FPU17/02715; and the University of Valladolid, predoctoral grant 2020.

Institutional Review Board Statement: The study was conducted in accordance with the Declaration of Helsinki and approved by the Ethics Committee of the Valladolid University Clinical Hospital (protocol code PI 21-2125 TESIS NO HCUV, 28 January 2021).

Informed Consent Statement: Informed consent was obtained from all subjects involved in the study.

Data Availability Statement: The original contributions presented in this study are included in the article and Supplementary Materials. Further inquiries can be directed to the corresponding author.

Acknowledgments: During the preparation of this manuscript/study, the authors used ChatGPT version 5 mini for the purposes of improving language and grammar. The authors have reviewed and edited the output and take full responsibility for the content of this publication.

Conflicts of Interest: The authors declare no conflicts of interest.

Abbreviations

The following abbreviations are used in this manuscript:

DED	Dry eye disease
IL	Interleukin
Ra	Receptor antagonist
MMP	Matrix metalloproteinase
MIP	Macrophage inflammatory protein
IFN	Interferon
miRNA	MicroRNA
TNF	Tumor necrosis factor
V1	First visit
V2	Follow-up visit
OSDI	Ocular Surface Disease Index
IVCM	In vivo confocal microscopy
EGF	Epidermal growth factor
MCP	Monocyte chemoattractant protein
GRO	Growth-related oncogene
SP	Substance P
RANTES	Regulated on activation, normal T cell expressed and secreted
NGF	Nerve growth factor
BDKRB1	Bradykinin receptor B1
CALCA	Calcitonin-related polypeptide alpha
CCL2	Chemokine (C-C motif) ligand 2
ITGAM	Integrin, alpha M (complement component 3 receptor 3 subunit)
TAC1	Tachykinin, precursor 1
CD200	CD200 molecule
TACR1	Tachykinin receptor 1
CX3CR1	Chemokine (C-X3-C motif) receptor 1
BDNF	Brain-derived neurotrophic factor
NTRK1	Neurotrophic tyrosine kinase, receptor, type 1
PENK1	Proenkephalin 1
OPRM1	Opioid receptor, mu 1

OPRD1	Opioid receptor, delta 1
OPRK1	Opioid receptor, kappa 1
TRPV3	Transient receptor potential cation channel, subfamily V, member 3
TRPA1	Transient receptor potential caption channel 1
TRPV1	Transient receptor potential cation channel, subfamily V, member 1
CNR2	Cannabinoid receptor 2 (macrophage)
PTGS1	Prostaglandin-endoperoxide synthase 1 (prostaglandin G/H synthase and cyclooxygenase)
CDES-Q	Change in Dry Eye Symptoms Questionnaire
TBUT	Fluorescein tear break-up time
CELab	Controlled Environment Laboratory
mSIDEQ	Modified Single-Item Dry Eye Questionnaire
Ct	Cycle threshold
GAPDH	Glyceraldehyde-3-phosphate dehydrogenase

References

1. Wolffsohn, J.S.; Benítez-Del-Castillo, J.; Loya-Garcia, D.; Inomata, T.; Iyar, G.; Liang, L.; Pult, H.; Sabater, A.L.; Starr, C.E.; Vehof, J.; et al. TFOS DEWS III Diagnostic Methodology. *Am. J. Ophthalmol.* 2025, *ahead-of-print*. [CrossRef]
2. Britten-Jones, A.C.; Wang, M.T.M.; Samuels, I.; Jennings, C.; Stapleton, F.; Craig, J.P. Epidemiology and Risk Factors of Dry Eye Disease: Considerations for Clinical Management. *Medicina* **2024**, *60*, 1458. [CrossRef]
3. Stapleton, F.; Argüeso, P.; Asbell, P.; Azar, D.; Bosworth, C.; Chen, W.; Ciolino, J.; Craig, J.P.; Gallar, J.; Galor, A.; et al. TFOS DEWS III Digest Report. *Am. J. Ophthalmol.* 2025, *ahead-of-print*. [CrossRef]
4. Benítez-del-Castillo, J.M.; Burgos-Blasco, B. Prevalence of Dry Eye Disease in Spain: A Population-Based Survey (PrevEOS). *Ocul. Surf.* **2025**, *36*, 126–133. [CrossRef]
5. Belmonte, C.; Acosta, M.C.; Merayo-Lloves, J.; Gallar, J. What Causes Eye Pain? *Curr. Ophthalmol. Rep.* **2015**, *3*, 111–121. [CrossRef]
6. Galor, A.; Levitt, R.C.; Felix, E.R.; Martin, E.R.; Sarantopoulos, C.D. Neuropathic Ocular Pain: An Important yet Underevaluated Feature of Dry Eye. *Eye* **2015**, *29*, 301–312. [CrossRef]
7. Mangwani-Mordani, S.; Goodman, C.F.; Galor, A. Novel Treatments for Chronic Ocular Surface Pain. *Cornea* **2023**, *42*, 261–271. [CrossRef] [PubMed]
8. Fong, P.; Shih, K.; Lam, P.; Chan, T.Y.; Jhanji, V.; Tong, L. Role of Tear Film Biomarkers in the Diagnosis and Management of Dry Eye Disease. *Taiwan J. Ophthalmol.* **2019**, *9*, 150. [CrossRef] [PubMed]
9. Blanco-Vázquez, M.; Vázquez, A.; Fernández, I.; Novo-Diez, A.; Martínez-Plaza, E.; García-Vázquez, C.; González-García, M.J.; Sobas, E.M.; Calonge, M.; Enríquez-de-Salamanca, A. Inflammation-Related Molecules in Tears of Patients with Chronic Ocular Pain and Dry Eye Disease. *Exp. Eye Res.* **2022**, *219*, 109057. [CrossRef] [PubMed]
10. López-Miguel, A.; Tesón, M.; Martín-Montañez, V.; Enríquez-de-Salamanca, A.; Stern, M.E.; González-García, M.J.; Calonge, M. Clinical and Molecular Inflammatory Response in Sjögren Syndrome–Associated Dry Eye Patients Under Desiccating Stress. *Am. J. Ophthalmol.* **2016**, *161*, 133–141.e2. [CrossRef]
11. Huang, J.-F.; Zhang, Y.; Rittenhouse, K.D.; Pickering, E.H.; McDowell, M.T. Evaluations of Tear Protein Markers in Dry Eye Disease: Repeatability of Measurement and Correlation with Disease. *Investig. Ophthalmol. Vis. Sci.* **2012**, *53*, 4556. [CrossRef] [PubMed]
12. Liang, H.; Kessal, K.; Rabut, G.; Daull, P.; Garrigue, J.S.; Melik Parsadaniantz, S.; Docquier, M.; Baudouin, C.; Brignole-Baudouin, F. Correlation of Clinical Symptoms and Signs with Conjunctival Gene Expression in Primary Sjögren Syndrome Dry Eye Patients. *Ocul. Surf.* **2019**, *17*, 516–525. [CrossRef]
13. Vergés, C.; Giménez-Capitán, A.; Ribas, V.; Salgado-Borges, J.; March de Ribot, F.; Mayo-de-las-Casas, C.; Armiger-Borras, N.; Pedraz, C.; Molina-Vila, M.Á. Gene Expression Signatures in Conjunctival Fornix Aspirates of Patients with Dry Eye Disease Associated with Meibomian Gland Dysfunction. A Proof-of-Concept Study. *Ocul. Surf.* **2023**, *30*, 42–50. [CrossRef]
14. Cocho, L.; Fernández, I.; Calonge, M.; Martínez, V.; González-García, M.J.; Caballero, D.; López-Corral, L.; García-Vázquez, C.; Vázquez, L.; Stern, M.E.; et al. Gene Expression–Based Predictive Models of Graft Versus Host Disease–Associated Dry Eye. *Investig. Ophthalmol. Vis. Sci.* **2015**, *56*, 4570. [CrossRef]
15. Sato, F.; Tsuchiya, S.; Meltzer, S.J.; Shimizu, K. MicroRNAs and Epigenetics. *FEBS J.* **2011**, *278*, 1598–1609. [CrossRef]
16. Rassi, D.M.; De Paiva, C.S.; Dias, L.C.; Módulo, C.M.; Adriano, L.; Fantucci, M.Z.; Rocha, E.M. Review: MicroRNAS in Ocular Surface and Dry Eye Diseases. *Ocul. Surf.* **2017**, *15*, 660–669. [CrossRef]

17. Yin, L.; Zhang, M.; He, T.; Chen, S. The Expression of miRNA-146a-5p and Its Mechanism of Treating Dry Eye Syndrome. *J. Clin. Lab. Anal.* **2021**, *35*, e23571. [CrossRef]
18. Kakan, S.S.; Edman, M.C.; Yao, A.; Okamoto, C.T.; Nguyen, A.; Hjelm, B.E.; Hamm-Alvarez, S.F. Tear miRNAs Identified in a Murine Model of Sjögren's Syndrome as Potential Diagnostic Biomarkers and Indicators of Disease Mechanism. *Front. Immunol.* **2022**, *13*, 833254. [CrossRef]
19. Pucker, A.D.; Ngo, W.; Postnikoff, C.K.; Fortinberry, H.; Nichols, J.J. Tear Film miRNAs and Their Association With Human Dry Eye Disease. *Curr. Eye Res.* **2022**, *47*, 1479–1487. [CrossRef] [PubMed]
20. Blanco-Vázquez, M.; Novo-Diez, A.; Vázquez, A.; Enríquez-de-Salamanca, A.; González-García, M.J.; Calonge, M. Clinical Characterization of the Lacrimal Functional Unit in Patients with Chronic Ocular Pain with Dry Eye Disease. *J. Clin. Med.* **2025**, *14*, 5250. [CrossRef] [PubMed]
21. Craig, J.P.; Nichols, K.K.; Akpek, E.K.; Caffery, B.; Dua, H.S.; Joo, C.K.; Liu, Z.; Nelson, J.D.; Nichols, J.J.; Tsubota, K.; et al. TFOS DEWS II Definition and Classification Report. *Ocul. Surf.* **2017**, *15*, 276–283. [CrossRef] [PubMed]
22. Guerrero-Moreno, A.; Liang, H.; Moreau, N.; Luzu, J.; Rabut, G.; Melik Parsadaniantz, S.; Labbé, A.; Baudouin, C.; Réaux-Le Goazigo, A. Corneal Nerve Abnormalities in Painful Dry Eye Disease Patients. *Biomedicines* **2021**, *9*, 1424. [CrossRef]
23. Galor, A.; Zlotcavitch, L.; Walter, S.D.; Felix, E.R.; Feuer, W.; Martin, E.R.; Margolis, T.P.; Sarantopoulos, K.D.; Levitt, R.C. Dry Eye Symptom Severity and Persistence Are Associated with Symptoms of Neuropathic Pain. *Br. J. Ophthalmol.* **2015**, *99*, 665–668. [CrossRef]
24. Patel, S.; Mittal, R.; Sarantopoulos, K.D.; Galor, A. Neuropathic Ocular Surface Pain: Emerging Drug Targets and Therapeutic Implications. *Expert Opin. Ther. Targets* **2022**, *26*, 681–695. [CrossRef] [PubMed]
25. Valencia-Sandonís, C.; Vázquez, A.; Valencia-Nieto, L.; Martínez-Plaza, E.; Blanco-Vázquez, M.; Sobas, E.M.; Calonge, M.; Ortega, E.; Enríquez-de-Salamanca, A.; González-García, M.J. Long-Term Evolution of Chronic Neuropathic Ocular Pain and Dry Eye Following Corneal Refractive Surgery. *J. Clin. Med.* **2025**, *14*, 4406. [CrossRef] [PubMed]
26. De Paiva, C.S.; Pflugfelder, S.C. Corneal Epitheliopathy of Dry Eye Induces Hyperesthesia to Mechanical Air Jet Stimulation. *Am. J. Ophthalmol.* **2004**, *137*, 109–115. [CrossRef]
27. Bourcier, T.; Acosta, M.C.; Borderie, V.; Borra's, F.; Gallar, J.; Bury, T.; Laroche, L.; Belmonte, C. Decreased Corneal Sensitivity in Patients with Dry Eye. *Investig. Ophthalmol. Vis. Sci.* **2005**, *46*, 2341. [CrossRef]
28. Belmonte, C.; Nichols, J.J.; Cox, S.M.; Brock, J.A.; Begley, C.G.; Bereiter, D.A.; Dartt, D.A.; Galor, A.; Hamrah, P.; Ivanusic, J.J.; et al. TFOS DEWS II Pain and Sensation Report. *Ocul. Surf.* **2017**, *15*, 404–437. [CrossRef]
29. Labbé, A.; Alalwani, H.; Van Went, C.; Brasnu, E.; Georgescu, D.; Baudouin, C. The Relationship between Subbasal Nerve Morphology and Corneal Sensation in Ocular Surface Disease. *Investig. Ophthalmol. Vis. Sci.* **2012**, *53*, 4926. [CrossRef]
30. Adatia, F.A.; Michaeli-Cohen, A.; Naor, J.; Caffery, B.; Bookman, A.; Slomovic, A. Correlation between Corneal Sensitivity, Subjective Dry Eye Symptoms and Corneal Staining in Sjögren's Syndrome. *Can. J. Ophthalmol.* **2004**, *39*, 767–771. [CrossRef]
31. Hoşal, B.M.; Örnek, N.; Zilelioğlu, G.; Elhan, A.H. Morphology of Corneal Nerves and Corneal Sensation in Dry Eye: A Preliminary Study. *Eye* **2005**, *19*, 1276–1279. [CrossRef]
32. Spierer, O.; Felix, E.R.; McClellan, A.L.; Parel, J.M.; Gonzalez, A.; Feuer, W.J.; Sarantopoulos, C.D.; Levitt, R.C.; Ehrmann, K.; Galor, A. Corneal Mechanical Thresholds Negatively Associate With Dry Eye and Ocular Pain Symptoms. *Investig. Ophthalmol. Vis. Sci.* **2016**, *57*, 617. [CrossRef] [PubMed]
33. Hamrah, P.; Liu, Y.; Zhang, Q.; Dana, R. Alterations in Corneal Stromal Dendritic Cell Phenotype and Distribution in Inflammation. *Arch. Ophthalmol.* **2003**, *121*, 1132. [CrossRef]
34. Hao, R.; Ding, Y.; Li, X. Alterations in Corneal Epithelial Dendritic Cell in Sjogren's Syndrome Dry Eye and Clinical Correlations. *Sci. Rep.* **2022**, *12*, 11167. [CrossRef]
35. Villani, E.; Galimberti, D.; Viola, F.; Mapelli, C.; Ratiglia, R. The Cornea in Sjögren's Syndrome: An In Vivo Confocal Study. *Investig. Ophthalmol. Vis. Sci.* **2007**, *48*, 2017. [CrossRef]
36. Lin, H.; Li, W.; Dong, N.; Chen, W.; Liu, J.; Chen, L.; Yuan, H.; Geng, Z.; Liu, Z. Changes in Corneal Epithelial Layer Inflammatory Cells in Aqueous Tear–Deficient Dry Eye. *Investig. Ophthalmol. Vis. Sci.* **2010**, *51*, 122. [CrossRef]
37. Ross, A.R.; Al-Aqaba, M.A.; Almaazmi, A.; Messina, M.; Nubile, M.; Mastropasqua, L.; Dua, H.S.; Said, D.G. Clinical and in Vivo Confocal Microscopic Features of Neuropathic Corneal Pain. *Br. J. Ophthalmol.* **2020**, *104*, 768–775. [CrossRef]
38. Kumar, N.R.; Praveen, M.; Narasimhan, R.; Khamar, P.; D'Souza, S.; Sinha-Roy, A.; Sethu, S.; Shetty, R.; Ghosh, A. Tear Biomarkers in Dry Eye Disease: Progress in the Last Decade. *Indian J. Ophthalmol.* **2023**, *71*, 1190–1202. [CrossRef]
39. Lam, H.; Bleiden, L.; de Paiva, C.S.; Farley, W.; Stern, M.E.; Pflugfelder, S.C. Tear Cytokine Profiles in Dysfunctional Tear Syndrome. *Am. J. Ophthalmol.* **2009**, *147*, 198–205.e1. [CrossRef] [PubMed]
40. Pflugfelder, S.C.; Jones, D.; Ji, Z.; Afonso, A.; Monroy, D. Altered Cytokine Balance in the Tear Fluid and Conjunctiva of Patients with Sjögren's Syndrome Keratoconjunctivitis Sicca. *Curr. Eye Res.* **1999**, *19*, 201–211. [CrossRef] [PubMed]

41. Fernández, I.; Enríquez-de-Salamanca, A.; Portero, A.; García-Vázquez, C.; Calonge, M.; Herreras, J.M. Age- and Sex-Adjusted Reference Intervals in Tear Cytokine Levels in Healthy Subjects. *Appl. Sci.* **2021**, *11*, 8958. [CrossRef]
42. Johnston, I.N.; Milligan, E.D.; Wieseler-Frank, J.; Frank, M.G.; Zapata, V.; Campisi, J.; Langer, S.; Martin, D.; Green, P.; Fleshner, M.; et al. A Role for Proinflammatory Cytokines and Fractalkine in Analgesia, Tolerance, and Subsequent Pain Facilitation Induced by Chronic Intrathecal Morphine. *J. Neurosci.* **2004**, *24*, 7353–7365. [CrossRef] [PubMed]
43. Clark, A.K.; Malcangio, M. Fractalkine/CX3CR1 Signaling during Neuropathic Pain. *Front. Cell. Neurosci.* **2014**, *8*, 121. [CrossRef]
44. Enríquez-de-Salamanca, A.; Castellanos, E.; Stern, M.E.; Fernández, I.; Carreño, E.; García-Vázquez, C.; Herreras, J.M.; Calonge, M. Tear Cytokine and Chemokine Analysis and Clinical Correlations in Evaporative-Type Dry Eye Disease. *Mol. Vis.* **2010**, *16*, 862–873.
45. Lu, B.; Rutledge, B.J.; Gu, L.; Fiorillo, J.; Lukacs, N.W.; Kunkel, S.L.; North, R.; Gerard, C.; Rollins, B.J. Abnormalities in Monocyte Recruitment and Cytokine Expression in Monocyte Chemoattractant Protein 1–Deficient Mice. *J. Exp. Med.* **1998**, *187*, 601–608. [CrossRef]
46. Kwiatkowski, K.; Popiolek-Barczyk, K.; Piotrowska, A.; Rojewska, E.; Ciapała, K.; Makuch, W.; Mika, J. Chemokines CCL2 and CCL7, but Not CCL12, Play a Significant Role in the Development of Pain-Related Behavior and Opioid-Induced Analgesia. *Cytokine* **2019**, *119*, 202–213. [CrossRef]
47. Gao, Y.-J.; Zhang, L.; Samad, O.A.; Suter, M.R.; Yasuhiko, K.; Xu, Z.-Z.; Park, J.-Y.; Lind, A.-L.; Ma, Q.; Ji, R.-R. JNK-Induced MCP-1 Production in Spinal Cord Astrocytes Contributes to Central Sensitization and Neuropathic Pain. *J. Neurosci.* **2009**, *29*, 4096–4108. [CrossRef]
48. Ferrari, G.; Bignami, F.; Giacomini, C.; Capitolo, E.; Comi, G.; Chaabane, L.; Rama, P. Ocular Surface Injury Induces Inflammation in the Brain: In Vivo and Ex Vivo Evidence of a Corneal–Trigeminal Axis. *Investig. Ophthalmol. Vis. Sci.* **2014**, *55*, 6289. [CrossRef]
49. Wang, S.; Naderi, A.; Kahale, F.; Ortiz, G.; Forouzanfar, K.; Chen, Y.; Dana, R. Substance P Regulates Memory Th17 Cell Generation and Maintenance in Chronic Dry Eye Disease. *J. Leukoc. Biol.* **2024**, *116*, 1446–1453. [CrossRef] [PubMed]
50. Yang, T.; Zhou, Y.; Ma, B.; Duan, H.; Liu, R.; Zhao, L.; Qi, H. Elevated Neuropeptides in Dry Eye Disease and Their Clinical Correlations. *Cornea* **2023**, *42*, 557–564. [CrossRef] [PubMed]
51. Zhang, Y.; Zhang, H.; Zhu, X.; Ye, H.; Yang, K.; Zhou, X.; Hong, J. Tear Neuropeptides Are Associated with Clinical Symptoms and Signs of Dry Eye Patients. *Ann. Med.* **2025**, *57*, 2451194. [CrossRef] [PubMed]
52. Bartlett, J.; Keith, M.; Sudharshan, L.; Snedecor, S. Associations between Signs and Symptoms of Dry Eye Disease: A Systematic Review. *Clin. Ophthalmol.* **2015**, *9*, 1719–1730. [CrossRef] [PubMed]
53. Goyal, S.; Hamrah, P. Understanding Neuropathic Corneal Pain—Gaps and Current Therapeutic Approaches. *Semin. Ophthalmol.* **2016**, *31*, 59–70. [CrossRef] [PubMed]
54. Rong, H.; Yang, H.; Liu, Q.; Zhang, H.; Wang, S. Substance P and Neurokinin 1 Receptor Boost the Pathogenicity of Granulocyte-macrophage Colony-stimulating Factor-producing T Helper Cells in Dry Eye Disease. *Scand. J. Immunol.* **2025**, *101*, e13434. [CrossRef]
55. Yu, M.; Lee, S.-M.; Lee, H.; Amouzegar, A.; Nakao, T.; Chen, Y.; Dana, R. Neurokinin-1 Receptor Antagonism Ameliorates Dry Eye Disease by Inhibiting Antigen-Presenting Cell Maturation and T Helper 17 Cell Activation. *Am. J. Pathol.* **2020**, *190*, 125–133. [CrossRef]
56. Üçeyler, N.; Sommer, C. Cytokine-Induced Pain: Basic Science and Clinical Implications. *Rev. Analg.* **2007**, *9*, 87–103. [CrossRef]
57. Lewin, G.R.; Lechner, S.G.; Smith, E.S.J. Nerve Growth Factor and Nociception: From Experimental Embryology to New Analgesic Therapy. *Handb. Exp. Pharmacol.* **2014**, *220*, 251–282.
58. Pan, Y.; Liu, F.; Qi, X.; Hu, Y.; Xu, F.; Jia, H. Nerve Growth Factor Changes and Corneal Nerve Repair after Keratoplasty. *Optom. Vis. Sci.* **2018**, *95*, 27–31. [CrossRef]
59. Lee, H.K.; Lee, K.S.; Kim, H.C.; Lee, S.H.; Kim, E.K. Nerve Growth Factor Concentration and Implications in Photorefractive Keratectomy vs Laser In Situ Keratomileusis. *Am. J. Ophthalmol.* **2005**, *139*, 965–971. [CrossRef]
60. Roda, M.; Corazza, I.; Bacchi Reggiani, M.L.; Pellegrini, M.; Taroni, L.; Giannaccare, G.; Versura, P. Dry Eye Disease and Tear Cytokine Levels—A Meta-Analysis. *Int. J. Mol. Sci.* **2020**, *21*, 3111. [CrossRef]
61. Reichardt, L.F. Neurotrophin-Regulated Signalling Pathways. *Philos. Trans. R. Soc. B Biol. Sci.* **2006**, *361*, 1545–1564. [CrossRef]
62. Pezet, S.; McMahon, S.B. NEUROTROPHINS: Mediators and Modulators of Pain. *Annu. Rev. Neurosci.* **2006**, *29*, 507–538. [CrossRef]
63. Barker, P.A.; Mantyh, P.; Arendt-Nielsen, L.; Viktrup, L.; Tive, L. Nerve Growth Factor Signaling and Its Contribution to Pain. *J. Pain Res.* **2020**, *13*, 1223–1241. [CrossRef] [PubMed]
64. O-Sullivan, I.; Kc, R.; Singh, G.; Das, V.; Ma, K.; Li, X.; Mwale, F.; Votta-Velis, G.; Bruce, B.; Natarajan Anbazhagan, A.; et al. Sensory Neuron-Specific Deletion of Tropomyosin Receptor Kinase A (TrkA) in Mice Abolishes Osteoarthritis (OA) Pain via NGF/TrkA Intervention of Peripheral Sensitization. *Int. J. Mol. Sci.* **2022**, *23*, 12076. [CrossRef] [PubMed]

65. Pezet, S.; Onténiente, B.; Grannec, G.; Calvino, B. Chronic Pain Is Associated with Increased TrkA Immunoreactivity in Spinoreticular Neurons. *J. Neurosci.* **1999**, *19*, 5482–5492. [CrossRef] [PubMed]
66. Hirose, M.; Kuroda, Y.; Murata, E. NGF/TrkA Signaling as a Therapeutic Target for Pain. *Pain Pract.* **2016**, *16*, 175–182. [CrossRef]
67. Li, M.; Zhang, S.; Qiu, Y.; He, Y.; Chen, B.; Mao, R.; Cui, Y.; Zeng, Z.; Chen, M. Upregulation of miR-665 Promotes Apoptosis and Colitis in Inflammatory Bowel Disease by Repressing the Endoplasmic Reticulum Stress Components XBP1 and ORMDL3. *Cell Death Dis.* **2017**, *8*, e2699. [CrossRef]
68. Lu, X.; Lv, S.; Mi, Y.; Wang, L.; Wang, G. Neuroprotective Effect of miR-665 against Sevoflurane Anesthesia-Induced Cognitive Dysfunction in Rats through PI3K/Akt Signaling Pathway by Targeting Insulin-like Growth Factor 2. *Am. J. Transl. Res.* **2017**, *9*, 1344–1356.
69. Lin, Y.; Li, M.; Rao, G.; Zhang, W.; Chen, X. Inhibition of miR-665 Alleviates Neuropathic Pain by Targeting SOCS1. *Trop. J. Pharm. Res.* **2020**, *19*, 1591–1597. [CrossRef]
70. Lemp, M.A.; Baudouin, C.; Baum, J.; Dogru, M.; Foulks, G.N.; Kinoshita, S.; Laibson, P.; McCulley, J.; Murube, J.; Plugfelder, S.C.; et al. The Definition and Classification of Dry Eye Disease: Report of the Definition and Classification Subcommittee of the International Dry Eye WorkShop (2007). *Ocul. Surf.* **2007**, *5*, 75–92. [CrossRef]
71. Xu, K.-P. Tear Function Index. *Arch. Ophthalmol.* **1995**, *113*, 84. [CrossRef]
72. Satitpitakul, V.; Kheirkhah, A.; Crnej, A.; Hamrah, P.; Dana, R. Determinants of Ocular Pain Severity in Patients with Dry Eye Disease. *Am. J. Ophthalmol.* **2017**, *179*, 198–204. [CrossRef]
73. Schug, S.A.; Lavand'homme, P.; Barke, A.; Korwisi, B.; Rief, W.; Treede, R.-D. The IASP Classification of Chronic Pain for ICD-11: Chronic Postsurgical or Posttraumatic Pain. *Pain* **2019**, *160*, 45–52. [CrossRef]
74. Calonge, M.; Pinto-Fraga, J.; González-García, M.J.; Enríquez-de-Salamanca, A.; López-de la Rosa, A.; Fernández, I.; López-Miguel, A. Effects of the External Environment on Dry Eye Disease. *Int. Ophthalmol. Clin.* **2017**, *57*, 23–40. [CrossRef]
75. Tesón, M.; González-García, M.J.; López-Miguel, A.; Enríquez-de-Salamanca, A.; Martín-Montañez, V.; Benito, M.J.; Mateo, M.E.; Stern, M.E.; Calonge, M. Influence of a Controlled Environment Simulating an In-Flight Airplane Cabin on Dry Eye Disease. *Investig. Ophthalmol. Vis. Sci.* **2013**, *54*, 2093. [CrossRef]
76. Miller, K.L. Minimal Clinically Important Difference for the Ocular Surface Disease Index. *Arch. Ophthalmol.* **2010**, *128*, 94. [CrossRef]
77. Ferreira-Valente, M.A.; Pais-Ribeiro, J.L.; Jensen, M.P. Validity of Four Pain Intensity Rating Scales. *Pain* **2011**, *152*, 2399–2404. [CrossRef] [PubMed]
78. Wong-Baker FACES Foundation. *Wong-Baker FACES Foundation Wong-Baker FACES® Pain Rating Scale 2025*; Wong-Baker FACES Foundation: Oklahoma City, OK, USA, 2025.
79. Quintana, J.M.; Padierna, A.; Esteban, C.; Arostegui, I.; Bilbao, A.; Ruiz, I. Evaluation of the Psychometric Characteristics of the Spanish Version of the Hospital Anxiety and Depression Scale. *Acta Psychiatr. Scand.* **2003**, *107*, 216–221. [CrossRef] [PubMed]
80. Zigmond, A.S.; Snaith, R.P. The Hospital Anxiety and Depression Scale. *Acta Psychiatr. Scand.* **1983**, *67*, 361–370. [CrossRef] [PubMed]
81. Pinto-Fraga, J.; Calonge, M.; Enríquez-de-Salamanca, A.; Fernández, I.; González-García, M.J.; Steven, P. Development of a Questionnaire for Detecting Changes in Dry Eye Disease–Related Symptoms. *Eye Contact Lens Sci. Clin. Pract.* **2021**, *47*, 8–14. [CrossRef]
82. Wolffsohn, J.S.; Arita, R.; Chalmers, R.; Djalilian, A.; Dogru, M.; Dumbleton, K.; Gupta, P.K.; Karpecki, P.; Lazreg, S.; Pult, H.; et al. TFOS DEWS II Diagnostic Methodology Report. *Ocul. Surf.* **2017**, *15*, 539–574. [CrossRef]
83. Höh, H.; Schirra, F.; Kienecker, C.; Ruprecht, K.W. Lid-Parallel Conjunctival Folds Are a Sure Diagnostic Sign of Dry Eye. *Ophthalmol. Z. Dtsch. Ophthalmol. Ges.* **1995**, *92*, 802–808.
84. Bron, A.J.; Evans, V.E.; Smith, J.A. Grading Of Corneal and Conjunctival Staining in the Context of Other Dry Eye Tests. *Cornea* **2003**, *22*, 640–650. [CrossRef]
85. Korb, D.R.; Herman, J.P.; Greiner, J.V.; Scaffidi, R.C.; Finnemore, V.M.; Exford, J.M.; Blackie, C.A.; Douglass, T. Lid Wiper Epitheliopathy and Dry Eye Symptoms. *Eye Contact Lens Sci. Clin. Pract.* **2005**, *31*, 2–8. [CrossRef]
86. Bron, A.J.; Benjamin, L.; Snibson, G.R. Meibomian Gland Disease. Classification and Grading of Lid Changes. *Eye* **1991**, *5*, 395–411. [CrossRef] [PubMed]
87. Shimazaki, J.; Goto, E.; Ono, M.; Shimmura, S.; Tsubota, K. Meibomian Gland Dysfunction in Patients with Sjögren Syndrome. *Ophthalmology* **1998**, *105*, 1485–1488. [CrossRef]
88. Tesón, M.; Calonge, M.; Fernández, I.; Stern, M.E.; González-García, M.J. Characterization by Belmonte's Gas Esthesiometer of Mechanical, Chemical, and Thermal Corneal Sensitivity Thresholds in a Normal Population. *Investig. Ophthalmol. Vis. Sci.* **2012**, *53*, 3154–3160. [CrossRef] [PubMed]

89. Kamper, S.J.; Maher, C.G.; Mackay, G. Global Rating of Change Scales: A Review of Strengths and Weaknesses and Considerations for Design. *J. Man. Manip. Ther.* **2009**, *17*, 163–170. [CrossRef]
90. Oliveira-Soto, L.; Efron, N. Morphology of Corneal Nerves Using Confocal Microscopy. *Cornea* **2001**, *20*, 374–384. [CrossRef]
91. Lagali, N.; Bourghardt, B.; Germundsson, J.; Eden, U.; Danyali, R.; Rinaldo, M.; Fagerholm, P. Laser-Scanning in Vivo Confocal Microscopy of the Cornea: Imaging and Analysis Methods for Preclinical and Clinical Applications. In *Confocal Laser Microscopy—Principles and Applications in Medicine, Biology, and the Food Sciences*; InTech: London, UK, 2013.
92. Britten-Jones, A.C.; Rajan, R.; Craig, J.P.; Downie, L.E. Quantifying Corneal Immune Cells from Human in Vivo Confocal Microscopy Images: Can Manual Quantification Be Improved with Observer Training? *Exp. Eye Res.* **2022**, *216*, 108950. [CrossRef]
93. Vázquez, A.; Blanco-Vázquez, M.; Martínez-Plaza, E.; Sobas, E.M.; González-García, M.J.; López-Miguel, A.; Ortega, E.; Enríquez-de-Salamanca, A.; Calonge, M. Corneal Sensory Changes and Nerve Plexus Abnormalities in Chronic Neuropathic Ocular Pain and Dry Eye Postrefractive Surgery. *Am. J. Ophthalmol.* **2025**, *276*, 170–185. [CrossRef] [PubMed]
94. Vandesompele, J.; De Preter, K.; Pattyn, F.; Poppe, B.; Van Roy, N.; De Paepe, A.; Speleman, F. Accurate Normalization of Real-Time Quantitative RT-PCR Data by Geometric Averaging of Multiple Internal Control Genes. *Genome Biol.* **2002**, *3*, research0034.1. [CrossRef]
95. Livak, K.J.; Schmittgen, T.D. Analysis of Relative Gene Expression Data Using Real-Time Quantitative PCR and the $2^{-\Delta\Delta CT}$ Method. *Methods* **2001**, *25*, 402–408. [CrossRef] [PubMed]
96. Galor, A.; De Lott, L.B. A Call to Abandon the Term Dry Eye When We Really Mean Pain. *Ophthalmology* **2025**, *in press*. [CrossRef] [PubMed]

International Journal of *Molecular Sciences*

MDPI

Review

The Immunobiology of Dry Eye Disease: A Review of the Pathogenesis, Regulation and Therapeutic Implications

Sarah Jacqueline Saram [1], Maya Natasha Thomas [2], Leo Feinberg [3,4], Harry W. Roberts [3,4], Conor M. Ramsden [3,4], Małgorzata Woronkowicz [2,5] and Piotr Skopiński [6,7,*]

1 Ministry of Health, 16 College Road College of Medicine Building and Singapore, Singapore 169854, Singapore; sarah.saram@mohh.com.sg
2 North Devon District Hospital, Royal Devon University Healthcare NHS Foundation Trust, Barnstaple EX31 4JB, UK; mayanatasha.thomas@nhs.net (M.N.T.); malgorzata.woronkowicz.14@alumni.ucl.ac.uk (M.W.)
3 West of England Eye Unit, Royal Devon University Healthcare NHS Foundation Trust, Exeter EX2 5DW, UK; leo.feinberg@nhs.net (L.F.); conor.ramsden@nhs.net (C.M.R.)
4 Faculty of Health and Life Science, University of Exeter Medical School, Exeter EX1 2HZ, UK
5 Moorfields Eye Hospital NHS Foundation Trust, London EC1V 2PD, UK
6 Department of Ophthalmology, SPKSO Ophthalmic University Hospital, Medical University of Warsaw, 00-576 Warsaw, Poland
7 Department of Histology and Embryology, Medical University of Warsaw, 02-004 Warsaw, Poland
* Correspondence: pskopin@wp.pl

Abstract: Dry eye disease (DED) is increasingly recognized as a condition driven by immune dysregulation at the ocular surface (OS). Chronic inflammation, mediated by aberrant activation of both innate and adaptive immune pathways, underlies disease progression and symptom persistence. Neuroimmune interactions further amplify OS inflammation, contributing to epithelial damage and impaired homeostatic regulation. This review summarizes current literature on the immunopathogenesis of DED, highlighting the complex interplay of molecular mechanisms of innate and adaptive immune activation, neuroimmune-mediated inflammation, and emerging molecular and cellular biomarkers. In addition, we examine existing and emerging therapeutic strategies that target these immune-molecular pathways, including precision immunomodulatory approaches, to inform future management of DED. By integrating mechanistic insights with clinical findings, this review aims to provide a comprehensive overview of the molecular mechanisms underlying the dysregulated immune response associated with DED.

Keywords: dry eye disease; ocular surface; immunopathogenesis; innate immunity; adaptive immunity; T cells; tear biomarkers

1. Introduction

Dry eye disease (DED) is a prevalent and multifactorial disorder impacting the ocular surface (OS), and is characterized by tear film instability, hyperosmolarity, and inflammation, affecting approximately 10–20% of people over the age of 40 globally [1,2]. Once primarily viewed as a disorder of tear deficiency or excessive evaporation, this perspective has evolved to recognize the significant role of the loss of immune homeostasis and dysregulation of the innate and adaptive immune system in driving disease progression and symptom persistence [2,3].

Over the past decade, advances in immunology, molecular profiling, and animal models have reshaped our understanding of DED pathogenesis. Accumulating evidence has elucidated complex immunoregulatory dysfunction at the OS, including aberrant activation of epithelial stress pathways, innate immune triggers, T cell polarization, and impaired regulatory networks [2,4–6]. A better understanding of the molecular mechanisms underlying DED has facilitated the identification of potential precision immunomodulatory techniques to mitigate disease progression.

This review underscores the central role of immune dysregulation in DED, reframing it as a complex disorder of disrupted immune homeostasis rather than just a binary deficiency–evaporation paradigm. We discuss evidence from human and preclinical models implicating aberrant innate and adaptive immune responses and neuroimmune interactions as key drivers of disease initiation and persistence, and highlight how these insights are shaping the development of emerging targeted immunomodulatory therapies.

2. Methodology

In this narrative review, a comprehensive search strategy was developed to identify relevant publications focusing on the role of the immune system in the pathogenesis of DED. Literature searches were performed using electronic databases, including PubMed, Google Scholar, Web of Science, and Scopus, covering the period from January 2000 to July 2025. The following combinations of Medical Subject Headings (MeSH) terms and keywords were used: *"dry eye disease," "dry eye syndrome," "ocular surface immunology," "innate immunity," "adaptive immunity," "T cells," "dendritic cells," "cytokines," "chemokines," "tear biomarkers,"* and *"immunopathogenesis."* To ensure comprehensive coverage of the literature, the reference lists of the included articles were screened to identify further relevant publications. No limitations were placed on study type, but we excluded those that did not focus specifically on immune dysregulation at the OS.

3. OS Immune Homeostasis

The OS in healthy eyes is actively kept in a strict immune homeostasis by various regulatory mechanisms that, when disrupted, can lead to uncontrolled inflammation seen in DED [3,7]. The tear film components, produced by the lacrimal glands, meibomian glands, and OS epithelia, act as an immunologically active barrier that preserves corneal clarity through lubrication, suppresses local inflammation, and promotes wound healing [8,9] (Figure 1). It contains a diverse array of growth factors, antimicrobial peptides, and antibodies, including immunoglobulin A (IgA) and G (IgG), which help to defend the OS from microorganisms and maintain homeostasis [9,10].

The lacrimal gland produces the aqueous component of the tear film along with antimicrobial proteins, immunoglobulins, and cytokines that regulate lubrication, epithelial integrity, and immune tolerance [11–17].

Complementing the aqueous layer, the meibomian glands supply the lipid layer that prevents tear evaporation. The meibomian glands have immune-regulatory functions, helping maintain OS homeostasis by controlling lipid secretion and limiting microbial overgrowth. Dysregulation of this immune balance, particularly through pathogenic Th17 responses and IL-17A–driven neutrophil recruitment, contributes to glandular obstruction, inflammation, and dysfunction [18].

The cornea has a unique immune-privileged status maintained through several mechanisms. Its avascular and alymphatic structure prevents the infiltration of circulating leukocytes and migration of antigen presenting cells (APCs) to regional lymphoid tissues, thereby dampening the adaptive immune response [3,5]. Furthermore, the cornea lacks mature resident APCs, which express low levels of major histocompatibility complex class II (MHC II) and lack co-stimulatory molecules such as CD80, CD86, and CD40, further contributing to corneal immunosenescence [3,19].

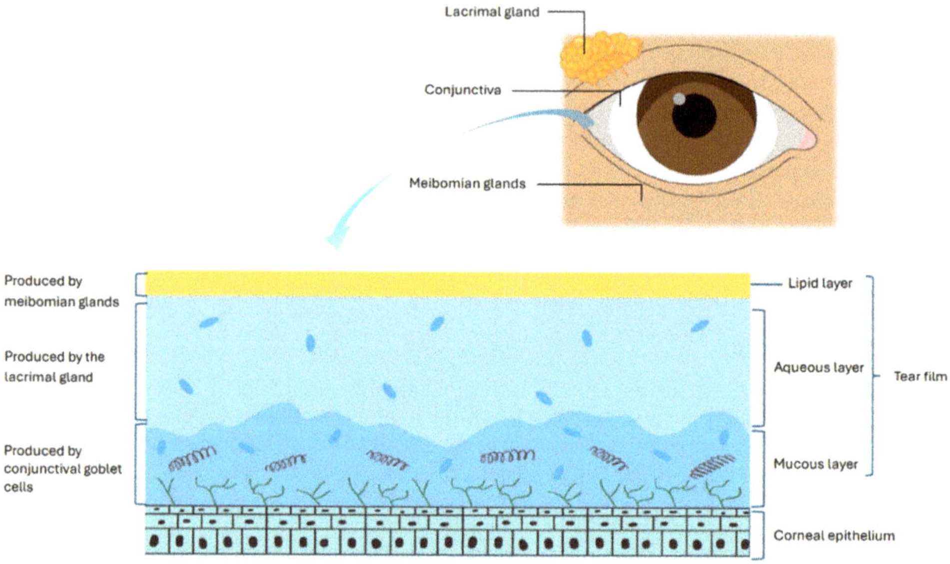

Figure 1. The components of the tear film.

The corneal epithelium serves as a physical barrier (with glycocalyx and tight junctions) against microorganisms and environmental insults. It actively participates in immunoregulation by expressing immunomodulatory molecules such as programmed death ligand 1 (PD-L1), which promote apoptosis of active effector T cells [3,20]. Corneal and conjunctival epithelial cells express functional toll-like (TLR) and NOD-like receptors (NLR), enabling pathogen detection and recognition of danger-associated molecular patterns (DAMPs) to initiate appropriate immune responses [20].

The cornea is a highly innervated surface and relies on neuropeptides derived from nerves such as substance P to help with immunoregulation by regulating virus and bacteria-induced inflammation and maintaining corneal epithelial homeostasis [3,21]. However, oversecretion of neuropeptides seen in DED can lead to pathological amplification of the immune response and propagation of the 'vicious cycle' of inflammation [3].

4. Definition and Classification of DED

The classification of DED has evolved to aid diagnostic precision and guide targeted therapy by identifying the suspected etiology of the disease [22]. Originally divided into tear-deficient and evaporative types, this was refined in 2007 to distinguish between aqueous-deficient dry eye (ADDE) and evaporative dry eye (EDE), with ADDE often further subclassified into Sjögren's syndrome (SS) and non-Sjögren's etiologies [5,23,24]. ADDE is characterized by insufficient or reduced tear volume, whilst EDE is due to over-evaporation of the tear film despite normal tear production. However, it is recognized that many patients exhibit overlapping features of both subtypes, with co-existing disturbance in tear quantity and quality, underscoring the complex and multifactorial nature of DED [2,22].

5. Pathophysiology of DED

5.1. The Role of Tear Hyperosmolarity in DED

Tear hyperosmolarity has been identified as a key feature of DED and underlies both reduced aqueous production and increased evaporation. It may represent the initiating insult, driving a cascade of OS damage wherein inflammation and immune dysregulation establish a dynamic, self-sustaining cycle that disrupts normal homeostatic control (Figure 2) [2,4]. This hyperosmolar state activates an epithelial stress response, causing the release of proinflammatory cytokines and matrix metalloproteinases (MMP), which promote marked recruitment and activation of both innate and adaptive immune cells to the OS [2,25]. Type 1 helper (Th1) and type 17 helper (Th17) lymphocytes are the predominant T cell subtypes in DED and cause IFN-γ and IL-17–mediated epithelial damage [5,26]. This immune-driven disruption of the homeostasis of the OS further destabilizes the tear film, increases evaporation, and perpetuates the 'vicious cycle' that characterizes chronic DED [22,26]. Other extrinsic (e.g., contact lens wear, LASIK surgery, use of systemic anticholinergics) and intrinsic factors (e.g., age, female sex, autoimmune conditions such as SS) can contribute to the cycle and further the chronicity of the disease [26]. While this 'vicious cycle' is dynamic and multifactorial, with overlap between innate and adaptive immune responses, for simplicity and clarity's sake, the authors felt it important to break down each structure in turn, while reflecting the complex interplay between the two.

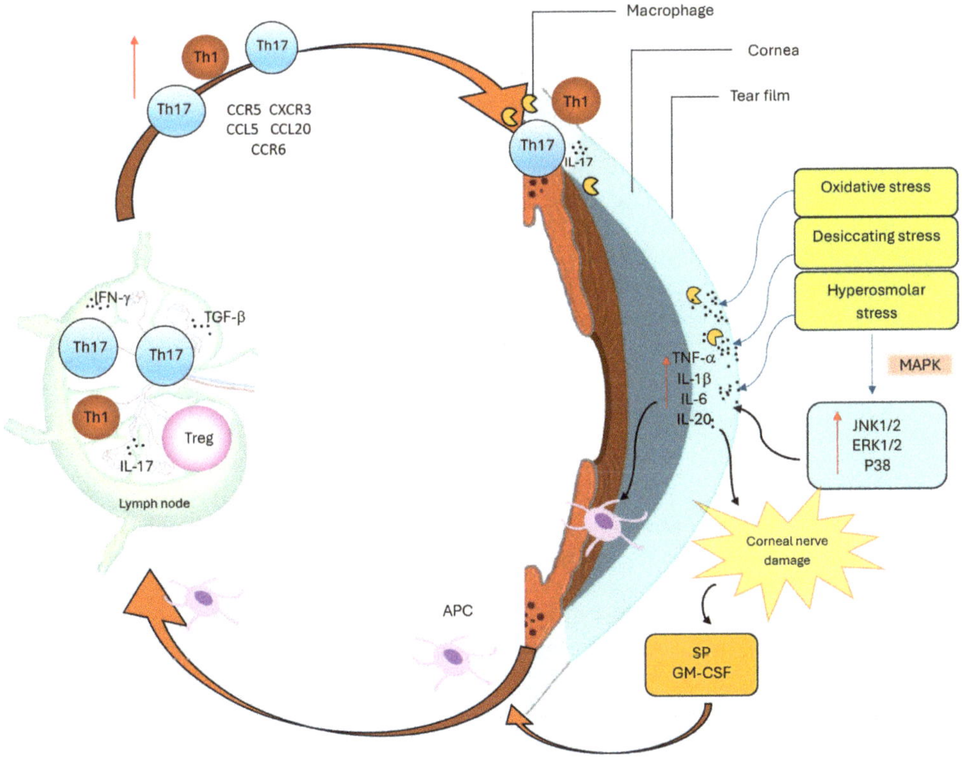

Figure 2. The vicious cycle of dry eye disease.

This cycle is driven by oxidative, desiccating, and hyperosmolar stress at the ocular surface, which activates mitogen-activated protein kinase (MAPK) pathways, including c-Jun N-terminal kinase 1/2 (JNK1/2), extracellular signal-regulated kinase 1/2 (ERK1/2), and p38 [27,28], and induces proinflammatory mediators, such as tumor necrosis factor-alpha (TNF-α), interleukin-1 beta (IL-1β), interleukin-6 (IL-6), and interleukin-20 (IL-20) [27,29]. These cytokines promote antigen-presenting cell (APC) maturation and migration via lymphatics to regional lymph nodes, where effector T helper 1 (Th1) and T helper 17 (Th17) cells are activated. Dry eye disease (DED)-primed Th1 cells expressing C-C chemokine receptor type 5 (CCR5) and C-X-C chemokine receptor type 3 (CXCR3), and Th17 cells expressing CCR6, are recruited back to the ocular surface (OS) through corresponding chemokine gradients, including C-C motif chemokine ligand 5 (CCL5) and C-C motif chemokine ligand 20 (CCL20) [30]. Interferon-gamma (IFN-γ) enhances APC maturation, while transforming growth factor-beta (TGF-β) promotes Th17 differentiation and weakens immune regulation [22,26]. At the OS, IL-1β and TNF-α amplify inflammation and barrier disruption, IL-20 enhances macrophage recruitment and signaling, and interleukin-17 (IL-17) induces matrix metalloproteinase (MMP) production, epithelial damage, and apoptosis. Neuroimmune dysregulation further amplifies this cycle: proinflammatory cytokines damage peripheral nerves, triggering substance P (SP) and granulocyte-macrophage colony-stimulating factor (GM-CSF) release from sensory nerve endings, which enhances major histocompatibility complex class II (MHC-II) expression and promotes T cell priming, further exacerbating ocular surface inflammation [31]. Together, these immune and neuroimmune interactions perpetuate chronic inflammation and sustain the vicious cycle of DED.

5.2. *Aging and Immune Dysregulation in DED*

Aging is a major risk factor for DED, driving both immune dysregulation and structural changes across the OS [32]. Aged C57BL/6 mice serve as a particularly informative model, developing meibomian gland dysfunction, corneal staining, GC depletion, and lymphocytic infiltration of the conjunctiva and lacrimal glands [33,34]. Aging promotes the generation of autoreactive $CD4^+$ T cells that infiltrate ocular tissues, contributing to chronic inflammation and goblet cell loss [35]. While DC density and morphology remain largely unchanged, age-related immune dysregulation may instead reflect functional alterations in APCs. IFN-γ plays a central role in this process, mediating GC depletion, while aged regulatory T cells (Tregs) lose their suppressive function and instead secrete IFN-γ and IL-17, further amplifying inflammation [36–38]. Furthermore, aged mice models demonstrate higher levels of memory Th-17 cells compared with their younger counterparts, which correlate with disease severity upon re-exposure to desiccating stress [39].

5.3. *The Role of the Microbiome in DED*

Whilst the OS is a site of low bacterial load, both preclinical and clinical studies suggest that the ocular and gut microbiome are interlinked in sustaining immune tolerance and preventing OS inflammation in DED [40]. In CD25KO mice (lacking CD25, the α-chain of the IL-2 receptor, resulting in Treg deficiency), absence of commensal bacteria at the OS amplified autoreactive $CD4^+IFN\text{-}\gamma^+$ T-cell responses and accelerated SS-like dacryoadenitis, whereas fecal transplantation restored immune regulation, highlighting a key microbiome–T cell axis in DED pathogenesis [41]. Complementary evidence from de Paiva and colleagues showed in murine models exposed to antibiotics and desiccating stress that loss of *Firmicutes/Bacteroidetes* and expansion of *Proteobacteria* promotes pathogenic $CD4^+$ effector T-cell responses, diminishes regulatory T-cell and IL-13–mediated goblet cell support, and exacerbates OS inflammation [42].

Clinical studies further support a link between microbiome dysbiosis and immune dysregulation in DED. Liang et al. reported heterogeneous conjunctival dysbiosis in DED patients, with depletion of commensals, reduced α-diversity, and overabundance of specific bacterial and fungal species (e.g., Staphylococcus aureus, Malassezia globosa), potentially disrupting mucosal tolerance and OS immune homeostasis [43].

In the gut, dysbiosis is also prevalent in SS and correlates with OS disease severity, characterized by loss of protective taxa such as *Bifidobacterium* and *Actinobacteria* and enrichment of *Prevotella* and *Veillonella*. These microbial shifts are thought to be mechanistically linked to altered short-chain fatty acid (butyrate) production, impaired epithelial barrier integrity, and skewed Th1/Th17 versus Treg balance, suggesting a gut–eye axis role in DED [44]. Additionally, enrichment of proinflammatory taxa such as *Corynebacterium tuberculostearicum* and *Propionibacteriaceae* has been observed at the OS in DED with postulated activation of NF-κB/TLR2 signaling and ROS-mediated cytokine release, further driving OS inflammation [45].

Overall, whilst these findings underscore the potential immune regulatory role of commensal microbiota in maintaining homeostasis at the OS, mechanistic studies remain limited, and small cohort sizes constrain generalizability.

6. Innate Immune System in DED

In response to stressors such as tear hyperosmolarity, the innate immune system at the OS mounts a rapid, non-specific defense [46]. In DED, however, this protective response can become maladaptive, triggering proinflammatory signaling cascades, promoting an influx of immune cells, and priming the adaptive immune response, thus impairing immune homeostasis at the OS [6,47–49].

6.1. Epithelial Cells' Stress Response and the Inflammatory Cascade

Stressed corneal epithelial cells release a rapid and high concentration of proinflammatory cytokines, which contribute to local inflammation [6,27]. Direct hyperosmolar stress to these cells rapidly activates mitogen-activated protein kinases (MAPKs), causing sustained activation of their three signaling pathways: c-Jun N-terminal kinase 1/2 (JNK1/2), extracellular signal-regulated kinase 1/2 (ERK1/2), and p38 [27,28]. These pathways transduce extracellular signals to intracellular responses, which upregulate inflammation, apoptosis, and immune response through the expression of cytokines and MMPs [50,51].

MMP-9, a key proteolytic enzyme upregulated by proinflammatory cytokines IL-1β and TNF-α, contributes to OS damage by degrading epithelial basement membrane components and disrupting tight junction proteins such as Zonula Occludens-1 (ZO-1) and Occludin, thereby weakening corneal barrier integrity in DED [27,50,52]. Moreover, increased nuclear transcription factors like Nuclear Factor kappa-light-chain-enhancer of activated B cells (NF-κB) and Nuclear Factor of Activated T cells 5 (NFAT5), drive the early upregulation of cytokines such as TNF-α, IL-1β, IL-6, and IL-20, creating a microenvironment conducive to immune cell activation and recruitment [27,29].

Wang et al. demonstrated, using multiple murine models of DED, alongside analyses of human tear samples, that IL-20 is upregulated and may act pathogenically by promoting macrophage recruitment, epithelial apoptosis, and Th17 responses [29]. While this study provides important translational insight by linking IL-20 elevation to human disease, the mechanistic evidence is largely derived from animal and in vitro models.

Further T cell recruitment to the OS is promoted by C-C motif chemokine ligand 5 (CCL5), C-X-C motif chemokine ligand 9 (CXCL9), CXCL10 chemokines, as well as Th17-inducing cytokines such as IL-6, TGF-β, IL-23, and IL-17A [6,37]. Recent work by Liu et al. demonstrated through murine DED models that basal epithelial cells, particularly fibroblast-like subtypes generated via epithelial–mesenchymal transition, can act as 'non-professional APCs' at the OS. These cells upregulate MHC class II and secrete chemokines such as CCL2, promoting macrophage recruitment and activating adaptive immune responses, thereby linking innate and adaptive immunity. This proinflammatory microenvironment persists in the chronic phase, with enduring fibrotic changes in epithelial cells and polarization of macrophages toward an inflammatory subtype, contributing to sustained immune-driven inflammation in DED [53]. However, these findings are again based solely on murine models, and whether the same immunopathological mechanisms occur in chronic human DED remains uncertain.

Toll-like receptor 4 (TLR4) is expressed on various corneal and conjunctival epithelial cells and requires co-receptors CD14 and myeloid differentiation factor 2 (MD2) to detect bacterial lipopolysaccharide (LPS) [46]. Under normal conditions, oversignaling is regulated through low TLR4 expression on apical cells and the absence of MD2, which prevents unnecessary immune responses to commensal bacteria [46]. Redfern et al. observed reduced TLR 4 and 9 protein expression in human corneal epithelial cells in vitro when exposed to dry eye conditions, whilst TLR 5 levels were increased or unchanged [54]. The same group also reported elevated levels of DAMPs, such as high mobility group box 1 (HMGB1) and heat shock protein (HSP-60), in the tear films of DED patients, which are associated with activation of the innate immune response via TLRs (especially TLR4) and increased cytokine and MMP-9 production, perpetuating OS inflammation [55]. This apparent discrepancy, low receptor protein yet high ongoing DAMP-driven activation, may be a reflection that in vitro findings may not fully capture the dynamics of in vivo chronic human DED pathogenesis or indicate that the mechanism of TLR dysregulation is not yet fully understood.

6.2. The Complement System

The complement system, a central arm of the innate immune defense, has been increasingly implicated in the pathogenesis of DED. Several clinical studies have shown that both the classical and alternative complement pathways and their regulatory proteins are present and functionally active in the normal eye, including the cornea, aqueous humor, and tears [56–59]. In murine eyes, complement was found to be constitutively active at a low basal level, with C3 cleavage fragments and terminal complex deposition detectable in ocular tissues, providing continuous immune surveillance. This activity is tightly regulated by complement regulatory proteins, where inhibition of decay-accelerating factor (DAF) or membrane cofactor protein (MCP) precipitated severe intraocular inflammation. Regulation at the level of C3 convertase has been identified as a critical checkpoint in preventing complement-driven injury [60]. Human studies corroborate these findings, showing that complement regulatory proteins, including DAF, MCP, CD59, factor H, and factor I, are widely distributed throughout ocular tissues, while aqueous and vitreous humor exhibit inhibitory activity against both the classical and alternative pathways in vitro [57,61–64].

In DED, clinical studies have demonstrated that tear fluid from DED patients with meibomian gland dysfunction contains elevated levels of complement activation products C3a and C5a compared with controls, indicating local complement activation and implicating innate immune dysregulation, particularly in elderly patients [65]. Preclinical models further support a mechanistic role for complement: DED-specific autoantibodies trigger OS inflammation in a complement-dependent manner, resulting in neutrophil infiltration, proinflammatory cytokine release, and GC loss. Complement depletion attenuates these effects, highlighting its function as a mediator linking humoral and T cell–driven immune responses in DED [66]. However, evidence for complement involvement in DED remains limited, mostly from small cohorts or murine models, whereas it is better characterized in other ocular diseases such as age-related macular degeneration [67].

6.3. Innate Immune Cells

6.3.1. Neutrophils

The increased release and production of proinflammatory cytokines and chemokines in DED causes abnormal immune cell infiltration and functioning [27,47]. Neutrophils contribute to inflammation not only through phagocytosis and reactive oxygen species (ROS) production but also by releasing neutrophil extracellular traps (NETs) in response to tear hyperosmolarity [47,68]. These NETs can form in the absence of infection, perpetuating sterile inflammation and promoting chronic OS damage through sustained cytokine expression and type I IFN signaling [68,69]. Kwon et al. identified the presence of anti-citrullinated protein autoantibodies (ACPA) in the OS wash of 40% of patients with DED, likely generated through peptidylarginine deiminase 4 (PAD4)-mediated citrullination of proteins during neutrophil NETosis. These ACPAs were found to subsequently induce OS inflammation in murine models [70].

6.3.2. Macrophages

Macrophages are versatile innate immune cells involved in pathogen clearance, tissue repair, and immune regulation. Differing activation states exist, including Classically activated (M1) proinflammatory macrophages and alternatively activated (M2) anti-inflammatory macrophages, depending on their environment [47]. In DED, hyperosmolar stress skews macrophage polarization toward a proinflammatory M1 state while suppressing anti-inflammatory M2 activity, promoting Th1 and Th17 infiltration, and amplifying OS immune dysregulation.

A recent study by Alam et al. using single-cell RNA sequencing in murine models of DED showed a three-fold increase in resident macrophages. Moreover, the phenotypic shift in macrophages towards pain sensitization via gene expression of CXCL1 and loss of homeostatic gene expression was observed. Increased production of neurosensitizing factors such as CXCL1 can activate transient receptor potential vanilloid 1 (TRPV-1), A disintegrin, and metalloproteinase 17 (ADAM17), contributing to ocular pain and epithelial barrier disruption associated with DED [71]. Complementing these findings, recent single-cell transcriptomic and epigenomic profiling has revealed distinct conjunctival macrophage subsets in DED mouse models, including a regulatory retinoid X receptor alpha (RXRα), a nuclear receptor modulating immune gene expression that suppresses inflammation via IL-10 signaling, the depletion of which exacerbates goblet cell loss and Th17-mediated pathology [72]. This highlights the capacity of macrophages to serve as a conduit between innate and adaptive immunity, where hyperosmolarity-driven M1 polarization not only amplifies local inflammation but also orchestrates T cell recruitment and activation, thereby propagating immune dysregulation in DED.

6.3.3. Natural Killer (NK) Cells

NK cells play a pivotal role in OS immunity by secreting large amounts of IFN-γ, which activates surrounding macrophages and T cells. In addition to their immunomodulatory function, NK cells exhibit cytotoxic activity via granzyme and perforin release, contributing to tissue damage [47]. The role of NK cells in the early stages of DED pathogenesis has been suggested, as their activation promotes IFN-γ–mediated inflammation and drives APC maturation, ultimately priming adaptive immune responses [73]. In murine models of DED, conjunctival NK and natural killer T cells (NKT) produce IL-6 and IL-23, activating DCs and enhancing Th17 responses [74]. Notably, NK cell depletion reduces cytokine levels and preserves corneal integrity, underscoring a critical NK–DC–Th17 axis in early DED. Similarly to macrophages, this evidence supports the role of NK cells not only in sustaining local inflammation at the OS but also in contributing to the oversensitization of the adaptive immune system seen in DED.

7. Adaptive Immune System in DED

Once primed, the adaptive immune system plays a central role in the chronicity of DED. Autoreactive T cells drive sustained inflammation of the OS, in particular, $CD4^+$ T helper subsets Th1 and Th17 cells. These mediate further cytokine-driven epithelial damage and perpetuate immune dysregulation and are unimpeded by impaired T regulatory cells [25].

The activation, migration, and interaction of APCs with naive T cells is central to the initiation of the adaptive immune response in DED and has been well established [27,75]. In murine models, the migration of APCs towards draining lymph nodes is facilitated by the upregulated expression of C-C chemokine receptor-7 (CCR7), which guides their exit from the OS to lymph nodes by responding to specific ligands CCL19 and CCL21, found in high density in corneal lymphatics and draining lymph nodes [76,77]. Within the lymph node microenvironment, APCs prime naive T cells by MHC–antigen interaction and costimulatory engagement (e.g., CD80/CD86 with CD28) towards $CD4^+$ Th1 and Th17 effectors [78,79].

7.1. Th1 Cells

The effect of Th1 cells in DED was initially noted to be more pronounced in the acute phase, as evidenced by the presence of its related cytokine IFN-γ in murine models of early DED and its reduced prominence later in disease progression [80]. DED-primed Th1 cells upregulate chemokine receptors CCR5 and CXCR3, facilitating their targeted migration from the lymph nodes back to the inflamed OS via corresponding chemokine gradients, as demonstrated in murine models [30].

IFN-γ was initially thought to amplify its own production by upregulating IL-12 receptor expression, promoting further Th1 differentiation and inducing chemokines (CXCL9, CXCL10, CXCL11), which recruit and retain Th1 cells in inflamed tissues [81]. IFN-γ itself exerts its effects in DED by inducing GC loss and reducing mucin production, thus worsening tear film instability and perpetuating the vicious cycle of inflammation [82]. Moreover, loss of conjunctival GC likely disrupts local immune tolerance by impairing APC tolerance, leading to enhanced IL-12 production and pathogenic Th1/Th17 polarization as evidenced in murine models [83]. However, a review by Chen et al., scrutinizing the varied roles of Th-17 cells in DED, concluded that the exact source of IFN-γ in the acute phase of DED may be associated with NK cells, and its continued secretion throughout the course of the disease may be related to IFN-γ^+IL-17^+ "double-positive" Th17/1 cells [27].

7.2. Th17 Cells

The role of Th-17 cells in DED is significant and central to the pathogenesis of DED. Differentiation of Th-17 cells is largely dependent on the microenvironment and is initiated by the signal transducer and activator of transcription 3 (STAT3) signaling pathway after exposure to IL-6 and TGF-β secreted by APCs [84,85]. This is further regulated and promoted by the transcription factor retinoic acid–related orphan receptor gamma t (RORγt), which was found to be significantly upregulated in the OS tissues after exposure to desiccating stress in murine models [86]. Th17 cells then migrate back to the OS, specifically the conjunctiva, via chemokine receptors CCR6 and CCL20, where they undergo further differentiation following exposure to IL-1 and IL-23 [87].

A key cytokine produced by Th17 is IL-17, found in greater concentrations in tears of both non-SS and SS-DED patients, which stimulates MMP production and causes damage to the corneal epithelium [81,88]. However, there are several other key Th-17 subsets, including IL-10 producing Th17 cells, Th17/Th1 cells which co-produce IL-17 and IFN gamma, Th-17 producing Granulocyte-macrophage colony-stimulating factor (Th17GM-CSF), and more recently interleukin 17 receptor E (IL-17RE) and CCR10 producing Th17 cells in murine models [31,89–91].

Whilst IL-10 producing Th-17 cells may potentially play a regulatory role in DED (as seen in murine models), other subsets are more detrimental [89]. Co-producing IL-17 and IFNγ Th-17 cells are significantly pathogenic and drive epithelial apoptosis, lymphangiogenesis, APC maturation and potentially IFNγ production seen in chronic DED [27,89,90].

Granulocyte-macrophage colony-stimulating factor (GM-CSF) exerts its role in DED through stimulation of monocytic cells to produce proinflammatory cytokines such as IL-1β, IL-6, and IL-23. IL-6 and IL-23 further perpetuate Th17 differentiation [31]. In a murine model of DED, the IL-17RE^highCCR10$^+$ Th17 subset exhibited enhanced JNK and p38 MAPK signaling. This is likely mediated through IL-17C/IL-17RE interaction, which reinforces and perpetuates their Th17 phenotype by sustaining IL-17A expression in vitro [91]. The presence of multiple subsets of Th-17 cells and their more hybrid phenotypes such as Th17/Th1 and CCR10 expression (typically found on T helper 22 cells) may suggest plasticity of Th17 cells which can transdifferentiate depending on the microenvironment as seen in murine models [91].

Alam et al. identified γδ T cells as a significant source of IL-17 in RXRα-deficient Pinkie mouse models, with elevated IL-17A and IL-17F expression that exacerbated DED [92]. They also demonstrated that 9-cis retinoic acid, the natural ligand for RXRα, suppresses IL-17 production from both γδ T cells and monocytes in vitro, suggesting that RXRα may act as a negative regulator of IL-17-driven inflammation [92].

7.3. Memory T Cells

Chronic DED is predominantly driven by a persistent Th17 response, particularly by effector memory Th17 cells [80]. Chen et al. used murine models to demonstrate that OS inflammation persists despite the absence of desiccating stress and is largely driven by continued IL-17 secretion from this population of cells [62]. Th17 memory cells also continue to promote further migration of effector T cells from lymph nodes (LN) to the OS via pathological lymphangiogenesis [80]. The same group also identified in pre-clinical models that IL-7 and IL-15 are critical for the maintenance of Th17 memory cells and promote continued survival via STAT5 and phosphoinositide 3-kinase–Akt (PI3K-Akt) pathways [93]. Moreover, IL-23 was found to promote the transition of Th17 effector cells into memory cells whilst IL-2 had an inhibiting effect on this pathway as demonstrated in murine models [94].

7.4. Tregs

Several studies examined Treg cells in DED, reporting various results. CD25$^+$CD4$^+$Foxp3$^+$ Tregs are peripheral Tregs with important mechanisms of action, including: (1) granzyme-B and perforin mediated cytolysis, (2) the release of immunosuppressive cytokines including IL-10, TGF-β and IL-35, (3) the inhibition of DC maturation and function via the transendocytosis of co-stimulatory molecules (CD80/86) and (4) suppression via metabolic competition [37,95,96]. In DED murine models, their reduction led to increased severity of SS-like DED [97]. Conversely, the transfer of in vitro expanded Tregs into two different strains of DED murine models, BALB/c and C57BL/6, showed suppression of pathogenic CD4$^+$ effector T cell-mediated inflammation [98].

In contrast, other reports demonstrated that Treg levels may remain unchanged in DED, but their suppressive function is compromised. Chauhan et al. noted preserved Treg numbers but impaired ability to restrain Th17 cells, likely due to IL-17A secretion by effector cells [99]. Similarly, the proinflammatory IL-6–rich microenvironment of DED inhibits Treg differentiation [100].

In patients with SS-associated DED, conjunctival biopsies showed marginally increased Treg counts without correlation to clinical severity, further suggesting that dysfunction rather than numerical deficit drives pathology [101]. This was further evidenced in stromal interaction molecule 1/2 (STIM1/2) Foxp3$^+$ mice, where targeted deletion of calcium-sensing proteins STIM1/2 in Foxp3$^+$ Tregs resulted in a fulminant SS-like phenotype characterized by lacrimal gland inflammation, lymphocytic infiltration, and IFN-γ–dominated transcriptional signatures [102]. Moreover, transcriptomic analyses revealed downregulation of core memory Treg genes in both mouse and human SS, suggesting that functional Treg impairment, not mere reduction, is a conserved and critical step in disease development [102].

The apparent discrepancies in Treg data across DED studies likely reflect differences in disease models, tissue compartments assessed, and methodological approaches to Treg identification, as well as the dynamic nature of Treg function across disease stages. This highlights the need for standardized methods to assess both Treg frequency and suppressive capacity in order to clarify their role in human DED pathogenesis.

7.5. B Cells and Humoral Dysfunction

B cells contribute to immune dysregulation in DED, but their role differs markedly between SS-associated DED and non-SS forms. In primary SS-associated DED, B cells are a central driver of pathology. Historically, glandular infiltrates were considered to be primarily CD4$^+$ T cell–mediated, but recent studies show that B cells play a dominant role across both early and late disease stages [103,104]. In murine models such as the NOD.H-2h4 strain, B cells are the predominant immune infiltrates within lacrimal glands, with T cells providing additional contributions to the inflammatory milieu [105].

Within the salivary and lacrimal glands of SS patients, periductal lymphocytic infiltrates and ectopic germinal centers are often B-cell-dominated. Their hyperactivity is sustained by chemokines such as CXCL12, CXCL13, CCL19, and CCL21, as well as cytokine axes involving BAFF, IL-6, and IL-21 [106]. This dysregulated signaling drives clonal expansion, the production of autoantibodies (SSA/Ro, SSB/La, rheumatoid factor), and, in severe cases, malignant transformation into B-cell lymphomas. Beyond antibody secretion, B cells also function as APC and cytokine producers (IL-2, IL-12, TNF-α, IFN-γ), amplifying autoreactive T-cell responses and promoting tissue destruction [107]. Animal studies further support their pathogenic role, as passive transfer of autoantibodies alone can induce disease features [66].

By contrast, evidence for B-cell involvement in non-SS DED is far more limited. While B cells and plasma cells are detectable in the conjunctiva and OS tissues, their proportions do not differ significantly between non-SS DED patients and healthy controls [108]. Some data suggest that autoantibodies, such as those against kallikrein-13, can induce complement-dependent OS inflammation in murine DED models, pointing to a potential but secondary role for B-cell–mediated autoimmunity [66]. Activated B cells may also contribute indirectly by producing proinflammatory cytokines such as IL-6 and TNF-α [107]. However, unlike SS-associated DED, ectopic germinal center formation within lacrimal glands is rare in non-SS disease, underscoring the limited role of B cells in its pathogenesis.

In summary, B-cell dysregulation is a hallmark of SS-associated DED, driving autoantibody production, cytokine amplification, and tissue damage. In non-SS forms however, B cells appear to play a minor, context-dependent role, with disease pathogenesis being more strongly linked to T-cell–mediated mechanisms.

8. Neuroimmune Mediated Inflammation in DED

Neuroimmune dysregulation significantly contributes to the pathogenesis of DED by aberrantly modulating both innate and adaptive immune responses. As proposed in a review by Huang et al., this may be due to a bidirectional feedback loop in which proinflammatory cytokines released by immune cells damage peripheral nerves, triggering excessive neuropeptide release [109]. These neuropeptides, in turn, further activate immune pathways, amplifying OS inflammation and perpetuating chronic disease [109]. Yu et al. have underscored the role of the neuropeptide substance P (SP) from sensory nerve endings in enhancing MHC-II expression on DCs, thereby promoting subsequent T cell priming [75]. Moreover, the SP–neurokinin 1 receptor (NK1R) axis directly acts on pathogenic Th17GM-CSF cells, significantly increasing GM-CSF production and exacerbating dry eye disease severity in murine models [110]. This highlights a novel neuroimmune pathway through which neuropeptides enhance effector T cell activity and OS inflammation [110].

In addition, SP/NK1R signaling has been implicated in pathological lymphangiogenesis in DED, where it upregulates Vascular Endothelial Growth Factor (VEGF)-C, VEGF-D, and VEGFR-3 expression, promoting lymphatic vessel growth and facilitating APC trafficking to draining lymph nodes [111]. Moreover, whilst Tregs expressing NK1R are found in increased quantities in DED, their abnormal expression of critical immunomodulatory markers CTLA-4, PD-1, TGF-β, and IL-10 demonstrates an impaired suppressive capacity against effector T cells, suggesting a compromised regulatory phenotype [112,113]. SP may also be implicated in the promotion and maintenance of memory Th17 cells [80]. In vitro studies have shown increased conversion of effector T cells to memory Th17 cells when cultured with SP [80]. Further, when cultured with Th17 memory cells, SP continued to preserve the cells [114].

Calcitonin gene-related peptide (CGRP) plays a potentially more complex and unclear role in DED, exhibiting both immunosuppressive and proinflammatory roles depending on the microenvironment [109,115]. Its immunosuppressive activity includes the inhibition of APCs by Langerhans cells and attenuation of contact hypersensitivity through the suppression of mast cell-derived tumor necrosis factor [116]. However, clinical data on CGRP and SP remain conflicting. Some studies report reduced tear concentrations of CGRP and SP, particularly in severe or chronic DED, where corneal nerve loss may impair neuropeptide production and secretion, thereby diminishing their homeostatic and immunomodulatory functions [115–117]. Conversely, other studies demonstrate increased neuropeptide levels, particularly in DED subtypes with prominent neuroinflammation or post-surgical neuropathic pain, suggesting upregulation in response to inflammatory stimuli or nerve sensitization [112,118]. These discrepancies possibly reflect underlying disease heterogeneity, variation in nerve integrity, and/or stage-specific dynamics (early inflammatory vs. late neurodegenerative disease).

Experimental models further underscore the complexity of neuroimmune interactions. In murine studies, tear hyperosmolarity alone disrupted neuroimmune homeostasis via TRPV1, NF-κB activation in conjunctival epithelium, leading to DC maturation, memory $CD4^{+}$ T cell priming, corneal nerve loss, and impaired mucosal tolerance [119]. Adoptive transfer of these T cells induced DED in naive mice, establishing hyperosmolarity as a direct pathogenic trigger [119]. Complementing these findings, studies in guinea pig models of aqueous tear deficiency demonstrate that chronic dryness also sensitizes TRPV1-expressing corneal nociceptors, enhancing blink reflexes and neuronal calcium responses to capsaicin [120]. This neuroplasticity likely contributes to the ocular hyperalgesia and discomfort characteristic of DED [120].

9. Tear Biomarkers of DED

The pathophysiology of dry eye disease involves a complex interplay of immune, epithelial, and neuronal factors at the OS. Numerous biomarkers have been identified that reflect distinct aspects of disease activity, including inflammatory mediators, chemokines, cytokines, matrix metalloproteinases, and regulatory molecules (Table 1). They play roles in promoting or modulating OS inflammation, epithelial barrier disruption, and immune cell recruitment.

Table 1. Up (↑) and downregulated (↓) biomarkers in DED and their role in disease activity.

Category	Biomarker	Response in DED	Functional/Pathophysiological Role	Ref.
Chemokines	CCL2	↑	Drives basal epithelial cells to act as 'non-professional APCs' in further activating immune response	[53]
	CCL20	↑	Aids migration of Th17 cells back to OS, specifically the conjunctiva	[87]
	CCL5	↑	Promotes T cell recruitment	[6,37]
	CXCL10	↑	Recruits Th1 cells to the OS through CXCR3 signaling, amplifying local inflammation	[6,37]
	CXCL9	↑	Activates T cells and sustains chronic inflammatory responses via CXCR3	[6,37]
	CXCL1	↑	Activates TRPV1 and ADAM17 which contribute to ocular pain and epithelial barrier disruption	[71]
Cytokines	ACPA	↑	Generated during neutrophil NETosis, induces OS inflammation in murine models	[70]
	GM-CSF	↑	Stimulates monocytic cells to produce proinflammatory cytokines such as IL-1β, IL-6, and IL-23 with IL-6 and IL-23 further perpetuating Th17 differentiation	[31]
	IFN-γ	↑ in early DED ↓ in later disease progression	Induces epithelial damage and disrupts homeostasis of OS NK activation promotes IFN-γ-mediated inflammation and drives APC maturation which primes adaptive immune response. Induces GC loss and reduces mucin production	[40,47,50]
	IL-1	↑	Allows Th17 cells to undergo further differentiation at the conjunctiva.	[87]
	IL-10	↓	Exacerbates goblet cell loss and Th17-mediated pathology contribute to impaired suppressive capacity against effector T cells.	[39,78,79]
	IL-12	↑	Leads to further Th1 polarization	[83]
	IL-15	↑	Maintains Th17 memory cells and promotes continued survival	[93]
	IL-17	↑	Disrupts corneal epithelium barrier integrity, stimulates MMP production, and promotes inflammation and apoptosis	[81,88]
	IL-17C	↑	Enhances JNK and p38 MAPK signaling though IL-17C/IL17RE interaction therefore reinforces and perpetuates Th17 phenotype	[91]
	IL-1β	↑	Promotes epithelial damage, upregulates proinflammatory mediators, and enhances immune cell activation	[27,50,52]

Table 1. *Cont.*

Category	Biomarker	Response in DED	Functional/Pathophysiological Role	Ref.
Cytokines	IL-2	-	Inhibits differentiation of Th17 effector cells into memory cells	[94]
	IL-20	↑	Promotes macrophage recruitment and increases inflammatory signaling in OS	[29]
	IL-23	↑	Allows Th17 cells to undergo further differentiation at the conjunctiva and promotes transition into memory cells	[6,13,41,55,64]
	IL-6	↑	Activates DCs and enhances Th17 responses; Initiates Th-17 cell differentiation via STAT3 signaling pathways; Exhibits inhibitory effect on Treg differentiation.	[6,13,41,52,53]
	IL-7	↑	Helps maintain Th17 memory cells and promotes continued survival	[93]
	IL17A	↑	Promotes neutrophil recruitment, epithelial barrier disruption, and proinflammatory cytokine production at OS	[61,70]
	IL17F	↑	Stimulates epithelial cells and immune cells to release inflammatory mediators and chemokines	[92]
	TGF-β	↑	Induces Th17 cells and contributes to impaired suppressive capacity against effector T cells.	[6,37]
	TNF-β	↑	Initiates Th-17 cell differentiation via STAT3 signaling pathways.	[84,85]
	TNF-α	↑	upregulates proinflammatory cytokines, disrupting epithelial barrier integrity, and amplifying immune cell infiltration	[27,50,52]
Chemokine receptors	CCR6	↑	Aids migration of Th17 cells back to OS, specifically the conjunctiva	[87]
	CXCR3	↑	Facilitates migration of DED-primed Th1 cells from lymph nodes back to inflamed OS	[30]
Damage-Associated Molecules (DAMPS)	HMGB1	↑	Activates TLR pathways and induces proinflammatory cytokine and MMP-9 release	[55]
	HSP-60	↑	Activates TLR pathways, leading to cytokine release and immune cell recruitment	[55]
Enzymes/receptors related to pain and epithelial integrity	ADAM17	↑	Contributes to ocular pain and epithelial barrier disruption	[71]
	TRPV1	↑	Contributes to ocular pain and epithelial barrier disruption	[71]

Table 1. *Cont.*

Category	Biomarker	Response in DED	Functional/Pathophysiological Role	Ref.
Growth/Neuroimmune factors	CGRP	↑ and ↓	Exhibits both an immunosuppressive and proinflammatory role depending on the microenvironment; Inhibits APCs through suppression of mast cell-derived TNF; upregulated in response to inflammatory stimulation or nerve sensitization.	[75,81,82,85]
	VEGF, VEGF-D, VEGFR-3	↑	Promotes lymphatic vessel growth and facilitates APC trafficking to draining lymph nodes.	[111]
Immune checkpoint molecules	CTLA-4	↑	Impairs suppressive capacity against effector T cells	[112,113]
	PD-1	↑	Impairs suppressive capacity against effector T cells	[112,113]
Matrix-degrading enzymes	MMP-9	↑	Degrades epithelial basement membrane components and disrupts tight junction proteins	[27,50,52]
Signaling molecules	NF-κB	↑	Drives early upregulation of proinflammatory cytokines, promoting immune cell activation	[27,29]
	NFAT5	↑	Promotes early cytokine upregulation and immune cell activation	[27,29]
Toll-Like Receptors	TLR4	ITLR mRNA ↑ TLR protein levels ↓	Recognizes DAMPs (like HMGB1) and microbial products, activating NF-κB and driving cytokine/chemokine release	[46]
	TLR9	TLR9 mRNA ↓ TLR9 protein ↓	Impairs local immune regulatory function at OS	[54]
Transcription factors	RORγt	↑	Regulates and promotes Th-17 cell differentiation	[86]
	RXRa	↓	Exacerbates goblet cell loss and Th17-mediated pathology.	[72]

10. Therapeutic Implications

While the initiating events in DED remain unclear, sustained immune dysregulation, marked by aberrant activation of innate and adaptive immune pathways, plays a central role in perpetuating OS inflammation. This understanding has driven a shift from symptomatic treatments to targeted immunomodulation, aimed at disrupting specific molecular mediators of inflammation and restoring immune homeostasis. Despite advances in targeted immunotherapies, the mainstay of DED management remains tear supplementation. Sodium hyaluronate, particularly when combined with pranoprofen, alleviates hyperosmolar stress on the OS but does not directly modulate immunity [121]. Diquafosol, recommended in the TFOS DEWS III report, acts primarily by stimulating fluid and mucin secretion; however, proteomic analyses suggest it may also exert indirect immunoregulatory effects by stabilizing the tear film and thereby supporting OS immune homeostasis [121–123].

Several currently approved agents exert immunomodulatory effects, albeit with variable efficacy [124]. Cyclosporine A, a topical calcineurin inhibitor, suppresses IL-2–mediated T cell activation, reduces epithelial apoptosis, and has been shown to restore GC density in DED. Lifitegrast, a lymphocyte function-associated antigen-1 (LFA-1) antagonist, blocks T cell adhesion and migration through competitive inhibition of the LFA-1/intercellular adhesion molecule 1 (ICAM-1) interaction on the OS. Topical corticosteroids, though effective in rapidly reducing inflammatory mediators such as MMP-9, IL-1β, and TNF-α via suppression of NF-κB and activator protein 1 (AP-1), carry well-documented risks with prolonged use, including ocular hypertension, cataract formation, and susceptibility to infection [125]. Recently, Tacrolimus, a macrolide immunomodulator that inhibits T cell activation through calcineurin blockade, has been compared with Cyclosporine A in a randomized controlled trial and showed equally effective outcomes in reducing the need for artificial tear supplementation compared with placebo. No significant difference between treatments, however, has been observed in patients with severe DED secondary to SS [123].

Therapeutic advances have shifted focus toward precision immunomodulation targeting the upstream molecular and cellular drivers of innate immune dysregulation in DED. Modulating macrophage polarization is a potential therapeutic target, with murine studies demonstrating that shifting macrophages from a proinflammatory M1 phenotype to an anti-inflammatory M2 phenotype can contribute to a reduction in proinflammatory cells and an increase in anti-inflammatory factors. In a benzalkonium chloride (BAC)-induced murine model of DED, treatment with M2 macrophage–derived extracellular vesicles (M2-EVs) improved tear production, preserved corneal integrity, and downregulated inflammatory cytokines [126]. Zhou et al. highlighted the α7 nicotinic acetylcholine receptor (α7nAChR) as a regulator of macrophage-driven inflammation; activation of this receptor reduced OS inflammation via neuroimmune crosstalk in DED murine models [127].

Endogenous counter-regulatory molecules such as pigment epithelium-derived factor (PEDF) have also demonstrated immunosuppressive effects [128]. In both murine and human cells, elevated PEDF expression in the corneal epithelium and tear film suppressed key proinflammatory cytokines, including IL-1β, IL-6, TNF-α, and IL-17A, and reduced Th17 cell density through inhibition of the p38 MAPK and JNK pathways [128]. A ROS-responsive microneedle patch (CE-MN), loaded with cyclosporin A and the antioxidant epigallocatechin gallate (EGCG), enabled sustained periocular delivery to the lacrimal gland. In an SS-DED model, CE-MN suppressed macrophage activation and oxidative stress, while attenuating downstream Th1 and Th17-mediated inflammation more effectively than conventional eye drops [129].

Several potential strategies that target the adaptive immune response have emerged. A number of murine studies have shown that neutralizing IL-17A or blocking its upstream regulators improves OS quality. Local CCL20 neutralization reduces Th17 cell infiltration and inflammation in vitro and in vivo, while RXRα agonism with 9-cis retinoic acid attenuates Th17-driven inflammation and preserves goblet cells in the Pinkie mouse model [87,92]. Topical inhibition of phosphodiesterase type-4 (PDE4) with Cilomilast significantly suppressed IL-17 and IL-23 expression in conjunctival tissue and draining lymph nodes, reduced $CD11b^+$ APC infiltration, and downregulated IL-1β, IL-6, and TNF-α [130]. This improved clinical outcomes, with therapeutic efficacy comparable or superior to both dexamethasone and cyclosporine in DED murine models [130]. However, when Secukinumab (a human monoclonal antibody that neutralizes IL-17A) was utilized systemically in patients with DED, it showed no significant amelioration of DED symptoms [131]. A phase II clinical trial focusing on the topical administration of an IL-17A antagonist has yet to release its results [132]. The apparent disparity between the promising pre-clinical data and clinical trial results of IL-17A neutralization further emphasizes the importance of delivery route, target engagement in the relevant tissue, and endpoint selection in translating cytokine-targeted therapies.

In chronic DED, targeting IL-7 and IL-15 with topical anti-IL-7 and anti-IL-15 antibody treatments in vivo murine models showed amelioration of disease severity; however, this could not target memory Th17 cells in draining lymph nodes [93]. Moreover, a murine study employing CCL22-releasing microspheres demonstrated increased recruitment of endogenous Tregs to the lacrimal gland, leading to improved epithelial integrity, reduced IFN-γ–mediated inflammation, and a restored Treg:effector T cell ratio [133].

Targeting neuroimmune signaling in DED is another therapeutic avenue that has been explored in the last decade. Topical blockade of NK1R using antagonists such as spantide and CP-99,994 significantly suppressed Th17 responses, reduced corneal lymphangiogenesis, and improved clinical outcomes [75,111]. Pyroptosis, a form of proinflammatory programmed cell death, and its associated polo-like kinase 1–cell division cycle 25C–cyclin-dependent kinase 1 (Plk1–Cdc25c–Cdk1) axis, can also be targeted using CP-99,994. This has led to reduced IL-6, IL-1β, and TNF-α levels, and further ameliorated OS inflammation in the murine DED model [134].

More recently, mesenchymal stem cell (MSC) therapy has emerged as a promising immunomodulatory strategy for the treatment of DED. MSCs derived from bone marrow, adipose tissue, and umbilical cord modulate ocular inflammation through both cell-mediated and paracrine mechanisms [135]. In a murine T cell–driven model of DED, local infusion of human or mouse MSCs suppressed $CD4^+$ T cell proliferation and IFN-γ production, reducing OS inflammation and restoring GC density and tear secretion. These effects occurred independently of Treg induction or indoleamine 2,3-dioxygenase (IDO)-mediated tryptophan metabolism, suggesting alternative regulatory pathways, including transient recruitment of other immunosuppressive cells or species-specific mechanisms such as inducible nitric oxide synthase in murine MSCs [136]. Similarly, in a murine SS-DED model, bone marrow–derived mouse MSCs improved lacrimal gland secretory function and increased aquaporin 5 expression, while reducing lymphocytic foci size without significant changes in $Foxp3^+$ Tregs or stromal cell-derived factor 1 (SDF-1)/CXCR4 signaling [137].

MSC-derived extracellular vesicles (MSC-EVs) demonstrate comparable efficacy: umbilical cord MSC-EVs downregulated the IRAK1/TAB2/NF-κB pathway via miRNAs, including miR-125b and let-7b, suppressing proinflammatory cytokines in murine DED models [138]. Adipose-derived MSC exosomes (mADSC-Exos) attenuated hyperosmotic stress–induced inflammation by reducing IL-1β, IL-6, and NOD-, LRR- and Pyrin domain-containing protein 3 (NLRP3) inflammasome activation in murine models, while promoting tear film stability and epithelial repair [139]. Additionally, human umbilical cord MSC–derived exosomal microRNA-146a (miR-146a) suppressed apoptosis and inflammation in hyperosmotic-stressed human corneal epithelial cells and a murine DED model by upregulating sequestosome 1 (SQSTM1), revealing a novel miRNA-mediated protective axis [140].

11. Conclusions

Our understanding of DED has shifted from a purely symptomatic perspective to one that recognizes dysregulated innate, adaptive, and neuroimmune pathways as central drivers of OS inflammation, highlighting the pivotal role of immune mechanisms in disease perpetuation and progression.

12. Future Directions

Advances in molecular and translational research have identified promising targeted immunomodulatory strategies such as Th17 inhibition, macrophage modulation, neuropeptide receptor blockade, and stem cell therapies. However, clinical translation remains limited by disease heterogeneity, lack of robust biomarkers, and incomplete understanding of human ocular immunopathology. Preclinical models, particularly murine systems, have provided critical mechanistic insight into immune dysregulation, yet their relevance to human disease is constrained, as evidenced by differences in outcomes between animal models and clinical trials. Moreover, studying large human populations is challenging due to variability in disease severity, phenotype, and access to standardized immunological assays. Future research should therefore prioritize precise immunophenotyping to enable personalized treatment and the development of reliable biomarkers for diagnosis and monitoring. Moreover, well-designed clinical trials exploring novel topical and cell-free immunotherapies are needed to bridge mechanistic insights from preclinical studies to human DED in order to restore immune homeostasis and improve patient outcomes.

Author Contributions: Conceptualization: M.W., H.W.R., C.M.R., P.S.; Methodology: S.J.S., M.N.T., L.F.; Writing—original draft preparation: S.J.S., M.N.T. Writing—review and editing: S.J.S., M.N.T., M.W., L.F., C.M.R., H.W.R. and P.S.; Illustrations: M.N.T. All authors have read and agreed to the published version of the manuscript.

Funding: This research received no external funding.

Institutional Review Board Statement: Not applicable.

Informed Consent Statement: Not applicable.

Data Availability Statement: No new data were created or analyzed in this study. Data sharing is not applicable to this article.

Conflicts of Interest: The authors declare no conflict of interest.

Abbreviations

ACPA	Anti-citrullinated protein autoantibodies
ADAM17	A Disintegrin And Metalloproteinase 17
ADDE	Aqueous-deficient dry eye
AP-1	Activator Protein 1
α7nAChR	α7 Nicotinic Acetylcholine Receptor
BAC	Benzalkonium Chloride
BALB/c	BALB/c mouse strain
CCL5	C-C motif chemokine ligand 5
CCR7	C-C chemokine receptor 7
CGRP	Calcitonin Gene-Related Peptide
CE-MN	Reactive Oxygen Species (ROS)-responsive Microneedle Patch
CP-99,994	N1KR antagonist
CXCL9	C-X-C motif chemokine ligand 9
DC	Dendritic Cell
DAMPs	Danger Associated Molecular Patterns
EDE	Evaporative Dry Eye
EGCG	Epigallocatechin Gallate
FoxP3	Forkhead Box Protein P3
HMGB1	High Mobility Group Box 1
HSP-60	Heat Shock Protein 60

ICAM-1	Intercellular Adhesion Molecule 1
IDO	Indoleamine 2,3-dioxygenase
IL	Interleukin
IL-17C	Interleukin 17C
IL-17RE	Interleukin 17 Receptor E
JNK1/2	c-Jun N-terminal kinase 1/2
LFA-1	Lymphocyte Function-Associated Antigen-1
LN	Lymph Nodes
MAPKs	Mitogen-Activated Protein Kinases
M1	Classically activated (proinflammatory) macrophage
M2	Alternatively activated (anti-inflammatory) macrophage
M2-EVs	M2 Macrophage–Derived Extracellular Vesicles
MD2	Myeloid Differentiation Factor 2
MHC	Major Histocompatibility Complex
miR-146a	MicroRNA-146a
MSC	Mesenchymal Stem Cell
MSC-EVs	MSC-Derived Extracellular Vesicles
mADSC-Exos	Adipose-Derived Mesenchymal Stem Cell Exosomes
mRNA	Messenger Ribonucleic Acid
NF-κB	Nuclear Factor kappa-light-chain-enhancer of activated B cells
NFAT5	Nuclear Factor of Activated T Cells 5
NK	Natural Killer Cells
NKT	Natural Killer T Cells
NETs	Neutrophil Extracellular Traps
NLRP3	NOD-, LRR- and Pyrin Domain-Containing Protein 3
PAD4	Peptidylarginine Deiminase 4
PEDF	Pigment Epithelium-Derived Factor
PI3K-Akt	Phosphoinositide 3-Kinase–Akt
Plk1–Cdc25c–Cdk1	Polo-Like Kinase 1—Cell Division Cycle 25C—Cyclin-Dependent Kinase 1
PDE4	Phosphodiesterase Type-4
PD-L1	Programmed Death Ligand 1
RASγt	Retinoic Acid–Related Orphan Receptor Gamma t
RXRα	Retinoid X Receptor Alpha
ROS	Reactive Oxygen Species
RORγt	Retinoic Acid–Related Orphan Receptor Gamma t
SDF-1	Stromal Cell-Derived Factor 1
SP	Substance P
STIM1/2	Stromal Interaction Molecule 1/2
SQSTM1	Sequestosome 1
STAT3	Signal Transducer and Activator of Transcription 3
Th17GM-CSF	Th-17 Producing Granulocyte-Macrophage Colony-Stimulating Factor
TGF	Tumor Growth Factor
Tregs	T Regulatory Cells
TRPV1	Transient Receptor Potential Vanilloid 1
ZO-1	Zonula Occludens-1

References

1. Britten-Jones, A.C.; Wang, M.T.M.; Samuels, I.; Jennings, C.; Stapleton, F.; Craig, J.P. Epidemiology and Risk Factors of Dry Eye Disease: Considerations for Clinical Management. *Medicina* **2024**, *60*, 1458. [CrossRef]
2. Bron, A.J.; de Paiva, C.S.; Chauhan, S.K.; Bonini, S.; Gabison, E.E.; Jain, S.; Knop, E.; Markoulli, M.; Ogawa, Y.; Perez, V.; et al. TFOS DEWS II Pathophysiology Report. *Ocul. Surf.* **2017**, *15*, 438–510. [CrossRef]

3. Chen, Y.; Wang, S.; Alemi, H.; Dohlman, T.; Dana, R. Immune Regulation of the Ocular Surface. *Exp. Eye Res.* **2022**, *218*, 109007. [CrossRef]
4. Stapleton, F.; Argüeso, P.; Argüeso, A.; Asbell, P.; Azar, D.; Bosworth, C.; Chen, W.; Ciolino, J.; Craig, J.P.; Gallar, J.; et al. TFOS DEWS III Digest Report. *Am. J. Ophthalmol.* **2025**, *279*, 451–553. [CrossRef] [PubMed]
5. Barabino, S.; Chen, Y.; Chauhan, S.; Dana, R. Ocular Surface Immunity: Homeostatic Mechanisms and Their Disruption in Dry Eye Disease. *Prog. Retin. Eye Res.* **2012**, *31*, 271–285. [CrossRef] [PubMed]
6. Periman, L.M.; Perez, V.L.; Saban, D.R.; Lin, M.C.; Neri, P. The Immunological Basis of Dry Eye Disease and Current Topical Treatment Options. *J. Ocul. Pharmacol. Ther.* **2020**, *36*, 137–146. [CrossRef] [PubMed]
7. Galletti, J.G.; de Paiva, C.S. Age-related Changes in Ocular Mucosal Tolerance: Lessons Learned from Gut and Respiratory Tract Immunity. *Immunology* **2021**, *164*, 43–56. [CrossRef]
8. Stern, M.E.; Schaumburg, C.S.; Pflugfelder, S.C. Dry Eye as a Mucosal Autoimmune Disease. *Int. Rev. Immunol.* **2013**, *32*, 19–41. [CrossRef]
9. Zhou, L.; Beuerman, R.W. Tear Analysis in Ocular Surface Diseases. *Prog. Retin. Eye Res.* **2012**, *31*, 527–550. [CrossRef]
10. de Paiva, C.S.; Leger, A.J.S.; Caspi, R.R. Mucosal Immunology of the Ocular Surface. *Mucosal Immunol.* **2022**, *15*, 1143–1157. [CrossRef]
11. Tsai, P.S.; Evans, J.E.; Green, K.M.; Sullivan, R.M.; Schaumberg, D.A.; Richards, S.M.; Dana, M.R.; Sullivan, D.A. Proteomic Analysis of Human Meibomian Gland Secretions. *Br. J. Ophthalmol.* **2006**, *90*, 372–377. [CrossRef] [PubMed]
12. Mathers, W.D. Why the Eye Becomes Dry: A Cornea and Lacrimal Gland Feedback Model. *CLAO J.* **2000**, *26*, 159–165. [PubMed]
13. He, X.; Wang, S.; Sun, H.; He, H.; Shi, Y.; Wu, Y.; Wu, H.; Liu, Z.; Zhuang, J.; Li, W. Lacrimal Gland Microenvironment Changes After Obstruction of Lacrimal Gland Ducts. *Investig. Ophthalmol. Vis. Sci.* **2022**, *63*, 14. [CrossRef] [PubMed]
14. Zhang, M.; Tian, X.; Wu, Y.; Zhang, L.; Zhang, L.; Zheng, X.; Ou, S.; Gu, H. Establishment of A Mouse Model of Aqueous Deficiency Dry Eye. *J. Visualized Exp.* **2024**, *213*, e67317. [CrossRef]
15. Fan, Q.; Yan, R.; Li, Y.; Lu, L.; Liu, J.; Li, S.; Fu, T.; Xue, Y.; Liu, J.; Li, Z. Exploring Immune Cell Diversity in the Lacrimal Glands of Healthy Mice: A Single-Cell RNA-Sequencing Atlas. *Int. J. Mol. Sci.* **2024**, *25*, 1208. [CrossRef]
16. Kumar, N.R.; Praveen, M.; Narasimhan, R.; Khamar, P.; D'Souza, S.; Sinha-Roy, A.; Sethu, S.; Shetty, R.; Ghosh, A. Tear Biomarkers in Dry Eye Disease: Progress in the Last Decade. *Indian J. Ophthalmol.* **2023**, *71*, 1190–1202. [CrossRef]
17. Ji, Y.W.; Mittal, S.K.; Hwang, H.S.; Chang, E.-J.; Lee, J.H.; Seo, Y.; Yeo, A.; Noh, H.; Lee, H.S.; Chauhan, S.K.; et al. Lacrimal Gland–Derived IL-22 Regulates IL-17-Mediated Ocular Mucosal Inflammation. *Mucosal Immunol.* **2017**, *10*, 1202–1210. [CrossRef]
18. Beatty, C.J.; Ruiz-Lozano, R.E.; Quiroga-Garza, M.E.; Perez, V.L.; Jester, J.V.; Saban, D.R. The Yin and Yang of Non-Immune and Immune Responses in Meibomian Gland Dysfunction. *Ocul Surf.* **2024**, *32*, 81–90. [CrossRef]
19. Forrester, J.V.; McMenamin, P.G. Evolution of the Ocular Immune System. *Eye* **2024**, *39*, 468–477. [CrossRef]
20. Galletti, J.G.; Guzmán, M.; Giordano, M.N. Mucosal Immune Tolerance at the Ocular Surface in Health and Disease. *Immunology* **2017**, *150*, 397–407. [CrossRef]
21. Jastrzębska-Miazga, I.; Machna, B.; Wyględowska-Promieńska, D.; Smędowski, A. The Role of *Substance P* in Corneal Homeostasis. *Biomolecules* **2025**, *15*, 729. [CrossRef]
22. Craig, J.P.; Nichols, K.K.; Akpek, E.K.; Caffery, B.; Dua, H.S.; Joo, C.K.; Liu, Z.; Nelson, J.D.; Nichols, J.J.; Tsubota, K.; et al. TFOS DEWS II Definition and Classification Report. *Ocul. Surf.* **2017**, *15*, 276–283. [CrossRef]
23. Lemp, M.A.; Baudouin, C.; Baum, J.; Dogru, M.; Foulks, G.N.; Kinoshita, S.; Laibson, P.; McCulley, J.; Murube, J.; Pflugfelder, S.C.; et al. The Definition and Classification of Dry Eye Disease: Report of the Definition and Classification Subcommittee of the International Dry Eye WorkShop (2007). *Ocul. Surf.* **2007**, *5*, 75–92. [CrossRef]
24. Report of the National Eye Institute/Industry Workshop on Clinical Trials in Dry Eyes—PubMed. Available online: https://pubmed.ncbi.nlm.nih.gov/8565190/ (accessed on 8 June 2025).
25. Baudouin, C.; Messmer, E.M.; Aragona, P.; Geerling, G.; Akova, Y.A.; Benítez-Del-Castillo, J.; Boboridis, K.G.; Merayo-Lloves, J.; Rolando, M.; Labetoulle, M. Revisiting the Vicious Circle of Dry Eye Disease: A Focus on the Pathophysiology of Meibomian Gland Dysfunction. *Br. J. Ophthalmol.* **2016**, *100*, 300–306. [CrossRef] [PubMed]
26. Pflugfelder, S.C.; de Paiva, C.S. The Pathophysiology of Dry Eye Disease: What We Know and Future Directions for Research. *Ophthalmology* **2017**, *124*, S4–S13. [CrossRef] [PubMed]
27. Chen, Y.; Dana, R. Autoimmunity in Dry Eye Disease—An Updated Review of Evidence on Effector and Memory Th17 Cells in Disease Pathogenicity. *Autoimmun Rev.* **2021**, *20*, 102933. [CrossRef] [PubMed]
28. Moustardas, P.; Aberdam, D.; Lagali, N. MAPK Pathways in Ocular Pathophysiology: Potential Therapeutic Drugs and Challenges. *Cells* **2023**, *12*, 617. [CrossRef]
29. Wang, H.H.; Chen, W.Y.; Huang, Y.H.; Hsu, S.M.; Tsao, Y.P.; Hsu, Y.H.; Chang, M.S. Interleukin-20 Is Involved in Dry Eye Disease and Is a Potential Therapeutic Target. *J. Biomed. Sci.* **2022**, *29*, 36. [CrossRef]

30. Annan, J.E.; Chauhan, S.K.; Ecoiffier, T.; Zhang, Q.; Saban, D.R.; Dana, R. Characterization of Effector T Cells in Dry Eye Disease. *Investig. Ophthalmol. Vis. Sci.* **2009**, *50*, 3802. [CrossRef]
31. Dohlman, T.H.; Ding, J.; Dana, R.; Chauhan, S.K. T Cell–Derived Granulocyte-Macrophage Colony-Stimulating Factor Contributes to Dry Eye Disease Pathogenesis by Promoting CD11b+ Myeloid Cell Maturation and Migration. *Investig. Ophthalmol. Vis. Sci.* **2017**, *58*, 1330. [CrossRef]
32. Parfitt, G.J.; Xie, Y.; Geyfman, M.; Brown, D.J.; Jester, J.V. Absence of Ductal Hyper-Keratinization in Mouse Age-Related Meibomian Gland Dysfunction (ARMGD). *Aging* **2013**, *5*, 825–834. [CrossRef]
33. de Paiva, C.S. Effects of Aging in Dry Eye. *Int. Ophthalmol. Clin.* **2017**, *57*, 47–64. [CrossRef]
34. McClellan, A.J.; Volpe, E.A.; Zhang, X.; Darlington, G.J.; Li, D.-Q.; Pflugfelder, S.C.; de Paiva, C.S. Ocular Surface Disease and Dacryoadenitis in Aging C57BL/6 Mice. *Am. J. Pathol.* **2014**, *184*, 631–643. [CrossRef] [PubMed]
35. De Silva, M.E.H.; Hill, L.J.; Downie, L.E.; Chinnery, H.R. The Effects of Aging on Corneal and Ocular Surface Homeostasis in Mice. *Investig. Ophthalmol. Vis. Sci.* **2019**, *60*, 2705. [CrossRef] [PubMed]
36. de Souza, R.G.; de Paiva, C.S.; Alves, M.R. Age-Related Autoimmune Changes in Lacrimal Glands. *Immune Netw.* **2019**, *19*, e3. [CrossRef] [PubMed]
37. Foulsham, W.; Marmalidou, A.; Amouzegar, A.; Coco, G.; Chen, Y.; Dana, R. The Function of Regulatory T Cells at the Ocular Surface: Review. *Ocul. Surf.* **2017**, *15*, 652. [CrossRef]
38. Coursey, T.G.; Bian, F.; Zaheer, M.; Pflugfelder, S.C.; Volpe, E.A.; De Paiva, C.S. Age-Related Spontaneous Lacrimal Keratoconjunctivitis Is Accompanied by Dysfunctional T Regulatory Cells. *Mucosal Immunol.* **2016**, *10*, 743. [CrossRef]
39. Foulsham, W.; Mittal, S.K.; Taketani, Y.; Chen, Y.; Nakao, T.; Chauhan, S.K.; Dana, R. Aged Mice Exhibit Severe Exacerbations of Dry Eye Disease with an Amplified Memory Th17 Cell Response. *Am. J. Pathol.* **2020**, *190*, 1474. [CrossRef]
40. Trujillo-Vargas, C.M.; Schaefer, L.; Alam, J.; Pflugfelder, S.C.; Britton, R.A.; de Paiva, C.S. The Gut-Eye-Lacrimal Gland-Microbiome Axis in Sjögren Syndrome. *Ocul. Surf.* **2019**, *18*, 335. [CrossRef]
41. Zaheer, M.; Wang, C.; Bian, F.; Yu, Z.; Hernandez, H.; de Souza, R.G.; Simmons, K.T.; Schady, D.; Swennes, A.G.; Pflugfelder, S.C.; et al. Protective Role of Commensal Bacteria in Sjögren Syndrome. *J. Autoimmun.* **2018**, *93*, 45–56. [CrossRef]
42. De Paiva, C.S.; Jones, D.B.; Stern, M.E.; Bian, F.; Moore, Q.L.; Corbiere, S.; Streckfus, C.F.; Hutchinson, D.S.; Ajami, N.J.; Petrosino, J.F.; et al. Altered Mucosal Microbiome Diversity and Disease Severity in Sjögren Syndrome. *Sci. Rep.* **2016**, *6*. [CrossRef]
43. Liang, Q.; Li, J.; Zou, Y.; Hu, X.; Deng, X.; Zou, B.; Liu, Y.; Wei, L.; Liang, L.; Wen, X. Metagenomic Analysis Reveals the Heterogeneity of Conjunctival Microbiota Dysbiosis in Dry Eye Disease. *Front. Cell Dev. Biol.* **2021**, *9*, 731867. [CrossRef]
44. Moon, J.; Choi, S.H.; Yoon, C.H.; Kim, M.K. Gut Dysbiosis Is Prevailing in Sjögren's Syndrome and Is Related to Dry Eye Severity. *PLoS ONE* **2020**, *15*, e0229029. [CrossRef] [PubMed]
45. Schlegel, I.; De Goüyon Matignon de Pontourade, C.M.F.; Lincke, J.B.; Keller, I.; Zinkernagel, M.S.; Zysset-Burri, D.C. The Human Ocular Surface Microbiome and Its Associations with the Tear Proteome in Dry Eye Disease. *Int. J. Mol. Sci.* **2023**, *24*, 14091. [CrossRef] [PubMed]
46. Bolaños-Jiménez, R.; Navas, A.; López-Lizárraga, E.P.; de Ribot, F.M.; Peña, A.; Graue-Hernández, E.O.; Garfias, Y. Ocular Surface as Barrier of Innate Immunity. *Open Ophthalmol. J.* **2015**, *9*, 49–55. [CrossRef] [PubMed]
47. Reyes, J.L.; Vannan, D.T.; Eksteen, B.; Avelar, I.J.; Rodríguez, T.; González, M.I.; Mendoza, A.V. Innate and Adaptive Cell Populations Driving Inflammation in Dry Eye Disease. *Mediators Inflamm.* **2018**, *2018*, 2532314. [CrossRef]
48. Luo, L.; Li, D.Q.; Doshi, A.; Farley, W.; Corrales, R.M.; Pflugfelder, S.C. Experimental Dry Eye Stimulates Production of Inflammatory Cytokines and MMP-9 and Activates MAPK Signaling Pathways on the Ocular Surface. *Investig. Ophthalmol. Vis. Sci.* **2004**, *45*, 4293–4301. [CrossRef]
49. Li, D.Q.; Luo, L.; Chen, Z.; Kim, H.S.; Song, X.J.; Pflugfelder, S.C. JNK and ERK MAP Kinases Mediate Induction of IL-1β, TNF-α and IL-8 Following Hyperosmolar Stress in Human Limbal Epithelial Cells. *Exp. Eye Res.* **2006**, *82*, 588–596. [CrossRef]
50. Li, S.; Lu, Z.; Huang, Y.; Wang, Y.; Jin, Q.; Shentu, X.; Ye, J.; Ji, J.; Yao, K.; Han, H. Anti-Oxidative and Anti-Inflammatory Micelles: Break the Dry Eye Vicious Cycle. *Adv. Sci.* **2022**, *9*, 2200435. [CrossRef]
51. De Paiva, C.S.; Corrales, R.M.; Villarreal, A.L.; Farley, W.J.; Li, D.Q.; Stern, M.E.; Pflugfelder, S.C. Corticosteroid and Doxycycline Suppress MMP-9 and Inflammatory Cytokine Expression, MAPK Activation in the Corneal Epithelium in Experimental Dry Eye. *Exp. Eye Res.* **2006**, *83*, 526–535. [CrossRef]
52. Li, D.Q.; Lokeshwar, B.L.; Solomon, A.; Monroy, D.; Ji, Z.; Pflugfelder, S.C. Regulation of MMP-9 Production by Human Corneal Epithelial Cells. *Exp. Eye Res.* **2001**, *73*, 449–459. [CrossRef]
53. Liu, Z.; Xie, H.; Li, L.; Jiang, D.; Qian, Y.; Zhu, X.; Dai, M.; Li, Y.; Wei, R.; Luo, Z.; et al. Single-Cell Landscape Reveals the Epithelial Cell-Centric pro-Inflammatory Immune Microenvironment in Dry Eye Development. *Mucosal Immunol.* **2024**, *17*, 491–507. [CrossRef]

54. Redfern, R.L.; Barabino, S.; Baxter, J.; Lema, C.; McDermott, A.M. Dry Eye Modulates the Expression of Toll-Like Receptors on the Ocular Surface. *Exp. Eye Res.* **2015**, *134*, 80–89. [CrossRef]
55. Alven, A.; Lema, C.; Redfern, R.L. Impact of Low Humidity on Damage Associated Molecular Patterns at the Ocular Surface during Dry Eye Disease. *Optom. Vis. Sci.* **2021**, *98*, 1231–1238. [CrossRef]
56. Willcox, M.D.P.; Morris, C.A.; Thakur, A.; Sack, R.A.; Wickson, J.; Boef, W. Complement and Complement Regulatory Proteins in Human Tears. *Investig. Ophthalmol. Vis. Sci.* **1997**, *38*, 1–8.
57. Bora, N.S.; Gobleman, C.L.; Atkinson, J.P.; Pepose, J.S.; Kaplan, H.J. Differential Expression of the Complement Regulatory Proteins in the Human Eye. *Investig. Ophthalmol. Vis. Sci.* **1993**, *34*, 3579–3584.
58. Mondino, B.J.; Rao, H. Complement Levels in Normal and Inflamed Aqueous Humor. *Investig. Ophthalmol. Vis. Sci.* **1983**, *24*, 380–384.
59. Mondino, B.J.; Brady, K.J. Distribution of Hemolytic Complement in the Normal Cornea. *Arch Ophthalmol.* **1981**, *99*, 1430–1433. [CrossRef] [PubMed]
60. Sohn, J.H.; Kaplan, H.J.; Suk, H.J.; Bora, P.S.; Bora, N.S. Chronic Low Level Complement Activation within the Eye Is Controlled by Intraocular Complement Regulatory Proteins. *Investig. Ophthalmol. Vis. Sci.* **2000**, *41*, 3492.
61. Vogt, S.D.; Barnum, S.R.; Curcio, C.A.; Read, R.W. Distribution of Complement Anaphylatoxin Receptors and Membrane-Bound Regulators in Normal Human Retina. *Exp. Eye. Res.* **2006**, *83*, 834–840. [CrossRef]
62. McLaughlin, B.J.; Fan, W.; Zheng, J.J.; Cai, H.; Del Priore, L.V.; Bora, N.S.; Kaplan, H.J. Novel Role for a Complement Regulatory Protein (CD46) in Retinal Pigment Epithelial Adhesion. *Investig. Ophthalmol. Vis. Sci.* **2003**, *44*, 3669–3674. [CrossRef] [PubMed]
63. Anderson, D.H.; Radeke, M.J.; Gallo, N.B.; Chapin, E.A.; Johnson, P.T.; Curletti, C.R.; Hancox, L.S.; Hu, J.; Ebright, J.N.; Malek, G.; et al. The Pivotal Role of the Complement System in Aging and Age-Related Macular Degeneration: Hypothesis Re-Visited. *Prog Retin Eye Res.* **2010**, *29*, 95–112. [CrossRef] [PubMed]
64. Sohn, J.H.; Kaplan, H.J.; Suk, H.J.; Bora, P.S.; Bora, N.S. Complement Regulatory Activity of Normal Human Intraocular Fluid Is Mediated by MCP, DAF, and CD59. *Investig. Ophthalmol. Vis. Sci.* **2000**, *41*, 4195.
65. Maehara, H.; Norikawa, K.; Tanaka, K.; Kato, Y.; Kasai, A.; Mukai, R.; Omori, T.; Machida, T.; Sekine, H.; Sekiryu, T. Complement Activation Products in Tears of Dry Eye and Meibomian Gland Dysfunction. *Sci. Rep.* **2024**, *14*, 43. [CrossRef]
66. Stern, M.E.; Schaumburg, C.S.; Siemasko, K.F.; Gao, J.; Wheeler, L.A.; Grupe, D.A.; De Paiva, C.S.; Calder, V.L.; Calonge, M.; Niederkorn, J.Y.; et al. Autoantibodies Contribute to the Immunopathogenesis of Experimental Dry Eye Disease. *Investig. Ophthalmol. Vis. Sci.* **2012**, *53*, 2062. [CrossRef]
67. Wilke, G.A.; Apte, R.S. Complement Regulation in the Eye: Implications for Age-Related Macular Degeneration. *J. Clin. Investig.* **2024**, *134*, e178296. [CrossRef]
68. Tibrewal, S.; Ivanir, Y.; Sarkar, J.; Nayeb-Hashemi, N.; Bouchard, C.S.; Kim, E.; Jain, S. Hyperosmolar Stress Induces Neutrophil Extracellular Trap Formation: Implications for Dry Eye Disease. *Investig. Ophthalmol. Vis. Sci.* **2014**, *55*, 7961. [CrossRef]
69. Sonawane, S.; Khanolkar, V.; Namavari, A.; Chaudhary, S.; Gandhi, S.; Tibrewal, S.; Jassim, S.H.; Shaheen, B.; Hallak, J.; Horner, J.H.; et al. Ocular Surface Extracellular DNA and Nuclease Activity Imbalance: A New Paradigm for Inflammation in Dry Eye Disease. *Investig. Ophthalmol. Vis. Sci.* **2012**, *53*, 8253–8263. [CrossRef]
70. Kwon, J.; Surenkhuu, B.; Raju, I.; Atassi, N.; Mun, J.; Chen, Y.F.; Sarwar, M.A.; Rosenblatt, M.; Pradeep, A.; An, S.; et al. Pathological Consequences of Anti-Citrullinated Protein Antibodies in Tear Fluid and Therapeutic Potential of Pooled Human Immune Globulin-Eye Drops in Dry Eye Disease. *Ocul. Surf.* **2020**, *18*, 80–97. [CrossRef]
71. Alam, J.; Yaman, E.; Silva, G.C.V.; Chen, R.; de Paiva, C.S.; Stepp, M.A.; Pflugfelder, S.C. Single Cell Analysis of Short-Term Dry Eye Induced Changes in Cornea Immune Cell Populations. *Front. Med.* **2024**, *11*, 1362336; Erratum in *Front. Med.* **2024**, *11*, 1414997. [CrossRef]
72. Alam, J.; Yaman, E.; de Paiva, C.S.; Li, D.Q.; Villalba Silva, G.C.; Zuo, Z.; Pflugfelder, S.C. Changes in Conjunctival Mononuclear Phagocytes and Suppressive Activity of Regulatory Macrophages in Desiccation Induced Dry Eye. *Ocul. Surf.* **2024**, *34*, 348–362. [CrossRef] [PubMed]
73. Chen, Y.; Chauhan, S.K.; Saban, D.R.; Sadrai, Z.; Okanobo, A.; Dana, R. Interferon-γ-Secreting NK Cells Promote Induction of Dry Eye Disease. *J. Leukoc. Biol.* **2011**, *89*, 965–972. [CrossRef] [PubMed]
74. Zhang, X.; Volpe, E.A.; Gandhi, N.B.; Schaumburg, C.S.; Siemasko, K.F.; Pangelinan, S.B.; Kelly, S.D.; Hayday, A.C.; Li, D.Q.; Stern, M.E.; et al. NK Cells Promote Th-17 Mediated Corneal Barrier Disruption in Dry Eye. *PLoS ONE* **2012**, *7*, e36822. [CrossRef] [PubMed]
75. Yu, M.; Lee, S.M.; Lee, H.; Amouzegar, A.; Nakao, T.; Chen, Y.; Dana, R. Neurokinin-1 Receptor Antagonism Ameliorates Dry Eye Disease by Inhibiting Antigen-Presenting Cell Maturation and T Helper 17 Cell Activation. *Am. J. Pathol.* **2020**, *190*, 125–133. [CrossRef]

76. Wang, T.; Li, W.; Cheng, H.; Zhong, L.; Deng, J.; Ling, S. The Important Role of the Chemokine Axis CCR7-CCL19 and CCR7-CCL21 in the Pathophysiology of the Immuno-Inflammatory Response in Dry Eye Disease. *Ocul. Immunol. Inflamm.* **2021**, *29*, 266–277. [CrossRef]
77. Kodati, S.; Chauhan, S.K.; Chen, Y.; Dohlman, T.H.; Karimian, P.; Saban, D.; Dana, R. CCR7 Is Critical for the Induction and Maintenance of Th17 Immunity in Dry Eye Disease. *Investig. Ophthalmol. Vis. Sci.* **2014**, *55*, 5871–5877. [CrossRef]
78. Hamrah, P.; Huq, S.O.; Liu, Y.; Zhang, Q.; Dana, M.R. Corneal Immunity Is Mediated by Heterogeneous Population of Antigen-Presenting Cells. *J. Leukoc. Biol.* **2003**, *74*, 172–178. [CrossRef]
79. Lee, H.S.; Amouzegar, A.; Dana, R. Kinetics of Corneal Antigen Presenting Cells in Experimental Dry Eye Disease. *BMJ Open Ophthalmol.* **2017**, *1*, e000078. [CrossRef]
80. Chen, Y.; Chauhan, S.K.; Soo Lee, H.; Saban, D.R.; Dana, R. Chronic Dry Eye Disease Is Principally Mediated by Effector Memory Th17 Cells. *Mucosal Immunol.* **2013**, *7*, 38–45. [CrossRef]
81. Pflugfelder, S.C.; Corrales, R.M.; de Paiva, C.S. T Helper Cytokines in Dry Eye Disease. *Exp. Eye Res.* **2013**, *117*, 118–125. [CrossRef]
82. Jackson, D.C.; Zeng, W.; Wong, C.Y.; Mifsud, E.J.; Williamson, N.A.; Ang, C.S.; Vingrys, A.J.; Downie, L.E. Tear Interferon-Gamma as a Biomarker for Evaporative Dry Eye Disease. *Investig. Ophthalmol. Vis. Sci.* **2016**, *57*, 4824–4830. [CrossRef] [PubMed]
83. Ko, B.Y.; Xiao, Y.; Barbosa, F.L.; de Paiva, C.S.; Pflugfelder, S.C. Goblet Cell Loss Abrogates Ocular Surface Immune Tolerance. *JCI Insight* **2018**, *3*, e98222. [CrossRef] [PubMed]
84. Mills, K.H.G. Induction, Function and Regulation of IL-17-Producing T Cells. *Eur. J. Immunol.* **2008**, *38*, 2636–2649. [CrossRef] [PubMed]
85. Chu, L.; Wang, C.; Zhou, H. Inflammation Mechanism and Anti-Inflammatory Therapy of Dry Eye. *Front. Med.* **2024**, *11*, 1307682. [CrossRef]
86. Zheng, X.; de Paiva, C.S.; Li, D.Q.; Farley, W.J.; Pflugfelder, S.C. Desiccating Stress Promotion of Th17 Differentiation by Ocular Surface Tissues through a Dendritic Cell-Mediated Pathway. *Investig. Ophthalmol. Vis. Sci.* **2010**, *51*, 3083–3091. [CrossRef]
87. Dohlman, T.H.; Chauhan, S.K.; Kodati, S.; Hua, J.; Chen, Y.; Omoto, M.; Sadrai, Z.; Dana, R. The CCR6/CCL20 Axis Mediates Th17 Cell Migration to the Ocular Surface in Dry Eye Disease. *Investig. Ophthalmol. Vis. Sci.* **2013**, *54*, 4081–4091. [CrossRef]
88. Tan, X.; Sun, S.; Liu, Y.; Zhu, T.; Wang, K.; Ren, T.; Wu, Z.; Xu, H.; Zhu, L. Analysis of Th17-Associated Cytokines in Tears of Patients with Dry Eye Syndrome. *Eye* **2014**, *28*, 608–613. [CrossRef]
89. Hong, Q.; Chen, Y.; Inomata, T.; Liu, R.; Dana, R. Potential Role of IL-10-Producing Th17 Cells in Pathogenesis of Dry Eye Disease. *Investig. Ophthalmol. Vis. Sci.* **2017**, *58*, 1022.
90. Chen, Y.; Chauhan, S.K.; Shao, C.; Omoto, M.; Inomata, T.; Dana, R. Interferon-γ-Expressing Th17 Cells Are Required for Development of Severe Ocular Surface Autoimmunity. *J. Immunol.* **2017**, *199*, 1163–1169. [CrossRef]
91. Wang, J.; Gong, J.; Yang, Q.; Wang, L.; Jian, Y.; Wang, P. Interleukin-17 Receptor E and C-C Motif Chemokine Receptor 10 Identify Heterogeneous T Helper 17 Subsets in a Mouse Dry Eye Disease Model. *Am. J. Pathol.* **2022**, *192*, 332–343. [CrossRef]
92. Alam, J.; Yazdanpanah, G.; Ratnapriya, R.; Borcherding, N.; de Paiva, C.S.; Li, D.Q.; Guimaraes de Souza, R.; Yu, Z.; Pflugfelder, S.C. IL-17 Producing Lymphocytes Cause Dry Eye and Corneal Disease With Aging in RXRα Mutant Mouse. *Front. Med.* **2022**, *9*, 849990. [CrossRef] [PubMed]
93. Chen, Y.; Chauhan, S.K.; Tan, X.; Dana, R. Interleukin-7 and -15 Maintain Pathogenic Memory Th17 Cells in Autoimmunity. *J. Autoimmun.* **2016**, *77*, 96–103. [CrossRef] [PubMed]
94. Chen, Y.; Shao, C.; Fan, N.W.; Nakao, T.; Amouzegar, A.; Chauhan, S.K.; Dana, R. The Functions of IL-23 and IL-2 on Driving Autoimmune Effector T-Helper 17 Cells into the Memory Pool in Dry Eye Disease. *Mucosal Immunol.* **2020**, *14*, 177–186. [CrossRef] [PubMed]
95. Shevach, E.M.; Thornton, A.M. TTregs, PTregs, and ITregs: Similarities and Differences. *Immunol. Rev.* **2014**, *259*, 88–102. [CrossRef]
96. Sakaguchi, S.; Ono, M.; Setoguchi, R.; Yagi, H.; Hori, S.; Fehervari, Z.; Shimizu, J.; Takahashi, T.; Nomura, T. $Foxp3^+CD25^+CD4^+$ Natural Regulatory T Cells in Dominant Self-Tolerance and Autoimmune Disease. *Immunol. Rev.* **2006**, *212*, 8–27. [CrossRef]
97. Niederkorn, J.Y.; Stern, M.E.; Pflugfelder, S.C.; De Paiva, C.S.; Corrales, R.M.; Gao, J.; Siemasko, K. Desiccating Stress Induces T Cell-Mediated Sjögren's Syndrome-Like Lacrimal Keratoconjunctivitis. *J. Immunol.* **2006**, *176*, 3950–3957. [CrossRef]
98. Siemasko, K.F.; Gao, J.; Calder, V.L.; Hanna, R.; Calonge, M.; Pflugfelder, S.C.; Niederkorn, J.Y.; Stern, M.E. In Vitro Expanded $CD4^+CD25^+Foxp3^+$ Regulatory T Cells Maintain a Normal Phenotype and Suppress Immune-Mediated Ocular Surface Inflammation. *Investig. Ophthalmol. Vis. Sci.* **2008**, *49*, 5434–5440. [CrossRef]
99. Chauhan, S.K.; El Annan, J.; Ecoiffier, T.; Goyal, S.; Zhang, Q.; Saban, D.R.; Dana, R. Autoimmunity in Dry Eye Is Due to Resistance of Th17 to Treg Suppression. *J. Immunol.* **2009**, *182*, 1247–1252. [CrossRef]

100. Fan, N.W.; Dohlman, T.H.; Foulsham, W.; McSoley, M.; Singh, R.B.; Chen, Y.; Dana, R. The Role of Th17 Immunity in Chronic Ocular Surface Disorders. *Ocul. Surf.* **2020**, *19*, 157–168. [CrossRef]
101. Kuklinski, E.J.; Yu, Y.; Ying, G.S.; Asbell, P.A. Association of Ocular Surface Immune Cells With Dry Eye Signs and Symptoms in the Dry Eye Assessment and Management (DREAM) Study. *Investig. Ophthalmol. Vis. Sci.* **2023**, *64*, 7. [CrossRef]
102. Wang, Y.-H.; Li, W.; McDermott, M.; Son, G.-Y.; Maiti, G.; Zhou, F.; Tao, A.Y.; Raphael, D.; Moreira, A.L.; Shen, B.; et al. IFN-γ-Producing Th1 Cells and Dysfunctional Regulatory T Cells Contribute to the Pathogenesis of Sjögren's Disease. *Sci. Transl. Med.* **2024**, *16*, eado4856. [CrossRef]
103. Doyle, M.E.; Boggs, L.; Attia, R.; Cooper, L.R.; Saban, D.R.; Nguyen, C.Q.; Peck, A.B. Autoimmune Dacryoadenitis of NOD/LtJ Mice and Its Subsequent Effects on Tear Protein Composition. *Am. J. Pathol.* **2007**, *171*, 1224–1236. [CrossRef] [PubMed]
104. Ibrahem, H.M. B Cell Dysregulation in Primary Sjögren's Syndrome: A Review. *Jpn. Dent. Sci. Rev.* **2019**, *55*, 139–144. [CrossRef] [PubMed]
105. Li, L.; Jasmer, K.J.; Camden, J.M.; Woods, L.T.; Martin, A.L.; Yang, Y.; Layton, M.; Petris, M.J.; Baker, O.J.; Weisman, G.A.; et al. Early Dry Eye Disease Onset in a NOD.H-2 h4 Mouse Model of Sjögren's Syndrome. *Investig. Ophthalmol. Vis. Sci.* **2022**, *63*, 18. [CrossRef] [PubMed]
106. Kroese, F.G.; Abdulahad, W.H.; Haacke, E.; Bos, N.A.; Vissink, A.; Bootsma, H. B-Cell Hyperactivity in Primary Sjögren's Syndrome. *Expert. Rev. Clin. Immunol.* **2014**, *10*, 483–499. [CrossRef]
107. Stern, M.E.; Schaumburg, C.S.; Dana, R.; Calonge, M.; Niederkorn, J.Y.; Pflugfelder, S.C. Autoimmunity at the Ocular Surface: Pathogenesis and Regulation. *Mucosal. Immunol.* **2010**, *3*, 425–442. [CrossRef]
108. Nair, A.P.; D'Souza, S.; Khamar, P.; Nuijts, R.M.M.A.; Sethu, S.; Shetty, R. Ocular Surface Immune Cell Diversity in Dry Eye Disease. *Indian J. Ophthalmol.* **2023**, *71*, 1237–1247. [CrossRef]
109. Huang, D.; Li, Z. Multidimensional Immunotherapy for Dry Eye Disease: Current Status and Future Directions. *Front. Ophthalmol.* **2024**, *4*, 1449283. [CrossRef]
110. Rong, H.; Yang, H.; Liu, Q.; Zhang, H.; Wang, S. Substance P and Neurokinin 1 Receptor Boost the Pathogenicity of Granulocyte-Macrophage Colony-Stimulating Factor-Producing T Helper Cells in Dry Eye Disease. *Scand. J. Immunol.* **2025**, *101*, e13434. [CrossRef]
111. Lee, S.J.; Im, S.T.; Wu, J.; Cho, C.S.; Jo, D.H.; Chen, Y.; Dana, R.; Kim, J.H.; Lee, S.M. Corneal Lymphangiogenesis in Dry Eye Disease Is Regulated by Substance P/Neurokinin-1 Receptor System through Controlling Expression of Vascular Endothelial Growth Factor Receptor 3. *Ocul. Surf.* **2021**, *22*, 72–79. [CrossRef]
112. Singh, R.B.; Naderi, A.; Cho, W.; Ortiz, G.; Musayeva, A.; Dohlman, T.H.; Chen, Y.; Ferrari, G.; Dana, R. Modulating the Tachykinin: Role of Substance P and Neurokinin Receptor Expression in Ocular Surface Disorders. *Ocul. Surf.* **2022**, *25*, 142–153. [CrossRef]
113. Taketani, Y.; Marmalidou, A.; Dohlman, T.H.; Singh, R.B.; Amouzegar, A.; Chauhan, S.K.; Chen, Y.; Dana, R. Restoration of Regulatory T-Cell Function in Dry Eye Disease by Antagonizing Substance P/Neurokinin-1 Receptor. *Am. J. Pathol.* **2020**, *190*, 1859–1866. [CrossRef] [PubMed]
114. Wang, S.; Naderi, A.; Kahale, F.; Ortiz, G.; Forouzanfar, K.; Chen, Y.; Dana, R. Substance P Regulates Memory Th17 Cell Generation and Maintenance in Chronic Dry Eye Disease. *J. Leukoc. Biol.* **2024**, *116*, 1446–1453. [CrossRef] [PubMed]
115. Zhang, Y.; Zhang, H.; Zhu, X.; Ye, H.; Yang, K.; Zhou, X.; Hong, J. Tear Neuropeptides Are Associated with Clinical Symptoms and Signs of Dry Eye Patients. *Ann. Med.* **2025**, *57*, 2451194. [CrossRef] [PubMed]
116. Yoon, H.-J.; Jang, W.-H.; An, S.; Ji, Y.S.; Yoon, K.C. Tear Neuromediators in Subjects with and without Dry Eye According to Ocular Sensitivity. *Chonnam Med. J.* **2022**, *58*, 37–42. [CrossRef]
117. Lambiase, A.; Micera, A.; Sacchetti, M.; Cortes, M.; Mantelli, F.; Bonini, S. Alterations of Tear Neuromediators in Dry Eye Disease. *Arch. Ophthalmol.* **2011**, *129*, 981–986. [CrossRef]
118. Blanco-Vázquez, M.; Vázquez, A.; Fernández, I.; Novo-Diez, A.; Martínez-Plaza, E.; García-Vázquez, C.; González-García, M.J.; Sobas, E.M.; Calonge, M.; Enríquez-de-Salamanca, A. Inflammation-Related Molecules in Tears of Patients with Chronic Ocular Pain and Dry Eye Disease. *Exp. Eye Res.* **2022**, *219*, 109057. [CrossRef]
119. Guzmán, M.; Miglio, M.; Keitelman, I.; Shiromizu, C.M.; Sabbione, F.; Fuentes, F.; Trevani, A.S.; Giordano, M.N.; Galletti, J.G. Transient Tear Hyperosmolarity Disrupts the Neuroimmune Homeostasis of the Ocular Surface and Facilitates Dry Eye Onset. *Immunology* **2020**, *161*, 148–161. [CrossRef]
120. Masuoka, T.; Yamashita, Y.; Nakano, K.; Takechi, K.; Niimura, T.; Tawa, M.; He, Q.; Ishizawa, K.; Ishibashi, T. Chronic Tear Deficiency Sensitizes Transient Receptor Potential Vanilloid 1-Mediated Responses in Corneal Sensory Nerves. *Front. Cell Neurosci.* **2020**, *14*, 598678. [CrossRef]
121. Yin, J.; Wu, Z. Sodium Hyaluronate and Pranoprofen Improve Visual Function and Reduce Inflammation in Patients with Dry Eye. *Immunopharmacol. Immunotoxicol.* **2024**, *46*, 627–634. [CrossRef]

122. Ji, Y.W.; Kim, H.M.; Ryu, S.Y.; Oh, J.W.; Yeo, A.; Choi, C.Y.; Kim, M.J.; Song, J.S.; Kim, H.S.; Seo, K.Y.; et al. Changes in Human Tear Proteome Following Topical Treatment of Dry Eye Disease: Cyclosporine A Versus Diquafosol Tetrasodium. *Investig. Ophthalmol. Vis. Sci.* **2019**, *60*, 5035–5044. [CrossRef]
123. Jones, L.; Craig, J.P.; Markoulli, M.; Karpecki, P.; Akpek, E.K.; Basu, S.; Bitton, E.; Chen, W.; Dhaliwal, D.K.; Dogru, M.; et al. TFOS DEWS III: Management and Therapy. *Am. J. Ophthalmol.* **2025**, *279*, 289–386. [CrossRef]
124. Sheppard, J.; Shen Lee, B.; Periman, L.M. Dry Eye Disease: Identification and Therapeutic Strategies for Primary Care Clinicians and Clinical Specialists. *Ann. Med.* **2022**, *55*, 241–252. [CrossRef]
125. Jones, L.; Downie, L.E.; Korb, D.; Benitez-del-Castillo, J.M.; Dana, R.; Deng, S.X.; Dong, P.N.; Geerling, G.; Hida, R.Y.; Liu, Y.; et al. TFOS DEWS II Management and Therapy Report. *Ocul. Surf.* **2017**, *15*, 575–628. [CrossRef] [PubMed]
126. Yang, C.; Gao, Q.; Liu, J.; Wu, Y.; Hou, X.; Sun, L.; Zhang, X.; Lu, Y.; Yang, Y. M2 Macrophage-Derived Extracellular Vesicles Ameliorate Benzalkonium Chloride-Induced Dry Eye. *Exp. Eye Res.* **2024**, *247*, 110041. [CrossRef] [PubMed]
127. Zhou, X.; Wu, Y.; Zhang, Y.; Chu, B.; Yang, K.; Hong, J.; He, Y. Targeting A7 Nicotinic Acetylcholine Receptor for Modulating the Neuroinflammation of Dry Eye Disease Via Macrophages. *Investig. Ophthalmol. Vis. Sci.* **2025**, *66*, 13. [CrossRef] [PubMed]
128. Ma, B.; Zhou, Y.; Liu, R.; Zhang, K.; Yang, T.; Hu, C.; Gao, Y.; Lan, Q.; Liu, Y.; Yang, X.; et al. Pigment Epithelium-Derived Factor (PEDF) Plays Anti-Inflammatory Roles in the Pathogenesis of Dry Eye Disease. *Ocul. Surf.* **2021**, *20*, 70–85. [CrossRef]
129. Mu, J.; Ding, X.; Song, Y.; Mi, B.; Fang, X.; Chen, B.; Yao, B.; Sun, X.; Yuan, X.; Guo, S.; et al. ROS-Responsive Microneedle Patches Enable Peri-Lacrimal Gland Therapeutic Administration for Long-Acting Therapy of Sjögren's Syndrome-Related Dry Eye. *Adv. Sci.* **2025**, *12*, 2409562. [CrossRef]
130. Sadrai, Z.; Stevenson, W.; Okanobo, A.; Chen, Y.; Dohlman, T.H.; Hua, J.; Amparo, F.; Chauhan, S.K.; Dana, R. PDE4 Inhibition Suppresses IL-17–Associated Immunity in Dry Eye Disease. *Investig. Ophthalmol. Vis. Sci.* **2012**, *53*, 3584–3591; Erratum in *Investig. Ophthalmol. Vis. Sci.* **2012**, *53*, 6291. [CrossRef]
131. Grosskreutz, C.L.; Hockey, H.U.; Serra, D.; Dryja, T.P. Dry Eye Signs and Symptoms Persist during Systemic Neutralization of IL-1b by Canakinumab or IL-17A by Secukinumab. *Cornea* **2015**, *34*, 1551–1556. [CrossRef]
132. Study Details | A Study to Evaluate the Safety, Tolerability, and Efficacy of A197 in Subjects with Dry Eye Disease | ClinicalTrials.Gov. Available online: https://clinicaltrials.gov/study/NCT05238597 (accessed on 2 July 2025).
133. Ratay, M.L.; Glowacki, A.J.; Balmert, S.C.; Acharya, A.P.; Polat, J.; Andrews, L.P.; Fedorchak, M.V.; Schuman, J.S.; Vignali, D.A.A.; Little, S.R. Treg-Recruiting Microspheres Prevent Inflammation in a Murine Model of Dry Eye Disease. *J. Control Release* **2017**, *258*, 208–217. [CrossRef]
134. Zhang, R.; Zou, Y.; Li, H.; Li, D.; Liu, Y.; Gong, B.; Yu, M. NK1R Antagonist, CP-99,994 Ameliorates Dry Eye Disease via Inhibiting the Plk1-Cdc25c-Cdk1 Axis. *J. Biochem. Mol. Toxicol.* **2025**, *39*, e70177. [CrossRef] [PubMed]
135. Surico, P.L.; Barone, V.; Singh, R.B.; Coassin, M.; Blanco, T.; Dohlman, T.H.; Basu, S.; Chauhan, S.K.; Dana, R.; Zazzo, A. Di Potential Applications of Mesenchymal Stem Cells in Ocular Surface Immune-Mediated Disorders. *Surv. Ophthalmol.* **2025**, *70*, 467–479. [CrossRef] [PubMed]
136. Joung Lee, M.; Young Ko, A.; Hwa Ko, J.; Ju Lee, H.; Kum Kim, M.; Ryang Wee, W.; In Khwarg, S.; Youn Oh, J. Mesenchymal Stem/Stromal Cells Protect the Ocular Surface by Suppressing Inflammation in an Experimental Dry Eye. *Mol. Ther.* **2015**, *23*, 139–146. [CrossRef] [PubMed]
137. Aluri, H.S.; Samizadeh, M.; Edman, M.C.; Hawley, D.R.; Armaos, H.L.; Janga, S.R.; Meng, Z.; Sendra, V.G.; Hamrah, P.; Kublin, C.L.; et al. Delivery of Bone Marrow-Derived Mesenchymal Stem Cells Improves Tear Production in a Mouse Model of Sjögren's Syndrome. *Stem Cells Int.* **2017**, *2017*, 3134543. [CrossRef]
138. Wang, L.; Wang, X.; Chen, Q.; Wei, Z.; Xu, X.; Han, D.; Zhang, Y.; Chen, Z.; Liang, Q. MicroRNAs of Extracellular Vesicles Derived from Mesenchymal Stromal Cells Alleviate Inflammation in Dry Eye Disease by Targeting the IRAK1/TAB2/NF-KB Pathway. *Ocul. Surf.* **2023**, *28*, 131–140. [CrossRef]
139. Wang, G.; Li, H.; Long, H.; Gong, X.; Hu, S.; Gong, C. Exosomes Derived from Mouse Adipose-Derived Mesenchymal Stem Cells Alleviate Benzalkonium Chloride-Induced Mouse Dry Eye Model via Inhibiting NLRP3 Inflammasome. *Ophthalmic Res.* **2022**, *65*, 40–51. [CrossRef]
140. Chen, L.; Gu, C.; Yang, Y.; He, T.; Zhang, Q. Exosomal MiR-146a Derived from Human Umbilical Cord Mesenchymal Stem Cells Alleviates Inflammation and Apoptosis in Dry Eye Disease by Targeting SQSTM1. *Exp. Eye Res.* **2025**, *258*, 110490. [CrossRef]

MDPI AG
Grosspeteranlage 5
4052 Basel
Switzerland
Tel.: +41 61 683 77 34

International Journal of Molecular Sciences Editorial Office
E-mail: ijms@mdpi.com
www.mdpi.com/journal/ijms

www.ingramcontent.com/pod-product-compliance
Lightning Source LLC
Chambersburg PA
CBHW061832210926
51850CB00006B/865
* 9 7 8 3 7 2 5 8 6 7 8 4 4 *